Women's Health in Sports and Exercise

American Academy of Orthopaedic Surgeons Symposium

Women's Health in Sports and Exercise

Edited by
William E. Garrett, Jr, MD, PhD
Frank C. Wilson Professor
Chair, Department of Orthopaedic Surgery
University of North Carolina at Chapel Hill
Chapel Hill, North Carolina

Gayle E. Lester, PhD
Research Professor
Department of Orthopaedic Surgery
University of North Carolina at Chapel Hill
Chapel Hill, North Carolina

Joan McGowan, PhD
Chief
Musculoskeletal Diesases Branch NIAMS/NIH
Bethesda, Maryland

Donald T. Kirkendall, PhD
Clinical Assistant Professor
Department of Orthopaedic Surgery
University of North Carolina at Chapel Hill
Chapel Hill, North Carolina

Supported by the
American Academy of Orthopaedic Surgeons

and the
National Institutes of Health

Workshop
Hunt Valley, Maryland
June 1999

American Academy of Orthopaedic Surgeons
6300 North River Road
Rosemont, IL 60018

2000 – 2010

American Academy of Orthopaedic Surgeons

Women's Health in Sports and Exercise

The material presented in *Women's Health in Sports and Exercise* has been made available by the American Academy of Orthopaedic Surgeons for educational purposes only. This material is not intended to present the only, or necessarily best, methods or procedures for the medical situations discussed, but rather is intended to represent an approach, view, statement, or opinion of the author(s) or producer(s), which may be helpful to others who face similar situations.

Some drugs or medical devices demonstrated in Academy courses or described in Academy print or electronic publications have not been cleared by the Food and Drug Administration (FDA) or have been cleared for specific uses only. The FDA has stated that it is the responsibility of the physician to determine the FDA clearance status of each drug or device he or she wishes to use in clinical practice.

Furthermore, any statements about commercial products are solely the opinion(s) of the author(s) and do not represent an Academy endorsement or evaluation of these products. These statements may not be used in advertising or for any commercial purpose.

First Edition

ISBN 0-89203-224-3

Contributors and Participants

Julie Agel, MA, ATC†‡
Minneapolis, Minnesota

Rosemary Agostini, MD†
Virginia Mason Medical Center
Seattle, Washington

Elizabeth A. Arendt, MD*†‡
Associate Professor Orthopedic Surgery
Medical Director Men's and Women's Varsity Athletics
Department of Orthopedic Surgery
University of Minnesota
Minneapolis, Minnesota

Leslie S. Beasley, MD*
Orthopaedic Resident
Orthopaedics
Hospital for Special Surgery
New York, New York

Steven N. Blair, PEd*†
Director of Research
Cooper Institute
Dallas, Texas

Marybeth Brown, PT, PhD*†
Associate Professor
Program in Physical Therapy
Washington University School of Medicine
St. Louis, Missouri

Lisa R. Callahan, MD*†
Medical Director
Women's Sports Medicine Center
Hospital of Special Surgery
New York, New York

Michelle Canham-Chervak, MPH*
Epidemiologist
Epidemiology and Disease Surveillance
US Army Center for Health Promotion and Preventive Medicine
Aberdeen Proving Ground, Maryland

James F. Clapp III, MD*†
Professor of Reproductive Biology, Obstetrics, and Gynecology
MetroHealth Campus of Case Western Reserve University
Cleveland, Ohio

Randall W. Dick, MS, FACSM*†‡
Senior Assistant Director of Health and Safety
National Collegiate Athletic Association
Indianapolis, Indiana

Susan N. DiGrazia, BS*
Medical Student
University of Nevada School of Medicine
Reno, Nevada

Deborah A. Faryniarz, MD*
Shoulder and Sports Medicine Fellow
Orthopaedic Surgery
Hospital for Special Surgery
New York, New York

Roger A. Fielding, PhD*†
Associate Professor of Health Sciences
Department of Health Sciences
Boston University
Boston, Massachusetts

William E. Garrett, Jr, MD, PhD*†‡
Frank C. Wilson Professor
Chair, Department of Orthopaedic Surgery
University of North Carolina at Chapel Hill
Chapel Hill, North Carolina

James G. Garrick, MD*†‡
Director
Center for Sports Medicine
Saint Francis Memorial Hospital
San Francisco, California

Letha Y. Griffin, MD, PhD*†‡
Team Physician
Georga State University
Atlanta, Georga

Jo A. Hannafin, MD, PhD*†‡
Associate Professor
Department of Orthopaedic Surgery
Hospital for Special Surgery, Cornell University Medical College
New York, New York

Timothy E. Hewett, PhD‡
Cincinnati, Ohio

Janet Howard†
Writer/Editor
Office of Communications and Public Liaison
National Institute of Arthritis and Musculoskeletal and Skin Diseases/NIH
Bethesda, Maryland

Cheryl Hug-English, MD, MPH*
Medical Director
Student Health Center
University of Nevada, Reno
Assistant Dean Admissions
University of Nevada School of Medicine
Reno, Nevada

Laura J. Huston, MS*†‡
Senior Research Associate
Section of Orthopaedic Surgery
University of Michigan
Ann Arbor, Michigan

Mary Lloyd Ireland, MD*†‡
Orthopaedic Surgeon
Orthopaedic Consultant, Shriner's Hospital
Kentucky Sports Medicine
Lexington, Kentucky

Robert J. Johnson, MD‡
Burlington, Vermont

Bruce Jones, MD, MPH*†
Supervisory Medical Officer
Division of Unintentional Injury Prevention
National Center for Injury Prevention and Control
Centers for Disease Control and Prevention
Atlanta, Georgia

Stephen Katz MD, PhD†
Director
NIAMS
Bethesda, Maryland

Kenton R. Kaufmann, PhD, PE*†
Director
Biomechanics Laboratory
Department of Orthopaedics
Mayo Foundation/Mayo Clinic
Rochester, Minnesota

W. Benjamin Kibler, MD*†‡
Medical Director
Lexington Sports Medicine Center
Lexington, Kentucky

Donald T. Kirkendall, PhD*†
Clinical Assistant Professor
Department of Orthopaedic Surgery
University of North Carolina at Chapel Hill
Chapel Hill, North Carolina

Joseph J. Knapik, ScD*
Research Physiologist
Epidemiology and Disease Surveillance
U.S. Army Center for Health Promotion and Preventative Medicine
Aberdeen Proving Ground, Maryland

Wendy M. Kohrt, PhD*†
Professor of Medicine
Division of Geriatric Medicine
University of Colorado Health Sciences Center
Denver, Colorado

Scott Lephart, PhD, ATC‡
Pittsburgh, Pennsylvania

Gayle E. Lester, PhD*†
Research Professor
Department of Orthopaedic Surgery
University of North Carolina at Chapel Hill
Chapel Hill, North Carolina

Jack Lewis, PhD‡
Minneapolis, Minnesota

Thomas Lindenfeld, MD‡
Cincinnati, Ohio

Stefan Lohmander, MD, PhD*
Professor
Department of Orthopedics
Lund University Hospital
Lund, Sweden

Donna A. Lopiano, PhD*†
Executive Director
Women's Sports Foundation
East Meadow, New York

Terry R. Malone, EdD, PT, ATC*†
Professor and Director of Physical Therapy
University of Kentucky
Lexington, Kentucky

Bert R. Mandelbaum, MD*†‡
Fellowship Director
Santa Monica Orthopaedic and Sports Medicine Group
Orthopaedic Surgery
Santa Monica, California

Patty Marchak†‡
Lake Mary, Florida

Anthony Margherita, MD*†
Associate Professor and Section Head
Sports, Spine, and Musculoskeletal Medicine
Division of Physical Medicine and Rehabilitation
Washington University
St. Louis, Missouri

Jerry R. May, PhD*†
Associate Dean
Professor of Psychiatry and Behavioral Sciences
University of Nevada School of Medicine
Reno, Nevada

Joan McGowan, PhD†
Chief
Musculoskeletal Diseases Branch
NIAMS/NIH
Bethesda, Maryland

Jill L. McNitt-Gray, PhD*†
Associate Professor
Director of the Biomechanics Research Lab
Department of Exercise Sciences
University of Southern California
Los Angeles, California

Frederick O. Mueller, PhD*†
Chairman
Exercise and Sport Science
University of North Carolina at Chapel Hill
Chapel Hill, North Carolina

Aurelia Nattiv, MD*†
Associate Professor
Department of Family Medicine,
Division of Sports Medicine and
Department of Orthopaedic Surgery
University of California, Los Angeles
Los Angeles, California

Bradley J. Nelson, MD*
Chief
Sports Medicine
Orthopaedic Surgery Service
Eisenhower Army Medical Center
Fort Gordon, Georgia

Jim Panagis, MD†
Musculoskeletal Diseases Branch
NIAMS/NIH
National Institutes of Health
Bethesda, Maryland

Heidi Prather, DO*†
Assistant Professor
Physical Medicine and Rehabilitation
Washington University School of Medicine
St. Louis, Missouri

Margot Putukian, MD, FACSM*†
Team Physician
Associate Professor, Orthopaedics and
Rehabilitation
Penn State University
University Park, Pennsylvania

Constance Raab†
Public Liaison Officer
Office of Communications and Public Liaison
National Institute of Arthritis and
Musculoskeletal and Skin Diseases
Bethesda, Maryland

Ralph K. Requa, MSPH*†
Research Director
Center for Sports Medicine
Saint Francis Memorial Hospital
San Francisco, California

Harold Roos, MD, PhD*
Lund University Hospital
Lund, Sweden

Sally Rudicel, MD*†
Associate Professor of Orthopaedics
Tufts University
Boston, Massachusetts

Leena Sharma, MD†
Assistant Professor
Department of Internal Medicine
Northwestern University
Chicago, Illinois

Sandra J. Shulta, MS, ATC‡
Charlottesville, Virginia

Deborah L. Squire, MD†
Pediatric Sports Medicine
Duke University
Durham, North Carolina

Margaret E. Stone, BSc, MS, CSCS*†
Scottish Institute of Sport
Edinburgh, Scotland

Michael H. Stone, PhD, CSCS*†
Chair of Sport
Sport Science
Edinburgh University
Edinburgh, Scotland

LTC Dean C. Taylor, MD*†
Chief
Orthopaedic Surgery Service
Keller Army Community Hospital
West Point, New York

Carol C. Teitz, MD*†
Associate Professor
Orthopaedic Surgery
University of Washington
Seattle, Washington

Laura L. Tosi, MD†
Chairman, Children's National Medical Center
Associate Professor of Orthopaedics and Pediatrics
George Washington University Medical Center
Washington, DC

Travis Triplett-McBride, PhD, CSCS*†
Department of Exercise and Sport Science
University of Wisconsin, La Crosse
La Crosse, Wisconsin

Edward M. Wojtys, MD*‡
Professor
Department of Surgery
University of Michigan
Ann Arbor, Michigan

Debra Zillmer, MD†
Orthopaedic Surgeon
Medical Director
Gurderson Lutheran Medical Center
La Crosse, Wisconsin

* Contributor to Volume
† Workshop Participant
‡ ACL Consensus Symposium Participant

Contents

Preface

In 1972, Congress passed Title IX of the Educational Amendments Act, ensuring that girls and women would have equal opportunity to participate in interscholastic and intercollegiate sports. The dramatic increase in women's participation in sports and exercise since Title IX was passed is heartening because increased physical activity clearly provides many benefits to those who participate. The benefits of an active lifestyle are profound and well documented: a recent report by the President's Council on Physical Fitness and Sports notes that regular involvement in sports and fitness programs contributes not only to the physical health of girls, but also to their psychological and moral development. These benefits range from physiologic dimensions such as improved cardiovascular health, better motor skill development, and enhanced immune system functioning to psychosocial dimensions such as higher self-esteem, better emotional health, and more sophisticated social interaction skills.

There are many reasons to celebrate women's increasing participation in sports and fitness programs including the increased national visibility of strong role models for young girls and more mature women who wish to pursue sports and fitness programs. There is, however, a growing awareness of the physical injuries associated with the increased participation in sports by young women and the need to improve recognition of the risks and benefits of exercise as well as to explore factors that might allow prediction and prevention of injuries. Therefore, along with the increased participation of women in sports and fitness come several challenges. One such challenge is the need to better scrutinize injury patterns in female athletes. Another is to assess and address the differences that exist between men and women as well as among women of different racial and ethnic groups with regard to the effects and benefits of and access to exercise. In 1990, four of the 10 leading causes of death in American women were chronic diseases directly associated with modifiable behavioral factors—including physical inactivity. Thus, researchers and health care providers must emphasize the importance of women's engaging in physical activity and sports to help prevent premature death and unnecessary illness and disability and to improve the quality of life.

The purpose of the workshop on Women's Health in Sports and Exercise was to explore ways to encourage physical activity while trying to understand more clearly what can be done to prevent activity-related injuries. This workshop was organized by the National Institute of Arthritis and Musculoskeletal and Skin Diseases (NIAMS) and the Office of Research on

Women's Health (ORWH) of the National Institutes of Health (NIH), and by the American Academy of Orthopaedic Surgeons (AAOS). The workshop was supported by an NIH grant, the AAOS, and a grant from AirCast.

The idea for this workshop originated from the Committee on Research of the AAOS. Committee members, the workshop editors, and several other authors envisioned a workshop that would coincide with the Women's World Cup, the largest women's sporting event ever held. This timing would capitalize on the excitement and significance of the World Cup to highlight for all American women that physical activity can be an integral part of their everyday lives, not just an "add on." The joint sponsorship of the workshop by the AAOS and by the NIAMS and ORWH of the NIH emphasizes the twin goals of increasing musculoskeletal fitness and improving treatment and prevention of injury.

This workshop addressed differences between men and women of all ages in health and injury associated with sports and exercise participation. It included not only the physical but also the psychological and psychosocial aspects of participation in sports on both the amateur and professional levels. This daunting task was accomplished through a highly qualified team of participants who presented "state-of-the-science" reviews of sports participation by children and seniors, and included both organized sports and recreational activities. The goal was to establish the status of current research in these areas and to identify issues and questions that need to be addressed with future research. Participants ranged from orthopaedic surgeons to clinical psychologists and included individuals in private practice as well as those engaged in full-time research. This book is based on manuscripts prepared specifically for this workshop and includes the synthesis of discussions held during the workshop.

We greatly appreciate the input and efforts of our Program Committee: Jo Hannafin, MD; Elizabeth Arendt, MD; Cynthia Shewan, PhD; and James Panagis, MD, MPH. We would like to thank many individuals at the AAOS, including Cynthia Shewan, PhD, for help in organizing and securing funding for this workshop; Jennifer Misius and Anita Cooper for help in organizing conference logistics; Marilyn Fox, PhD, Director of Publications; and Laurie Braun, Lisa Moore, Sophie Tosta, Joan Abern, and Sharon O'Brien in the Department of Publications for organizing and managing the publication of this project.

William E. Garrett, Jr, MD, PhD
Gayle E. Lester, PhD
Joan McGowan, PhD
Donald T. Kirkendall, PhD

Introduction

William E. Garrett, Jr, MD, PhD
Gayle E. Lester, PhD
Donna Lopiano, PhD

Current Trends and Perspectives in Sports Participation by Women

The participation in sports and exercise by women, from young girls to elderly women, has substantially increased in the last four decades and has become a more prominent part of public life than ever before. National interest received a substantial boost in 1972 with the passage of Title IX, federal legislation prohibiting sex discrimination in educational settings. The effect has been an increase in the participation of women in interscholastic sports from approximately 300,000 to greater than 2.2 million in 1998.[1] Women's participation in Olympic sports, World Cup soccer, professional basketball leagues, professional golf, and professional tennis receives widespread media attention. More than 3,800 women participated in the 1996 Olympics alone, representing a 27% increase over 1992 participation.[2] However, this is just the tip of the iceberg, in that there is widespread serious participation in nonprofessional sports and exercise programs by women of all ages and skill levels. Additionally, women of all ages are being encouraged to engage in regular exercise programs to improve overall health and prevent diseases.[3,4]

General Fitness and Training Response

In the US Public Health Service (PHS) release "Healthy People 2000," one of the top recommendations was to increase the physical fitness of all women in an effort to reduce the health disparities between men and women and among differing ethnic and racial groups.[5] Data collected subsequent to that report show that fewer than half of US women have a regular, sustained activity program that would be sufficient to reduce risks for chronic disease.[6] However, some investigators report that current physical activity surveys misclassify activity patterns in women because they were developed for and validated by studies on men. Thus, they imply that the data collected do not accurately reflect the activities performed by women, especially those in midlife and not of European descent.[6] The potential upsurge in physical activity among women of all ages and races in response to the PHS recommendations raises substantial questions about gender-related differences in response to training and injury susceptibility.

Physical training studies among both civilian and military women have shown high rates of injury.[7] Although the patterns for injuries are similar, actual injury rates among female military recruits have been reported to be 2.9 times higher than comparable rates for male recruits.[8] Among civilian populations, Koplan and associates[9] reported that 27% of an initial cohort of female runners temporarily or permanently stopped running over a 10-year period as a result of injuries. However, the actual risk factors that predispose women to increased injury rates have not been precisely identified, nor have means to prevent such injuries. One factor that has been closely associated with higher rates of injury is decreased cardiorespiratory fitness or aerobic capacity;[10] increased injury risk ranged from 1.6 to 4.3 relative to level of aerobic capacity. However, many other factors must be considered to prevent exercise- and sports-related injuries. It has been shown in several studies that women respond differently to training than do men.[7] Women, given the same training program as men, develop less aerobic capacity, less strength, and less endurance. Thus, women may require very different types of training programs to acquire fitness levels comparable to those of men.

To prevent injuries and maximize response to training, it is necessary to know the types of training programs and amounts of activities needed to achieve levels of fitness equivalent to those of men. To accomplish this, it is necessary to understand the biomechanical or muscular differences between men and women and how they impact the development of fitness. Gender-specific differences in body composition and size are obvious and have been attributed to differences in the effect of sex hormones on muscular and skeletal development.[11] However, both women and men benefit in a similar manner from short-term physical training.[12] Women appear to use fat as a substrate for energy, which might indicate that they have increased capacity for endurance exercises. Men and women with similar training programs show similar cardiovascular responses;[13] however, significant differences between men and women have been reported in the hemodynamic responses to strenuous exercise.[14] Results differ from study to study when evaluating gender-related differences in strength. Fuster and associates[15] evaluated overall static and dynamic strength in 100 men and 203 women in relation to body height and weight. They found that for men, static strength was closely related to body weight, whereas in women it was more related to body height. In another study, O'Hagan and associates[16] explored gender differences in strength in response to resistance training. They reported that men and women showed similar increases in muscle size but women had relatively greater increases in strength after a 20-week training program. Thus, it appears that there may be specific, gender-related differences in the response to training and in physiology that would be important to understand to achieve maximal performance with minimal injury

General Health

The emphasis on increased physical activity for women not only relates to overall health concerns that equally affect men and women but also to diseases and conditions that are specific to women. Although women live longer than men, the health of older women has been reported to be disproportionately characterized by disease and disability compared to that of older men.[17] This is especially true for musculoskeletal conditions such as arthritis, fractures, and low back pain. The course and severity of some of these diseases, such as cardiovascular disease, osteoporosis, arthritis, and breast cancer, have been shown to be impacted by physical activity.[18–22] There are also concerns about the impact of increased physical activity on the reproductive health of women.[23] In general, there is a consensus that moderate exercise is beneficial rather than harmful at all stages of reproductive life; however, there is considerable concern as to the short- and long-term effects of high levels or excessive physical activity on both general and reproductive health of girls and women.

Increased physical activity in girls and women can have both positive and negative effects on health and well-being. To quote LK Bunker,[1] "Involvement in sport and physical activity contributes to the physical movement capacities of girls, the health status of their bodies, the values and ethical behaviors they develop and their personal, unique identit[ies]." Physical activity, or the lack thereof, plays a critical role in the development of peak bone mass during development and osteoporosis in later life.[24] However, it is clear that abrupt changes in activity level can contribute to or cause menstrual disturbances[25] and in combination with disorders of eating and low body weight result in osteoporosis as manifest in the "female athlete triad."[2] In the absence of other physiologic or psychological stress, exercise alone must significantly exceed the usual recreational levels to disrupt hypothalamic, ovarian, or menstrual function in normal women.[23]

Response to Exercise and Injuries

Although extensive studies have been carried out on exercise effects and sports-related injuries, most have been focused on the male athlete, both elite and nonelite. There is a significant body of evidence indicating that there are differences in both the response to exercise and the types of injuries incurred by female athletes. In general, injuries to the musculoskeletal system tend to be sport specific rather than sex specific. However, injuries to the knee provide an interesting exception to this generalization. Data collected on injuries to the knee among collegiate basketball and soccer players by Arendt and Dick[26] present interesting differences between both general knee injuries and more specifically, injuries to the anterior cruciate ligament (ACL). The incidence of ACL injuries for soccer players during a 5-year period was reported to average 0.31/1,000 athletic exposures for women and 0.13/1,000 athletic exposures for men. Basketball-related ACL injuries followed the same pattern, with rates of 0.26 for women and 0.07 for men. These data were collected from 92 men's and 56 women's teams throughout the country. This increased rate of ACL injuries in women has been observed in numerous other studies,[2,27–32] with some reporting rates of 4 times that in men.[33] However, the actual basis for the increased incidence of ACL ruptures has not been identified. It has been observed that women have a smaller femoral notch width than men;[30,34] this has been shown to correlate with ACL tears in one study[30] but not in another.[34] There are also studies that describe significant differences in the recruitment of muscles in female versus male athletes during dynamic loading[32,35,36] and differences in the muscle strength and development of the quadriceps femoris and hamstrings in response to training and fatigue.[32,34] Other possible causative factors that have been suggested include both extrinsic (body movement, muscular strength, shoe/surface interface) and intrinsic (joint laxity, limb alignment, notch dimensions, and ACL size) factors.[26] Whatever the causative factors, it is clear that ACL and knee injuries result in high cost and the chance of long-term disability in female elite and nonelite athletes. In summary, although overall injury patterns are similar in men and women, there are some sports that attract more women than men, such as gymnastics and volleyball. Thus, injuries related to these sports tend to have a higher incidence in women due to participation statistics and not vulnerability.

Social and Economic Importance

Widespread participation by women in sports and exercise has had very significant occupational and economic ramifications as well. Sporting goods and apparel manufacturers have seen tremendous market increases. The number of women playing professional sports is only a small portion of individuals involved with coaching, training, and support staff for these teams. Health club and fitness center staffing and administration and a host of other exercise-related career choices for men and women now exist. Perhaps an obvious example is the change seen in one of the most widespread, organized, and successful sports in the world, soccer (to Americans and football to the rest of the world). The international governing body for the sport, Federation Internationale de Football Associations (FIFA), is represented by more nations than are represented in the United Nations. The president of FIFA, Mr. Sepp Blatter, said recently in a personal communication, "The future of football is feminine." It is no secret that our American society realizes the influence of its "soccer moms."

Summary

The purpose of this volume is to examine the participation of women in sports and exercise from the standpoint of current and potential effects on health and fitness. The effects of training on fitness levels, general health, and quality of life and the risks of injury or other adverse health effects will be evaluated. Emphasis will be placed on known differences between men and women with respect to sport and exercise and areas where particular gaps exist in knowledge of gender differences or similarities. We will, finally, identify valuable areas for future research in this field.

References

1. Bunker LK: Psycho-physiological contributions of physical activity and sports for girls. *Phys Activity Fitness Res Digest* 1998;3:1–8.
2. Wiggins DL, Wiggins ME: The female athlete. *Clin Sports Med* 1997;16:593–612.
3. National Leadership Conference on Physical Activity and Women's Health. *Womens Health Issues* 1998;8:69–97.
4. Smith AD: The fit woman of the 21st century: Making lifelong exercise the norm. *Phys Sportsmed* 1998;26:23–30.

5. Public Health Service: *Healthy People 2000: National Health Promotion and Disease Prevention Objectives. Full Report, With Commentary.* Washington, DC, US Department of Health and Human Services, 1990, DHHS publication (PHS) 91-50212.
6. Masse LC, Ainsworth BE, Tortolero S, et al: Measuring physical activity in midlife, older, and minority women: Issues from an expert panel. *J Womens Health* 1998;7:57–67.
7. Deuster PA, Jones BH, Moore J: Patterns and risk factors for exercise-related injuries in women: A military perspective. *Mil Med* 1997;162:649–655.
8. Reinker KA, Ozburne S: A comparison of male and female orthopaedic pathology in basic training. *Mil Med* 1979;144:532–536.
9. Koplan JP, Powell KE, Sikes RK, Shirley RW, Campbell CC: An epidemiologic study of the benefits and risks of running. *JAMA* 1982;248:3118–3121.
10. Amoroso PJ, Bell NS, Jones BH: Injury among female and male army parachutists. *Aviat Space Environ Med* 1997;68:1006–1011.
11. Aulin KP: Gender-specific issues. *J Sports Sci* 1995;13:S35–S39.
12. Levesque M, Boulay MR, Bouchard C, Simoneau JA: Time course of training-induced changes in maximal exercise of short duration in men and women. *Int J Sports Med* 1997;18:464–469.
13. Mier CM, Domenick MA, Wilmore JH: Changes in stroke volume with beta-blockade before and after 10 days of exercise training in men and women. *J Appl Physiol* 1997;83:1660–1665.
14. Ben-Sira D, Sagiv M: The effect of gender on left ventricular function immediately after the wingate test. *Eur J Appl Physiol* 1997;75:549–553.
15. Fuster V, Jerez A, Ortega A: Anthropometry and strength relationship: Male-female differences. *Anthropol Anz* 1998;56:49–56.
16. O'Hagan FT, Sale DG, MacDougall JD, Garner SH: Response to resistance training in young women and men. *Int J Sports Med* 1995;16:314–321.
17. La Croix AZ, Newton KM, Leveille SG, Wallace J: Healthy aging: A women's issue. *West J Med* 1997;167:220–232.
18. Limacher MC: Exercise and rehabilitation in women: Indications and outcomes. *Cardiol Clin* 1998;16:27–36.
19. Cummings SR, Nevitt MC, Browner WS, et al: Risk factors for hip fracture in white women: Study of Osteoporotic Fractures Research Group. *N Engl J Med* 1995;332:767–773.
20. Cummings SR: Prevention of hip fractures in older women: A population-based perspective. *Osteoporos Int* 1998;8(suppl 1):S8–S12.
21. Ainsworth BE, Sternfeld B, Slattery ML, Daguise V, Zahm SH: Physical activity and breast cancer: Evaluation of physical activity assessment methods. *Cancer* 1998;83(suppl 3):611–620.
22. Friedenreich CM, Thune I, Brinton LA, Albanes D: Epidemiologic issues related to the association between physical activity and breast cancer. *Cancer* 1998;83(suppl 3):600–610.
23. Clapp JF III, Little KD: The interaction between regular exercise and selected aspects of women's health. *Am J Obstet Gynecol* 1995;173:2–9.
24. Kano K: Relationship between exercise and bone mineral density among over 5,000 women aged 40 years and above. *J Epidemiol* 1998;8:28–32.
25. Loucks AB, Vaitukaitis J, Cameron JL, et al: The reproductive system and exercise in women. *Med Sci Sports Exerc* 1992;24(suppl 6):S288–S293.

26. Arendt E, Dick R: Knee injury patterns among men and women in collegiate basketball and soccer: NCAA data and review of literature. *Am J Sports Med* 1995;23:694–701.
27. Levy AS, Wetzler MJ, Lewars M, Laughlin W: Knee injuries in women collegiate rugby players. *Am J Sports Med* 1997;25:360–362.
28. Bjordal JM, Arnly F, Hannestad B, Strand T: Epidemiology of anterior cruciate ligament injuries in soccer. *Am J Sports Med* 1997;25:341–345.
29. Baker MM: Anterior cruciate ligament injuries in the female athlete. *J Womens Health* 1998;7:343–349.
30. Shelbourne KD, Facibene WA, Hunt JJ: Radiographic and intraoperative intercondylar notch width measurements in men and women with unilateral and bilateral anterior cruciate ligament tears. *Knee Surg Sports Traumatol Arthrosc* 1997;5:229–233.
31. Traina SM, Bromberg DF: ACL injury patterns in women. *Orthopedics* 1997;20:545–549.
32. Lund-Hanssen H, Gannon J, Engebretsen L, Holen K, Hammer S: Isokinetic muscle performance in healthy female handball players and players with a unilateral anterior cruciate ligament reconstruction. *Scand J Med Sci Sports* 1996;6:172–175.
33. Bieze J: Editorial: Somebody should just do it. *BioMechanics* 1998;8:5.
34. Teitz CC, Lind BK, Sacks BM: Symmetry of the femoral notch width index. *Am J Sports Med* 1997;25:687–690.
35. Huston LJ, Wojtys EM: Neuromuscular performance characteristics in elite female athletes. *Am J Sports Med* 1996;24:427–436.
36. Nyland JA, Caborn DN, Shapiro R, Johnson DL: Fatigue after eccentric quadriceps femoris work produces earlier gastrocnemius and delayed quadriceps femoris activation during crossover cutting among normal athletic women. *Knee Surg Sports Traumatol Arthrosc* 1997;5:162–167.

Section One

The Epidemiology of Musculoskeletal Injuries

Section Editor:
Jo A. Hannafin, MD, PhD

Michelle Canham-Chervak, MPH
Randall W. Dick, MS, FACSM
James G. Garrick, MD
Bruce Jones, MD, MPH
Joseph J. Knapik, ScD
Frederick O. Mueller, PhD
Bradley J. Nelson, MD
Ralph K. Requa, MSPH
LTC Dean C. Taylor, MD

Overview

Participation in sports and fitness activities by girls and women of all ages has increased dramatically over the past 20 years. Opportunities for team and individual sports for girls are available in grade school in many communities around the country. The expansion of gymnastics, soccer, swimming, and baseball for young girls has clearly changed the face of Saturday mornings. High school participation in sports continues to expand with opportunities present in a variety of sports that may result in significant college sports scholarships for talented female athletes. Title IX legislation has resulted in a marked expansion of opportunities for sports participation by women in college, and women's participation in postcollegiate professional, amateur, and Olympic sports continues to expand. In addition to this very visible participation in sports by women, there is widespread participation by women of all ages and activity levels in noncompetitive sports and fitness activities.

It appears clear that both musculoskeletal and cardiovascular health are potential benefits of exercise and that injury is a potential risk of exercise and competition. It is possible to ask what factors play a role in the design of a musculoskeletal health maintenance program and what factors are needed to prevent injury. Musculoskeletal health maintenance should include resistance and endurance training, flexibility and balance training, cardiovascular training, and avoidance of overuse injuries. Data currently available suggest that sport-specific injuries occur, and it has been recognized that gender may play a role in the etiology of specific injuries in high school and collegiate athletes. These groups of injuries have been studied in a limited way to date, and broader studies must be performed to further elucidate the role of gender in injury and injury prevention.

It is unknown at the present time whether the differences seen in male and female injury profiles are intrinsic to gender. It is known that the single most important factor influencing the type and location of sports injuries is the sport itself. Injury to the anterior cruciate ligament of the knee appears to be one of the notable exceptions. Injuries are also common in activities in which most participants are preadolescent and adolescent girls. These activities include gymnastics, ballet dancing, and figure skating. It is not known how common these injuries are on a national level because the question has not been studied to date.

The number of female participants in high school sports has expanded dramatically since 1972. In 1971, there were 14 female sports with approximately 300,000 participants in the nation's high schools. In 1997 those numbers increased to 37 sports with 2.5 million participants. Limited data are available to describe injury types and patterns seen in high school sports. Studies performed in North Carolina, New Jersey, and Connecticut have demonstrated an increase in anterior cruciate ligament injuries in female participants in soccer and basketball. The National College Athletic Association (NCAA) Injury Surveillance System was established in 1982 to collect data on traumatic injury in collegiate sports. Soccer and basketball have been shown to have the highest game injury risk among women's sports, with an increased risk of injury noted when compared with men's sports. Stress fractures were also noted to occur with increased frequency in the female athletes. No published data are available on overuse injuries in competitive sports or on the risk of injury to women participating in professional or post-collegiate amateur sports. It is clear that women's sports injury issues exist; however, significant, physical and psychological benefits come with participation in athletic activities.

It is unknown at this time whether the differences in injury profiles seen in men and women are intrinsic to gender. It is not known whether methods of training and coaching, the risks of injury, and the physical and emotional response to exercise are the same for men and women. To help to answer these questions investigators will need to determine whether the differences in injury profiles are present prior to puberty, whether they increase with the hormonal changes seen during puberty, and whether they persist with increasing age.

The first step in answering these questions is to define the groups of interest because these groups may require different methods of study. The groups to be studied must include a range from children through the elderly. Injury data currently are available for traditional adolescent and young adult sports but must be expanded to include information on the noncompetitive athlete population and athletes involved in nontraditional and less studied sports. In addition, the role of gender and age in both acute and overuse injuries must be critically evaluated.

Surveillance strategies must be created that will allow the study of the populations at risk. These strategies must include the creation and maintenance of a broad-based health surveillance system that tracks and links gender, physical activity, exercise, and other health behaviors with adverse medical outcomes such as injury and disease. These data should be used to establish normative data for each decade of life.

A standardized sports surveillance system that links injury and exposure data is necessary. Such a system should be available for use at a team, school, local, state, or national level. This system should include minimum basic data sets for use in making health policy decisions, developing sports rules and regulations to prevent injuries, and assisting coaches in making decisions about training to optimize performance and prevent injury.

The risk and benefit of participation must be defined in competitive sport, vigorous exercise, and exercise designed for maintenance of musculoskeletal health. It is not known at the present time whether early experience in sports or fitness activities plays a role in the development or prevention of injury. Do gender and age play significant roles in defining the risks and benefits of sports participation in different stages of life? Once an injury occurs, is there a gender-specific or gender-modified response to conservative or surgical treatment of the injury? Does attempted maintenance of musculoskeletal health diminish the development of frailty in the later stages of life?

With the aging of the American population, it will be critical to study the effect of higher physical fitness and activity levels on the risk of injury and functional disability among middle-aged and older women and men. The effect of physical fitness and activity on costs associated with musculoskeletal functional impairment must be critically assessed, and studies need to be conducted to identify risk factors for injury and discontinuation of exercise/activity among women and men of different ages.

JO A. HANNAFIN, MD, PHD

Chapter 1

Sports Injuries in Adolescent and Preadolescent Girls

James G. Garrick, MD

The recent furor surrounding documentation of the enhanced incidence of anterior cruciate ligament injuries among female athletes in selected sports has raised questions concerning the existence of other gender-specific injuries in sports. Of particular concern is the identification of such problems in children, not only because the sequelae of childhood injuries have many years to develop but also because children depend on adults for their protection.

When considering young female athletes, spondylolysis in gymnasts and scoliosis in ballet dancers come immediately to mind. Both represent well-documented musculoskeletal problems that are almost unique to young female participants. Unfortunately, the activities with which these conditions are associated are also almost unique to young female participants. In order to gather information useful in making sports activities safer for these young female participants, the potentially causative roles played by both the activity and the participant must be defined. This chapter is an attempt to define how gender, a relatively young age, and activity influence the incidence of injuries.

Problems

Sports injuries occurring to older adolescents and young adults are theoretically easy to study. Most activities are institutionally-based (high schools and colleges) and organized into teams, making cohort members easy to identify. Team records usually facilitate calculation of time at risk. The presence of athletic trainers and team physicians eases the identification and measurement of the consequences (time-loss) of injuries. Adequate injury records are routinely kept and often can be mined for data used in retrospective studies. Both demographic and past medical information can be gleaned from the preparticipation examinations.

Unfortunately, studying injuries among athletes under high school age is almost the antithesis of the situation described above. Most activities are extra- rather than inter- or intrascholastic; thus, team membership varies throughout the season, record-keeping is more casual, and medical care is not readily available. Often the only records of injuries are those available through medical insurers of the teams, resulting in only the most severe injuries being recorded.

Children participating in individual sports and activities such as ballet and gymnastics are even more difficult to study. Although injury studies have been reported in these activities, they invariably involve only the most elite, and older, participants, a group teeming with selection bias. The injuries that preclude entry into the elite ranks are not systematically recorded, and thus are available only in the form of case reports, the epitome of identification bias. But injuries requiring surgical intervention are rare among children participating in sports, so even case reports are sparse in number.

The ideal means of identifying problems that are both gender and age specific involves surveillance of sports and activities with male and female participants of similar (in this case, young) ages. Although fairly common at the high school level, such investigations of younger participants are rare, and data concerning these children must often be gleaned from case-type studies carried out at medical care facilities. Unfortunately, studies such as these rarely contain sufficient information regarding time at risk, thus injury rates, which are necessary for age and gender comparisons, are rarely available.

Studies

Perhaps the most extensive, recent report of injuries encountered among youthful participants is that of Beachy and associates.[1] In a study of athletic injuries sustained over an 8-year period by students in grades 7 through 12 of a private school, they recorded 11,184 injuries among 14,318 participants. Overall injury rates were higher among boys (0.90 injuries per athlete) than girls (0.64). Removing the injuries sustained in football and wrestling yielded a boys' rate of 0.58, essentially identical to that seen in girls. Examination of comparative rates for the 12 sports in which both boys and girls participated failed to reveal any substantive gender differences. Analysis of injuries by anatomic region revealed seven areas (knee, shoulder, foot, neck, wrist, head, and toe) in which days-lost injury rates among boys exceeded that of girls by more than 20% compared to four (gastrocnemius muscle, hand, forearm, and upper arm) in which girls had higher days-lost injury rates. None of the latter were among the 12 most frequently injured anatomic regions. Injury rates based on team level (intermediate grades 7–9, junior varsity grades 9–11, and so forth) also failed to reveal significant gender and/or age differences.

Surveys of schoolchildren from countries other than the United States also fail to reveal higher injury rates for girls. Watson[2] reported 116 injuries in 6,799 Irish schoolchildren between the ages of 10 and 18 years during a single academic year. Overall, the injury rate for boys was 0.025 (injuries/ participant) compared with 0.0068 for girls. The probability of injury was similar for boys and girls 11 to 14 years of age but increased significantly among boys 15 years and older. Among girls only sprains exceeded the proportion expected based on the ratio of boys' and girls' injuries.

Twelve years later Weir and Watson[3] again studied 266 adolescents who sustained 230 sports injuries over the course of a year in an Irish school. Injury rates (based on hours of participation) and average age at the time of injury were similar for boys and girls.

More common are studies looking at injuries rather than participants. Melding these data with population demographics allows calculation of rates by age or sex but does not account for levels of participation in the activities resulting in the injuries. An example of such a system is that of Bienefeld and associates[4] who reviewed injury reports from 7,572 injury events among children 0 to 19 years of age, gathered by a regional surveillance program in Kingston, Ontario. Overall injury rates were higher among boys (202/1,000) than girls (143.7/1,000). Athough these investigators created categories including sports injuries among 10- to 19-year-old children and youth and playground injuries of children aged 5 to 14 years, the lack of time-at-risk data precluded meaningful age or gender comparisons.

In a similar fashion, acute sports injuries treated in a hospital emergency department in Oslo, Norway, were studied by Maehlum and Daljord.[5] Of 4,673 injuries, 70% were sustained by boys and men. Noteworthy among gender differences were the facts that the girls and women were younger than the boys and men (55% versus 41% younger than 20 years of age) and more likely to sustain their injuries pursuing recreational sports (52% females versus 36% males) rather than competitive activities. Unfortunately, the relative frequency of recreational versus competitive sports participation and the ages of the participants are unknown. Were Norway similar to the United States, however, these conclusions would come as no surprise because opportunities for both sports participation and competitive team membership are generally more available for older men than women.

Surveillance studies originating from hospital facilities are characterized by diagnostic information and severity determinations of the highest quality. Unfortunately, reporting biases based on severity are an integral part of such studies, with both acute and relatively severe injuries making up the bulk of the cases. The gradual-onset, overuse injuries so typical in most sports rarely find their way into such data sets.

Case studies originating from facilities primarily responsible for the care of athletes reverse the severity reporting bias and, if anything, oversample the gradual-onset, overuse injuries. Watkins and Peabody,[6] in a 3-year study of 394 patients (5 to 17 years old) treated in a sports medicine clinic in Glasgow, Scotland, over a 3-year period also noted that injured girls were younger than injured boys. Of the 394 injuries, 45.2% occurred in girls. Girls' injuries peaked at 13 to 14 years of age and boys' injuries were highest at 15 to 16 years.

An indirect, retrospective, and imaginative means of comparing boys'and girls' injury rates was used by DuRant and associates[7] in a study of the results of preparticipation examinations in 1,259 high school athletes. They found that the girls had significantly fewer orthopaedic problems as determined by both the health history and physical examination. These findings were a reflection of a lower percentage of abnormalities involving the hips, knees, and ankles. Presumably these data are a reflection of previous athletic injuries, but the lack of time-at-risk information precludes comparing rates.

Another approach common in the orthopaedic literature is to look at both an activity and a specific injury or medical condition. One of the earliest such sports injury surveys was reported by Jackson and associates[8] in 1976. In a radiographic survey of the lumbar spines of 100 competitive gymnasts, they demonstrated an incidence of spondylolysis of 11% in gymnasts averaging 15.1 years of age. The comparable incidence in a control population of white, nonathletic females of a similar age is 2.3%.

In a similar survey of 75 female professional ballet dancers (average age 24.3 years), Warren and associates[9] found a prevalence of scolioisis of 24%. Among these, 83% had experienced delayed menarche (14 years or older) compared with only 54% of those without scoliosis. The presence of stress fractures also rose with increasing age at menarche.

Both the spondylolysis and scoliosis surveys had in common the fact that they surveyed only the tip of the competitive pyramid. Elite gymnasts make up no more than 10% of the sport's participants, and ballet dancers who have successfully gained employment with a professional company represent a far smaller proportion of those involved in that activity. Because either of these conditions could preclude successful advancement in the activity, it requires no particular leap of faith to imagine that the conditions could be even more prevalent in the less successful participants.

Case studies are the final source of information concerning sport-, gender-, and age-specific injuries. Elbow injuries in gymnasts provide an excellent example of this type of report. Among the earliest was that of Priest and Weise,[10] who described 32 injuries in 30 female gymnasts averaging 13.6 years of age. The injuries were severe. All but two were fractures and/or dislocations, and many carried with them long-term consequences. Similar consequences could be expected from the 10 cases of osteochondritis dissecans in high-performance female gymnasts, ages 10 to 17 years, reported by Jackson and associates[11] and the seven cases of the same condition (ages 11 to 13 years) reported by Singer and Roy.[12] Although the long-term effects are less clearly defined, stress injury of the distal radial epiphysis as typified by Caine and associates[13] appears as another nearly unique injury associated with young gymnasts.

The literature provides reports of other gender-related sports injuries of both the acute and overuse varieties. The former are typified by anterior cruciate ligament sprains[14] and the latter by an apparently gender-related higher incidence of stress fracture among women runners, such as that reported by Paty and Swafford.[15] The relationship of these conditions to age has yet to be clearly defined, although the study of indoor soccer injuries by Lindenfeld and associates[16] perhaps comes the closest. Their study included both boys and girls, the two youngest groups being younger than 12 years and 12 to 15 years. The girls in both groups experienced higher injury rates (5.6 versus 2.8 and 6.3 versus 4.4 injuries/100 player hours). Total injuries were four and 10 for the two groups respectively, too small to be indicative of specific patterns. The gender issue regarding these conditions permits examination because both boys and girls participate in the activities with which the injuries are associated.

Gender comparisons cannot be made with some other problems commonly experienced by young girls. For example, posterior ankle impingement is a condition seen frequently among midteenage female ballet dancers.[17] Whether this apparent predilection for girls is a function of the fact that (only) girls dance en pointe, and thus constantly use the ankle in an excessively plantarflexed position, or the fact that pre- and midteenage ballet students are predominantly girls cannot be ascertained with the information currently available.

Summary

Epidemiologic studies of sports injuries among boys and girls encompassing participants from childhood through adolescence are rare. The studies that do exist suggest that among prepubertal athletes involved in similar activities, gender plays little or no role regarding risk of injury.

The conventional wisdom suggesting that the activity, rather than age or gender of the participants, plays the biggest role in producing both the type and frequency of injuries makes gender comparisons particularly difficult. Among the most extensively studied activities, many are gender-specific (for example, football and ballet) and thus allow no opportunity for gender comparisons. Studies of those activities that allow legitimate comparisons have revealed significant, gender-related differences in but a few injuries such as stress fractures and anterior cruciate ligament sprains.

The lack of recognition, or perhaps acknowledgment, of the most glaring gender-related injury, that of the anterior cruciate ligament, for so long would suggest that the currently available epidemiologic data concerning sports may lack the precision and detail necessary to identify other important gender-related problems. There appears to be a need for comprehensive, prospective studies of sports with both male and female participants, focused on specific injuries and using consistent methods of injury recognition and reporting.

References

1. Beachy G, Akau CK, Martinson M, Olderr TF: High school sports injuries: A longitudinal study at Punahou School: 1988 to 1996. *Am J Sports Med* 1997;25:675–681.
2. Watson AW: Sports injuries during one academic year in 6799 Irish school children. *Am J Sports Med* 1984;12:65–71.
3. Weir MA, Watson AW: A twelve month study of sports injuries in one Irish school. *Ir J Med Sci* 1996;165:165–169.
4. Bienefeld M, Pickett W, Carr PA: A descriptive study of childhood injuries in Kingston, Ontario, using data from a computerized injury surveillance system. *Chronic Dis Can* 1996;17:21–27.
5. Maehlum S, Daljord OA: Acute sports injuries in Oslo: A one-year study. *Br J Sports Med* 1984;18:181–185.
6. Watkins J, Peabody P: Sports injuries in children and adolescents treated at a sports injury clinic. *J Sports Med Phys Fitness* 1996;36:43–48.
7. DuRant RH, Linder CW, Sanders JM Jr, Jay S, Brantley G, Bedgood R: Adolescent females' readiness to participate in sports: Sex and race differences in the preparticipation athletic examination. *J Adolesc Health Care* 1988;9:310–314.
8. Jackson DW, Wiltse LL, Cirincione RJ: Spondylolysis in the female gymnast. *Clin Orthop* 1976;117:68–73.

9. Warren MP, Brooks-Gunn J, Hamilton LH, Warren LF, Hamilton WG: Scoliosis and fractures in young ballet dancers: Relation to delayed menarche and secondary amenorrhea. *N Engl J Med* 1986;314:1348–1353.

10. Priest JD, Weise DJ: Elbow injury in women's gymnastics. *Am J Sports Med* 1981;9:288–295.

11. Jackson DW, Silvino N, Reiman P: Osteochondritis in the female gymnast's elbow. *Arthroscopy* 1989;5:129–136.

12. Singer KM, Roy SP: Osteochondrosis of the humeral capitellum. *Am J Sports Med* 1984;12:351–360.

13. Caine D, Roy S, Singer K, Broekhoff J: Stress changes of the distal radial growth plate: A radiographic survey of 60 young competitive gymnasts and an epidemiologic review of the related literature. *Am J Sports Med* 1992;20:290–298.

14. Arendt E, Dick R: Knee injury patterns among men and women in collegiate basketball and soccer: NCAA data and review of literature. *Am J Sports Med* 1995;23:694–701.

15. Paty JG Jr, Swafford D: Adolescent running injuries. *J Adolesc Health Care* 1984;5:87–90.

16. Lindenfeld TN, Schmitt DJ, Hendy MP, Mangine RE, Noyes FR: Incidence of injury in indoor soccer. *Am J Sports Med* 1994;22:364–371.

17. Marotta JJ, Micheli LJ: Os trigonum impingement in dancers. *Am J Sports Med* 1992;20:533–536.

Chapter 2

Athletic Injuries in High School Girls

Frederick O. Mueller, PhD

Introduction

Organized interscholastic athletics are an integral part of the educational program at most high schools in the United States. During the past 28 years there has been a tremendous increase in both the number of participants and the number of sports offered at the high school level.[1] During the 1970–1971 academic year, there were 26 high school boys' sports with 3,666,917 participants, and 14 girls' sports with 294,015 participants. In the 1997–1998 academic year, there were 36 high school boys' sports with 3,763,120 participants and 37 girls' sports with 2,570,120 participants. An example of the increase in girls' participation is high school soccer, with 700 participants in 1970 and 246,687 in 1997 (an increase of over 35,000%).[2] The most significant event that influenced this increase in girls' participation was the enactment in 1972 of Title IX of the Federal Educational Assistance Act, which prohibited sex discrimination in all education programs, including sports, that received federal funds.

With this growing popularity in sports and their inclusion in more public high schools, it becomes increasingly apparent that additional consideration must be given to the injury problem associated with sports.[1] The possibility of a high school athlete being injured during a season ranged from a low of 21% to a high, in football, of 81%.[3] An average injury percentage of 50% would amount to 3,166,726 (1,881,560 boys and 1,285,166 girls) high school athletic injuries each year. Most athletic injuries are not accidents and are preventable.[4] A study in Michigan revealed that 74% of the high schools in Michigan had neither a physician nor an athletic trainer present at any time during the year.[5] To protect the athlete, high school administrators must take a greater role in evaluating the risk of involvement in sports participation, develop preventive measures, and enforce accepted safe practices with respect to participation.

Background

There is a general lack of research investigating athletic injuries in the female athlete, and some of the best research at the high school level dates back to the late 1970s. In 1978, Garrick and Requa[6] studied 4 girls' high school athletic programs, with certified athletic trainers collecting the data. The 870 participant-seasons in 9 sports resulted in 192 injuries. The type and frequency of injuries were comparable with those seen in noncontact boys' interscholastic sports. Garrick and Requa[7] also looked at girls' gymnastics injuries in 4 Seattle-area high schools for 1 year, and in the second year expanded to include an additional 12-team high school league, 2 college teams, and 3 private clubs. The total time-loss injury rate was 39.8 injuries per 100 participant seasons. The authors concluded that there was a need for improvement in conditioning and other preventive programs in girls' gymnastics. A study by Young and Cohen[8] of high school girls participating in the 1977 or 1978 Minnesota State High School Girls Basketball Tournament found that the injured female high school basketball player possessed a higher overall level of self-esteem.

According to McLemore and Grana,[9] the increase in the female orthopaedic patient population has been directly associated with the increase in women's athletic participation. Research also has shown that female athletes have a much higher rate of anterior cruciate ligament (ACL) injuries than do male athletes. In 1982 Wirtz[10] reported that female basketball players in 22 Iowa public schools had more injuries than did male athletes, and that high school girls sustained 15 out of the 16 ACL injuries. National Collegiate Athletic Association (NCAA) research shows that women playing soccer have twice as many ACL injuries per exposure as do men over 5 years, and in basketball women's ACL injuries numbered 122 compared with 24 for men (unpublished data, 1993). In 1994, Lindenfeld and associates[11] reported that female soccer players were 5.75 times as likely to have serious knee ligament injuries as are male soccer players. Research on Alpine skiing showed that 1 in 5 women reported an ACL injury, and that women were 3.1 times as likely to sustain an ACL injury as were their male counterparts.[12] The accumulation of these data shows that women have a significantly greater risk than men of sustaining an ACL injury.

In 1988 Durant and associates[13] conducted a standardized preparticipation physical evaluation (PPE) on 1,259 high school athletes and found that girls reported significantly fewer orthopaedic problems than boys on both the health history and the physical examination. A higher percentage of boys were referred for further evaluation before athletic participation. In a 12-month prospective study of male and female athletes aged 17 to 26 years, Bennell and associates[14] found that there were no risk factors that predicted the occurrence of stress fractures in male athletes. However, in female athletes, significant risk factors included lower bone density, a history of menstrual disturbance, less lean mass in the lower limbs, and a lower-fat diet.

Certain conditions are unique to the female athlete, one of which is the female triad of disordered eating, amenorrhea, and osteoporosis. Related to this triad, the bone density of young women with several years of amenorrhea may be the same as that of postmenopausal women without estrogen replacement.[9]

It is apparent that there is a need for more in-depth epidemiologic research with female athletes. Along with the dramatic increase in girls' and women's sports participation there have also been dramatic changes in conditioning and coaching. There is a need for data on injury patterns and strategies for prevention.

Catastrophic Injuries: National Center for Catastrophic Sports Injury Research, 1982–1997

The National Center for Catastrophic Sports Injury Research started collecting data on catastrophic football injuries in 1966. Due to the success of the football project, the center expanded its efforts in 1982 to cover all sports on a national level for both high school and college. Data presented in this chapter include high school sports only from the fall of 1982 through the spring of 1997. The term "catastrophic" is defined as any severe injury incurred during participation in a school-sponsored sport. Catastrophic is divided into the following three categories: (1) fatal; (2) nonfatal, permanent severe functional disability; and (3) serious, no permanent functional disability but severe injury. An example of the latter would be a fractured cervical vertebra with no paralysis.

Injuries are also described as direct or indirect. Direct injuries are those injuries that resulted directly from participation in the skills of the sport. Indirect injuries are those injuries that were caused by systemic failure as a result of exertion while participating in a sport activity or by a complication that was secondary to a nonfatal injury.

Data Collection

Data were collected with the assistance of coaches, athletic directors, state and national organizations, a national newspaper clipping service, and professional associates of the researchers. Upon receiving information concerning a possible catastrophic injury, contact by telephone, letter, and questionnaire was made with the injured player's coach or athletic director. Data collected included demographic information on the athlete (eg, age, height, weight, experience, previous injury), incident information, immediate and postevent medical care, type of injury, and equipment involved. Autopsy reports were used when available and applicable.

Catastrophic Injuries to Female Athletes

Catastrophic injuries to female high school athletes have increased over the years. As an example, in the 1982–1983 academic year there was 1 catastrophic injury to a girl, and during the past 14 years there has been an average of 6.1 per year. A major factor in this increase has been the change in cheerleading activity, which now involves gymnastic-type stunts. High school cheerleading accounted for 46% of all direct catastrophic injuries to female high school athletes. The high school female athlete population experienced 39 direct catastrophic injuries from the fall of 1992 through the spring of 1997. In addition, there were 23 indirect injuries to female athletes.

As indicated in Tables 1 and 2, there were 389 direct and 118 indirect catastrophic injuries in high school fall sports from the fall of 1982 through the fall of 1996. Female athletes were associated with only 2 of the direct injuries and 2 of the indirect injuries. The 2 direct injuries were in field hockey and were nonfatal permanent disability injuries. The injuries occurred in 1996 and resulted in permanent disability brain and eye injuries. The direct injury rate for field hockey was 0.26 per 100,000 participants.

Table 1 Direct catastrophic injuries in fall sports, 1982–1996

Sport	Fatal	Nonfatal	Serious	Total
Boys				
Cross-country	0	1	0	1
Football	61	147	166	374
Soccer	4	2	6	12
Total	65	150	172	387
Girls				
Field hockey	0	2	0	2
Combined totals	**65**	**152**	**172**	**389**

Table 2 Indirect catastrophic injuries in fall sports, 1982–1996

Sport	Fatal	Nonfatal	Serious	Total
Boys				
Cross-country	9	1	0	9
Football	88	0	1	89
Soccer	15	0	0	15
Water polo	3	0	0	3
Total	115	0	1	116
Girls				
Cross-country	1	0	0	1
Soccer	1	0	0	1
Total	2	0	0	2
Combined totals	**117**	**0**	**1**	**118**

The catastrophic indirect injuries to female athletes were associated with the sports of cross-country and soccer. The cross-country death was heart related, and the soccer death was listed as natural causes. The indirect injury rate for cross-country was 0.06 per 100,000, and the rate for soccer was 0.05 per 100,000.

As indicated in Tables 3 and 4, there were a total of 71 direct and 76 indirect catastrophic injuries in high school winter sports from 1982 through 1997. Female athletes were associated with 14 of the direct and 14 of the indirect injuries. As would be expected, 9 of the 14 direct injuries were associated with gymnastics. There were no fatalities. The direct nonfatal injury rate for gymnastics was 1.44 per 100,000 participants, and for serious injuries it was 0.72 per 100,000 participants. The gymnastics injuries included 6 permanent disability injuries and 3 serious injuries. All of the gymnastics injuries involved trauma to the spinal cord. Three of the injured gymnasts were injured from falls off the uneven bars, 2 from vaulting, 1 from tumbling, and the activity of 1 was unknown. Two of the direct injuries were in swimming, and both involved permanent disability. The athletes were performing a racing dive in the shallow end of the pool in practice, with the result being cervical vertebrae damage. The nonfatal direct injury rate for swimming was 0.15 per 100,000 participants. Basketball was associated with 1 nonfatal and 1 serious injury, and volleyball was asociated with 1 nonfatal injury. Girls' basketball, swimming, and volleyball were associated with 14 indirect injuries, and 12 of those resulted in death.

As shown in Tables 5 and 6, there were 70 direct and 29 indirect catastrophic injuries in high school spring sports from 1982 through the spring

Table 3 Direct catastrophic injuries in winter sports, 1982–1997

Sport	Fatal	Nonfatal	Serious	Total
Boys				
Basketball	0	1	4	5
Gymnastics	1	1	1	3
Ice hockey	2	4	5	11
Swimming	0	2	3	5
Wrestling	2	20	11	33
Total	5	28	24	57
Girls				
Basketball	0	1	1	2
Gymnastics	0	6	3	9
Swimming	0	2	0	2
Volleyball	0	1	0	1
Total	0	10	4	14
Combined totals	**5**	**38**	**28**	**71**

Table 4 Indirect catastrophic injuries in winter sports, 1982–1997

Sport	Fatal	Nonfatal	Serious	Total
Boys				
Basketball	47	0	0	47
Ice hockey	2	0	0	2
Wrestling	13	0	0	13
Total	62	0	0	62
Girls				
Basketball	7	0	1	8
Swimming	4	0	1	5
Volleyball	1	0	0	1
Total	12	0	2	14
Combined totals	**74**	**0**	**2**	**76**

of 1997. Female high school athletes accounted for 5 of the direct injuries, with 3 in track and 2 in softball. One of the track accidents resulted in death, and the other 2 were listed as serious. Two of the injured athletes were struck by a discus and 1 by a javelin. The fatality and serious direct injury rates per 100,000 participants were 0.02 and 0.04, respectively. Both of the softball injuries were nonfatal and happened when the athlete was struck by a batted ball. The injury rate per 100,000 participants was 0.05. Female spring sports were also associated with 4 indirect deaths, all of which were in track.

Table 5 Direct catastrophic injuries in spring sports, 1982–1997

Sport	Fatal	Nonfatal	Serious	Total
Boys				
Baseball	6	11	11	28
Lacrosse	1	0	1	1
Track	15	10	11	36
Total	22	21	22	65
Girls				
Track	1	0	2	3
Softball	0	2	0	2
Total	1	2	2	5
Combined totals	**23**	**23**	**24**	**70**

Table 6 Indirect catastrophic injuries in spring sports, 1982–1997

Sport	Fatal	Nonfatal	Serious	Total
Boys				
Baseball	7	0	0	7
Lacrosse	2	0	0	2
Track	15	0	0	15
Tennis	1	0	0	1
Total	25	0	0	25
Girls				
Track	4	0	0	4
Total	2	0	0	2
Combined totals	**29**	**0**	**0**	**29**

Cheerleading has changed dramatically during the past 15 years and now involves more gymnastic-type stunts. As the stunts became more difficult, there has been an increase in the number of catastrophic injuries. A number of states have implemented safety rules in cheerleading, and the cheerleading squad has become a part of the athletic program. There is no doubt that cheerleading should be considered a sport and that schools should treat it accordingly. From the fall of 1982 through the spring of 1997, high school cheerleading accounted for 18 direct catastrophic injuries: 1 fatality, 7 nonfatal injuries, and 10 serious injuries. In addition, there were 3 indirect deaths.

North Carolina High School Athletic Injury Study

The North Carolina High School Athletic Injury Study (NCHSAIS)[1] was conducted to delineate the magnitude and scope of the injury problem among male and female athletes in North Carolina high schools. This 4-year prospective research study included 12 sports: soccer (male and female), track (male and female), basketball (male and female), baseball, softball, volleyball, cheerleading, wrestling, and football. A 2-stage cluster sample of 100 North Carolina high schools was selected for this project. The first stage of the sampling included the 100 schools that were invited to participate, and the second stage involved randomly selecting existing sports teams at each of the study schools. Specific aims were to measure the incidence, severity, and etiology of injuries; to study the relationship of coaches' training and experience to injury occurrence; and to compare the incidence and severity of injury among female and male athletes in the same or comparable sports. A reportable injury was one that occurred as a result of participation in a high school sport and either limited the student's full participation in the sport the day following the injury or required medical attention by a medical professional.[1] This chapter discusses the first 2 years of the project, fall of 1996 through the spring of 1998. The data used for this chapter are preliminary.

From the fall of 1996 through the spring of 1998 there were a total of 16,008 male and female athletes in the 100 study schools. Boys accounted for 9,266 (57.9%) and girls accounted for 6,742 (42.1%). During this same time period, there were a total of 2,222 injuries. Boys experienced 1,648 (74.2%), and girls experienced 574 (25.8%). One reason for boys being associated with a greater number of injuries is that only boys participated in the contact sports of football and wrestling. Both of these sports are associated with higher injury rates.

The injury rate for the girls' sports was 8.5 injuries per 100 participants, and the injury rate for the boys' sports was 17.8 injuries per 100 participants. The combined injury rate was 13.8 injuries per 100 participants. A discussion of injuries in various sports follows.

Basketball

There were 334 injuries in basketball during the first 2 years of the study, with girls accounting for 141 (42.2%) and boys for 193 (57.8%). During this time period, 958 girls, resulting in an injury rate of 14.7 per 100 participants, and 1,068 boys, resulting in an injury rate of 18.1 per 100 participants, took part in the sport. Consistent with the literature in this area, girls sustained 28 knee injuries while their male counterparts had only 17. The knee injury rate per 100 participants for girls was 2.92 and for boys 1.59. Girls also sustained more ankle injuries than boys (61 to 51). Sixty-three percent of the girls' injuries affected the foot and ankle, compared with only 35% of the boys' injuries. Concussions are not a major concern in basketball; girls sustained only 2 and boys 3.

Injury severity was measured by time missed from competition or practice. Girls and boys were almost identical when looking at missing 1 to 3 weeks, but boys had a greater number of injuries that involved missing 3 or more weeks.

Soccer

A total of 2,124 athletes participated in soccer in the first 2 years of the study: 826 girls with 87 injuries and 1,298 boys with 212 injuries. The girls' injury rate was 10.5 per 100 participants, and the boys' injury rate was 16.3 per 100 participants. Girls accounted for 29.1% of the total injuries, and boys for 70.9%. Female soccer players had 18 knee injuries and male players had 38. The knee injury rate for girls was 2.2 per 100 participants, and for boys it was 2.9 per 100 participants. More ankle injuries occurred in boys (57) than in girls (27). When knee and ankle injuries are combined, they account for 51.7% of the total girls' injuries and 44.8% of the total boys' injuries. Because soccer is more of a contact sport than basketball, concussion injuries are slightly higher: 5 for girls and 6 for boys.

When evaluating injury severity, male soccer players missed more practice and game time than did female soccer players.

Track

During the 1997 and 1998 track seasons there were 1,445 female and 1,437 male participants in the study schools. These 2,882 athletes experienced only 128 injuries: 69 for girls and 59 for boys. This was the only school sport studied in which the girls had more injuries than the boys. The injury rate per 100 participants was 4.8 for the girls and 4.1 for the boys. The combined injury rate was 4.4 injuries per 100 participants. Female track athletes had a greater number of knee injuries than their male counterparts: 19 for girls and 2 for boys. This was also true for ankle injuries, with the girls having 15 and the boys 6. Injury severity was fairly equal between the girls and boys.

Softball and Baseball

During the 1997 and 1998 seasons there were 1,193 female softball players and 1,182 male baseball players in the study schools. Softball was associated with 76 injuries and an injury rate of 6.4 per 100 participants. Baseball was associated with 105 injuries and an injury rate of 8.9 per 100 participants. Each sport had 6 knee injuries, but softball had 16 ankle injuries compared to 10 in baseball. Injury severity was fairly equal; however, baseball participants had more injuries that involved missing more than 3 weeks of practices and games.

Most of the injuries in both softball and baseball were caused by being struck with a batted ball, being struck with a thrown ball, or sliding into a fixed base. The baseball pitchers sustained 19 injuries while the softball pitchers had only 5.

Volleyball

For the first 2 years of data collection, the injury rate among female volleyball players was 6.9 per 100 participants. There were a total of 1,023 girls with 71 injuries. The most common sites of injury were the ankle, with

40.8% of the total injuries, and the knee, with 16.9% of the total injuries. Most of the athletes missed 1 or 2 days of practice or competition due to their injury, but 10% missed 1 to 3 weeks and 8.5% missed more than 3 weeks. Twenty-six percent of the injuries were caused by diving for the ball, and 15.4% were caused by being hit with the ball.

Cheerleading

There were 1,281 cheerleaders in the study schools, and 130 were injured. The cheerleading injury rate was 10.2 per 100 participants. These numbers do not include the 16 male participants who did not sustain any injuries. Two thirds of the injured participants missed from 1 to 6 days of practice or competition, but 22.9% missed from 1 to 3 weeks and 11.5% missed more than 3 weeks. Most of the injuries were sprains and strains, and 12.3% of the injuries were fractures. There were also 2 concussion injuries. Cheerleading injuries involved a number of different body parts, but two thirds of the injuries were to the knee and ankle. Twenty-six percent of the injured cheerleaders fell from a pyramid or some other activity that involved height, 16.8% were injured from contact with another cheerleader, and 16% were injured while tumbling.

Summary

It is obvious from the available information that there has been a tremendous increase in the number of high school female athletes, and that with this increase in participation there has also been an increase in girls' athletic injuries. It is also quite obvious that research to define female athletic injury risk is in its infancy. Although there is compelling evidence that female athletes have a greater number of ACL knee injuries than their male counterparts, the reasons for this difference are unknown. Both epidemiologic and clinical research are needed to help solve this dilemma.

References

1. Weaver NL, Mueller FO, Kalsbeek WD, Bowling JM: The North Carolina high school athletic injury study: Design and methodology. *Med Sci Sports Exerc* 1999;31:176–182.
2. *National Federation of State High School Associations Handbook 1998-99*. Kansas City, MO, 1998, pp 54–55.
3. Garrick JG, Requa RK: Injuries in high school sports. *Pediatrics* 1978;61:465–469.
4. Landry GL: Sports injuries in childhood. *Pediatr Ann* 1992;21:165–168.
5. Lindaman LM: Physician care for interscholastic athletes in Michigan. *Am J Sports Med* 1991;19:82–87.
6. Garrick JG, Requa RK: Girls' sports injuries in high school athletics. *JAMA* 1978;239:2245–2248.

7. Garrick JG, Requa RK: Epidemiology of women's gymnastics injuries. *Am J Sports Med* 1980;8:261–264.
8. Young ML, Cohen DA: Self-concept and injuries among female high school basketball players. *J Sports Med Phys Fitness* 1981;21:55–61.
9. McLemore E, Grana WA: Women's orthopedic problems: A review of their occurrence and management. *J Okla State Med Assoc* 1998;91:393–398.
10. Wirtz PD: High school basketball knee ligament injuries. *J Iowa Med Soc* 1982;72:105–106.
11. Lindenfeld TN, Schmitt DJ, Hendy MP, Mangine RE, Noyes FR: Incidence of injury in indoor soccer. *Am J Sports Med* 1994;22:364–371.
12. Stevenson H, Webster J, Johnson R, Beynnon B: Gender differences in knee injury epidemiology among competitive alpine ski racers. *Iowa Orthop J* 1998;18:64–66.
13. Durant RH, Linder CW, Sanders JM Jr, Jay S, Brantley G, Bedgood R: Adolescent females' readiness to participate in sports: Sex and race differences in the preparticipation athletic examination. *J Adolesc Health Care* 1988;9:310–314.
14. Bennell KL, Malcolm SA, Thomas SA, et al: Risk factors for stress fractures in track and field athletes: A twelve-month prospective study. *Am J Sports Med* 1996;24:810–818.

Chapter 3

Epidemiology of Women's Collegiate Sports Injuries

Randall W. Dick, MS, FACSM

Benefits of physical activity have been well documented in the literature; the 1996 Surgeon General's report on Physical Activity and Health is a current representative example.[1] This report also noted that a significant percentage of the US population do not incorporate exercise into their daily routine, leaving them at higher risk for health problems. It also stated that physical inactivity was more common in girls and women than it was in boys and men.

However, in college athletics, data on participation by women are more encouraging. Since the incorporation of women's athletics into the National Collegiate Athletic Association (NCAA) in 1982, participation by women has increased by over 50% to 129,000 in 1996[2] (Fig. 1). Soccer participation alone has increased 441% in 14 years, while softball, volleyball, lacrosse, and basketball also have shown significant gains[2] (Table 1). Although these participants should reap health benefits that extend well beyond their years in college athletics, increased participation brings with it issues such as sport injuries, which have not been well documented.

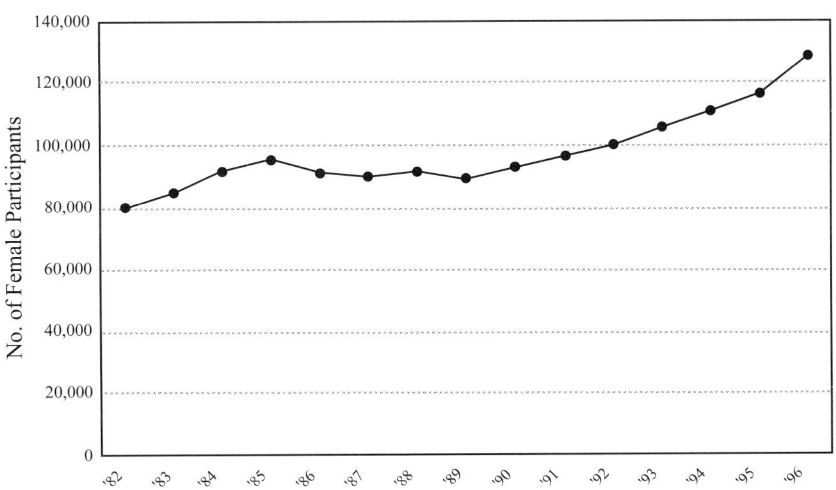

***Fig. 1** Participation by women in NCAA sports.*

Table 1 Participation in women's sports

	1982–1983		1990–1991		1996–1997		% Change from 1982–1983 season to 1996–1997 season
	Teams	Athletes	Teams	Athletes	Teams	Athletes	
Basketball	747	10,242	786	10,551	966	13,392	31
Field hockey	262	5,644	217	4,714	228	4,857	–14
Gymnastics	170	1,934	103	1,348	91	1,311	–32
Lacrosse	113	2,887	118	2,821	182	4,068	41
Soccer	103	2,743	318	6,781	691	14,829	441
Softball	441	8,035	580	9,724	770	13,167	64
Volleyball	638	8,656	741	9,713	923	12,284	42

The purpose of this chapter is to examine the epidemiology of sports injuries in collegiate women. Specific injury rates will be established initially for 7 sports in which women take part and for comparable men's activities using data from the NCAA Injury Surveillance System (ISS). Selected injury types and mechanisms within each sport then will be examined. Injury trends across time and between genders also will be reviewed. Finally, recommendations for future research will be presented.

NCAA Injury Surveillance System

The NCAA ISS was developed in 1982 to provide current and reliable data on injury trends in intercollegiate athletics. Injury data are collected yearly from a representative sample of NCAA member institutions, and the resulting data summaries are reviewed by the NCAA Committee on Competitive Safeguards and Medical Aspects of Sports and by appropriate sports committees. The information provides a foundation for health and safety policy development and for modification of rules and equipment at the NCAA and individual school levels. This function is consistent with the NCAA's principle of student-athlete welfare, which states that member institutions have a responsibility to protect the health of and provide a safe environment for each of its participating student-athletes.[3]

During the 1982–1983 academic year, injury data were collected only for the sport of football. Since that time, the ISS has been expanded to include 4 additional fall sports (men's soccer, women's soccer, field hockey, and women's volleyball), 6 winter sports (men's gymnastics, women's gymnastics, wrestling, ice hockey, men's basketball, and women's basketball), and 5 spring sports (spring football, baseball, softball, men's lacrosse, and women's lacrosse).

Sampling

Participation in the NCAA ISS is voluntary and limited to the 964 member institutions (as of August 1998). ISS participants are selected from the population of schools sponsoring a given sport. Selections are random within the constraints of having a minimum 10% representation of each NCAA division (I, II, and III) and region (East, South, Midwest, West). This sampling scheme assures a cross section of NCAA institutions that can be used to express injury rates representative of the total population of NCAA institutions sponsoring a particular sport.

Gathering Data

Injury and exposure data are recorded by certified and student athletic trainers from participating institutions. Information is collected from the first official day of preseason practice to the final tournament contest.

A reportable injury in the ISS is defined as one that (1) occurs as a result of participation in an organized intercollegiate practice or game, (2) requires medical attention by a team athletic trainer or physician, and (3) results in restriction of the student-athlete's participation for 1 or more days beyond the day of injury. A separate report is submitted for each injury by the athletic trainer. Each injury is described in detail including type of injury, body part injured, severity of injury, field type, field condition, and special equipment worn.

To establish an injury rate, data are expressed as the number of injuries per unit of participation or risk. An athlete exposure (A-E), the unit of risk in the ISS, is defined as 1 athlete participating in 1 practice or game where he or she is exposed to the possibility of athletic injury.

A 1-page exposure form, submitted weekly, summarizes the number of practices and games, types of playing surfaces, and numbers of participants. For example, 5 practices, each involving 60 participants, and 1 game involving 40 participants, would result in 300 practice A-Es, 40 game A-Es, and 340 total A-Es for a particular week.

Determining Injury Rate

An injury rate is a ratio of the number of injuries in a particular category to the number of A-Es in that category. In the ISS, this value is expressed as injuries per 1,000 A-Es. For example, 6 reportable injuries during 563 A-Es result in an injury rate of $(6/563) \times 1{,}000$ or 10.7 injuries/1,000 A-Es.

In the above example, 10.7 injuries would be anticipated if 1 athlete participated in 1,000 practices and/or games, if 50 athletes participated in 20 practices and/or games, or if 100 athletes participated in 10 practices and/or games. Expressing injuries in the form of a rate allows comparison within and across sports on a variety of variables.

Injury Rates in Practices and Games

Injury rates during the 1997–1998 academic year for 16 NCAA activities are shown in Figures 2 (practice) and 3 (game). In most women's sports, the injury rate in games was 2 to 3 times higher than the injury rate in practice.

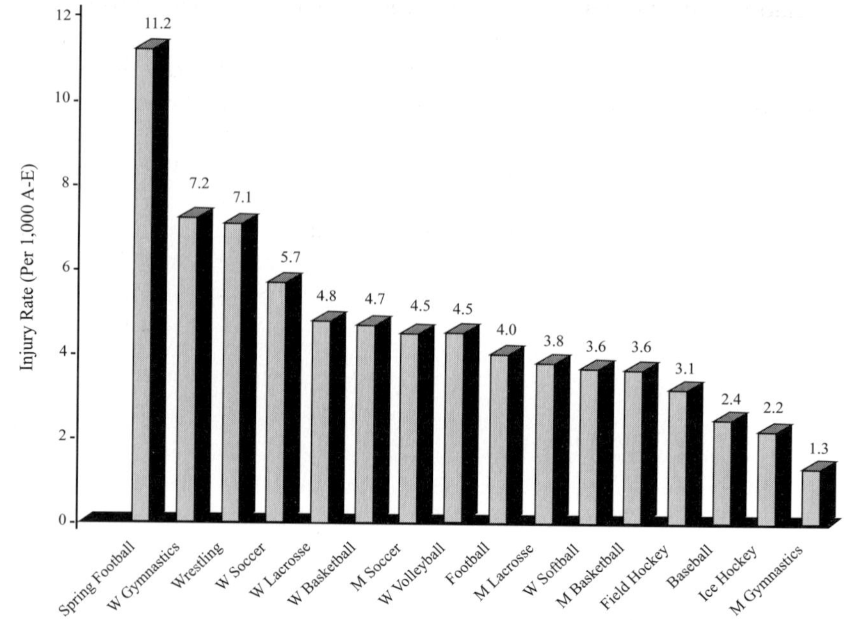

Fig. 2 Practice injury rate summary, 1997–1998 season.

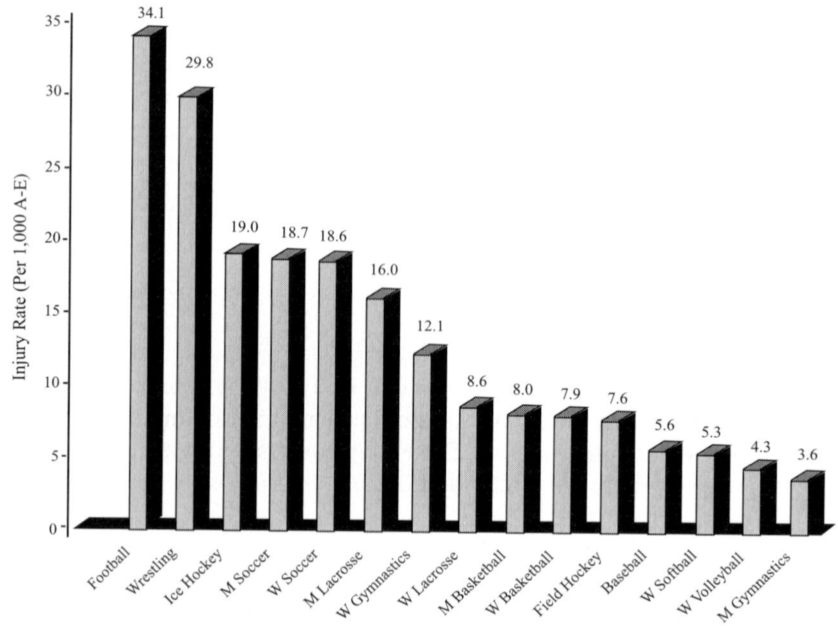

Fig. 3 Game injury rate summary, 1997–1998 season.

This finding was not surprising given the increased intensity level usually associated with a game situation. Women's soccer had the highest game to practice injury ratio at 3.3:1, whereas women's softball and volleyball had similar injury rates in practice and games. Women's practice injuries were higher than comparable men's practice injuries in soccer, gymnastics, and basketball; however, women's game injury rates in these activities were comparable to those of men. Practice injury rates and game injury rates have shown a slight increasing trend in women's basketball, women's lacrosse, and field hockey over the last 10 years. Game injury rates have shown slight decreasing trends in women's gymnastics and women's basketball over the past 5 years.[4]

Measures of Severity

There are 2 basic measures of severity found in the ISS: time loss and injuries requiring surgery. Figures 4 (practice) and 5 (game) reflect rates for injuries requiring 7 days or more time loss for the 1997–1998 season. Figures 6 and 7 show 1997–1998 rates for injuries requiring surgery. Rates for women's sports were similar or higher than rates for comparable men's activities in these categories. Although most sports analyzed showed stable rates of 7-day time loss or surgery across time, rates of game injuries requiring surgery increased slightly in women's lacrosse and basketball over the last 5 years.[4]

Another way to analyze severity across sport is to quantify specific injury types such as fractures, concussions, and surgeries. Table 2 shows these injury categories in 7 women's collegiate sports and 2 corresponding men's sports. This analysis reveals 3 levels of serious game injury risk: soccer in the highest risk category; field hockey, lacrosse, gymnastics, and basketball in the moderate risk category; and softball and volleyball in the lowest risk category. Table 2 also shows that the risk of serious injury was higher in women's soccer and basketball than in comparable men's sports, primarily because of greater concussion and surgery rates.

Injuries Involving Player Contact

Sports that are traditionally considered noncontact in nature, such as basketball and soccer, do, in fact, have a significant number of injuries resulting from contact with another player. Table 3 shows player contact injury rates for 6 collegiate women's sports and 3 comparable men's sports for the 1997–1998 season. Women's rates in soccer, basketball, and lacrosse were lower than the men's rates; this finding should not be surprising in lacrosse because the men's game allows player contact, which is prohibited in the women's game. The sport of soccer, in particular, had a surprisingly high player contact injury rate relative to other sports. The women's soccer rate of 9.05 contact injuries per 1,000 A-Es translates into 1 player contact injury/team every 7 games, assuming 15 game participants.

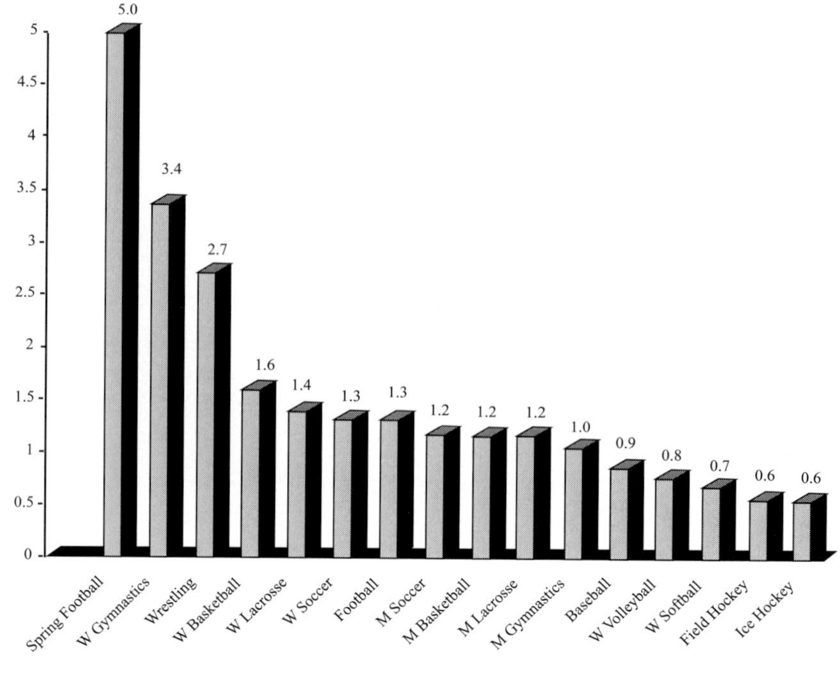

Fig. 4 *Severity: > 7 days' time loss injury rate in practice, 1997–1998 season.*

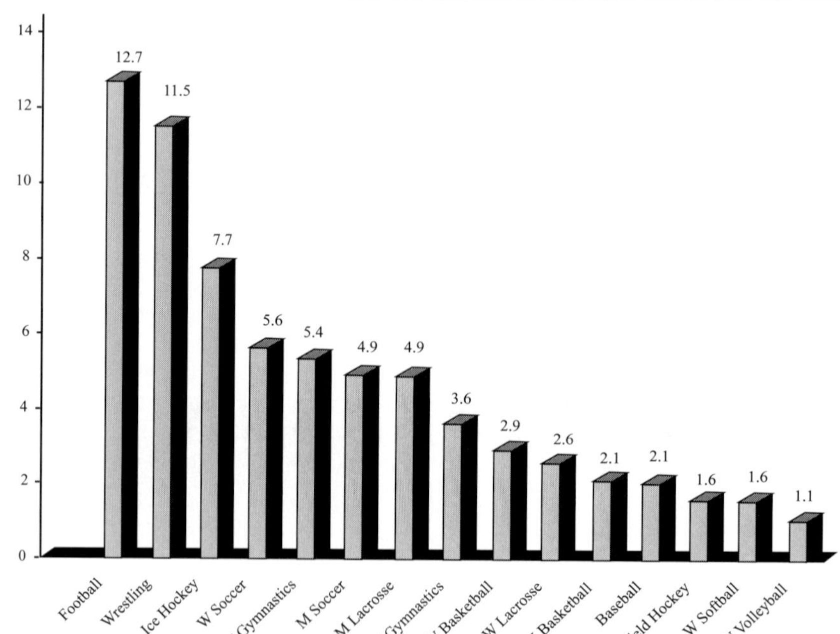

Fig. 5 *Severity: > 7 days' time loss injury rate in games, 1997–1998 season.*

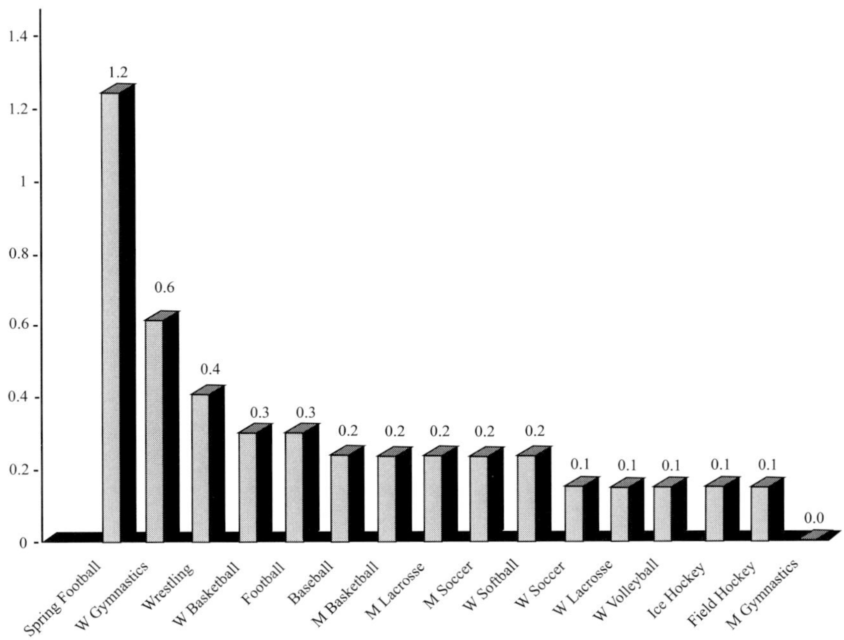

Fig. 6 *Severity: surgery injury rate in practice, 1997–1998 season.*

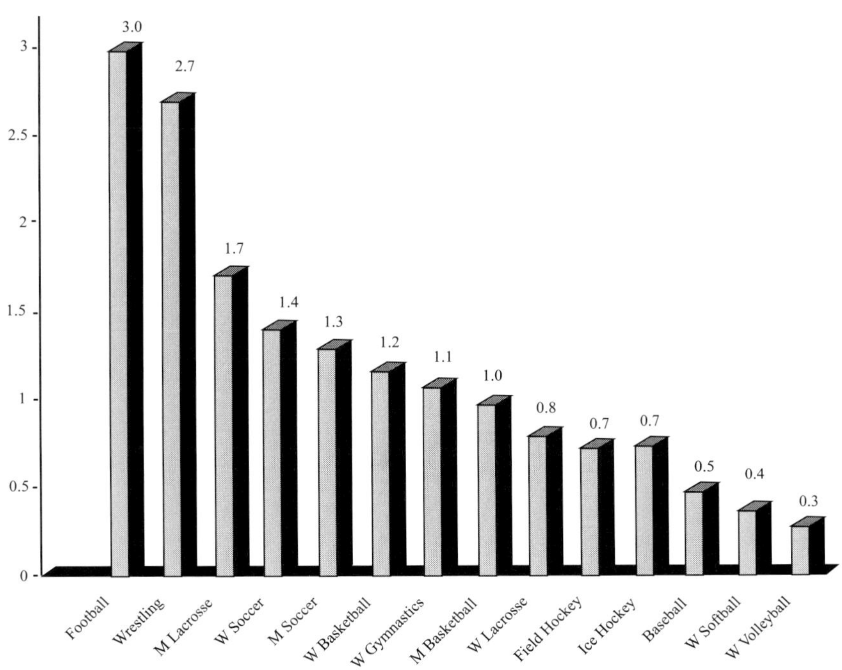

Fig. 7 *Severity: surgery injury rate in games, 1997–1998 season.*

Table 2 Serious game injury rates (injuries per 1,000 A-Es), 1997–1998

	Women				Men			
	Fracture	Concussion	Surgery	Total	Fracture	Concussion	Surgery	Total
Soccer	0.92	1.92	1.40	**4.24**	1.16	1.19	1.29	**3.64**
Field hockey	1.45	0.36	0.72	**2.53**				
Lacrosse	0.46	1.26	0.80	**2.52**				
Gymnastics	1.07	0.36	1.07	**2.50**				
Basketball	0.75	0.51	1.15	**2.41**	0.97	0.22	0.98	**2.17**
Softball	0.37	0.22	0.45	**1.04**				
Volleyball	0.04	0.12	0.28	**0.44**				

Table 3 Contact game injury rates (injury rates per 1,000 A-Es), 1997–1998

	Women	Men
Soccer	9.05	10.92
Basketball	3.84	4.55
Lacrosse	2.05	6.53
Volleyball	1.81	
Softball	1.27	
Field hockey	0.72	

Figure 8 shows the percent of game injuries in men's and women's soccer resulting from player contact over a 10-year period. Although the injury percentage appears to be stable over time in both men's and women's soccer, it is interesting to note that over 50% of all game injuries in both sports result from contact with another player.

Figure 9 shows the percent of game injuries in men's and women's basketball resulting from player contact over a 10-year period. Both sports show approximately a 10% rise in injuries resulting from player contact over this period, and almost 50% of women's basketball injuries result from this mechanism.

Figure 10 shows the percent of game injuries in men's and women's lacrosse resulting from player contact over a 9-year period. As noted above, the men's game specifically allows player contact, whereas the women's game strictly prohibits it. Yet the percentage of player contact injuries in the women's game has accounted for at least 10% of all game injuries and has shown an increasing trend over the last few years. In addition, injuries resulting from contact with the ball or stick exceed the rates of player contact injuries in both women's lacrosse and field hockey.

Specific Injuries

Concussions

Head trauma, particularly concussion, has received increased interest in the sports medicine community over the past few years. Current research is focused on the frequency of head trauma in sport,[5] particularly in professional

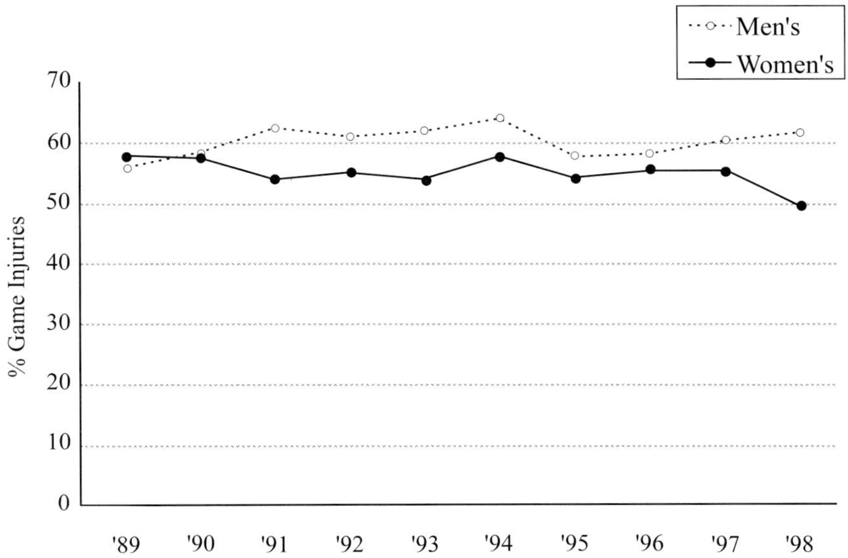

***Fig. 8** Men's and women's soccer: percent of game injuries from contact.*

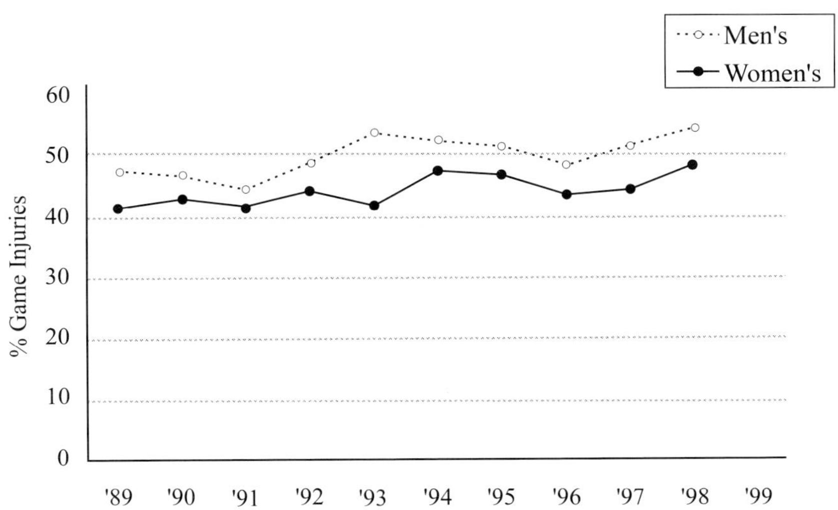

***Fig. 9** Men's and women's basketball: percent of game injuries from contact.*

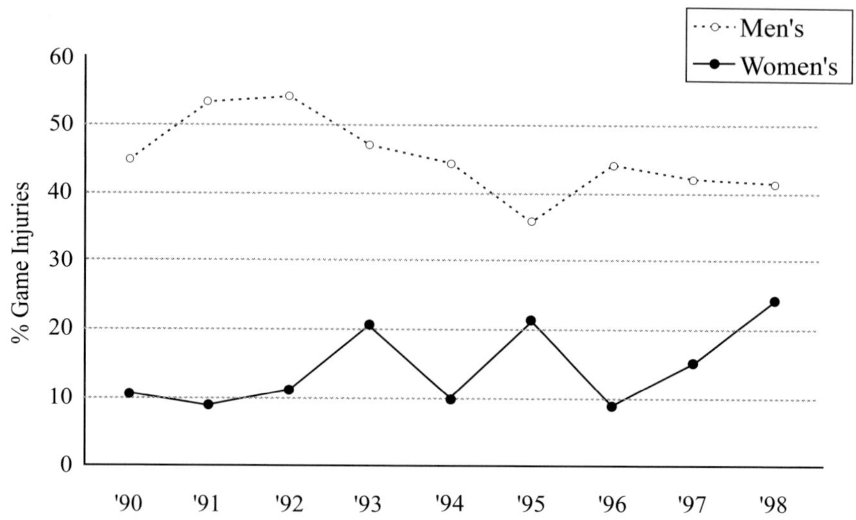

***Fig. 10** Men's and women's lacrosse: percent of game injuries from contact.*

football and ice hockey. These issues were recently highlighted in the American Medical Society for Sports Medicine Head-Injured Athlete symposium at the 1998 XXVI International Sports Medicine Federation World Congress of Sports Medicine. Other efforts, such as the 1997 Concussion in Sports Workshop sponsored by the American Orthopaedic Society for Sports Medicine, focused on developing consensus on severity categories and return to play criteria. However, little has been published on head trauma in women's sports. Given the unexpected magnitude of contact injuries associated with women's collegiate sports, this is an area worthy of further research.

A reportable concussion in the ISS meets the injury definition reported previously. Tables 4 and 5 compare concussions in sports with and without head protection. Concussions accounted for a higher percentage of game injuries in women's soccer than in men's, although the sports had a similar game concussion rate (1.1 per 1,000 A-Es). Women's soccer also showed increases in the game concussion rate across time, especially over the last few years (Fig. 11). All other women's sports analyzed show relatively stable game concussion rates over the 10-year period. Although women's lacrosse had a relatively low game injury and concussion rate, the percent of game injuries that were concussions rivaled that in men's ice hockey and exceeded that found in football.

Knee Injuries

One joint that has received significant attention in the sports medicine literature is the knee. Table 6 shows the 1997–1998 season game knee injury rates in 7 collegiate women's sports and 3 comparable men's sports. Women's knee injury rates were highest in soccer and gymnastics. Compared to men's sports, knee injuries were significantly higher in

Table 4 Concussions in sports that require head protection: % of all game injuries, 1989–1998

Ice hockey*	7.5%
Men's lacrosse*	5.2%
Football*	4.5%
Spring football*	3.9%
Softball	3.6%
Baseball	2.7%

*Requires mouthguard

Table 5 Concussions in sports without head protection: % of all game injuries, 1989–1998

Women's lacrosse*	8.5%
Women's soccer	6.5%
Men's soccer	5.4%
Field hockey	5.2%
Women's basketball	4.9%
Wrestling	4.3%
Men's basketball	3.1%

*Requires mouthguard

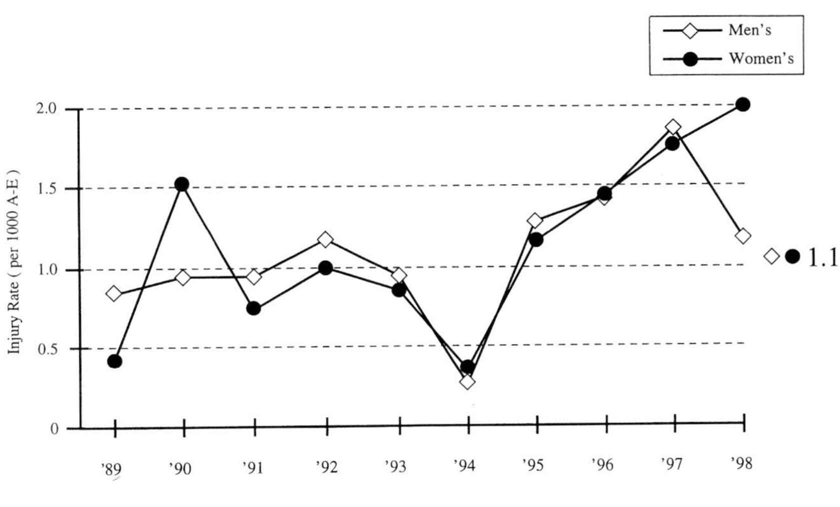

Fig. 11 Men's and women's soccer: game concussion injury rates.

women's soccer and basketball. The anterior cruciate ligament (ACL) is a specific knee structure that shows real gender differences in injury risk. A 1995 study reviewing ACL injuries in collegiate soccer and basketball players over a 5-year period showed that the women's soccer ACL injury rate was 2.4 times higher and the women's basketball ACL rate was 4.1 times higher than the rates for their male counterparts.[6]

Table 6 Game injury rates for the knee (injuries per 1,000 A-Es), 1997–1998

	Women	Men
Soccer	3.64	2.78
Gymnastics	2.85	
Lacrosse	1.83	3.42
Basketball	1.56	0.76
Softball	1.23	
Field hockey	1.08	
Volleyball	0.68	

Table 7 Stress fractures in practice and game (injuries per 1,000 A-Es), 1997–1998

	Women	Men
Basketball	0.45	0.18
Lacrosse	0.36	0.00
Soccer	0.20	0.05
Gymnastics	0.16	
Volleyball	0.12	
Field hockey	0.05	
Softball	0.02	

This trend has been maintained through 1998. ACL injury rates for soccer and basketball from 1995 to 1998 were 1.8 (practice) and 2.8 (game) times higher, respectively, for female soccer players compared with their male counterparts and 2.5 (practice) and 2.7 (game) times higher for female basketball players. In addition, results of a recent study suggested that ACL injury risk did not differ by skill level, as measured by division of collegiate participation.[7]

Noncontact Injuries

Table 7 shows the 1997–1998 season stress fracture injury rates in 7 collegiate women's sports and 3 men's sports. Because acute injuries are most readily captured by the ISS, these data may be an underestimation of the frequency of such overuse injuries. However, these results did show that the stress fracture injury rate was 2 to 3 times higher in the women's sports that have comparable men's sports.

The opposite is true when evaluating arm injuries in women's collegiate fastpitch softball and men's collegiate baseball. In the 1997–1998 season, the percentage of arm injuries resulting from pitching in men's baseball (17%) was significantly higher than that of arm injuries resulting from pitching in women's softball (6%). This result may seem surprising because softball pitchers normally throw more innings with less rest than baseball pitchers. For example, the top 10 (as determined by earned run average) 1999 NCAA Division I softball pitchers appeared in an average 37 games and threw an average 210 innings, while their counterparts in baseball appeared in 25 games and averaged 82 innings pitched. One Division III softball player pitched an amazing 77% of all innings played by her team in 1999 (52 games). It is not yet known whether those differences are related to the greater biomechanical stresses put on the arm in throwing overhand or whether they are influenced by techniques or gender differences.

Summary

Women's participation in college athletics has increased dramatically since 1982. This participation boom has brought increased opportunities for physical fitness and competition. It also has created a new area of research in sports medicine—the female athlete. The NCAA ISS is one tool available to study some of the factors involved in injury risk. Annual data collection and review have allowed injury trends to be monitored as sports evolve, with subsequent modification of rules and equipment.

Comparisons of injury rates in various sports are difficult because of the unique schedules and characteristics of each activity. However, if such comparisons are necessary, it may be best to use the game data for which the intensity variable is more consistent. Although injury patterns within specific women's sports are relatively stable across time, there are interesting comparisons across sports. For example, soccer and basketball have the highest game injury rates among women's sports; they also have a higher risk of serious injury relative to comparable men's sports. Measures of severity have not been agreed on in the medical literature; however, such measures may provide a more practical application of medical resources than basic practice or game injury rates. Limitations to measures such as time loss or required surgery include: (1) injuries that restrict participation in one sport may not restrict participation in another; (2) the importance of the athlete to the team or the upcoming game, which may influence return to play decisions in a nonsystematic way; (3) injuries that carry over beyond the end of the season, which may be estimated; (4) the changing nature of surgical techniques; and (5) the assumption that all sports have access to a similar quality of medical evaluation and intervention. The latter 2 issues are of particular interest to this chapter.

Gender differences in comparable sports are also apparent in knee injuries, especially ACL injuries, and stress fractures. These findings are consistent with a study of high school sports injuries that reported girls' sports having higher injury rates than identical boys' sports (cross-country, soccer, basketball, track, and swimming).[9] There is significant opportunity for further research in this area. Contact injuries are surprisingly high in perceived noncontact sports such as soccer and basketball with a recent increasing trend for both men's and women's basketball. This is one area in which men's sports have higher injury rates than comparable women's sports, although women's basketball has rates approaching those of the men's game. It will be interesting to see how these rates change as the women's game continues to evolve.

Although significant research has been done to investigate concussions in men's contact sports such as football and ice hockey, this report indicates that head injuries also are a concern in women's sports. The change in concussion rate over time may be influenced by a variety of factors including greater sensitivity of data reporters, rules changes, and equipment. Concussion rates across sports may differ because of gender, protective equipment, or rules of the game. While sports such as women's lacrosse and field hockey have a relatively low injury rate, 6% to 8% of the injuries that do occur result in head trauma and concussion. Such injuries primarily result from contact with a stick or ball rather than from contact with another player and raise questions about the value of protective equipment in these activities. Although helmets and masks do reduce head and facial lacerations,[10] some argue that the use of this equipment may increase head and neck injuries because players will perform more aggressively.

This study also showed a relatively low incidence of stress fractures in most monitored sports, although the current ISS system was not primarily designed to collect injuries that evolve gradually rather than having an acute onset. Overuse injury surveillance may need to be developed with a different surveillance tool because such injuries result primarily from practice techniques rather than playing rules or equipment. If the goal of overuse injury surveillance is to quantify injury and bring about change, variables such as surface type (where applicable), conditioning time, mileage run (or swum), and menstrual history should be considered. Such research may better quantify overuse issues in currently monitored sports such as volleyball, basketball, and gymnastics, as well as provide new insights on sports such as cross-country, track, and swimming, which accounted for almost 40% of NCAA female athlete participants in 1996.

References

1. US Department of Health and Human Services*: Physical Activity and Health: A Report of the Surgeon General*. Atlanta, GA, US Department of Health and Human Services, Centers for Disease Control and Prevention, National Center for Chronic Disease Prevention and Health Promotion, 1996.
2. *NCAA Participation Statistics Report 1982–97*. Indianapolis, IN, National Collegiate Athletic Association, 1998, pp 5, 99, 115, 127.
3. Principles for conduct of intercollegiate athletics: 2.2.3–student-athlete welfare health and safety, in *1998–99 NCAA Division I, II and III Manuals*. Indianapolis, IN, National Collegiate Athletic Association, 1998, p 3.
4. *NCAA Injury Surveillance System*. Indianapolis, IN, National Collegiate Athletic Association, 1988–1998.
5. Hoerner EF (ed): *Head and Neck Injuries in Sports*. Philadelphia, PA, American Society for Testing and Materials, 1994.
6. Arendt E, Dick R: Knee injury patterns among men and women in collegiate basketball and soccer: NCAA data and review of literature. *Am J Sports Med* 1995;23:694–701.
7. Harmon KG, Dick R: The relationship of skill level to anterior cruciate ligament injury. *Clin J Sport Med* 1998;8:260–265.
8. *NCAA 2000 Baseball and Softball Records Book*. Indianapolis, IN, National Collegiate Athletic Association, 2000, pp 102, 254.
9. Rice SG: An injury surveillance system. *Sports Med Digest* 1991;13:1–2.
10. LaPrade RF, Burnett QM, Zarzour R, Moss R: The effect of the mandatory use of face masks on facial lacerations and head and neck injuries in ice hockey: A prospective study. *Am J Sports Med* 1995;23:773–775.

Chapter 4

Health, Exercise, and Injury in Women: Military Academy Experience

LTC Dean C. Taylor, MD
Bradley J. Nelson, MD

Cadets and Midshipmen at the US Service Academies always have been challenged physically in their athletic and military training requirements. In 1976, women were admitted for the first time to the US Service Academies (United States Military Academy, United States Naval Academy, United States Air Force Academy, United States Coast Guard Academy, and the United States Merchant Marine Academy). United States Public Law 94-106 mandated the admission of women and stated that "the academic and other relevant standards required for appointment, admissions, training, graduation, and commissioning of female individuals shall be the same as those required for male individuals, except for those minimal essential adjustments in such standards required because of physical differences between male and female individuals."

Since 1976, through extensive study, and through trial and error, much has been learned about the physical capabilities of women in the service academy environment, and how this environment affects the health of women. This chapter will examine the issues of health, exercise, and injury for the women at the service academies, with specific focus on the US Military Academy (USMA) at West Point. We will outline the requirements in the physical and military programs, examine the physiologic differences between men and women, and show how the physically challenging environment of the service academies affects the health of women.

Requirements for Physical and Military Training

Athletic participation at the United States Military Academy has a higher purpose than just the playing of games. General of the Army Douglas A. MacArthur probably said it best: "Upon the fields of friendly strife, are sown the seeds that, upon other fields, on other days, will bear the fruits of victory." As such, all cadets are required to participate in athletics at either the intramural, club, or intercollegiate level, and this requirement has led to the dictum, "Every cadet an athlete, every athlete challenged."[1]

Cadets are required to participate in a competitive sport each semester. Until recently, during their cadet careers, all cadets competed in at least one team sport that involved contact or collision. Most intramural sports are mixed gender (Table 1). Competitive clubs also are largely mixed gender, with exclusively female teams in lacrosse and team handball, and exclusively male teams in volleyball, boxing, rugby, squash, water polo, and team handball. Intercollegiate athletic teams in basketball, soccer, track, cross-country, swimming and diving, and tennis exist for both men and women. In addition, women have varsity intercollegiate teams in volleyball and softball. Women make up approximately 15% of the United States Corps of Cadets; however, the number of women cadets in intercollegiate athletics is disproportionately greater than the number of men, approximately 45% of women versus 30% of men.

In addition to competitive athletics, all cadets are required to complete a rigorous, physical development program (Table 1). In the combatives program, women take required self-defense courses in lieu of boxing and wrestling. Additionally, both men and women are required to complete the Army Physical Fitness Test (2-mile run, push-ups, and sit-ups) twice a year, and the Indoor Obstacle Course Test 3 of the 4 years. These tests have the same events for both men and women cadets, but grading scales are normalized by gender, as will be discussed.

Military training is another physically demanding requirement for cadets at USMA. All cadets must successfully complete Cadet Basic Training (CBT), previously known as "Beast Barracks," before starting their freshman academic year. CBT is a 6-week long physically and emotionally demanding program. Cadet Field Training, between their freshman and sophomore academic years, is another 6 weeks of intense military and physical training. During the summers between their sophomore and junior, and junior and senior years, cadets participate in a variety of military training programs, which include attending the Army's Airborne or Air Assault Schools. These military requirements and physical activities are the same for both male and female cadets.

Physical Differences Between Male and Female Cadets

Following the introduction of women into the United States Corps of Cadets in 1976, much has been learned about the physical differences between the sexes. Before the start of the first class of women, a study titled "Project 60" was conducted that examined 60 high-school girls to determine physical differences when compared with boys. The girls were noted to be more physically proficient than what was reported in the literature; however, even the best girls performed at a level below the average male cadet. The authors concluded that "in order to maintain the one-track cadet experience with minimal essential adjustments, a concerted effort must be made to identify and attract high-level female physical performers to become cadets."[2]

In a study of the female members of the Class of 1980, decreased upper-body strength, leg strength, power endurance, and grip strength were reported, but no significant difference was found in cardiorespiratory efficiency relative to body weight.[3] As expected, after 1976, these differences between

Table 1 Physical training and athletic team participation for cadets at the US Military Academy

	Intramurals		
Sport	**Men**	**Women**	**Coeducational**
Area hockey			X
Basketball			X
Boxing	X		
Cross country			X
Flickerball			X
Football	X		
Handball			X
Orienteering			X
Racquetball			X
Sandhurst			X
Soccer			X
Softball			X
Swimming			X
Team handball			X
Volleyball			X
Wallyball			X
Wrestling	X		

	Club Sports		
Sport	**Men**	**Women**	**Coeducational**
Boxing	X		
Crew			X
Cycling			X
Fencing			X
Judo			X
Lacrosse		X	
Marathon			X
Mountaineering			X
Rugby	X		
Sailing			X
Ski-Alpine			X
Ski-Nordic			X
Squash	X		
Team Handball	X	X	
Volleyball	X		
Water polo	X		
Wrestling	X		

Continued on next page

Table 1, continued

Varsity Intercollegiate Athletics		
Sport	**Men**	**Women**
Baseball	X	
Basketball	X	X
Cross country	X	X
Football	X	
Golf	X	
Gymnastics	X	
Hockey	X	
Lacrosse	X	
Soccer	X	X
Softball		X
Sprint football	X	
Swimming	X	X
Tennis	X	X
Track	X	X
Volleyball		X
Wrestling	X	

Physical Education Classes			
Sport	**Men**	**Women**	**Coeducational**
Advanced close quarters combat			X
Aerobic fitness			X
Basketball			X
Boxing	X		
Close quarters combat			X
Emergency water			X
Fitness foundations			X
Golf			X
Gymnastics			X
Handball			X
Ice skating			X
Racquetball			X
Self defense			X
Skiing			X
Squash			X
Soccer			X
Strength development			X
Swimming			X
Tennis			X
Volleyball			X
Wrestling	X		

the genders led to some changes in training and physical education. In her PhD thesis, Colonel Maureen LeBoeuf, the current head of the Department of Physical Education at USMA, identified several areas of change.[1] During CBT, all cadets were required to wear t-shirts at all times during athletic

Table 2 Changes in the Army physical fitness grading scales, 1981–1999

	Push-ups*		Sit-ups*		2 Mile Run Time*	
Year	Women	Men	Women	Men	Women	Men
1981	16/40	40/68	27/61	40/69	22:14/17:10	17:55/13:05
1999	19/67	42/96	53/100	53/100	18:54/13:06	15:54/11:54

*Values are listed as minimum passing score/maximum score

training, separate running groups were formed based on ability, fewer hills were included in runs, and women trained in the lighter rifles (M16 versus M14). In physical education, women now take two separate courses in self-defense and men take courses in boxing and wrestling. Also, in gymnastics class, balance beam and uneven bar training for women substitute for the parallel bar and high bar training that the men receive. On the Indoor Obstacle Course Test, the balance beam and tire run obstacles have replaced the parallel bar hand walk. In the intramural program, women are not allowed to participate in football, wrestling, boxing, and rugby.

Based on the physiologic differences between men and women, the Department of Physical Education at USMA uses the doctrine of comparable training, which emphasizes "equal effort" rather than "equal performance." This translates into different rating scales for various fitness tests. Over time, the rating scales have changed to keep up with increases in performance (Table 2). Both men and women have increased their performance on the Army Physical Fitness Test (APFT) in all three measures—push-ups, sit-ups, and the 2-mile run (Figs. 1 through 3). The rate of improvement has been similar for both male and female cadets. Physical differences remain, particularly for upper body strength, as indicated in the difference in push-ups, and also in run times; however, sit-up performance and grading scales are now equal for male and female cadets and throughout the US Army.

Injury Differences Between Women and Men

General

Several investigators have examined the epidemiology of injuries in women at the service academies. Cox and Lenz[4,5] reviewed injury data from the United States Naval Academy; they found a twofold increase in sick-call visits by female midshipman for blisters, sprains, and heat illness. There was a threefold increase in visits by women for overuse injuries such as shin splints, stress fractures, and tendinitis. The authors noted that sick-call visits tended to decrease over time for female midshipman, whereas visits by male midshipman remained the same. The authors attributed this to societal pressure on men to "tough it out" that was adopted by the female midshipman while they were at the Naval Academy. In their first study, the authors reported a decreased incidence in traumatic injuries among female midshipman. Five years later, they stated that the rate of traumatic injuries did not differ and for some sports, women were more susceptible to injuries

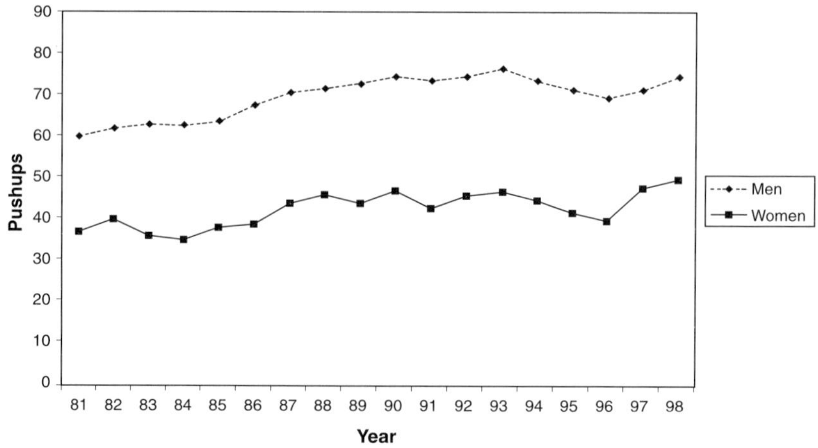

Fig. 1 *US Military Academy cadet scores for push-ups on the Army Physical Fitness Test, 1981–1998.*

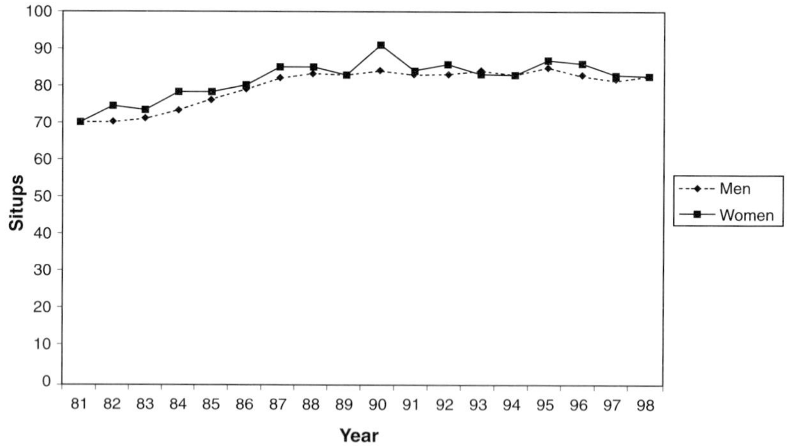

Fig. 2 *US Military Academy cadet scores for sit-ups on the Army Physical Fitness Test, 1981–1998.*

than men. The incidence of anterior cruciate ligament injuries in basketball was used as an example of higher injury risk in women.

In a 1989 study from the US Air Force Academy,[6] women had 2.5 times the number of injuries as men in coeducational intramural sports. There were similar injury rates in the activities of the general physical fitness program.

In a study of the first class of women at USMA, Protzman[7] noted that after 8 weeks of CBT, 25% of the women were not physically able to fully participate in the training because of injury compared to 5% of the men. However, Protzman noted that later in their cadet careers, there was no difference in

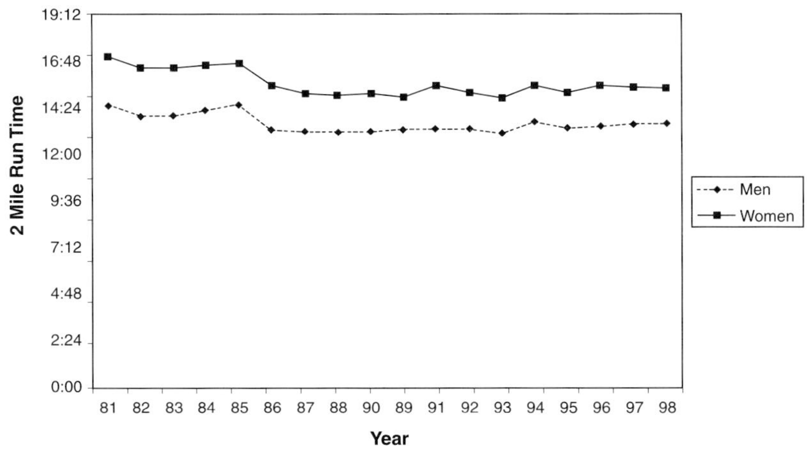

Fig. 3 US Military Academy cadet scores for the 2-mile run on the Army Physical Fitness Test, 1981–1998.

missed practice days between male and female intercollegiate athletes participating in the same sports.

McBride and associates[8] performed a retrospective review of randomly selected medical records from 74 male and female USMA cadets. The authors noted an increased incidence of lower extremity injuries in female cadets. Female cadets had a threefold increase in patellofemoral pain and shin splints compared to the male cadets. Female cadets also demonstrated a fourfold increase in ankle sprains and an increased incidence of low back pain. The 11 stress fractures in the study group all occurred in women. The time to recover from these injuries and return to full participation was the same for women and men, with the exception of low back pain. It took male cadets twice as long to recover from low back pain.

The male cadets demonstrated an increased incidence of shoulder instability. The authors postulated that this difference was a result of the high incidence of shoulder subluxation in boxing and wrestling. Female cadets do not participate in these sports. Additionally, there was an increased incidence of hand and wrist injuries in male cadets, which was thought to be secondary to participation in tackling sports such as football and rugby.

In a prospective study at USMA, we followed 133 female and 136 male cadets over a 47-month period and recorded injury rates (J. Ryan and D. Taylor, MD, unpublished data, 1993). Overall, there were 664 injuries to the extremities and spine, 316 in men and 328 in women. There were 254 traumatic injuries in male cadets compared to 167 in female cadets. We noted a threefold increase in shoulder injuries in the male cadets. There was a significant increase in overuse injuries in the female cadets with 167 injuries occurring in the women compared to 62 in the men. The most common injuries in both the female and male cadets were tendinitis, blisters, shin splints, patellofemoral pain, and iliotibial band friction syndrome.

We also looked at a subset of injuries that occurred during summer military training, which is essentially identical for women and men. The incidence of traumatic injuries was the same for female and male cadets; however, the incidence of overuse injuries was over twofold greater in the women.

In summary, these studies suggest that female cadets are at greater risk for injury than their male counterparts. This appears to be partly a result of more overuse injuries in the women. The traumatic injury rates appear to be similar when men and women are engaged in similar activities.

Stress Fractures

Of the overuse injuries seen in cadets, a stress fracture is perhaps the most serious. The stress fracture incidence rates in the early classes of women were very high. Protzman and Griffis[9] reviewed the incidence of stress fractures sustained by cadets at the USMA during summer CBT in 1976. The class consisted of 119 women and 1,366 men. Twelve male cadets (1%) and 10 female cadets (10%) sustained stress fractures during an 8-week period of intensive physical training; the difference was statistically significant ($p < 0.05$) (Table 3).

Over the next 10 years, several modifications were made to the training program. Running shoes were substituted for combat boots during daily distance and conditioning runs throughout the Army. A regimented pre-arrival training program was mailed to each new cadet candidate 3 months before summer training. Following an initial fitness test, cadets were placed in 3 different groups according to run times. Over the course of summer training the pace of each of these groups was gradually increased. Shorter cadets (men and women) were assigned to the front ranks during marching, thus setting the stride.

Reflecting these changes, the overall incidence rate of stress fractures during CBT decreased; however, women still had 10 times more stress fractures. During the summer of 1986, female members of the Class of 1990 had a 5.1% stress fracture incidence rate compared to 0.5% for males.[10]

Our experience in the 1990s continued to show a high rate of stress fractures in women. Over a 3-year period, from January 1994 to January 1997, there were 80 stress fractures in women and 105 in men. The incidence of stress fractures per year was 5.2% for women and 0.9% for men (J. Uhorchak, Beaumont Army Medical Center, El Paso, TX, personal communication, 1998).

Table 3 Stress fractures during cadet basic training (1976)

Fracture Location	No. of Fractures	
	Women	Men
Metatarsal	2	3
Calcaneus	2	2
Fibula	1	2
Tibia	2	5
Femur	3	0

Preliminary study of the USMA Class of 2002 has shown similar findings. Over the past year, 16 of the 136 women studied (11.8%) have had a total of 25 stress fractures, compared to 26 stress fractures in 21 of 744 men (2.8%). This is a statistically significant difference ($p < 0.001$, chi-square analysis) (J. Nieves, D. DeWitt, West Point, NY, personal communication, 1999).

In an attempt to examine stress fractures and potential causal relationships with hormonal changes and bone mineral density (BMD), a prospective, longitudinal study was performed at USMA by Wade and associates (unpublished data, 1999). Eighty-four female and 94 male cadets of the Class of 1993 were monitored over a 42-month period. Hormone levels, BMD, and the incidence of stress fractures were obtained biannually.

Estradiol and progesterone levels were decreased in female cadets over the first year. The levels remained low in 13% of the female cadets for the entire 42-month study period, with the lowest levels during the first 2 months of training. Testosterone levels remained low in 13% of the male cadets. Calcium and phosphate levels were greater in male cadets as were osteocalcin levels. Osteocalcin levels increased in both male and female cadets after 18 months.

BMD was lower in female cadets throughout the 42-month study period compared to BMD in the male cadets. Female cadets demonstrated a decrease in BMD over the first 6 months of training. This decrease persisted for the first year and then returned to baseline. There was an increase in BMD at a rate of 0.018g/cm^2/yr for the remaining 30 months. There was not a significant difference in BMD in women with low estradiol levels. However, female cadets with persistently low estradiol levels did not show gains in BMD.

Male cadets demonstrated no change in BMD over the first 6 months but did show an increase of 0.022 g/cm^2/yr for the next 30 months. BMD was significantly lower in men with persistently low testosterone levels.

There were 11 stress fractures in 10 study subjects for an overall incidence of 5.6%. The incidence of 2.1% in men and 9.5% in women was significantly different ($p = 0.035$). However, there was no statistically significant gender difference in the incidence of stress fractures during the first 2 months of intensive training, possibly because of the small number of stress fractures detected. The incidence of stress fractures was not related to BMD in either female or male cadets. No relationship was demonstrated between stress fractures and decreased gonadal hormones.

Menstrual irregularities were reported in 9.5% of female cadets. There was no difference demonstrated in BMD or the incidence of stress fractures in women with menstrual irregularities. Oral contraceptive use was reported by 62% of female cadets. No relationship was demonstrated between oral contraceptive use and BMD or the incidence of stress fractures.

This study suggests that both female and male cadets have hypogonadism and decreased BMD during periods of intense physical training and stress. Possibly because of the lower numbers of stress fractures detected, the incidence of stress fractures was not statistically related to this period of hypogonadism and decreased BMD; however, there was an increased incidence of stress fractures in female cadets over time, which may be related to decreased BMD in women compared to men.

Other studies have shown that most adolescents show an increase in BMD during the late teens and early twenties.[11,12] This is particularly true if moderate physical exercise is undertaken.[13] The long-term effect of a transient decrease in BMD in female and male cadets during a time when bone mass is supposed to be at its peak is unknown.

In summary, stress fractures occur 4 to 10 times more frequently in female cadets than in male cadets. There appears to be a relationship between periods of stress, sex hormone levels, and BMD. Women have lower levels of BMD than do men, but a statistically significant correlation with stress fractures has not been demonstrated.

Anterior Cruciate Ligament Injuries

In recent years, there has been a great deal of interest in anterior cruciate ligament (ACL) injuries in female athletes. Some studies have suggested that women involved in similar activities as men are at an increased risk for ACL injuries.[14–17] Similarly, data reported on ACL injury rates at the US Naval Academy have shown a higher incidence in women than in men. In a 6-year review of ACL injury data in midshipmen, the incidence of ACL injuries/yr was 0.005 for men and 0.0135 for women, for a relative risk of 2.44. There were relative risks of 3.96, 1.40, and 9.74 for women in comparisons of intercollegiate athletics, intramural athletics, and military training, respectively.[18]

At the USMA, the ACL injury rates for men and women are very similar. Examination of the ACL reconstructions at West Point over a 10-year period between 1987 and 1997, revealed an operation rate for ACL tears that was proportionate to the cadet male and female population at large (J. Uhorchak, unpublished data, 1998).

Data collected prospectively for the classes of 1994 until the present demonstrate similar findings. The average class size for the classes of 1994 through 1999 has been 1,089 (range 1,190 for 1994 to 1015 for 1998), with 134 women (12%) and 956 men (88%). Cadets in these six classes have sustained 223 complete ACL tears for an average of 37 injuries per class during the 4 years at USMA. There was an average of 4 ACL tears per class (1 to 7) in women, and 33 per class (23 to 42) in men. Based on these 6 classes, the probability of sustaining an ACL tear during a cadet career is 0.034; 0.030 for women and 0.036 for men, for a relative risk of 0.86. This difference was not statistically significant (chi-square analysis, $p = 0.22$). The greatest number of injuries occurred during varsity football and intramural football with 31 injuries each (Table 4). Intramural and club rugby accounted for 26 injuries. The greatest number of ACL injuries in women occurred during various levels of basketball with 5, followed by physical education gymnastics and club team handball with 4 each (Table 4).

To provide a better estimate of injury rates for male and female cadets involved in similar activities, we excluded football and rugby injuries and adjusted the male population downward to reflect time spent playing football and rugby. For example, intramural football occupies approximately one third to one fourth of the athletic time during a year. Therefore, the intramural football playing population of the class is estimated by multiplying the intramural football players of the class times 0.25. Similarly, the

Table 4 Anterior cruciate ligament injuries by activity (men/women), 1981–1998

Activity	Activity Level: Free Time	Organized Other	Physical Education Class	Intramural	Club Sports	Varsity Sports	Total
Football	1/0	0/0	NA	31/0	0/0	38/0*	70/0
Rugby	0/0	0/0	NA	18/0	8/0	0/0	26/0
Military training	0/0	6/2	11/1	NA	NA	NA	17/3
Soccer	0/0	0/0	0/0	9/1	NA	3/2	12/3
Basketball	7/0	0/0	2/1	6/2	NA	0/2	15/5
Skiing	11/0	0/0	2/1	NA	0/0	NA	13/1
Gymnastics	0/0	0/0	4/4	NA	0/0	0/0	4/4
Other	3/2	0/0	7/0	8/0	8/5	15/1	41/8
Total	22/2	6/2	26/7	72/3	16/5	56/5	198/24

*Includes 7 varsity lightweight football players
NA = Not Applicable

number of intramural and club rugby players are multiplied by 0.25, lightweight football by 0.50, and intercollegiate football by 1.0. These football and rugby populations are subtracted from the total class size to give an estimate of the non-football/rugby population. With these corrections, the probability that a cadet will sustain an ACL tear outside of football and rugby during a 4-year career is 0.022; 0.030 for women and 0.021 for men, for a relative risk of 1.43. This difference was statistically significant (chi-square analysis, $p = 0.05$)

The reason why the injury risk for female cadets is not as great as that of other collegiate women, or that of female midshipmen is unclear. Men at West Point have an ACL injury rate that is similar to their Annapolis peers, 0.006 versus 0.005, respectively. The incidence of ACL tears/year in women at Annapolis is 0.0135 versus 0.005 in women at West Point, almost three times as high. The relatively small numbers available may provide an explanation; however, the general experience at USMA over the last decade has been that, even if there is a difference in ACL injury rates for men and women, there is not a large difference. The discrepancy may be related to the emphasis placed on accepting only the most physically fit women in accordance with the Project 60 recommendations "…to identify and attract high-level women physical performers to become women cadets."[2] This "natural selection" of athletic females could account for the relatively lower ACL injury rates; however, there is no supporting evidence, it would be difficult to evaluate this premise, and it is unlikely that the students attending USNA and USMA are that different.

A better explanation could be differences in training. At USMA, there is a concerted effort to train cadets before testing or competition. For example, the Indoor Obstacle Course is given as a test only after cadets are instructed on the correct techniques for each obstacle during their first year physical education gymnastics course. They are then tested on the obstacle course during their final 3 years. This could help explain the large discrepancy between USMA and USNA women. At USNA, there is limited training before the obstacle course testing, which is conducted during military training. Female midshipmen have more than a tenfold increase in ACL injuries on the obstacle course relative to men. At USMA, the ACL injury relative risk for women and men during the Indoor Obstacle Course Test is approximately equal at 1.8.

In an effort to determine possible risk factors associated with ACL injuries, we initiated a prospective study of the USMA class of 1999. During their first summer, we evaluated cadets with multiple measures thought to be predictive of ACL injury. The study was completed in the summer of 1999. Preliminary analysis of the results suggests several interesting findings. First, review of radiographic analysis shows that measurements of the intercondylar eminence width index (EWI) and the intercondylar notch width index (NWI) correlate with ACL injuries. The EWI is believed to provide an estimate of ACL size, and the NWI is believed to provide an estimate of space for the ACL between the femoral condyles. Compared to their uninjured classmates, female cadets with ACL injuries had a significant decrease in NWI ($p < 0.05$), and male cadets with ACL injuries had a significant decrease in both NWI and EWI. There does not appear to be a significant gender difference in either measure (J. Uhorchak, personal communication, 1999).

Female cadets with ACL tears also had a greater average weight (67.2 versus 60.4 kg, $p < 0.05$) than uninjured women and were more likely to have hypermobility of other joints. There were no significant differences in KT2000 measurements, quadriceps or hamstring isokinetic strength measurements, or in quadriceps:hamstring strength ratios between injured and uninjured women. There were no significant differences in these measures between injured and uninjured men. In comparison, a study by Lysens and associates[19] found that men with greater flexibility and women with greater body weight were more prone to acute injuries of any kind, not just ACL injuries.

Conclusion

More than two decades of experience with women at the US Service Academies has demonstrated several things. First, women have adapted well to the demanding environment of the academies, with little change necessary in the physical development program. Second, physiologic differences are recognized; therefore, women do not participate in certain activities and are not evaluated using the same rating scale on fitness tests as men. Third, women are evaluated for injuries more often than are men. In particular, women sustain two to three times more overuse injuries, but have similar rates of traumatic injuries. Women have 4 to 10 times more stress fractures. Women at USMA have lower ACL injury rates than men overall, but slightly higher rates than men when the high-risk men's sports of football and rugby are eliminated.

Acknowledgments

The authors would like to acknowledge the following individuals for their contributions to this chapter: Jane Reddington for manuscript editing and technical advice; LTC Bill Maloney for statistical analysis; LTC John Uhorchak for data on stress fractures and ACL injuries at West Point, and for manuscript review; COL Maureen Leboeuf for helpful suggestions on describing the USMA physical development program; CPT Dave DeWitt for assistance with stress fracture data; CPT Matt Posner for organization and management of the ACL database; and Mr. Craig Yunker for assistance with sports participation information for the US Corps of Cadets.

References

1. LeBoeuf MK: *Effectiveness of the Physical Education Curriculum at the United States Military Academy in Preparing Its Women Graduates*. Athens, Georgia, University of Georgia, 1994. Dissertation.
2. Peterson JA, Vogel JA, Koval, et al: *Summary Report: Project 60: A Comparison of Two Types of Physical Training Programs on the Performance of 16–18 Year-Old Women*. West Point, NY, United States Military Academy, 1976.
3. Stauffer RW: *Comparison of United States Military Academy Men and Women on Selected Physical Performance Measures: "Project Summertime."* West Point, New York, United States Military Academy, 1976.
4. Cox JS, Lenz HW: Women in sports: The Naval Academy experience. *Am J Sports Med* 1979;7:355–357.
5. Cox JS, Lenz HW: Women midshipmen in sports. *Am J Sports Med* 1984;12:241–243.
6. Petosa S: Women in the military academies: US Air Force Academy (Part 2 of 3). *Phys Sports Med* 1989;17:133–142.
7. Protzman RR: Can women be overextended in physical conditioning programs? *Am J Sports Med* 1979;7:145–146.
8. McBride JT, Meade WC III, Ryan JB: Incidence and patterns of injury in female cadets at West Point Military Academy, in Pearl AJ (ed): *The Athletic Female*. Champaign, IL, Human Kinetics, 1993, pp 557–689.
9. Protzman RR, Griffis CG: Stress fractures in men and women undergoing military training. *J Bone Joint Surg* 1977;59A:825.
10. Welch MJ: Women in the military academies: US Army (Part 3 of 3). *Phys Sports Med* 1989;17:89–96.
11. Bailey DA, Faulkner RA, McKay HA: Growth, physical activity, and bone mineral acquisition. *Exerc Sport Sci Rev* 1996;24:233–266.
12. Bonjour JP, Theintz G, Buchs B, Slosman D, Rizzoli R: Critical years and stages of puberty for spinal and femoral bone mass accumulation during adolescence. *J Clin Endocrinol Metab* 1991;73:555–563.
13. Marcus R, Drinkwater B, Dalsky G, et al: Osteoporosis and exercise in women. *Med Sci Sports Exerc* 1992;24(suppl 6):S301–S307.
14. Arendt E, Dick R: Knee injury patterns among men and women in collegiate basketball and soccer: NCAA data and review of literature. *Am J Sports Med* 1995;23:694–701.
15. Bjordal JM, Arnly F, Hannestad B, Strand T: Epidemiology of anterior cruciate ligament injuries in soccer. *Am J Sports Med* 1997;25:341–345.
16. Ferretti A, Papandrea P, Conteduca F, Mariani PP: Knee ligament injuries in volleyball players. *Am J Sports Med* 1992;20:203–207.

17. Gray J, Taunton JE, McKenzie DC, Clement DB, McConkey JP, Davidson RG: A survey of injuries to the anterior cruciate ligament of the knee in female basketball players. *Int J Sports Med* 1985;6:314–316.

18. Gwinn DE, Wilckens JH, McDevitt ER, et al: The relative gender incidence of anterior cruciate ligament injury in men and women at the United States Naval Academy. *Am J Sports Med* 2000;28:98–102.

19. Lysens RJ, Ostyn MS, Vanden Auweele Y, Lefevre J, Vuylsteke M, Renson L: The accident-prone and overuse-prone profiles of the young athlete. *Am J Sports Med* 1989;17:612–619.

Chapter 5

Physical Fitness and Other Risk Factors for Physical Training–Related Injuries Among Young Women: Clues for Prevention From Military Research

Bruce Jones, MD, MPH
Joseph J. Knapik, ScD
Michelle Canham-Chervak, MPH

Introduction

Physical fitness is an essential component of military readiness. However, the physical training necessary to develop or improve the physical fitness of military trainees can result in high injury rates,[1–5] especially among women. A recent review indicates that over the last 20 years the incidence of injury for women during the 8 weeks of basic combat training (BCT) in the US Army has ranged from 42% to 67%.[5] The predominant category of injury is the overuse type.[3,4,6–8] Overuse injuries such as stress fractures, patellofemoral syndrome, and tendinitis result from incremental tissue damage (cumulative microtrauma) associated with successive bouts of repetitive physical activity, such as running, marching, or walking. These overuse injuries account for 75% of all injuries among women during BCT compared to about 25% for acute traumatic injuries such as sprains, fractures, and lacerations.[4] Eighty percent or more of military training injuries among women involve the lower body.[4,7] In order of most frequent occurrence, injury locations include: ankle, foot, knee, and lower leg.[3,4,6,7] Upper body/extremity injuries account for only about 20% of all injuries.

High rates of BCT injuries also lead to increases in limited duty. The incidence of injury-related "sick call" clinic visits among female basic trainees is about the same as for illness-related visits (25 per 100 trainees per month).[5,8] However, the rates of injury-related limited duty are substantially higher than illness-related limited duty (129 days per 100 trainees per month versus 6 days, respectively)[5,8] (Table 1). Clearly, injuries represent a significant loss of valuable training time and a threat to the health and performance of young women engaged in physically demanding military training activities.

Table 1 Rates of injury, illness, and limited duty among female Army trainees

Measure	Injury Rates	Illness Rates	Rate Ratio
≥ One Visit (trainees/100/mo)	25.2	24.2	1.0
Sick Call Visits (visits/100/mo)	39.6	37.2	1.1
Days of Limited Duty (days/100/mo)	129	6	22.0

(Adapted from Jones BH, Manikowski R, Harris JA, et al: *Incidence of, and Risk Factors for Injury and Illness Among Male and Female Army Basic Trainees*. Natick, MA, US Army Research Institute of Environmental Medicine, 1988.)

Risk Factors for Injuries

Prevention and control of military training injuries requires a knowledge of risk factors and causes of injury. Over the past decade, Army researchers have examined a variety of risk factors including demographic variables, physical characteristics, health risk behaviors, and physical fitness.[3,5,7–9] Studies of physical characteristics of women, such as height, weight, and body fat, have not shown consistent correlation with injury risks during basic military training.[4–7,9] Anecdotal reports suggested that the shortest women were at greater risk of injuries during BCT and early data from Jones and associates[7,8] seem to support this; however, in subsequent studies, stature has not been consistently associated with injury risks,[4,6] possibly because of changes in training guidance that recommend that the shortest individuals lead running and marching activities. In regard to body mass index (BMI) or direct measures of body fat, the data also are not consistent. Although some studies suggest women with higher BMI or body fat may be at higher injury risk, some also show a bimodal relationship, with the leanest and fatter individuals at greater risk.[4,7–9] The association of physical characteristics with injury deserves further study in larger populations.

Several components of physical fitness and behavioral factors (such as smoking) are well-established risk factors. The following section will examine association between injury risk and some physical fitness and behavioral factors.

Aerobic Fitness

The most consistently reported risk factor for training-related injuries among both women and men has been low levels of physical fitness—in particular, aerobic fitness.[4–7,9] Female and male trainees and infantry soldiers who run the 1 mile or 2 mile slower in the physical fitness test experience more injuries during BCT[4–7,9–11] (Figs. 1 and 2). Direct measures of maximal oxygen uptake (peak Vo_{2max}) also demonstrate that the least aerobically fit individuals, those with the lowest peak Vo_{2max} (mL/kg), are at the highest risks of injury.[4]

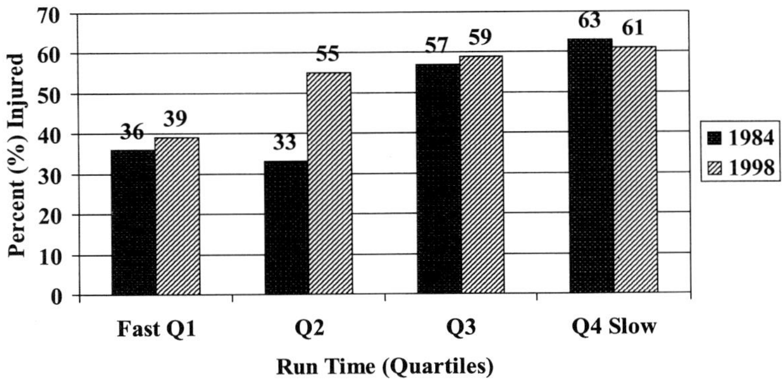

Fig. 1 *Run times on physical training test and risk (%) of injury among female trainees during 8 weeks of Army basic combat training at Ft. Jackson, South Carolina, in 1984 and 1998. One-mile run times in 1984: Mean time = 9.7 min ± 1.4 min.*[8] *Two-mile run times in 1998: Mean time = 21.5 min ± 3.0 min.*[4]

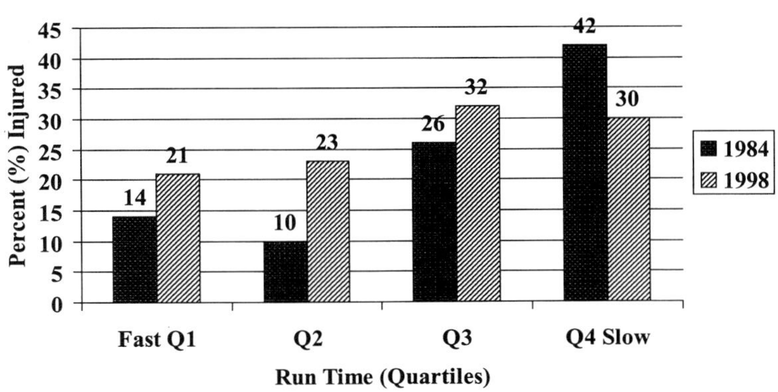

Fig. 2 *Run times on the physical training test and risk (%) of injury among male trainees during 8 weeks of Army basic combat training at Ft. Jackson, South Carolina, in 1984 and 1988. One-mile run times in 1984: Mean time = 7.2 min ± 1.0 min.*[8] *Two-mile run times in 1998: Mean time = 17.5 min ± 2.9 min.*[4]

Muscle Endurance

Several studies have demonstrated an association between increasing muscle endurance, as measured by push-ups and sit-ups, and lowered risk of injury during BCT. Specifically, these studies indicate that individuals who perform higher numbers of push-ups in 2 min may have a lowered risk of training-related injuries.[3–8] Muscle endurance for women, as measured by push-ups, showed a trend of decreasing incidence of injury for the successively more fit groups, those quartiles of women performing successively greater numbers in 2 min[4,7,8] (Fig. 3). In another study,[6] women who performed more than 16 push-ups in 2 min had the least injuries in BCT (65%); women who performed only one push-up in the same period had the highest injury incidence (72%). Men had overall lower incidences of injuries, but showed the same association between higher number of push-ups, ie, greater physical fitness, and lower rates of injuries.[4,7,8,10] Although trials with sit-ups have been less consistent, the overall trends have been in the same direction.[4,8] Women who could perform more than 48 sit-ups in 2 min had the least injuries in BCT (54%); women who performed fewer than 21 sit-ups in the same period had the highest incidence (70%).[6] More recently[4] it was found that the 25% (quartile) of men and women who performed the lowest number of push-ups were 1.6 and 1.4 times more likely, respectively, to suffer a time-loss injury (an injury resulting in 1 or more days of limited duty) compared with the 25% of trainees performing the highest number of push-ups. These relationships were even stronger for an injury requiring removal from training; here, the relative risk was 6.1 for men and 3.5 for women.

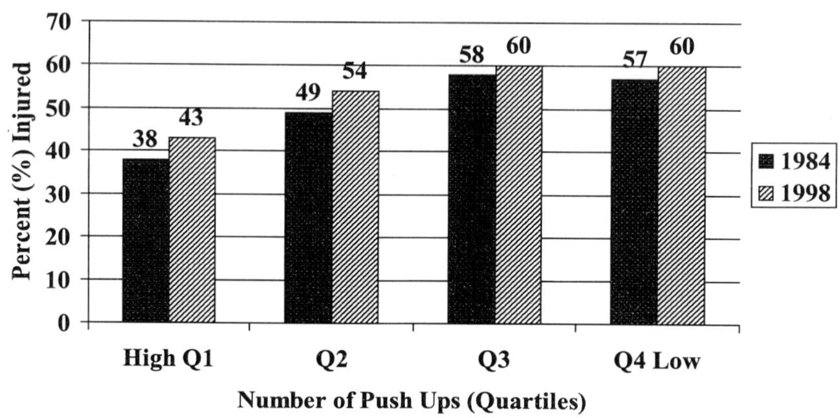

Fig. 3 *Push-up performance on the physical training test and risk (%) of injury among female trainees during 8 weeks of Army basic combat training at Ft. Jackson, South Carolina, in 1984 and 1998. 1984: Mean number of push-ups (± SD) = 12.4 (± 9.9).[8] 1998: Mean number of push-ups (± SD) = 10.6 (± 10.0).[4]*

Muscle Strength

Only a few studies have examined the association between muscle strength and injury risk during BCT or other military training. In a study of Army trainees, researchers[6] showed that women who could lift more weight on a "dynamic lift test" (ie, lifting a rack of weights on a machine from floor to chest height) experienced fewer injuries during 8 weeks of BCT. Muscle strength, as measured with the bench press, showed a similar (but less significant) association. Cowan and associates[12] and Knapik and associates[4] also showed a similar association between dynamic lift and injury rates among young men during infantry BCT, but the results were not statistically significant. Westphal and associates[6] studied a combined measure of muscle strength and muscle endurance known as a "timed load carriage task" (ie, lifting a 20-kg box and carrying it around a 90-m course for time). The researchers showed a highly significant trend of increasing injury risk with slower load carriage task performance.

Flexibility

Military studies have consistently demonstrated a bimodal relationship between injury risk and flexibility of the hamstring muscle group.[3–5] That is, those with the highest and lowest levels of flexibility are at the greatest risk while those of average or near average flexibility are at lower risk. Similar findings have been reported among female collegiate athletes.[5,13]

Gender and Aerobic Fitness

As noted earlier, the injury rates for women have been about twice as high as those for men in BCT[4–9,14–16] (Table 2). However, these studies have also shown that on entry into the military, women generally exhibit lower levels of physical fitness (Table 3). Women run slower and do fewer push-ups and sit-ups than men.[4–7,14,15] This raises the question of whether relative risks of

Table 2 Incidence of injury among women and men during Army basic training

Study	Year Data Collected	Risk Women %	Risk Men %	Ratio Women Versus Men (%)
Kowal[16]	1978	54	26	2.1 : 1
Bensel and Kish[1]	1982	42	23	1.8 : 1
Jones et al[7]	1984	50	28	1.8 : 1
Bell et al[15]	1988	57	27	2.1 : 1
Canham et al[14]	1995	65	41	1.6 : 1
Knapik et al[4]	1998	63	37	1.7 : 1

Table 3 Age and physical fitness characteristics of male and female trainees, 1988

	Mean	
Variable	**Women**	**Men**
Age (yrs)	20.2	20.1
Height (cm)	162.0*	175.2
Weight (kg)	58.3*	75.7
BMI (wt/ht^2)	22.2	24.6
Body fat (%)	26.8*	16.1
1-Mile run (min)	10.3*	7.6
2-Mile run (min)	20.3*	16.4
Sit-ups (N)	33.9*	44.3
Push-ups (N)	10.3*	30.5

(Adapted from Jones BH, Bovee MW, Knapik JJ: *Associations Among Body Composition, Physical Fitness, and Injury in Men and Women Army Trainees: Body Composition and Physical Performance*. Washington, DC, National Academy Press, 1992, pp 141–173.)

*Difference between men and women significant at $p < 0.05$

injury for men and women would be different if controlled for differences in physical fitness.

Results of two studies[9,14] of US Army trainees have been analyzed to compare injury risks of men and women during 8 weeks of BCT while controlling for differences in aerobic endurance performance (run time). In both of these studies, the crude (unadjusted) risks of injury for women were twice as high as for men, with risk of any injury showing significant differences as well as risks of overuse injuries such as stress fractures (Table 4). However, when a multilevel (stratified) analysis was performed to control for the effect of aerobic endurance performance capability (ie, run times), there were no statistically different risks of injury between men and women (ie, the risk ratios approached one), as shown in Table 5. In other words, when men and women who ran similar run times were compared, their risks of injuries were similar. Although these results were only partly confirmed in a more recent study,[4] this same study demonstrated that when men and women were stratified on the basis of peak Vo_{2max} (mL/kg), men and women of similar aerobic power had

Table 4 Risks of injury for female and male Army basic trainees[14]

Type of Injury	Risk Women (%)	Risk Men (%)	Risk Ratio Women/Men
Study Ft. Jackson, 1984			
All	50.5	27.4	1.8*
Stress fractures	12.3	2.4	5.1*
Study Ft. Leonard Wood, 1995			
All	55.8	34.8	1.6†
Stress fractures and stress reactions	17.9	5.2	3.5†

* $p < 0.05$
† $p = 0.001$

Table 5 Risks of injury compared for women and men of similar aerobic fitness level (stratified by run times on Army initial entry physical fitness test)[9]

Study Ft. Jackson, 1984[9*]				
Run Time Tertile	**Injury Risk Women (%)**	**Injury Risk Men (%)**	**Risk Ratio (Women/Men)**	**95% Confidence Interval**
1 (5.9 to 7.9 min)	20.0	17.5	1.1*	0.3 to 4.5
2 (> 7.9 to 9.7 min)	37.3	46.7	0.8*	0.4 to 1.5
3 (> 9.7 min)	57.7	0.0	—	—

Study Ft. Leonard Wood, 1995[14†]				
Run Time Quartiles	**Injury Risk Women (%)**	**Injury Risk Men (%)**	**Risk Ratio (Women/Men)**	**95% Confidence Interval**
1 (11.63 to 16.50 min)	0.0	25.0	—	—
2 (16.51 to 19.01 min)	50.0	34.5	1.4	0.7 to 3.2
3 (19.02 to 21.85 min)	54.5	44.8	1.2	0.7 to 2.0
4 (21.86 to 32.32 min)	59.6	63.6	0.9	0.6 to 1.5

[*]Mantel-Haenszal weighted risk ratio = 0.98; $p = 1.0$; NS, $p > 0.05$
[†]Summary Mantel-Haenszel weighted risk ratio = 1.1, $p = 0.7$

similar injury risks. Taken as a whole, these results suggest that men and women of similar aerobic fitness have similar injury risks.

Behavioral Risk Factors

Several recent studies have examined the association of behavioral risk factors (eg, physical activity level, alcohol consumption, and smoking habits) before entry into the Army with risks of injury during BCT.[3,4,6,7,9,12] Although a strong protective effect of a physically active lifestyle prior to BCT has been thoroughly documented in men,[3,4,7,9,12] such an association has not been proven for women.

One of the most consistently demonstrated behavioral risk factors for training injuries in the military is cigarette smoking. Westphal and associates[6] reported a 25% higher incidence of injury among women who smoked before entry into the military compared with nonsmokers (77% versus 62%). Altarac and associates[17] showed women who smoked were at 1.7 times greater risk of overuse injuries. The results on smoking were similar for male trainees, with the largest incidence of injury, 50%, occurring in those who smoked between 10 and 20 cigarettes a day before basic training, compared with 29% for nonsmokers.[3] More recently, Knapik and associates[4] have observed that the cumulative incidence of injuries over the 8 weeks of BCT among women who smoked cigarettes before basic training is 1.6 times higher than those who never smoked (60% versus 38%). This is similar to what has been observed among male trainees in BCT[3,4] and male infantry soldiers.[11] Male soldiers who smoked cigarettes had 1.5 times the risk of injury as nonsmokers even when differences in physical fitness were taken into consideration.

Commentary

The incidence of injury among women during Army basic training is high. A number of studies have shown unadjusted rates of injuries for women to be twice those for men. A variety of potentially modifiable risk factors for injury have been identified. Women and men share these factors that include, among others, aerobic fitness, muscle endurance, sedentary lifestyle (low levels of physical activity), and smoking. The data indicate that individuals who exhibit higher levels of physical fitness experience a protective effect from injuries. Likewise, those who have been most physically active prior to entering the military service have fewer injuries during basic training—a finding that makes sense given that physical activity and exercise are the means by which higher levels of fitness are achieved. The finding of an association of smoking with physical training–related injury rates among Army personnel is consistent with civilian studies that suggest that smoking may be a risk factor for occupational and other unintentional injuries.[18]

Of the risk factors identified by military studies, the level of aerobic fitness on entering the military is the most consistently significant factor for both men and women. The military data also show that during basic training, men and women of the same aerobic fitness level exhibit similar risks of injury. These findings suggest that the primary underlying risk factor for physical training–related injuries among both men and women is low aerobic fitness. The data further suggest that improvements in physical fitness should reduce risks of injury among the least fit women and men. Recent reviews[5,19,20] of physical training and injury risks in military populations indicate that it is possible to significantly lower training-related injury rates while maintaining fitness levels. One such strategy to prevent injuries is to reduce the total amount of high-intensity weight-bearing training (running) and replace it with lower intensity activities (eg, walking, marching, or hiking without loads). Military research suggests a number of ways training injuries might be prevented. However, systematic prevention of injuries will require further studies of the occurrence of injuries as they relate to physical training and fitness. Finally, as strategies to prevent training injuries are developed and implemented, their effectiveness should be evaluated.

References

1. Bensel CK, Kish RN (ed): *Lower Extremity Disorders Among Men and Women in Army Basic Training and Effects of Two Types of Boots*. Natick, MA, US Army Natick Research and Development Center, Technical Report No. TR-83/026, 1983. Available at: http://www.dtic.mil/.
2. Jones BH: Overuse injuries of the lower extremities associated with marching, jogging, and running: A review. *Mil Med* 1983;148:783–787.
3. Jones BH, Cowan DN, Tomlinson JP, Robinson JR, Polly DW, Frykman PN: Epidemiology of injuries associated with physical training among young men in the army. *Med Sci Sports Exerc* 1993;25:197–203.
4. Knapik JJ, Canham M, Hoedebecke E, et al: *Injury Incidence and Injury Risk Factors Among US Army Basic Trainees at Ft. Jackson, SC, 1998.* Aberdeen Proving Ground, MD, Army Center for Health Promotion and Preventive Medicine, EPICON Report No. 29-HE-8370-98, 1999. Available at: http://www.dtic.mil/.
5. Jones BH, Knapik JJ: Physical training and exercise-related injuries: Surveillance, research and injury prevention in military populations. *Sports Med* 1999;27:111–125.
6. Westphal KA, Friedl KE, Sharp MA, et al: *Health, Performance, and Nutritional Status of US Army Women During Basic Combat Training.* Natick, MA, US Army Research Institute of Environmental Medicine, Technical Report No. T96-2, 1995. Available at: http://www.dtic.mil/.
7. Jones BH, Bovee MW, Harris JM III, Cowan DN: Intrinsic risk factors for exercise-related injuries among male and female army trainees. *Am J Sports Med* 1993;21:705–710.
8. Jones BH, Manikowski R, Harris JA, et al: *Incidence of and Risk Factors for Injury and Illness Among Male and Female Army Basic Trainees.* Natick, MA, US Army Research Institute of Environmental Medicine, Technical Report No. T19/88, 1988. Available at: http://www.dtic.mil/.
9. Jones BH, Bovee MW, Knapik JJ: Associations among body composition, physical fitness, and injury in men and women army trainees, in Marriott BM (ed): *Body Composition and Physical Performance: Applications for the Military Services.* Washington, DC, National Academy Press, 1992, pp 141–173.

10. Knapik J, Ang P, Reynolds K, Jones B: Physical fitness, age, and injury incidence in infantry soldiers. *J Occup Med* 1993;35:598–603.

11. Reynolds KL, Heckel HA, Witt CE, et al: Cigarette smoking, physical fitness, and injuries in infantry soldiers. *Am J Prev Med* 1994;10:145–150.

12. Cowan DN, Jones BH, Tomlinson P, et al: *The Epidemiology of Physical Training Injuries in the US Army Infantry Trainees: Methodology, Population, and Risk Factors.* Natick, MA, US Army Research Institute of Environmental Medicine, Technical Report No. T4/89, 1988. Available at: http://www.dtic.mil/.

13. Knapik JJ, Bauman CL, Jones BH, Harris JM, Vaughan L: Preseason strength and flexibility imbalances associated with athletic injuries in female collegiate athletes. *Am J Sports Med* 1991;19:76–81.

14. Canham M, Knapik JJ, Smutock MA, Jones BH: Training, physical performances and injuries among men and women preparing for acceptation in the Army, in Kumar S (ed*): Advances in Occupational Ergonomics and Safety*. Amsterdam, The Netherlands, IOS Press, 1998, pp 711–714.

15. Bell NS, Mangione TW, Hemenway D, Amoroso PJ, Jones BH: Higher injury rates among female Army trainees: A function of gender? *Am J Prev Med* 2000;18:141–145.

16. Kowal DM: Nature and causes of injuries in women resulting from an endurance training program. *Am J Sports Med* 1980;8:265–269.

17. Altarac M, Gardner JW, Popovich RM, Potter R, Knapik JJ, Jones BH: Cigarette smoking and exercise-related injuries among young men and women. *Am J Prev Med* 2000;18:96–102.

18. Sacks JJ, Nelson DE: Smoking and injuries: An overview. *Prev Med* 1994;23:515–520.

19. Jones BH, Cowan DN, Knapik JJ: Exercise, training and injuries. *Sports Med* 1994;18:202–214.

20. Gilchrist J, Jones BH, Sleet DA, Kimsey CD: Exercise-related injuries among women: Strategies for prevention from civilian and military studies. *Morb Mort Wkly Rep* 2000;49:15–33.

Chapter 6

The Epidemiology of Injury in Adult Women's Recreational Activity

Ralph K. Requa, MSPH
James G. Garrick, MD

Introduction

It has been shown many times that the single most influential factor determining the overall pattern of injury arising from athletic activity for both men and women is the nature of the athletic activity itself. Variations in patterns of participation, particularly by gender but also by age, are so pronounced that their independent effects are exceedingly difficult to recognize.

This is not to say that there are not fascinating gender-related injury issues in sports. Women are at risk for certain activity-related injuries and illness, such as eating disorders and low bone density problems, that are largely absent among men and are at higher risk for others such as anterior cruciate ligament ruptures in certain activities. Although these injuries may well have significant long-term consequences, in sheer numbers they are greatly outnumbered by conventional sports injuries present in both genders.

To describe the features of conventional sports injuries in adult women, comparing sport to injury, we discuss injuries collected from a cohort of active adult recreational participants followed intensely for a 4-month period to document both the patterns of participation and injury compared to gender ("cohort"). Although the cohort was followed for significantly more than 200 person-years, relatively few serious or catastrophic injuries were recorded. The participants engaged primarily in conventional, reasonably low-risk sports activities. In addition we contrast 60,000+ injury records collected over a 20-year period in a specialty sports medicine clinic ("clinic"). These injury reports reveal patterns of injury by type, location, and age although they have no denominator and thus cannot yield rates.

Whatever the contribution of gender to these injuries versus that of activity selection, injuries occur in activities in which many if not most participants are women and should not be ignored. In addition, there are subtle features of the injury patterns that suggest that women may sustain somewhat different patterns of injury for reasons we do not yet understand.

It is generally accepted that a person can enhance health by regularly engaging in almost any type of fitness activity. Men and women are encouraged to increase their levels of physical activity to benefit their cardiovascular health as well as their general fitness, physical appearance, and mental attitude. And while attention is directed toward the safety of exercise from a cardiac risk standpoint, there is substantially less written about the musculoskeletal (injury) consequences of many common recreational/fitness activities for both men and women.

For many of the activities that take place regularly in health and fitness facilities across the country it is difficult to weigh the potential benefits against the risks of participation, because the risks have not been measured. Enthusiasts, physicians, and fitness professionals alike might benefit from information about the relative risks of participation among common fitness activities.

The omission of comparative risk is in large part the result of few investigations into the injury consequences of participation in adult fitness activities. For some activities, such as running, skiing, cycling, and aerobic dance, information is available.[1–7] Many popular activities, however, take place in unsupervised, unstructured settings and have largely escaped study.

Comparisons between studies, even if each is well done, must be done carefully because of differing study populations and injury definitions. A single prospective approach that follows a large group of participants through a variety of exposures allows comparisons to be made; whatever definitional, population, case ascertainment, and classification biases exist should at least be constant across activities.

A large group of adult fitness participants were followed, using consistent methods and definitions of injury, to document the consequences of adult fitness activities in active exercisers. The physician prescribing exercise or fitness enhancement programs for his or her adult patients may find such information of use.

Study Parameters

Sample

As reported elsewhere, participants were recruited from 15 Bay Area fitness clubs and exercise studios through fitness personnel and direct in-facility recruitment.[8] The focus of the study was active recreational participants of both genders. In order to participate, each volunteer had to indicate that he or she participated in aerobic dance for at least 3 sessions of at least 45 minutes each week or in more than a single major fitness activity for at least 4, 45-minute sessions per week.

As an inducement to sign up and continue to participate, those that continued to participate for the full 12 weeks were eligible to participate in a drawing, held at the close of the study, for prizes consisting of pairs of shoes and sports gear bags.

Prospective documentation of injuries occurring in a large group of recreational participants has several clear advantages over surveillance of a single sport or activity. Beginning with a large group of active adults makes it possible to examine a wide variety of recreational activities, both organized and unorganized. More importantly, injury rates arising from these various activities can be meaningfully compared.

This population may not be typical of all adult recreational athletes. The members of this population were relatively young, healthy, and possessed of sufficient economic means to purchase and maintain club memberships.

Because of club memberships, some activities that take place outside organized fitness facilities may be less frequent (eg, cycling, hiking, tennis, golf, and so forth) than in an active population not characterized by fitness club membership. At the same time it seems unlikely that the nature of the participation observed in these outside activities in this group would be radically different from that of club members.

Because the study was not based on a "season" or period of time in which participants were beginning a new activity, it also avoided the period wherein the highest injury rates are often observed. To the extent that this is true, the overall rates may better reflect ongoing activities rather than starting up an activity, and they may be somewhat lower than would otherwise be the case.

The sample was voluntary; participants had to agree to take part in the study and also to be called on a regular basis. This favors cooperative people who are willing to report on their experience. Perhaps this might also have tended to favor those with some interest in sports injuries, perhaps those who had experienced an injury in the past. By looking at the history of a previous injury in the analysis, this, at least, was investigated. The extent to which this history may have skewed the selection of the entire sample is unknown, but it seems unlikely to have had a major effect given that the rates of previous injury are not particularly high.

The participants had to state that they met the participation rule noted above, so it is likely that their activity levels may be somewhat higher than that of a group selected with no activity level requirement. In addition, because of the weekly phone calls, anecdotal evidence suggests that the activity levels, particularly in the less active, may have been encouraged. More than 1 participant apologized for their levels of participation in 1week or another. The degree to which the sample represents typical active recreational participants is unknown.

Data Collection

In addition to fulfilling the described activity level criteria, participants agreed to participate in a weekly telephone contact to document both athletic activities and injuries. Trained telephone interviewers called the volunteers once each week. All recreational and sports activity engaged in and the amount of time involved was recorded each week along with any injuries that occurred.

Enrollment data included items such as age, gender, prior physical activity, history of orthopaedic limitations, and previous injuries. Weekly data collected included nature and duration of physical activity and any injury or complaint. For an injury/complaint, the onset, severity, location, description, treatment, days of time-loss, and relation of exercise activity to injury were recorded.

The clinic data consist of injury reports filled out for new patients and existing patients who sustain new injuries. Type and location of injury and the patient's age will be examined for injuries resulting from sports participation.

Data Validation

To evaluate the validity of injury information acquired by telephone, the first 35 injuries reported and classified by the interviewers were examined in detail. Ten were either seen by a physician (and thus were by definition correctly classified) or obvious (for example, minor contusion). The 25 remaining athletes were interviewed in person by an athletic trainer. In 22 of 25 cases the anatomic/pathologic classifications were completely unchanged; in the remaining three the athletic trainer was able to glean additional detail through talking with the person face-to-face. A "forearm strain" for example was further classified as a wrist flexor strain on examination. There were no significant discrepancies between the diagnostic codes assigned by the telephone interviewers and those of the athletic trainer. In all, the athletic trainer talked to about 3 fourths of the participants (> 300) reporting injuries or complaints over the telephone and reviewed all of the injury forms. At the request of the interviewers, the athletic trainer also met with 12 injured participants whose symptoms could not be satisfactorily resolved over the telephone.

Using telephone interviewers to gather the major part of the injury information suggests the possibility of a certain lack of precision in injury classification. In fact, an initial comparison suggests just the opposite. We found no anatomic/pathologic errors, suggesting that the general accuracy of the data is acceptable.

Definition of Injury and Severity

Injury and injury severity were defined by the impact that they had on a person's activity level (Table 1). A given injury throughout its course may have varying levels of severity at different times. There were four levels of severity, ranging from a significant complaint (one that does not interfere with a participant's activities) to the fourth level, which occurs when a participant is unable to do his or her fitness activities and, in addition, the injury interferes with daily living (for example, by requiring the use of crutches). Whether medical care was sought is also a measure of severity and was noted. In addition to recording the number of days of activity affected at each level of severity for each injury, each injury was also assigned an overall level of severity equal to the highest level attained throughout its course. We encouraged each individual to continue participation in the study for 12 weeks, although some elected to withdraw before that time.

To provide some comparison between our study and others, we can place some injury rates in a similar context by comparing time-loss injuries among our runners using a definition similar to that used by Koplan and associates.[9] They noted that more than a third cited an injury that at least diminished mileage over a year of running. Our definition of time-loss injuries, those

Table 1 Definition: Severity of injury[8]

Level	Time Lost?	Description
Level I	No	Injury or pain not affecting sport and fitness activities
Level II	Yes	Injury or pain resulting in modifying duration or intensity of sport and fitness activities
Level III	Yes	Injury or pain resulting in missing part or all of any sport and fitness activity
Level IV	Yes	Injury or pain resulting in missing part or all of any sport and fitness activity and in alterations in daily life (eg, crutches)

that altered or stopped participation, was similar. The rate of time-loss injury among our participants who ran was 10.79/1,000 hours or 43.3/100 study-person-years; this is somewhat higher than the rate noted by Koplan and associates of slightly over one third injured per year. Our study participants may have differed from runners selected from participants in a road race because we required our subjects to engage in more than one major fitness activity. Few participated regularly in road races. Whether this had an effect on their rate of injury is not known. Even so, the comparison shows that the rates obtained from recreational runners with our methodology did not differ substantially from that obtained over 10 years ago from a completely different technique, a questionnaire survey of 10K race participants.

Our definition of injury distinguished between an action of the participant due to an injury (eg, altered or missed activity due to a flare up of a chronic condition) as opposed to an action taken simply as a result of the participant's choice (eg, stopped or modified an activity due to fear or conjecture that they might hurt themselves). Missing or altering sports participation had to be due to a new injury or flare-up on an old injury to qualify as a reportable time-loss injury event.

The easy availability of multiple activities, as well as variations within activities such as aerobic dance, means that these data should be viewed from a somewhat different perspective than used when looking at the conventional, single-sport epidemiologic study. Here, it was normal for the participants' athletic activities to vary from week to week. Unlike members of a football or gymnastic team, the participants in this investigation were neither rigidly supervised/coached nor held accountable for performing specific athletic tasks. With a myriad of different activities available, these tasks could be altered according to the participant's health or preferences on any given day. Although this creates a somewhat more complex accounting task for observers recording participation, it may be closer to how most adults participate in recreational activity.

In the traditional sports environment, time loss means the inability to perform the tasks associated with the activity (eg, the inability to run, throw, or catch the football), and some sort of time loss usually is reflected in the definition of an injury. In this group, because of the nature of their activity patterns, the inability to perform a specific task because of an injury may have meant only the cessation or alteration of that 1 activity. Applying the definition of an injury and accounting for time loss becomes somewhat more complicated with many activities involved. Indeed, the common pattern of engaging in specific activities only once, twice, or three times throughout the week reduces the possibility of having a one-day time loss injury. While this varying participation presented challenges from the standpoint of precisely accounting for participation and time loss, it may well have been of benefit to the participants.

Participation

The sample was taken from 1,089 recreational athletes who filled out an initial enrollment form. Eighteen elected not to participate when first contacted by telephone, 32 were disqualified (had a current injury, too few workouts/week, enrolled too late to participate, had moved out of the area), and 53 could not be reached or were never enrolled (were from out of town, had an answering machine only and could not be called, were students with no telephone) leaving 986 who were enrolled. Time recorded was 10,582 weeks of activity for an average of 10.7 weeks per participant. Female participants engaged in more hours of participation than did the men, 34,122 versus 26,507 (Table 2). The patterns of participation were quite different as well. About one third of the women's participation time was in various types of aerobic dance compared to approximately 10% of the men's participation. Within aerobic dance, the traditional style was most popular although together the other styles, low impact, step, jazz/funk, and so on, accounted for about twice the hours of traditional aerobic dance alone. The converse is true for strength training with free weights and weight machines where women spent only one third as much time as men. Free weights alone account for more than 1 in 5 of the men's total hours versus less than 1 in 10 of the women's. As might be expected, time spent in competitive team sports was also about three times less frequent for women. Table 2 also has the ratios of female/male hours by type of activity, each divided by the overall ratio of female to male hours to normalize for the overall excess of female participation.

Exercise using aerobic fitness equipment such as stair climbing and stationary bicycles was also popular in both genders, approximately 17% of the women's hours versus 19% of the men's. StairMasters (StairMaster, Tulsa, Oklahoma) and Lifecycles (Life Fitness, Chicago, Illinois) were the most popular specific types of exercise equipment used.

Running represented the most hours for individual activities outside the fitness facilities and was popular with both genders. The participants averaged seven to eight different activities each. Some accumulated as many as 25 different activities throughout the study period.

Injury Rates

The rates for all injuries (time-loss + complaints) and time-loss injuries alone in women were 7.27 and 5.22/1,000 hours of activity, respectively, or 2.17 and 1.56 injuries per year based on the observed average hours per week. Time-loss injuries (≥ level II) made up about 80% of all

Table 2 Hours and percent participation by gender and type of activity

	Women		Men		All		F/M
	Hours	%	Hours	%	Hours	%	Ratio*
Aerobic dance (jazz, funk, etc)	1,054.58	3.1%	486.58	1.8%	1,541.16	2.5%	1.68
Aerobic dance traditional (~ "high impact")	4,133.32	12.1%	714.50	2.7%	4,847.82	8.0%	4.49
Aerobic dance low impact	1,812.73	5.3%	363.53	1.4%	2,176.26	3.6%	3.87
Aerobic dance step	2,179.93	6.4%	474.65	1.8%	2,654.58	4.4%	3.57
Aerobic dance other	1,820.43	5.3%	559.67	2.1%	2,380.10	3.9%	2.53
Class, dance other	614.30	1.8%	366.52	1.4%	980.82	1.6%	1.30
Class, yoga	338.83	1.0%	77.83	0.3%	416.66	0.7%	3.38
Class, other	790.83	2.3%	285.80	1.1%	1,076.63	1.8%	2.15
Cycles	1,660.25	4.9%	1,726.52	6.5%	3,386.77	5.6%	0.75
Cross country ski exercise equipment	83.58	0.2%	131.13	0.5%	214.71	0.4%	0.50
Rowing machines	162.30	0.5%	404.20	1.5%	566.50	0.9%	0.31
Stair climbing equipment	3,126.42	9.2%	2,297.30	8.7%	5,423.72	8.9%	1.06
Treadmills	734.28	2.2%	366.22	1.4%	1,100.50	1.8%	1.56
Other cardio equipment	11.62	0.0%	19.38	0.1%	31.00	0.1%	0.47
Free weights	2,555.47	7.5%	5,903.88	22.3%	8,459.35	14.0%	0.34
Weights, other	45.17	0.1%	149.93	0.6%	195.10	0.3%	0.23
Cybex	703.58	2.1%	625.80	2.4%	1,329.38	2.2%	0.87
Gravitron	36.40	0.1%	79.13	0.3%	115.53	0.2%	0.36
Nautilus	969.62	2.8%	1,171.80	4.4%	2,141.42	3.5%	0.64
Universal	44.42	0.1%	91.55	0.3%	135.97	0.2%	0.38
Polaris	170.08	0.5%	165.75	0.6%	335.83	0.6%	0.80
Other weight equipment	56.05	0.2%	34.63	0.1%	90.68	0.1%	1.26
Individual cycling	1,223.33	3.6%	941.32	3.6%	2,164.65	3.6%	1.01
Individual roller skating	99.50	0.3%	43.75	0.2%	143.25	0.2%	1.77
Individual running	2,435.35	7.1%	2,382.83	9.0%	4,818.18	7.9%	0.79
Individual skiing alpine	1,301.22	3.8%	881.10	3.3%	2,182.32	3.6%	1.15
Individual walking	2,926.03	8.6%	1,056.48	4.0%	3,982.51	6.6%	2.15
Individual other	1,722.93	5.0%	2,076.18	7.8%	3,799.11	6.3%	0.64
Team basketball	177.42	0.5%	1,133.27	4.3%	1,310.69	2.2%	0.12
Team racquetball	145.25	0.4%	283.33	1.1%	428.58	0.7%	0.40
Team tennis	567.98	1.7%	595.35	2.2%	1,163.33	1.9%	0.74
Team other	418.75	1.2%	617.50	2.3%	1,036.25	1.7%	0.53
Total	34,121.95	100.0%	26,507.41	100.0%	60,629.36	100.0%	1.29†

*F/M Ratio = (women's hours divided by men's hours) divided by 1.29 (overall female/male ratio)
†Overall F/M ratio not normalized

injuries/complaints for women and 71.8% for men. Among time-loss injuries, about one fourth altered participation, almost two thirds stopped participation, and about one in 10 stopped participation and altered the activities of daily life for both genders.

Injury Rates by Major Categories of Activity

In aggregate, team/competitive activities had the highest overall and time-loss rates of injury for both genders, followed by individual recreation, strength exercise equipment, dance/aerobic dance, and aerobic fitness exercise equipment, that is, cardiovascular exercise equipment (exercise bicycles, ski machines, etc). There were differences according to gender as the aerobic dance/fitness classes category was higher for men and aerobic fitness exercise equipment was higher for women (Table 3).

The rates for time-loss injuries and complaints in activity categories with more than 250 hours (Table 4) were highest for both genders for team sports (basketball) and jazz/funk style aerobic dance classes; intermediate for running and most other styles of aerobic dance; and lowest for low-impact aerobic dance, exercise cycling, and individual walking. Injury rates varied in a remarkably similar way for both genders by the type of aerobic dance; dance-style aerobics (jazz/funk) had higher rates compared to other forms of aerobics. Differences in rates by gender stood out for a few activities: women's rates were higher for rowing machines, stair climbers, exercise cycles, and tennis; men's rates were higher for treadmills, Alpine skiing, and walking. Of these activities, only rowing had fewer than 1,000 hours of participation.

Individual recreation activities varied and included everything from mountaineering, jogging, swimming, and walking to wind surfing and scuba diving but had relatively few hours of participation.

Age

Most of our cohort group were in their 20s and 30s (17 years old being the youngest). The median age was 32 years. Over 150 were in their 40s and almost 60 were older than 50 years of age (76 years was the oldest). The women were slightly younger on average compared to the men.

The age distribution of the cohort study differed from that of the clinic dataset (Table 5). Although the 29 years and younger group made up similar proportions of both data sets, the rest of the cohort group was concentrated in the younger end of the age span: 39% of the cohort study was in the 30 to 39 years group versus only 26% for the clinic group; 99% of the cohort group was younger than 50 years of age compared to 88% for the clinic group.

Rates for complaints appear relatively constant for men and women across age groups (Fig. 1). Rates for injuries (> level I) were indistinguishable in those 29 years and younger but for ages 30 to 39 years, the male rate was 64% higher (8.43 versus 5.15, $p < 0.05$). While the rates appear to decrease slightly for men older than the 30 to 39 years group while staying higher than those for the women, there were no significant differences in those older than 30 to 39 years.

Table 3 Injuries and rates per 1,000 hours by gender and type of activity

Women

	Aerobic Dance/ Fitness Class	Aerobic Fitness Exercise Equipment	Strength Exercise Equipment	Individual Recreational Activities	Team-competitive
Hours	12,496.58	5,671.5	4,352.73	10,270.33	1,309.4
%	36.6	16.6	12.8	30.1	3.8
Injuries	85	25	28	93	17
Rate/1,000	6.80	4.41	6.43	9.06	12.98

Men

	Aerobic Dance/ Fitness Class	Aerobic Fitness Exercise Equipment	Strength Exercise Equipment	Individual Recreational Activities	Team-competitive
Hours	3,214.25	4,906.35	8,030.47	7,542.93	2,629.45
%	12.2	18.6	30.5	28.7	10.0
Injuries	32	9	53	85	46
Rate/1,000	9.96	1.83	6.60	11.27	17.49

F/M Ratio*

Aerobic Dance/ Fitness Class	Aerobic Fitness Exercise Equipment	Strength Exercise Equipment	Individual Recreational Activities	Team-competitive
0.68	2.40	0.97	0.80	0.74

*Ratio of female injury rate/male injury rate

Table 4 Injuries and rates for time-loss and nontime-loss injuries by gender and type of activity

	Women		Men		All		F/M
	Injuries	Rate	Injuries	Rate	Injuries	Rate	Ratio*
Aerobic dance (jazz, funk, etc)	19	18.02	11	22.61	30	19.47	0.80
Aerobic dance, traditional (~ "high impact")	24	5.81	4	5.60	28	5.78	1.04
Aerobic dance, low impact	4	2.21	1	2.75	5	2.30	0.80
Aerobic dance, step	11	5.05	3	6.32	14	5.27	0.80
Aerobic dance, other	9	4.94	3	5.36	12	5.04	0.92
Class, dance, other	12	19.53	6	16.37	18	18.35	1.19
Cycles	5	3.01	1	0.58	6	1.77	5.20
Rowing machines	2	12.32	1	2.47	3	5.30	4.98
Stair climbing equipment	14	4.48	2	0.87	16	2.95	5.14
Treadmills	3	4.09	4	10.92	7	6.36	0.37
Free weights	9	3.52	27	4.57	36	4.26	0.77
Weight machines, Universal, etc	7	3.64	9	4.22	16	3.94	0.89
Individual cycling	8	6.54	5	5.31	13	6.01	1.23
Individual running	35	14.37	36	15.11	71	14.74	0.95
Individual skiing, Alpine	4	3.07	14	15.89	18	8.25	0.19
Individual walking	1	0.34	2	1.89	3	0.75	0.18
Team basketball	4	22.55	20	17.65	24	18.31	1.28
Team racquetball	2	13.77	4	14.12	6	14.00	0.98
Team tennis	6	10.56	3	5.04	9	7.74	2.10
Total	**179**	**5.86**	**156**	**6.76**	**335**	**6.25**	**0.87**

*Ratio of female injury rate/male injury rate (time-loss and nontime-loss)

Table 5 Clinic versus cohort age of injury for women

	Clinic		Cohort	
Age, years	**%**	**No.**	**%**	**No.**
≤ 29	43.8	10,976	46.0	127
30–39	26.1	6,532	38.8	107
40–49	17.9	4,486	14.1	39
50–59	7.4	1,850	1.1	3
60–69	3.2	792	0.0	0
≥ 70	1.6	397	0.0	0
Total	**100.0**	**25,033**	**100.0**	**276**

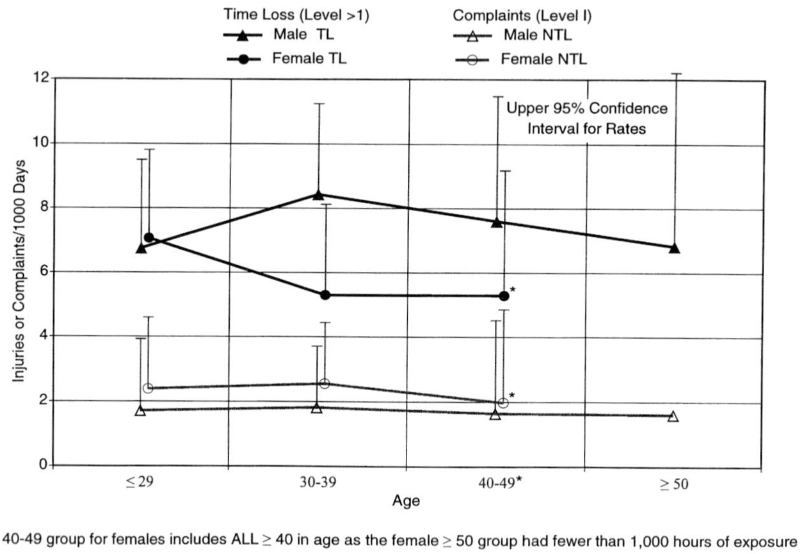

***Fig. 1** Rates by age and gender (time loss and complaints).*

Injury History

Almost three of four participants checked one or more "previous significant injuries" (70.6%, 696 of 986). Two or more sites were checked by 43%, and almost one in 10 (83) checked five or more locations. Ten anatomic areas were each checked "yes" for a previous injury more than 5% of the time. The knee was the clear leader for both genders with almost one in three indicating a previous injury to that area. The neck, upper back, and foot and toes were more often checked by women compared to men, the shoulder, fingers and leg less often (Fig. 2).

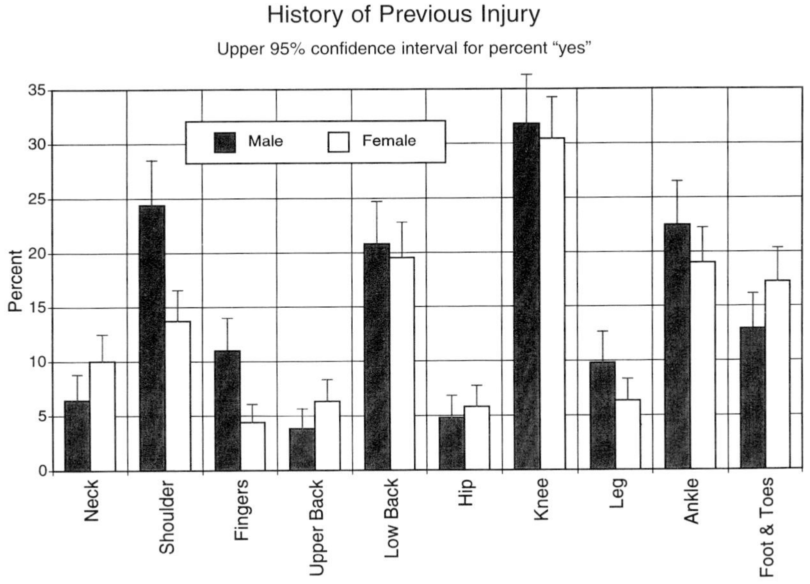

Fig. 2 Percent with positive history (areas with > 5% checking "yes"); N = 986. Each area is independent; participants checked as many as they wished.

Injury Characteristics

Injury Onset and Type

Onset was slightly different by gender; women had a higher rate of complaints and lower rate of time-loss injury (Table 6). The five most common types of injury are listed in Table 7.

Type by Severity The percentage of each type of injury that resulted in time loss varied from 69% for "pain-ache" injuries to 90% for strains. Another measure of severity is the use of medical care, whether an injury resulted in the participant consulting a physician. While only 2% of the strain and 3% of the pain-ache classifications resulted in a physician visit, the figure rose to more than one in four for sprains. Comparing severity indices by gender shows some differences (Table 8). There was a smaller proportion of contusions and a slightly higher percent of sprains that resulted in time loss. The proportion of injuries that resulted in a physician visit were strikingly less for women for sprains, contusions, inflammations, and pain/ache. Only for strains and other were the percents seeking medical care similar.

Type by Onset Comparing the injuries in terms of their onset, over 80% of the sprains and contusions, just over half of the strains, and about one fourth of the inflammations and "pain-ache" were acute. A greater percent of the women's inflammations were classified as acute.

Injury Location: Anatomic Location and Body Region

Percent Comparison of Injury Locations In the clinic and cohort, the knee led all other areas with over 31% and 21% to 23% of the injuries, respectively (Table 9). The shoulder made up only 6% for women in the cohort study versus 15% for the men. The shoulder made up almost the same proportion of the clinic data by gender, 6% and 11%. The converse was true for foot and toes, where the cohort percents for women and men were 12% and 6% versus 22% and 14% for the clinic data.

Location by Severity The percent that resulted in time loss by location varied from 61% to 96%, while those consulting a physician varied from 0% to 19% (Table 10). The foot and toes led for women, the ankle followed by the knee were the locations most often associated with a physician visit for men. The low back most often resulted in time loss for both genders, yet, along with the leg and hip/thigh, was least likely to require physician care.

Location by Onset The ankle suffered from an acute episode almost two out of three times but slightly less in women (57% versus 69%); conversely, the foot and toe area sustained a much smaller proportion of acute injuries for women (19%, Table 10).

Upper Extremity Injuries, Lower Extremity Injuries, and Spine/Trunk Injuries Collapsing anatomic location into three categories allows a simpler comparison to be made with activity groups. For the cohort study, almost two thirds of the injuries (62% to 73%) were to the lower extremity. About 16% of the injuries were to the upper extremity, while the remaining 12.4% were to the spine/trunk region. For the clinic series the pattern was very similar with 16% of injuries to the upper extremity and 11% to the spine/trunk. In both data sets the proportion of upper extremity injuries in women is approximately half that in men, 12% versus 20% in the clinic study and 8% versus 24% in the cohort study.

Table 6 Injuries and rates per 1,000 hours by gender and time loss

		Type of Injury	
	Complaint	Time Loss	Total
		Women	
No. of Injuries	70	178	248
Injuries/1,000 h	2.05	5.22	7.27
		Men	
No. of Injuries	45	180	225
Injuries/1,000 h	1.71	6.84	8.55
		All	
No. of Injuries	115	358	473
Injuries/1,000 h	1.90	5.92	7.83
		F/M Ratio*	
	1.20	0.76	0.85

*Ratio of female injury rate/male injury rate

Table 7 Percent time loss, MD/DO/DPM reported, and acute by type of injury

	Total	Time Loss (> Level I)		MD/DO/DPM Reported		Acute	
Type of Injury*	**No.**	**No.**	**%**	**No.**	**%**	**No.**	**%**
Sprain	47	38	80.9	13	27.7	38	80.9
Strain	84	76	90.5	2	2.4	46	54.8
Inflammation	77	60	77.9	10	13.0	17	22.1
Pain-ache	211	146	69.2	6	2.8	55	26.1
Contusion	29	23	79.3	3	10.3	25	86.2

*The top five types of injuries included 85.3% of the injuries
MD = medical doctor, DO = osteopathic doctor, DPM = podiatrist

Table 8 Percent time loss, MD/DO/DPM reported, and acute by type of injury and gender

	Time Loss (> Level I)				MD/DO/DPM Reported				Acute			
	Female		Male		Female		Male		Female		Male	
Type of Injury	**No.**	**%**	**No.**	**%**	**No.**	**%**	**No.**	**%**	**No.**	**%**	**No.**	**%**
Sprain	19	86.4	19	76.0	3	14.0	10	40.0	18	81.8	20	80.0
Strain	31	81.6	45	97.8	1	2.6	1	2.2	20	52.6	26	56.5
Inflammation	23	71.9	37	84.1	1	3.1	9	21.0	10	31.3	6	13.6
Pain-ache	93	67.9	52	71.2	2	1.5	4	5.5	34	24.8	20	27.4
Contusion	6	66.7	17	85.0	0	0.0	3	15.0	7	77.8	18	90.0
Other	28	73.7	31	79.5	9	24.0	8	21.0	14	36.8	24	61.5

MD = medical doctor, DO = osteopathic doctor, DPM = podiatrist

Table 9 Clinic versus cohort location of injury by gender

	Female				Male			
Location of Injury	**Clinic**		**Cohort**		**Clinic**		**Cohort**	
	%	**No.**	**%**	**No.**	**%**	**No.**	**%**	**No.**
Head	0.1	35	0.0	0	0.2	62	2.8	7
Neck	1.8	466	4.3	12	1.8	474	0.4	1
Shoulder	6.2	1,567	5.8	16	11.4	2,968	15.4	38
Arm	0.2	41	1.8	5	0.3	90	2.8	7
Elbow	2.9	725	0.4	1	4.7	1,215	2.8	7
Hand/wrist/fingers	2.4	614	5.1	14	3.5	905	6.5	16
Upper extremity, other	0.3	77	0.0	0	0.5	120	1.6	4
Chest/abdomen	1.5	366	1.4	4	1.8	461	2.0	5
Upper back	0.9	228	2.2	6	1.0	273	2.0	5
Lower back	6.4	1,608	10.5	29	6.9	1,804	8.9	22
Hip	5.5	1,398	4.7	13	3.7	974	6.1	15
Thigh	2.5	632	5.4	15	3.5	900	5.7	14
Knee	30.8	7,773	23.2	64	31.3	8,149	20.6	51
Lower leg	6.9	1,747	11.6	32	6.5	1,696	8.9	22
Ankle	9.5	2,408	10.9	30	8.1	2,116	6.5	16
Foot/toes	21.6	5,443	11.6	32	14.4	3,746	6.5	16
Other	0.4	111	1.1	3	0.4	109	0.4	1
Total	**100.0**	**25,239**	**100.0**	**276**	**100.0**	**26,062**	**100.0**	**247**

Table 10 Percent time loss, MD/DO/DPM reported, and acute injuries by location of injury and gender

	Time Loss (> Level I)				MD/DO/DPM Reported				Acute			
	Female		Male		Female		Male		Female		Male	
Injury Location*	No.	%	No.	%	No.	%	No.	%	No.	%	No.	%
Shoulder	13	81.3	34	89.5	1	6.3	4	10.4	8	50.0	14	36.8
Low back	26	89.7	21	95.5	1	3.4	2	9.1	10	34.5	8	36.4
Hip/thigh	18	60.7	25	86.2	0	0.0	1	3.4	12	42.9	16	55.2
Knee	45	70.3	37	72.5	3	4.7	8	15.7	23	35.9	16	31.4
Leg	25	78.1	18	81.8	1	3.1	2	9.1	10	31.3	7	31.8
Ankle	19	63.3	11	68.8	2	6.7	3	18.8	17	56.7	11	68.8
Foot/toes	22	68.8	10	62.5	4	13.0	2	12.5	6	18.8	6	37.5

*The top seven-plus locations of injury included 83.7% (women) and 78.5% (men) of the time-loss injuries

Lower extremity injuries were most frequent in dance/aerobic dance and aerobic fitness exercise equipment in women and were least frequent in strength exercise equipment in men, and intermediate in individual/recreational and team/competitive. The percent upper extremity injuries were most frequent in those using strength exercise equipment and much less frequent in the remaining groups. The rate of injuries to the spine/ trunk was highest in those using strength exercise equipment, intermediate for team/competitive, and lowest in the aerobic fitness exercise equipment and dance/aerobic dance groups.

Injury "Cause"

A great variety of causes for their injury were cited by the participants. Most men and women related that there were no special or unusual events associated with the injury, rather that injury arose out of normal activities (customary activity). Changes of activity, or mistakes in choosing activity levels, falls, equipment, collisions, and movements of various sorts were all cited as causes. Only collisions and falls seemed to have any gender relationship, with more among men.

Injury "Mechanism"

Once again, the mechanism of injury most often cited was "customary activity." Preexisting conditions, overuse/too much intensity, twisting or stretching, and direct blows were all noted at approximately the 10% level. Only direct blows seemed to vary by gender with the men mentioning it a bit less than twice as often as the women. Direct blow as a mechanism was most common in team/competitive and individual/recreational activities. Twist/stretch was also common in team/competitive activities.

Injury Severity

Time Loss

Injury severity as measured by time-loss versus nontime-loss injury rates varied somewhat by category of activity, as noted above. The activity groups with the highest overall rate, the team/competitive, had the highest rate of both time loss and nontime loss injuries for both genders, although it had the lowest percentage of total time-loss injury. Individual/recreational was second overall for both genders for both time-loss and nontime-loss rates.

Permanent Injury

As far as we know, our group had but one injury in this category, resulting in major permanent injury. One male cyclist was hit by a car, causing a head injury that produced permanent disability. At the close of the study, although there was significant improvement, the rehabilitation process not been completed. It was predicted, however, that there would be permanent and significant gait and mental sequelae.

Clinical Outcome/Medical Care

Overall almost one in 10 injuries/complaints (9.5%) sought medical attention with women seeking care less than half as often as men (Tables 7, 8, and 10). Another 9% (49) were seen by other health workers such as chiropractors, acupuncturists, physical therapists, or nurses with women seeking care as often as men. Although the overall percent seeking medical care was higher in team/competitive and individual recreation relative to the other groups, women were much less likely to seek medical care than men, whereas in strength exercise equipment there was essentially no gender difference. In dance/aerobic dance, the proportions seeking care were smaller, but the women still were less likely to seek medical care.

Identifying Risk Factors/Suggestions for Injury Prevention

The medical community is playing an increasingly active role in encouraging fitness enhancement. Whether by threats (the dangers of high cholesterol or too much low density lipoprotein, osteoporosis, or cardiovascular disease) or promises (enhanced competitive performance or lowered body fat), at least some portion of organized medicine appears to be encouraging the fitness movement. At the same time, such support might be applied more thoughtfully if it were possible to better predict the injury consequences of participation. It is useful to attempt to identify risk factors and suggest what might be done to alter these factors.

The injury rates did not seem to vary greatly by age. Although the 30 to 39 year age group had the highest injury rates, this was only in the men.

This is a significantly higher rate of injury in men and is primarily due to their participation in the higher risk team/competition activities. In addition to contact sports, which did contribute injuries to the male injury rate (some from relatively few hours of participation), basketball was also a significant contributor.

Extrinsic Factors

Generally, the rates of injury were highest for team and competitive sports compared to endeavors engaged in more for recreation, and this seemed to hold generally for both genders. Many noncompetitive activities also were engaged in at lower levels of intensity than were the competitive activities such as basketball, lacrosse, racquetball, rugby, and so on, so it is difficult to separate the degree of competition with the intensity of play.

Although the rates of injury generally were highest for team and competitive sports, it is impossible to say whether it was the team versus solo aspect of activity rather than the intensity that was actually influencing the rates of injury. Except for running, which resembled team activities in overall rates, most individual activities had relatively low rates of injury as did most forms of dance, aerobic dance, and working with exercise equipment of both the cardiovascular and weight variety.

More generally, in addition to an activity's solo versus individual character or its competitiveness or intensity, it is clear that what actually goes on in a particular sport or pastime strongly influences the patterns and severity of injury. Some sports are clearly lower extremity sports as are their injury patterns. However, because any activity may represent a particular package of characteristics, it is often difficult to see the contribution of a single element. Situations that allow comparisons, where men and women play in similar sports or where there are similar activities by participants of varying age are not always present in the team and competitive sports. However, for individual activities, participation is often not restricted to discrete categories.

Analysis and Recommendations

Players

Injuries occurred about twice as frequently to those with a history of a previous injury, without much regard to the part of the body injured, suggesting that the risks of sustaining injuries in recreational activities might be altered.

Recommendation The recreational athlete with a previous injury should engage in a suitable rehabilitation program, one aimed at eliminating any lack of strength or flexibility resulting from a past injury. It is hoped that this would reduce the risks of reinjury to an area shown to be vulnerable.

Sport

Relatively low rates of injury were found for most recreational sports activities, even using a sensitive definition of injury that included minor as well as major problems. Overall, the rate for injuries that caused an alteration in participation was less than two per person per year, based on the level of activity observed in the study. Although most individual activities appear to be relatively benign, running had a higher risk of injury than did many team/competitive sports. Most aerobic fitness activities (exercise cycling, step climbing, aerobic dance, etc.) carried low rates of injury, as did most weight activity, both free and machine. As might be expected, adults participating in competitive contact sports such as basketball fared worse.

Recommendation Avoiding more hazardous recreational activities is one important way to alter the risks. In addition, opting for a less competitive activity in place of a competitive contact sport would dramatically lower risk of injury.

External Environment

In an active adult population, the majority of the injuries seen will be of the nonacute variety, suggesting the external environment is not, at least in an obvious sense, hazardous. While it is recognized that many if not most injuries will be gradual onset or overuse in nature, conceptually the injury prevention model is often that of the acute injury.

Recommendation We need to consider injury prevention strategies in light of the demonstrated prevalence of gradual onset, chronic, acute exacerbations of chronic injuries, and reinjuries in the active adult population.

Health Support System

In a parallel way, since the majority of the injuries seen will be of the nonacute variety, the health support system must learn to better cope with these sorts of problems. The acute injury model also is still strong in the minds of many health care professionals as well as the participants. It is easy to fail with these injuries when we become frustrated from unrealistic expectations based on the acute injury recovery model.

Recommendation Both injury treatment and prevention strategies need to recognize these realities.

Definitions

The issue of injury definitions is difficult, particularly for recreational activities in which medical personnel are rarely anywhere about. Time loss and medical utilization data give information that can be compared to other studies since they are understood and commonly used.

Recommendation Collecting more detailed and sophisticated data should not preclude the collection of standard types of data as well. There are operational difficulties in applying a definition and, of course, there are great variations in time loss experienced and medical care used by different persons for the same injury. Whatever definition is employed should both serve the purposes of the study and as much as possible provide comparisons with previous work.

Research Design

A prospective cohort approach following a large group of participants in recreational activity, through a variety of exposures, has several advantages. Selecting the group in advance helps to minimize recall bias. Applying consistent methods and definitions of injury allows reasonable comparisons to be made between activities; whatever definitional, population, case ascertainment and classification biases exist should at least be constant across activities.

Recommendation Although rigorously following subjects using telephone callers as described is somewhat expensive, particularly compared to simple questionnaire methods, it offers a number of advantages as we have outlined. Activity is by our definition impure compared to an organized team sport, as all participants in this study were required to engage in a variety of recreational activities. This approach is very useful, however, when the interest is in multisport participation or where there is no organized structure to participation (no leagues, no registration) to identify participants.

Monitoring their experience on a weekly basis with trained callers helps to reduce memory errors since the information is collected quickly after the event. Injury information must be collected at some interval after the event, of course, but because of the frequent telephone contacts, little time had generally elapsed after an injury before the initial information was collected. The standard weekly calls would be used to document any time loss and medical care sought more or less as it occurred.

Acknowledgments

We wish to express sincere thanks to our interviewers Pamela Turner, Francine Cohen, Heidi Harrison, Alicia Head, and Jim Taylor, to our database supervisor Constance Foester-Bourges, and to our field supervisor, Bernetta Schadewald, ATC. Without their skill, dedication, and persistence this study would not have been possible.

We are also gratefully acknowledge the financial support provided by AVIA Athletic Footwear, Inc. We particularly wish to thank Todd Miller and Dan Richards for their consistent interest, support, and encouragement.

References

1. Walter SD, Hart LE, McIntosh JM, Sutton JR: The Ontario cohort study of running-related injuries. *Arch Intern Med* 1989;149:2561–2564.
2. Macera CA: Lower extremity injuries in runners: Advances in prediction. *Sports Med* 1992;13:50–57.
3. Macera CA, Pate RR, Powell KE, Jackson KL, Kendrick JS, Craven TE: Predicting lower-extremity injuries among habitual runners. *Arch Intern Med* 1989;149:2565–2568.
4. Bouter LM, Knipschild PG, Volovics A: Personal and environmental factors in relation to injury risk in downhill skiing. *Int J Sports Med* 1989;10:298–301.

5. Burns TP, Steadman JR, Rodkey WG: Alpine skiing and the mature athlete. *Clin Sports Med* 1991;10:327–342.
6. Thompson DC, Thompson RS, Rivara FP: Incidence of bicycle-related injuries in a defined population. *Am J Public Health* 1990;80:1388–1390.
7. Garrick JG, Requa RK: Aerobic dance: A review. *Sports Med* 1988;6:169–179.
8. Requa RK, Garrick JG: Adult recreational fitness, in Caine DJ, Caine CG, Lindner KJ (eds): *Epidemiology of Sports Injuries*. Champaign, IL, Human Kinetics, 1996.
9. Koplan JP, Powell KE, Sikes RK, Shirley RW, Campbell CC: An epidemiologic study of the benefits and risks of running. *JAMA* 1982;248:3118–3121.

Directions for Future Research

Study the epidemiology of ankle sprains, including the possible role of gender in their etiology.
The extent and types of injuries need to be well documented, and risk factors for both men and women need to be determined and evaluated. This information should be used to determine preventive measures.

Use the National Collegiate Athletic Association Injury Surveillance System to study medial ankle injuries, including the possible role of gender.
The diagnosis and treatment of these injuries in the younger population should be studied. Possible risk factors, including gender and anatomic alignment, need to be examined.

Collect epidemiologic data on women's athletic injuries.
Sports such as basketball, soccer, cheerleading, lacrosse, rowing, field hockey, and ice hockey have grown tremendously, especially among women. Injury data, exposure data, demographic data, and equipment information relating to women's participation in these sports is needed.

Evaluate the possible relationship between coaching background and training and incidence of injury by team.
Obtain information on playing experience, coaching experience, training, certification, safety education, and coaching courses taken by athletic coaches for both men and women.

Obtain data on female athletes regarding their history of physical activity from early childhood to the present.
The information should include sports played, injury history, physical education experience, and the type of family support received during sports participation. Data for female and male athletes should be compared.

Collect more data on athletic injuries in men and women and boys and girls participating in the same or similar sports.
This information should be used to determine whether the causes of injury are different, whether time missed as a result of the same types of injury differs by gender, and whether athletic equipment plays a role in the injury rate for both genders. The injury data should also include new women's sports such as ice hockey, lacrosse, rowing, and pole vaulting.

Section Two

Specific Injury Locations

Section Editor:
Elizabeth A. Arendt, MD

Leslie S. Beasley, MD
Lisa R. Callahan, MD
Deborah A. Faryniarz, MD
Letha Y. Griffin, MD, PhD
Jo A. Hannafin, MD, PhD
Stefan Lohmander, MD, PhD
Bert R. Mandelbaum, MD
Harold Roos, MD, PhD
Sally Rudicel, MD
Leena Sharma, MD

Overview

Exercise typically has a positive effect on the quality of life, improving a person's fitness and well-being. Its effect on the musculoskeletal system is also felt to be generally positive, with an increase in muscle strength, bone stock, and soft-tissue strength. Women and girls make up a greater percentage of active Americans than ever before. However, as women and girls enter the sporting arena in ever-increasing numbers, so, too, are they entering emergency rooms and doctors' offices. Injuries related to sports and exercise have significant impact on health care costs and time lost from work. In addition to the immediate consequences, sports-related injuries can have long-term consequences on the musculoskeletal system, resulting in pain, limb dysfunction, and reduced quality of life. US society has embraced sports and physical activity in the last half century. Although people in the health-care field have generally applauded this trend, they need to recognize the negative side of sports and exercise as it relates to their domain, and alter or modify its consequences when possible.

Injury prevention is the ultimate goal of improving the safety of sports and exercise. Prevention is predicated on knowledge of risk factors and injury mechanisms, but risk factors have been identified for very few common sports injuries. Sophisticated data are available on muscle activation and joint motion in a pitcher's throw, a golfer's swing, and a snow skier's turn, but such knowledge of body motion in sports performance far exceeds the knowledge of body motion during injury. There is increasing evidence, however, that some acute musculoskeletal injuries, such as noncontact injuries of the anterior cruciate ligament of the knee, have their etiology in disordered motor patterns. Early evidence suggests a gender difference in neuromuscular function and/or motor patterns, and these patterns correlate with known injuries that are more prevalent in girls and women. There also are limited data on whether improvement in motor/muscle patterns, proprioception, and strength decrease musculoskeletal injuries. This is a promising area of research, because it likely involves risk factors that can be modified. However, though gender has been scrutinized with regard to motor patterns, further research is needed to better understand the effect of variables such as body size, sport experience, or athleticism. If motor patterns and neuromuscular behavior do prove to be different in men than in women, there is a need to better understand how motor patterns in each variant may lead to injury.

Joint trauma can result from an acute injury or chronic overload. Sometimes joint injury can be occult, with the sequela of an acute injury leading to limb dysfunction at a time remote from the injury. Effects of macro and micro trauma to the joint are currently difficult to characterize and quantify. More information is needed regarding the relationship between acute joint trauma and chronic overuse joint injury and the subsequent development of degenerative joint disease, especially among women, who are disproportionately represented among those who have knee or hip osteoarthritis in the United States.

Improving neuromuscular control of a joint has been a strategy much used in orthopaedics as a nonsurgical approach to the treatment of clinical pain and joint dysfunction. Several musculoskeletal conditions that have primary symptoms of pain, including patellofemoral overuse syndrome and shoulder impingement syndrome, clinically improve with rehabilitation including a strengthening program. It appears that pain is related to loss of normal joint neuromuscular control. Regaining strength or neuromuscular control of the joint improves the clinical symptoms of pain with concomitant improvement of joint/limb function. Little is known about the strategy used by the body to restore normal neuromuscular control and whether this is performed at the central or local level.

Further exploration of neuromuscular motor control and motion patterns, leading to understanding the neuromuscular relationship with joint control, would greatly advance the treatment of many musculoskeletal conditions. This understanding might help to explain the difference between a cartilage defect in a joint that is pain free versus a cartilage defect in a joint that is painful. The strategies may be different for men than for women, and strategies may be different under different load conditions or joint alignment. Muscle strength and muscle fatigue play an important role in the transference of joint load. The relationship of neuromuscular control, muscle strength, and muscle fatigue to the appearance of clinical symptoms of pain and the development of long-term consequences of joint dysfunction needs to be better elucidated.

This is an exciting time for musculoskeletal research. There has been significant technological advancement in the ability to care for the injured athlete. Injured joints can be imaged in three planes, with and without motion. The degradation and synthesis of musculoskeletal tissue can be identified and traced with identified tissue markers. Joint ligaments can be reconstructed and joint pathology viewed through the arthroscope with minimal invasive damage to the joint. Technological communication allows physicians to share information with minimal physical or language barriers. These technological advances and explosion of basic science knowledge need to be pooled and redirected to injury and disease prevention.

Elizabeth A. Arendt, MD

Chapter 7

Upper Extremity Injuries: Shoulder

Jo A. Hannafin, MD, PhD
Deborah A. Faryniarz, MD
Leslie S. Beasley, MD

Introduction

Involvement and interest in women's athletics have exploded since the passage of Title IX legislation in 1972. Paralleling the advances in women's sports participation has been increased recognition of gender-specific variables that will impact training, injury, and recovery from injury in athletic women. In contrast to injuries to the anterior cruciate ligament, the role of gender in injuries to the shoulder has received minimal attention.

Shoulder Injuries

Shoulder injuries in athletic individuals can be classified as acute/traumatic or repetitive/microtraumatic. Traumatic injuries include fracture, glenohumeral dislocation or subluxation, labral injury, acromioclavicular (AC) joint separation, and traumatic injuries of the rotator cuff. Microtraumatic injuries include impingement syndrome, secondary impingement, and atraumatic or microtraumatic glenohumeral instability. Shoulder instability and impingement are by far the most common injuries seen in the athletic shoulder. The incidence of shoulder instability (traumatic and atraumatic) and impingement syndrome (primary and secondary) in active women is unknown. The National Collegiate Athletic Association Injury Surveillance System has included women's gymnastics and volleyball, and recently has expanded to include softball, but data are unavailable for swimming, tennis, and rowing. The focus to date has been on reporting acute injuries, whereas overuse or repetitive overuse injuries have not been evaluated.

Shoulder impingement can be divided into primary and secondary impingement. Primary impingement results from chronic wear to the rotator cuff tendons as they pass under the acromion and can also result from acute traumatic injury to the rotator cuff. Secondary impingement results from a functional decrease in the subacromial space because of fatigue or weakness of the rotator cuff in athletes with underlying gleno humeral instability. Repetitive stresses to the shoulder joint occurring in swimming, racquet sports, softball, gymnastics, and rowing may predispose the female athlete to development of primary or secondary impingement syndrome. Shoulder instability can also be described as acute/traumatic, repetitive/microtraumatic, and atraumatic/multidirectional instability. The characteristic of the type of instability demonstrated by athletic women is unknown.

Multidirectional Instability

Multidirectional instability (MDI) of the shoulder is a complex entity, characterized by symptomatic global laxity of the glenohumeral joint, and is believed to be more common in women than in men. Because symptoms vary widely, making the diagnosis of MDI is not always straightforward. In addition, relatively few series of patients with this disorder have been reported. The frequency of episodes of instability may range from a single event to multiple daily occurrences, and may be either acute or chronic. In hypermobile shoulders, there may or may not be an initial traumatic event as is often seen with unidirectional instability. Cumulative repetitive stress from athletic activities may be enough to cause symptomatic laxity. Common overuse syndromes result from swimming the butterfly or backstroke, gymnastics, and overhead throwing. Recurrent subluxation or an "unstable feeling" is more common than a locked dislocation, and most dislocations can be relocated with ease, often by the patient.

Neer and Foster[1] in 1980 defined MDI as an entity distinct from unidirectional instability. Since that time, only a few studies have reported the surgical outcome of shoulder stabilization in this population. In the published studies, women treated with an inferior capsular shift for MDI made up less than half of the total patients, and most of the patients were athletes.[1–8] Generalized ligamentous laxity was present in 25% to 100% of the patients in each study; however, laxity was not broken down by gender. It is known that women tend to have greater ligamentous laxity than men. It is interesting to note that in these studies of MDI, the percentage of female patients does not reach 50%. Do women with MDI respond better to conservative treatment than men, or are women undertreated for MDI and thus underreported? As athletes, women may be more prone to overuse syndromes and microtrauma, with an increased risk of converting global laxity to symptomatic instability. This has not been studied to date.

It is important to keep in mind that global laxity of the shoulder does not imply MDI. Laxity implies the ability to sublux or dislocate; instability refers to symptomatic laxity. MDI is distinguished from other types of instability by two features. First, symptoms are experienced in the midrange positions of glenohumeral motion, such as during normal activities of daily living. These symptoms are often severe enough to limit the extremes of glenohumeral motion. Second, clinical examination reveals the ability to dislocate or sublux the glenohumeral joint anteriorly, posteriorly, and inferiorly with concurrent reproduction of symptoms in one or more of these directions.[9]

With joint laxity, the rotator cuff muscles play an increasingly important role in stabilizing the glenohumeral joint, especially at midrange positions where the capsuloligamentous structures are slack. Although the surface areas of the larger humeral head and smaller glenoid fossa do not match, the joint is congruent. This congruence allows for a very secure concavity-compression effect as the rotator cuff compresses the humeral head into the matched concavity of the glenoid. Lippitt and Matsen[10] demonstrated that this effect is enhanced by an intact surrounding labrum, which deepens the glenoid socket by 50%. Additionally, the rotator cuff provides synchronous coordinated contraction of its muscle units to maintain the head of the humerus in the glenoid fossa during movement of the arm. Normal scapulothoracic motion is also essential for normal glenohumeral function. A failure of the scapula to rotate so that the glenoid remains underneath the rotating humeral head increases the tendency for instability because of loss of a stable glenoid platform. In addition, if the scapula is not effectively stabilized, the lateral scapula will droop, allowing inferior translation of the humeral head.[11] Many patients presenting with instability have significant abnormalities of scapulothoracic motion, with concomitant weakness of the posterior scapular stabilizers. This posterior weakness may be more common in women than in men, thus affecting response to conservative treatment.

There is some evidence that proprioception is diminished in athletes with recurrent anterior dislocation of the shoulder. Warner and associates[12] postulated that gradual development of shoulder instability may be the result of cumulative injury to the capsuloligamentous structures with loss of its proprioceptive feedback mechanism and subsequent loss of reflexive muscular protection against excessive humeral head translation and rotation.

Flexibility

There is a general perception that women have more flexible joints than men. However, there are few published data available that compare flexibility in men and women. Factors contributing to joint range of motion include joint structure, elasticity, muscle size, age, and activity patterns. There is some evidence to support an increased incidence of generalized ligamentous laxity in women.[13] Marshall and associates[14] reported that joint laxity in the elbow and hip is related to female gender. Normative data for sit and reach tests also appear to support this concept. Several recent studies have evaluated gender differences in shoulder laxity. An increase in posterior and inferior laxity was demonstrated in asymptomatic high school and college female athletes. Posterior subluxation of the glenohumeral joint was demonstrated in 65% of female athletes in contrast to 51% of male athletes. Also, a statistically increased incidence of generalized ligamentous laxity was noted in the female athletes studied.[15]

Epidemiology of Shoulder Injuries

In a study of Army parachutists from 1985 to 1994, the rates of injury between male and female subjects were not significantly different; however, the sites of injury were different. Upper body injuries were reported in 43% of the men versus 27% of the women.[16] A prevalence study of recurrent shoulder dislocation in the Israeli military demonstrated a similar male predominance with an incidence of 30% in men and 5% in women younger than age 21 years. The authors noted that this 6:1 ratio might reflect the importance of trauma in the etiology of recurrent dislocation.[17]

Aagaard and Jorgensen[18] reported data derived from a questionnaire study of elite Danish volleyball players during 1993 to 1994. The injury incidence was noted to be similar in men and women. Most injuries occurred during spiking and blocking and included injuries to the fingers (21%), ankles (18%), shoulders (15%), and knees (16%). Shoulder and knee injuries were predominantly overuse injuries, with a slight increase in shoulder injuries seen in female athletes. In a study of Alpine skiing and snowboarding, the demographics of ski injuries were related to both age and gender. Head, face, and shoulder injuries were more common in men, whereas knee injuries were more common in women.[19] Kocher and associates[20] reported a 3-year review of shoulder injuries from Alpine skiing. Shoulder injuries comprised 11% of the total injuries reported and 39% of the upper extremity injuries. A female:male ratio of 1:3 was noted for all shoulder injuries. The breakdown of the most common shoulder injuries is shown in Table 1. Rotator cuff strain and greater tuberosity fractures showed a male:female ratio of 1.7:1. In contrast, glenohumeral dislocations (5:1), AC separations (5:1), and clavicle fractures (7:1) were significantly more common in men. It is unclear whether these data reflect mechanism of injury, speed of fall, force of impact, or more gender-specific injury variables. It should be noted that this chapter reflects the largest series of shoulder injuries reported wherein gender is addressed as a specific variable. Shoulder injuries are common in male and female elite swimmers; however, in the published literature the role of gender as an independent variable in injury or response to treatment is not discussed.[21,22]

Treatment of Shoulder Injuries

Conservative and Surgical Treatment of Impingement Syndrome

Morrison and associates[23] evaluated the outcome of conservative treatment of impingement syndrome in 616 patients. The patients were of mixed age, activity level, and gender, but were treated with a uniform rehabilitation protocol. Sixty-seven percent of the patients had a satisfactory result, 28% failed to respond to conservative treatment and required surgical intervention, and 5% failed conservative treatment but refused surgery. In this study, gender did not appear to affect outcome: 68% of the 386 men and 66% of the 230 women had a satisfactory outcome. This is the only published study to our knowledge that critically evaluates the role of gender in response to treatment of impingement syndrome. Numerous studies report the results of surgical treatment of impingement syndrome or debridement of partial-thickness rotator cuff tears. Results of arthroscopic treatment of partial-thickness rotator cuff injury and impingement are more favorable in patients with a traumatic etiology.[24,25] Atraumatic development of impingement and rotator cuff pathology has been linked to glenohumeral instability, which responded poorly to subacromial decompression; however, the role of gender has not been evaluated in recently published studies.[25–27]

Table 1 Types and frequencies of shoulder injuries to Alpine skiers (*N* = 393)

			Age		Sex (%)	
Injury	**N**	**%**	**Mean**	**SD**	**M**	**F**
Rotator cuff	95	24.2	36.1	13.1	62.9	37.1
Anterior glenohumeral dislocation/subluxation	85	21.6	34.5	12.2	83.5	16.5
Acromioclavicular separation	77	19.6	35.4	12.9	83.1	16.9
Clavicle fracture	43	10.9	32.8	15.2	88.4	11.6
Greater tuberosity fracture	27	6.9	39.7	12.0	63.0	37.0
Trapezius muscle strain	25	6.4	32.5	10.0	60.0	40.0
Proximal humeral fracture	13	3.3	36.3	18.9	76.9	23.1
Biceps tendon strain	9	2.3	32.9	10.3	67.0	37.0
Glenoid fracture	6	1.5	38.5	12.3	66.7	33.3
Scapular body fracture	4	1.0	37.3	9.9	75.0	25.0
Humeral head fracture	4	1.0	46.0	9.7	50.0	50.0
Sternoclavicular separation	2	0.5	29.0	1.0	100	
Acromion fracture	1	0.3	46.0			
Posterior glenohumeral dislocation	1	0.3	44.0			
Biceps tendon dislocation	1	0.3	42.0			

(Reproduced with permission from Kocher MS, Dupre MM, Feagin JA Jr: Shoulder injuries from alpine skiing and snowboarding: Aetiology, treatment and prevention. *Sports Med* 1998;25:201–211.)

Conservative and Surgical Treatment of Shoulder Instability

MDI usually can be treated nonsurgically.[11,28,29] Nonsurgical management includes patient education, modification of activities, and physical rehabilitation using exercises that strengthen the rotator cuff musculature, scapular stabilizers, and deltoid muscles. The aim of treatment is to improve the patient's muscle tone and coordination and to increase the patient's general functional adaptation.[30]

Kronberg and associates[31] demonstrated a significant imbalance of shoulder muscular control in patients with generalized joint laxity and shoulder instability when compared with normal controls. These results suggest that muscle strengthening and coordination training may be more effective treatment than soft-tissue reconstruction to improve shoulder stability in this group of patients. A similar conclusion about conservative strengthening in the management of MDI can be drawn from the study performed by Burkhead and Rockwood.[32] They evaluated the treatment of shoulder instability with an exercise program, demonstrating that 88% of 33 patients with MDI had good or excellent results following treatment with a specific set of muscle-strengthening exercises. They concluded that muscle-strengthening exercises may be able to accommodate for ligamentous and capsular laxity. The role of gender in success or failure of conservative treatment was not addressed in these studies.

Surgical treatment should be offered for the compliant symptomatic patient who is unresponsive to nonsurgical management. Indications include pain, instability with activities of daily living, or persistent paresthesias in the involved extremity. Painless, nonlimiting laxity of the shoulder is not, in itself, an indication for capsular reconstruction and should always be distinguished from symptomatic instability.

Before the procedure, an examination of the shoulder should be performed under anesthesia to confirm direction and degree of instability that will dictate the surgical treatment. The most commonly performed procedure for MDI is the inferior capsular shift as described by Neer and Foster.[1] In addition, closure of the rotator interval capsule is recommended to decrease inferior instability in adduction and posterior instability in flexion.[33] The most commonly performed procedure for traumatic, recurrent anterior instability is the Bankart repair. Success of the repair depends not only on operative technique, but also on strict adherence to the postoperative rehabilitation protocol.

In light of the fact that capsular laxity and possibly MDI are more common in women than men, the literature review for open stabilization focuses on the surgical treatment of MDI. In the few existing surgical series on MDI, the short-term results are promising.[1–8] Of the 225 total MDI patients treated, 99 were women (45%) and 26% to 100% in each study had generalized ligamentous laxity. Results were not consistently stratified by either gender or laxity. To our knowledge, the following studies comprise the surgical literature on MDI.

Neer and Foster[1] were the first to recognize the importance of differentiating MDI from unidirectional instability because the treatment differs. Anterior instability can be treated by repairing the anterior labrum (Bankart repair) and/or tightening the anterior capsule. This procedure performed in a patient with MDI leaves the shoulder unstable inferiorly; moreover, tightening the capsule anteriorly may force the shoulder in the opposite direction posteriorly, resulting in severe arthritic changes. In their original study, only one out of 36 patients treated with an inferior capsular shift for MDI had recurrent subluxations (7 months postoperatively). This patient was treated with a posterior capsular shift and had undiagnosed anterior laxity secondary to a labral tear. However, only 17 patients had been followed for more than 2 years. This study included equal numbers of male and female patients, and 47% of these had generalized ligamentous laxity.[1]

Cooper and Brems[4] studied 38 patients with MDI with follow-up averaging 39 months (range, 24 to 71 months). This group included 22 women and 16 men treated with an inferior capsular shift through an anterior approach. Their results showed improvement in 86% of patients and recurrent instability in four (10%). Two of these four failures were in women who had excessive ligamentous laxity with a history of voluntary dislocations. Twenty-nine patients (76%) had generalized ligamentous laxity.

Altchek and associates[2] evaluated 40 patients with anterior inferior instability in which 90% had a Bankart lesion in addition to capsular laxity. They used a modified inferior capsular shift (medially based capsular incision) with a Bankart repair. Follow-up averaged 3 years (range, 2 to 7 years). The study included 10 female and 30 male patients. Fifty percent had excessive ligamentous laxity. Four patients had recurrent episodes of instability (two of which were considered to have generalized ligamentous laxity).

Bigliani and associates[3] reported their results of inferior capsular shifts in 63 athletes with anterior inferior shoulder instability. Additionally, 12 of these had concomitant posterior instability and 21 had a Bankart lesion that was repaired concurrently. They also noted frequent laxity of the anterosuperior capsule with spreading of the rotator interval. This was imbricated as part of the repair. This study consisted of 21 women and 42 men with average follow-up of 4 years (range, 1 to 9 years). Forty-three patients had some traumatic event, but all patients had some degree of inferior capsular laxity that was corrected at surgery. Unlike patients with generalized ligamentous laxity, these shoulders, subjected to the repetitive microtrauma of athletic use, were frequently lax out of proportion to other joints. Only two patients redislocated postoperatively after violent falls.

Several smaller studies have evaluated the outcome of capsular shifts in patients with MDI. Steinbeck and Jerosch[8] demonstrated excellent results in 17 out of 19 patients undergoing a modified inferior capsular shift with mean follow-up of 38 months (range, 30 to 54 months). Two patients had recurrent dislocations. Seventeen of their patients were women. Similarly, Lebar and Alexander[6] investigated the clinical results of 10 patients (including three women) for a mean of 28 months. All patients had generalized hyperlaxity, and one carried a diagnosis of Ehlers-Danlos syndrome. Eight of these 10 patients reported good results and two reported no improvement; one of the two had a second surgical procedure. McIntyre and associates[7] followed 19 patients for an average of 34 months following an arthroscopic inferior capsular shift. Eight of these patients were women, 14 were athletes, and five had generalized hyperlaxity. Eighteen reported good or excellent results; one experienced recurrent anterior subluxations but was then treated successfully with a second arthroscopic procedure. Finally, Duncan and Savoie[5] followed 10 patients 12 to 36 months after arthroscopic inferior capsular shift for MDI. All patients in this series reported satisfactory results, with only one complaining of some continued pain when swimming. None had recurrent subluxation or dislocation. Outcomes in this cohort were not stratified by gender.

Although these studies reveal satisfactory results for inferior capsular shift procedures in patients with MDI who fail conservative management, many shoulder surgeons suspect that results will deteriorate over time.[11] Many of these patients have generalized hyperlaxity and may have some form of collagen abnormality. Recent work by Rodeo and associates[34] demonstrated intrinsic biochemical and morphologic differences in stable and unstable shoulders. Capsules from unstable shoulders (both MDI and unidirectional instability) revealed increases in collagen cross-links, collagen fibril diameters, cysteine content, and elastin content when compared with normal shoulder capsules. The authors hypothesize that repetitive capsular deformation provided stimulus for adaptive changes that increase capsular strength in an attempt to diminish instability. Because of the likelihood of intrinsic collagen abnormalities, the capsule may have decreased resistance to deformation and warrant longer follow-up periods after both open and arthroscopic procedures. The role of gender in determination of the biochemical and mechanical properties of the shoulder capsule is unknown.

Numerous studies have been published on the role of arthroscopic stabilization in the treatment of anterior shoulder dislocation. Hayashida and associates[35] reported on the results of arthroscopic transglenoid suture repair for traumatic anterior shoulder instability. Eighty-two patients (63 men and 19 women) were included in the study. The authors reported 67% excellent, 17% good, and 16% poor results. All patients with a poor result had recurrence of anterior instability as defined by anterior dislocation. A multivariate analysis was performed to assess clinical parameters that might influence outcome. Gender was not found to be a statistically significant parameter. To our knowledge this is the only study that assesses gender as an independent variable in outcome. The remaining studies either do not report the gender of the patients evaluated or do not assess gender as a variable in outcome.[36–40] Thermal capsular shrinkage is a relatively new technique being advocated for the treatment of capsular laxity and symptomatic glenohumeral micro and macro instability. Several studies have shown that collagenous tissue can be shortened by the application of heat via laser energy.[41–45] This technique is being used to shrink the glenohumeral joint capsule in an attempt to reduce shoulder instability, thus reducing the need for an open capsular shift procedure. While initial clinical results of capsular shrinkage look promising, further research on the effects of heat and longer clinical follow-up must be performed. It is important to clarify the advantages and disadvantages of this procedure, to define its role in the treatment of MDI, and to determine if there is a gender-specific or tissue-specific response to treatment. Future investigations of MDI should include other modalities to tighten the capsule. This may include the use of biologic factors to promote capsular contracture or to increase collagen cross-linking.

References

1. Neer CS II, Foster CR: Inferior capsular shift for involuntary inferior and multidirectional instability of the shoulder: A preliminary report. *J Bone Joint Surg* 1980;62A:897–908.
2. Altchek DW, Warren RF, Skyhar MJ, Ortiz G: T-plasty modification of the Bankart procedure for multidirectional instability of the anterior and inferior types. *J Bone Joint Surg* 1991;73A:105–112.
3. Bigliani LU, Kurzweil PR, Schwartzbach CC, Wolfe IN, Flatow EL: Inferior capsular shift procedure for anterior-inferior shoulder instability in athletes. *Am J Sports Med* 1994;22:578–584.
4. Cooper RA, Brems JJ: The inferior capsular-shift procedure for multidirectional instability of the shoulder. *J Bone Joint Surg* 1992;74A:1516–1521.
5. Duncan R, Savoie FH III: Arthroscopic inferior capsular shift for multidirectional instability of the shoulder: A preliminary report. *Arthroscopy* 1993;9:24–27.
6. Lebar RD, Alexander AH: Multidirectional shoulder instability: Clinical results of inferior capsular shift in an active-duty population. *Am J Sports Med* 1992;20:193–198.
7. McIntyre LF, Caspari RB, Savoie FH III: The arthroscopic treatment of multidirectional shoulder instability: Two-year results of a multiple suture technique. *Arthroscopy* 1997;13:418–425.

8. Steinbeck J, Jerosch J: Surgery for atraumatic anterior-inferior shoulder instability: A modified capsular shift evaluated in 20 patients followed for 3 years. *Acta Orthop Scand* 1997;68:447–450.
9. Schenk TJ, Brems JJ: Multidirectional instability of the shoulder: Pathophysiology, diagnosis, and management. *J Am Acad Orthop Surg* 1998;6:65–72.
10. Lippitt S, Matsen F: Mechanisms of glenohumeral joint stability. *Clin Orthop* 1993:291:20–28.
11. Mallon WJ, Speer KP: Multidirectional instability: Current concepts. *J Shoulder Elbow Surg* 1995;4:54–64.
12. Warner JJ, Lephart S, Fu FH: Role of proprioception in pathoetiology of shoulder instability. *Clin Orthop* 1996;330:35–39.
13. Beighton P, Solomon L, Soskolne CL: Articular mobility in an African population. *Ann Rheum Dis* 1973;32:413–418.
14. Marshall JL, Johanson N, Wickiewicz TL, et al: Joint looseness: A function of the person and the joint. *Med Sci Sports Exerc* 1980;12:189–194.
15. McFarland EG, Campbell G, McDowell J: Posterior shoulder laxity in asymptomatic athletes. *Am J Sports Med* 1996;24:468–471.
16. Amoroso PJ, Bell NS, Jones BH: Injury among female and male army parachutists. *Aviat Space Environ Med* 1997;68:1006–1011.
17. Milgrom C, Mann G, Finestone A: A prevalence study of recurrent shoulder dislocations in young adults. *J Shoulder Elbow Surg* 1998;7:621–624.
18. Aagaard H, Jorgensen U: Injuries in elite volleyball. *Scand J Med Sci Sports* 1996;6:228–232.
19. Macnab AJ, Cadman R: Demographics of alpine skiing and snowboarding injury: Lessons for prevention programs. *Inj Prev* 1996;2:286–289.
20. Kocher MS, Dupre MM, Feagin JA Jr: Shoulder injuries from alpine skiing and snowboarding: Aetiology, treatment and prevention. *Sports Med* 1998;25:201–211.
21. Bak K, Magnusson SP: Shoulder strength and range of motion in symptomatic and pain-free elite swimmers. *Am J Sports Med* 1997;25:454–459.
22. Bak K, Fauno P: Clinical findings in competitive swimmers with shoulder pain. *Am J Sports Med* 1997;25:254–260.
23. Morrison DS, Frogameni AD, Woodworth P: Non-operative treatment of subacromial impingement syndrome. *J Bone Joint Surg* 1997;79A:732–737.
24. Stephens SR, et al: Arthroscopic acromioplasty: A 6- to 10-year follow-up. *Arthroscopy* 1998;14:382–388.
25. Payne LZ, et al: Arthroscopic treatment of partial rotator cuff tears in young athletes: A preliminary report. *Am J Sports Med* 1997;25:299–305.
26. Hartwig CH, Burkhard R: Operative release of the impingement syndrome: Indication, technique, results. *Arch Orthop Trauma Surg* 1996;115:249–254.
27. Roye RP, Grana WA, Yates CK: Arthroscopic subacromial decompression: Two- to seven-year follow-up. *Arthroscopy* 1995;11:301–306.
28. Dines DM, Levinson M: The conservative management of the unstable shoulder including rehabilitation. *Clin Sports Med* 1995;14:797–816.
29. Yamaguchi K, Flatow EL: Management of multidirectional instability. *Clin Sports Med* 1995;14:885–902.
30. Flatow EL, Warner JI: Instability of the shoulder: Complex problems and failed repairs: Part I. Relevant biomechanics, multidirectional instability, and severe glenoid loss, in Cannon WD Jr (ed): *Instructional Course Lectures 47*. Rosemont, IL, American Academy of Orthopaedic Surgeons, 1998, pp 97–112.

31. Kronberg M, Brostrom LA, Nemeth G: Differences in shoulder muscle activity between patients with generalized joint laxity and normal controls. *Clin Orthop* 1991;269:181–192.

32. Burkhead WZ Jr, Rockwood CA Jr: Treatment of instability of the shoulder with an exercise program. *J Bone Joint Surg* 1992;74A:890–896.

33. Harryman DT II, Sidles JA, Harris SL, Matsen FA III: The role of the rotator interval capsule in passive motion and stability of the shoulder. *J Bone Joint Surg* 1992;74A:53–66.

34. Rodeo SA, Suzuki K, Yamauchi M, Bhargava M, Warren RF: Analysis of collagen and elastic fibers in shoulder capsule in patients with shoulder instability. *Am J Sports Med* 1998;26:634–643.

35. Hayashida K, Yoneda M, Nakagawa S, Okamura K, Fukushima S: Arthroscopic Bankart suture repair for traumatic anterior shoulder instability: Analysis of the causes of a recurrence. *Arthroscopy* 1998;14:295–301.

36. Koss S, Richmond JC, Woodward JS Jr: Two- to five-year followup of arthroscopic Bankart reconstruction using a suture anchor technique. *Am J Sports Med* 1997;25:809–812.

37. Mologne TS, McBride MT, Lapoint JM: Assessment of failed arthroscopic anterior labral repairs. Findings at open surgery. *Am J Sports Med* 1997;25:813–817.

38. Geiger DF, Hurley JA, Tovey JA, Rao JP: Results of arthroscopic versus open Bankart suture repair. *Clin Orthop* 1997;337:111–117.

39. Arciero RA, Wheeler JH, Ryan JB, McBride JT: Arthroscopic Bankart repair versus nonoperative treatment for acute, initial anterior shoulder dislocations. *Am J Sports Med* 1994;22:589–594.

40. Segmuller HE, Hayes MG, Saies AD: Arthroscopic repair of glenolabral injuries with an absorbable fixation device. *J Shoulder Elbow Surg* 1997;6:383–392.

41. Schaefer SL, Ciarelli MJ, Arnoczky SP, Ross HE: Tissue shrinkage with the holmium:yttrium aluminum garnet laser: A postoperative assessment of tissue length, stiffness, and structure. *Am J Sports Med* 1997;25:841–848.

42. Hayashi K, Markel MD, Thabit G III, Bogdanske JJ, Thielke RJ: The effect of nonablative laser energy on joint capsular properties: An in vitro mechanical study using a rabbit model. *Am J Sports Med* 1995;23:482–487.

43. Hayashi K, Thabit G III, Vailas AC, Bogdanske JJ, Cooley AJ, Markel MD: The effect of nonablative laser energy on joint capsular properties: An in vitro histologic and biochemical study using a rabbit model. *Am J Sports Med* 1996;24:640–646.

44. Hayashi K, Thabit G III, Bogdanske JJ, Mascio LN, Markel MD: The effect of nonablative laser energy on the ultrastructure of joint capsular collagen. *Arthroscopy* 1996;12:474–481.

45. Vangsness CT Jr, Mitchell W III, Nimni M, Erlich M, Saadat V, Schmotzer H: Collagen shortening: An experimental approach with heat. *Clin Orthop* 1997;337:267–271.

Chapter 8

Foot and Ankle Injuries in Female Athletes

Sally Rudicel, MD

Introduction

Foot and ankle injuries are very common in athletes. In many sports, the ankle is the most frequently injured body part. Early epidemiologic studies on injury rates of female athletes, shortly after the passage of Title IX to the Education Amendments Act in 1972, found that they were higher than those of male athletes. However, follow-up work has shown that most injuries are sport specific rather than gender specific.[1] Women have now begun to train longer and to condition properly. Some foot and ankle injuries, however, may be more common in women because of anatomic or physiologic risk factors, because of improper footwear, or because more women participate in the sport.

Female anatomy may cause differences in the types or incidence of foot and ankle injuries. Women have a wider pelvis, more varus of the hips, more genu valgus, shorter lower extremities, and a lower center of gravity, which gives them an advantage in balance sports such as gymnastics. Women also have more mobile joints and are more flexible for sports such as gymnastics. Their lower extremity anatomy, however, may lead to more lower extremity overuse syndromes. Women also have less muscle mass and more fat, giving them less power and speed. Physiologic differences also place women at more risk of stress fractures, particularly at the distal fibula and metatarsals.[1]

Women have more problems with poorly fitting shoes. Various athletic shoes only recently have been specifically designed for women, and fit has not always been appropriate. Many athletic shoes are built on a man's last. Women's feet are not just a smaller version of men's feet; the heel of the shoe often needs to be narrower.[2,3] A split last or a shoe built on a woman's last may provide better fit and fewer foot problems. Women who wear high heels may get tight Achilles tendons with heel varus, predisposing the recreational athlete to lateral ankle sprains. Appropriate shoe wear and fit are thus important for foot health.

Some sports, dance in particular, have more female participants. Ballet, with women dancing en pointe, is a prime example of highly trained female athletes with injuries that are both gender specific and sport specific. Aerobic dance is another sport with many female participants and more foot and ankle injuries.

Ankle sprains are probably the most frequent injury across all sports, for both men and women.[4–6] There is a suggestion in the literature that ankle sprains may be more frequent in women when compared with men in the same sport.[7,8] They are certainly very common in female gymnasts, with an incidence as high as 27%.[1] Other foot and ankle injuries commonly seen in women are ankle impingement, posterior tibial tendinitis, stress fractures, flexor hallucis longus tendinitis in dancers, and bunions.

Epidemiology

Men and women are different, and it might be expected that rates and types of athletic injuries might be different as well. Women have less muscle mass and more fat per body weight. Wilmore[9] showed that men have greater absolute strength but little difference in strength relative to lean body weight. He also found little gender difference in the endurance of trained athletes.[9] Women have less power and speed, but their increased body fat is an advantage in long-distance swimming, for example.[1] Because men have relatively longer bones, they have a mechanical advantage in sports that require striking, hitting, or kicking. Thus, anatomic and physiologic differences create different spectrums of possible injury for the male and female athlete.

Various studies of female athletic injuries have been done since the passage of Title IX. A report by the US Department of Health, Education and Welfare estimated that injury rates of college and high school athletes in 1975–1976 were lower in women than in men. At that time, women made up approximately 29% of varsity teams and accounted for 16% of injuries. Soccer data showed an increase in women's injuries during the 1970s, but this equalized in later studies.[10]

Gillette surveyed varsity intercollegiate athletic injuries in 1973–1974 and reported that the most common injuries in women were to the ankles and knees.[11] Haycock and Gillette found that women sustain the same types of injuries as men, except women may have more patella and joint injuries.[12] In 1980, Whiteside[13] and Clarke and Buckley[14] each independently concluded that injuries were sport rather than gender specific. In Whiteside's study, the ankle and foot had the highest relative frequency of reportable injuries in women's and men's basketball. Ankle and foot and knee injuries had the highest relative frequency in women's gymnastics as well. The injury pattern in men was similar, but women had a higher relative frequency of ankle injuries.

Since 1982, the National Collegiate Athletic Association (NCAA) Injury Surveillance System has provided detailed injury information on 16 collegiate sports. Comparable sports for men and women include gymnastics, basketball, soccer, and lacrosse. The highest overall injury rate for women is in gymnastics, followed by soccer and basketball. Overall, the ankle was the most commonly injured joint, and gymnastics was the biggest offender.[15] Ritter and associates[16] found ankle injuries to be most common in a study at Indiana University during the 1977–1978 season as well.[16] Garrick and Requa[5] reported on injuries to girls in high school athletics in 1978, and they found the ankle to be the most common joint injured. Haycock and Gillette[12] found this as well in female college athletes.

Rose[17] examined field hockey injuries at California State University from 1976 to 1980. Ankle sprains were the most common injury. Shively and associates[18] used data from the Oklahoma Secondary Schools Sports Injury Registry to look at high school sports injuries reported in 1981. Although there was no difference in overall injury rate between boys and girls, girls had a significantly larger number of major ankle injuries and lost more playing time than boys.

DeHaven and Lintner[19] reported injury incidence and type in a university setting in 1986. The ankle was the second most common site of injury in women and men. Women who were injured were more likely than men to injure their ankle, foot, or toe.

Garrick and Requa[6] reported in 1988 that foot and ankle injuries accounted for 25.2% of all injuries treated at a sports center during a 9-year period. Ankle sprains were the single most common injury. The injuries were not distinguished by gender.

Clanton and Beaver recently conducted an as yet unpublished study of foot and ankle injuries in an NCAA Division I athletic program from 1983–1998 at the University of Texas. The overall incidence of foot or ankle injuries was 10.4%: 13.6% in women compared with 9.4% for men. Female basketball and volleyball players had the highest incidence of injuries. Ankle sprains were the most common injury.

Basketball seems to be very demanding on the ankle. Zelisko and associates[8] compared professional basketball injuries in men and women in 1982 and found that the injury frequency in women was 1.6 times that of men, and the ankle was the most frequently injured body part. Men had a slightly higher percentage of ankle injuries (17.9% compared with 20.3%), and women had a markedly higher percentage of foot injuries (6% compared with 0.7% of all injuries).[8]

Hosea, Carey, and Harrer recently conducted an as yet unpublished study of ankle injuries in scholastic and collegiate basketball players in New Jersey over a 2-year period. Women had a 25% greater risk of sustaining a grade I ankle sprain compared with men. There was no significant difference in the risk for grade II or III ankle sprains, fractures, or syndesmotic sprains. The risk of an ankle injury in intercollegiate level basketball was double that in interscholastic basketball for either gender.

Baumhauer and associates[20] published a prospective study of risk factors for ankle injury in college-aged athletes. Ten percent of the intercollegiate athletes in the study sustained an inversion ankle sprain during the sports season. They did not find a correlation between generalized joint laxity and the incidence of inversion ankle sprains. Nor were anatomic variants of feet (pes cavus, pes planus) found to correlate with ankle injury. They did find that individuals with muscle strength imbalance with an elevated eversion-to-inversion strength ratio had a higher incidence of inversion injury than did individuals with a greater plantar flexion strength and a smaller dorsiflexion-to-plantar flexion ratio. No differences between men and women were mentioned.[20] Given how common ankle sprains are in many sports, assessing these strength issues in all athletes may provide preventative clues for ankle injuries in both men and women. It may be that there are gender differences in these muscle ratios that make grade I sprains more common in certain women.

Ballet

Ballet is a highly demanding activity in which the foot and ankle are placed in extremes of position. Dancers must have marked external rotation of the hips and generalized ligamentous laxity to perform the maneuvers required. Most participants are women. The greatest amount of literature on women's athletic foot and ankle injuries centers on this discipline. The foot and ankle are the most commonly injured areas in dancers. Chronic injuries are more common than acute ones.[21]

Both gymnastics and ballet have specific aesthetic demands. They demand grace, strength, and flexibility.[22] Shoes associated with these activities have no cushioning or shock absorption, and dancing en pointe places large stresses on the forefoot and great toe, in particular. Not everyone has the necessary physical requirements for this activity, and thus more injuries may occur in those individuals trying to perform beyond their body capabilities.

The ankle sprain is the most common injury reported in the elite dancer. The plantar flexed position of the foot and ankle is fundamental to ballet. According to Hamilton,[23] the grade II sprain is the most common and occurs on demi pointe. The anterior talofibular ligament is almost vertical and is torn when an adduction-inversion force is applied. In the full pointe position, the posterior lip of the tibia rests against the os calcis, the subtalar joint is locked, and the ankle is stable. In this position, a sprain of the midfoot as described later more likely occurs. With a few degrees of dorsiflexion at the ankle rather than complete plantar flexion, the lateral ankle sprain may occur.[23]

Injuries to the ankle occur more commonly in the left foot, the working foot. They are more common during the fatigue of rehearsal. They also are found frequently in the cavus foot. Hamilton[23] described 17 ankle sprains in 100 dancers of the New York City Ballet during a 16-month period. Various instabilities can persist, including varus instability and rotatory instability. Peroneal strengthening is critical.

The midfoot commonly is not sprained, but a sprain can be caused by a valgus force applied to the foot with the toe shoe acting as a lever tearing the medial collateral ligament of the navicular-first cuneiform-first metatarsal. These tears are usually partial. An occasional forefoot sprain unique to toe dancing involves the bases of the fourth and fifth metatarsals, the most mobile metatarsals. The plantar ligaments are strong. If a ballet dancer en pointe goes "over the top," dancing on the dorsal side of the foot, the bases of the fourth and fifth metatarsals are sprained dorsally. This usually occurs in the high arched, hypermobile foot. Cuboid subluxation in ballet dancers has been described, as well.[24]

Dancers also may have posterior ankle pain. This may be either posterior impingement from an os trigonum, with pain posterolaterally or flexor hallucis longus tendinitis, with pain posteromedially. Hamilton and associates[25] reported on 37 dancers who required surgery for either of these problems. Twenty-two of the dancers were women.

The maneuver to the en pointe position can produce compression of the calcaneus with the posterior aspect of the tibia leading to posterior impingement.

The os trigonum, which occurs in 8% to 13% of the population, may impinge between the posterior lip of the tibia and the os calcis. In full plantar flexion, the os may get bruised, get a compression fracture, or actually fracture, if it is attached. An injection of a local anesthetic into the area may be diagnostic of the problem. Surgical exploration with excision of the os trigonum or osteophytes off of the tibia or calcaneus may be needed.

Flexor hallucis longus tendinitis is also rather unique to dance. The tendon is particularly stressed while en pointe. The tendon is strained as it passes through its fibro-osseous tunnel on the posterior aspect of the talus between the medial and lateral tubercles. A nodule may form on the tendon causing triggering of the great toe. Progressive inflammation can lead to stenosing tenosynovitis, and the tendon can become frozen in the sheath causing a "pseudo hallux rigidus."[26] Sammarco and Miller[27] reported on two cases of partial ruptures of the flexor hallucis longus in dancers. The condition may become chronic and tends to occur in relatively "tight" dancers, especially those with stiff feet and a poor point position. Anything that contributes to pronation of the foot and adds more strain to the medial side of the ankle may exacerbate the problem.[28] With the patient plantar flexed, flexing the great toe against resistance will hurt along the tendon sheath. This tendinitis must be differentiated from posterior ankle impingement.

Other than toe fractures, the most common fracture in dancers is the spiral fracture of the distal fifth metatarsal, the so-called "dancer's fracture." The fracture occurs when dancers lose their balance on demi pointe and roll over the outer border of their foot. Symptomatic treatment is indicated, and displaced fractures may need to be treated in a cast.[21] O'Malley and associates[29] reported on 35 such fractures in professional dancers. Twenty-five of these were in women.

Stress fractures are well described in ballet dancers, as well.[30–32] The base of the second metatarsal is the most common location. These fractures are characterized by an insidious onset of midfoot pain and require an average of 6.2 weeks until return to performance, and 14% of dancers still have occasional pain or stiffness at follow-up.[32]

Because of the lack of protection of the foot and the demands and position placed on it in dance, dancers, particularly women because they dance en pointe, have numerous problems in the forefoot, including hallux rigidus, hammer toes, calluses, and injuries. Oglivie-Harris and associates[33] investigated the importance of second toe length in dancers. They found that second toe length made no difference in men as far as calluses, pain, or injuries. However, women with a shorter second toe had fewer calluses, less pain, and less hallux rigidus. The incidence of hallux rigidus was 44% in women with a longer second toe. While not significant, the group of uninjured dancers had an overrepresentation of women with a second toe equal in length to that of the great toe. Pain, however, did not appear to be a significant factor in the dancers' ability to function, so the ideal second toe length could not be proven by this study.[33]

Hallux valgus can begin in adolescence and is much more common in women in our society, as a result of ill-fitting shoes. However, dancers may acquire a bunion perhaps as a result of increased loads on the medial collateral ligament of the hallux. Dancers spend a great deal of time in the demi pointe position and push off of the medial aspect of the great toe.[34] Teitz and associates[35] have stated that this type of axial pressure has not been shown to correlate with a hallux valgus deformity but the everted positioning may increase the possibility of the development of hallux rigidus. Baxter[36] does not believe dancers are more prone to hallux valgus, but if they have the tendency, the deformity may deteriorate more rapidly.

Two studies could be found on musculoskeletal injuries in theatrical dance. In a large survey of professional dancers published in 1978, the ankle was the third most common injury site and the foot the fourth. Injuries were not discussed by gender.[37] In a second article involving injuries in a dancing school during 1981–1982, 25% of the injuries involved the foot and ankle. Again, no gender specifications were made.[38]

Miscellaneous Foot and Ankle Problems

Anterior ankle impingement may result from repetitive axial loading sports. Gymnastics is a particular offender, with the frequency of maximal dorsiflexion in dismounts, for example.[1] Osteophyte formation may limit motion and cause pain. Arthroscopic removal and debridement may be necessary.

Posterior tibial tendinitis is more common in women in the general population, particularly those over age 40 years. It may be that it is related to increased femoral anteversion in women, which may result in a compensatory pronation of the foot. This increases hindfoot valgus and stresses the posterior tibial tendon. The tendon is stressed during the push-off phases of walking and running, so this problem may occur from sports such as basketball, soccer, and tennis. It is also seen in ballet.[39] There may be an association with an accessory navicular, as well. Treatment is generally conservative, and activity modifications may be necessary. Occasionally, the accessory navicular needs to be excised, or the posterior tibial tendon requires debridement or reconstruction.

Interdigital neuroma is 7 to 10 times more frequent in women than men. It is especially prevalent in runners and dancers. Interdigital neuroma may be associated with cavus feet and/or a tight Achilles tendon. The second and third interspaces are the most common, probably related to the small space between these metatarsal heads. Trauma to the nerve in the forefoot may be the main etiology, as well as tight-fitting shoes. Therefore, appropriately fitted and cushioned shoes plus metatarsal pads may be beneficial. Injections of cortisone may occasionally be needed. Surgical excision is done in intractable cases but is only 80% successful in the general population.[40]

Although these problems of the forefoot are in general more common among women, little is written about these issues in the female athlete. We can only speculate that their incidence continues to be higher in the female athlete.

Stress Fractures

Stress fractures are much more common in women because of a multifactorial etiology. Running probably causes the highest incidence of stress fractures, and women runners are 12 times more likely than men to have a stress fracture during their running career.[3] The distal tibia, lateral malleolus, navicular, metatarsals, os calcis, and sesamoids are frequently involved. Chapter 12 discusses stress fractures in the female athlete in detail.

Summary

Several studies have shown the high incidence of foot and ankle injuries in many sports for both men and women. Women have a different lower extremity anatomy than men and may be more likely to have a history of wearing poorly fitting shoes; also, some sports, such as ballet, have a higher percentage of female participants. Thus, some injuries and their incidence might be expected to be different in women.

Ankle sprains are probably the most common injury for both men and women across all sports. There is a suggestion that ankle sprains may be more frequent in women, particularly the grade I ankle sprain as discussed by Hosea (unpublished data). It is not yet known if or why this might be true. It may possibly relate to different strength ratios as discussed by Baumhauser and associates.[20]

Ballet, with a high percentage of female participants and the foot positioning en pointe, has the most literature on foot and ankle injuries. Posterior ankle impingement, the os trigonum syndrome, flexor hallucis longus tendinitis, the midfoot sprain, a spiral fracture of the fifth metatarsal, and the forefoot problems of hallux rigidus, hallux valgus, hammer toes, calluses, and neuroma are well described. In this particular population, these entities are all more common in women, because more participants are women.

Other problems such as posterior tibial tendinitis and forefoot conditions such as hallux valgus, neuromas, and metatarsalgia occur more often in women in the general population, but little is written on these conditions specifically in the female athlete. Certainly stress fractures, a frequent occurrence in the foot and ankle, are more common in women.

Entire books are written on foot and ankle injuries in the athlete, but very little is known or written about the female athlete, in particular. We do not know if certain injuries are different, occur with different frequencies, or have different manifestations in women. Anatomy is different between men and women so that the forces on the foot and ankle are applied differently, depending on the sport, and there are endocrine and physiologic differences all of which may lead to different injury results. We also do not know if certain anatomic alignment with more ligamentous laxity or more foot pronation, for example, either predisposes a woman to certain injuries or precludes her participation in sports at a highly competitive level. These questions are yet to be answered, and their solutions can hopefully help us better understand injury pattern and thus prevention.

References

1. Mitchell LA: Foot and ankle injuries in the female athlete, in Baxter DE (ed): *The Foot and Ankle in Sport.* St Louis, MO, Mosby-Year Book, 1995, pp 337–345.
2. Frey C: Shoes, in Teitz CC (ed): *The Female Athlete*. Rosemont, IL, American Academy of Orthopaedic Surgeons, 1997, pp 63–73.
3. Wiggins DL, Wiggins ME: The female athlete. *Clin Sports Med* 1997;16:593–612.
4. Garrick JG: The frequency of injury, mechanism of injury, and epidemiology of ankle sprains. *Am J Sports Med* 1977;5:241–242.
5. Garrick JG, Requa RK: Girls' sports injuries in high school athletics. *JAMA* 1978;239:2245–2248.
6. Garrick JG, Requa RK: The epidemiology of foot and ankle injuries in sports. *Clin Sports Med* 1988;7:29–36.
7. Wells CL: Athletic injuries, in Wells CL (ed): *Women, Sport and Performance: A Physiological Perspective.* Champaign, IL, Human Kinetics Publishers, Inc. 1985, pp 255–271.
8. Zelisko JA, Noble HB, Porter M: A comparison of men's and women's professional basketball injuries. *Am J Sports Med* 1982;10:297–299.
9. Wilmore JH: Inferiority of female athletes: Myth or reality. *J Sports Med* 1975;3:1–6.
10. Arendt EA: Orthopaedic issues for active and athletic women. *Clin Sports Med* 1994;13:483–503.
11. Gillette J: When and where women are injured in sports. *Phys Sports Med* 1975;2:12:61–63.
12. Haycock CE, Gillette JV: Susceptibility of women athletes to injury: Myth vs reality. *JAMA* 1976;236:163–165.
13. Whiteside PA: Men's and women's injuries in comparable sports. *Phys Sports Med* 1980;8:130–140.
14. Clarke KS, Buckley WE: Women's injuries in collegiate sports: A preliminary comparative overview of three seasons. *Am J Sports Med* 1980;8:187–191.
15. Ireland ML: Special concerns of the female athlete, in Fu FH, Stone DA (eds*):* *Sports Injuries: Mechanisms, Prevention, and Treatment*. Baltimore, MD, Williams & Wilkins, 1994, pp 153–187.
16. Ritter MA, Gioe TJ, Albohm M: Sport-related injuries in women. *J Am Coll Health Assoc* 1980;28:267–268.
17. Rose CP: Injuries in women's field hockey: A four-year study. *Phys Sports Med* 1981;9:97–100.
18. Shively RA, Grana WA, Ellis D: High school sports injuries. *Phys Sports Med* 1981;9:46–50.
19. DeHaven KE, Lintner DM: Athletic injuries: Comparison by age, sport, and gender. *Am J Sports Med* 1986;14:218–224.
20. Baumhauer JF, Alosa DM, Renström AF, Trevino S, Beynnon B: A prospective study of ankle injury risk factors. *Am J Sports Med* 1995;23:564–570.
21. Hamilton WG: Foot and ankle injuries in dancers. *Clin Sports Med* 1988;7:143–173.
22. Teitz CC: Sports medicine concerns in dance and gymnastics. *Clin Sports Med* 1983;2:571–593.
23. Hamilton WG: Sprained ankles in ballet dancers. *Foot Ankle Int* 1982;3:99–102.
24. Marshall P, Hamilton WG: Cuboid subluxation in ballet dancers. *Am J Sports Med* 1992;20:169–175.

25. Hamilton WG, Geppert MJ, Thompson FM: Pain in the posterior aspect of the ankle in dancers: Differential diagnosis and operative treatment. *J Bone Joint Surg* 1996;78A:1491–1500.
26. Hamilton WG: Stenosing tenosynovitis of the flexor hallucis longus tendon and posterior impingement upon the os trigonum in ballet dancers. *Foot Ankle Int* 1982;3:74–80.
27. Sammarco GJ, Miller EH: Partial rupture of the flexor hallucis longus tendon in classical ballet dancers: Two case reports. *J Bone Joint Surg* 1979;61A:149–150.
28. Hamilton WG: Tendonitis about the ankle joint in classical ballet dancers. *Am J Sports Med* 1977;5:84–88.
29. O'Malley MJ, Hamilton WG, Munyak J: Fractures of the distal shaft of the fifth metatarsal: "Dancer's fracture." *Am J Sports Med* 1996;24:240–243.
30. Kadel NJ, Teitz CC, Kronmal RA: Stress fractures in ballet dancers. *Am J Sports Med* 1992;20:445–449.
31. Micheli LJ, Sohn RS, Solomon R: Stress fractures of the second metatarsal involving Lisfranc's joint in ballet dancers: A new overuse injury of the foot. *J Bone Joint Surg* 1985;67A:1372–1375.
32. O'Malley MJ, Hamilton WG, Munyak J, DeFranco MJ: Stress fractures at the base of the second metatarsal in ballet dancers. *Foot Ankle Int* 1996;17:89–94.
33. Ogilvie-Harris DJ, Carr MM, Fleming PJ: The foot in ballet dancers: The importance of second toe length. *Foot Ankle Int* 1995;16:144–147.
34. Sammarco GJ, Miller EH: Forefoot conditions in dancers: Part I. *Foot Ankle Int* 1982;3:85–92.
35. Teitz CC, Harrington RM, Wiley H: Pressures on the foot in pointe shoes. *Foot Ankle Int* 1985;5:216–221.
36. Baxter DE: Bunion deformity in elite athletes, in Baxter DE (ed): *The Foot and Ankle in Sport*. St Louis, MO, Mosby-Year Book, 1995, pp 259–264.
37. Rovere GD, Webb LX, Gristina AG, Vogel JM: Musculoskeletal injuries in theatrical dance students. *Am J Sports Med* 1983;11:195–198.
38. Washington EL: Musculoskeletal injuries in theatrical dancers: Site, frequency, and severity. *Am J Sports Med* 1978;6:75–98.
39. Arendt EA, Teitz CC: The lower extremities, in Teitz CC (ed): *The Female Athlete*. Rosemont, IL, American Academy of Orthopaedic Surgeons, 1997, pp 45–62.
40. Mann RA, Reynolds JC: Interdigital neuroma: A critical clinical analysis. *Foot Ankle Int* 1983;3:238–243.

Chapter 9

The Female Athlete's Knee: Meniscus, Articular Cartilage, and Osteoarthritis

Bert R. Mandelbaum, MD
Harold Roos, MD, PhD
Stefan Lohmander, MD, PhD

Introduction

The 20th Century can be equated with tremendous evolution in medicine and science. The role of the woman in relation to exercise and sports has been a recent challenge, instigated by Title IX legislation in 1972. Since that time, girls and women have been training and competing in exercise and sports at levels previously unknown. As a consequence the medical field is challenged and confronted with developing new concepts, policies, and protocols for this population to optimize performance as well as treat and prevent injuries. The female athlete's knee joint response over time to sports and exercise differs from that of her male counterpart. Although the basic anatomy and physiology of articular cartilage, meniscal cartilage, and ligaments are similar in men and women, there are differences. The woman's knee has basic structural and biochemical variances and has a significantly greater incidence and severity of acute and chronic injury, chronic overuse syndromes, and osteoarthritis. Schnitzer and Runyan,[1] in an overview of orthopaedic injuries and disease in women, found that more women presently visit orthopaedic surgeons than do men. In addition, they point to changing trends in musculoskeletal disorders in women and the importance of developing strategies for intervention and prevention. The purpose of this chapter is to define structural and physiologic, epidemiologic injury differences and predilections, with the major objective to develop a strategy of prevention and preservation of the functioning knee joint over time.

Gender Differences in Incidence of Injury

The menstrual cycle and its relation to soccer injuries was prospectively studied by Möller-Nielsen and Hammar.2 The study showed that female soccer players were more susceptible to traumatic injuries during the premenstrual and menstrual period compared with the rest of the menstrual cycle ($p < 0.05$), especially among players with premenstrual symptoms such as irritability, swelling and discomfort in the breasts, and swelling and congestion in the abdomen. It was also found that women using contraceptive pills had a lower rate of traumatic injuries ($p < 0.05$) compared with women who were not on the pill. The results can be explained by the fact that oral contraceptives ameliorate some symptoms of the premenstrual and menstrual period that might also affect coordination and, hence, the risk of injury.2

Female soccer players show a higher rate of injuries than do males.[3–5] Sullivan and associates[5] found that young girls had a higher incidence of injury. Lindenfeld and associates[4] demonstrated that female players sustained a significantly higher rate of knee ligament injuries than did male players in a study of indoor soccer. The reason for the difference remains unclear, but some authors have discussed a relative lack of physical fitness in female athletes, compared to male athletes, as one possible cause. This may to some extent be caused by factors such as training background. The differences may also be a result of intensity during training sessions and/or the amount and quality of training. The training time for female elite players was approximately half of that of male elite players. Training habits have changed rapidly since the late 1980s, so this important question requires further investigation. Although there are similarities in the incidence and the type of injuries, there are also significant differences in comparison to male soccer players, especially regarding the knee.

Knee Injuries

Anterior Cruciate Ligament Tears: Epidemiology and Mechanisms

The epidemiology of knee injuries in soccer is well documented because the rate is between 17% and 23% in multiple studies.[3,6] The youth injury incidence is between 11.7% and 19%. In one National Collegiate Athletic Association study on knee injury, Arendt and Dick[3] in 1995 found a rate of 1.6 per 1,000 exposures in women as compared with 1.3 in age-matched men. In addition, the rate of anterior cruciate ligament (ACL) tears per 1,000 exposures in female soccer players is 0.31 as compared with 0.13 in male players. In fact, when all studies are analyzed simultaneously, the incidence of ACL injuries in women is two to six times greater than in men. The questions, therefore, are as follows: (1) How and why do these injuries occur? (2) What are the pathologic mechanisms? and (3) Can these injuries be prevented through education, training, skill development, or rule changes?

Noyes and associates[7] in 1983 indicated that 78% of ACL injuries occurred with a noncontact mechanism. Arendt and Dick[3] found that noncontact mechanisms were significantly greater than contact in the female soccer athlete ($p < 0.01$) but equal to contact mechanisms in the male athlete. The contact mechanisms, as demonstrated by Ekstrand and Gillquist[8] in 1983, include charge or block tackling and foul play, especially with tackles from behind. Boden and associates[9] further identified the mechanism of injury by evaluating 90 athletes with ACL tears and determined that 72% were noncontact with deceleration occurring at an average knee flexion of

23°. The exact mechanisms include deceleration in 53%, landing in 37%, hyperextension in 3%, and other in 7%. Shoemaker and associates[10] found that the anterior tibial force was maximized at 25° of flexion, internal torque, and a varus moment.

The risk factors for injury to the ACL are divided into intrinsic and extrinsic factors.[3] As an intrinsic factor, the quadriceps is the major antagonist of the ACL, and the hamstring is an agonist. During gait and heel strike, the quadriceps becomes activated, creating an eccentric contraction that limits flexion and facilitates extension, resulting in greater forces on the ACL.[11,12] Huston and Wotjys[13] demonstrated that, overall, female athletes have less quadriceps and hamstring isokinetic strength. In addition, in the female athlete the quadriceps is recruited first, which is in contradistinction to the male athlete in whom the hamstring is recruited first. Furthermore, the maximal hamstring torque and recruitment of that torque requires more time in female athletes than in male athletes.

The level of aerobic and anaerobic fitness is a possible risk factor and etiology for ACL injury. Garrick and Requa[14] believed that women, in general, are more novice at their respective sports. Huston and Wotjys[13] demonstrated that female athletes were significantly weaker. Limb alignment is another intrinsic factor that may be related to an ACL injury. Gray and associates[15] demonstrated that there is no correlation between Q-angle, femorotibial alignment, and ACL injury. In contradistinction, Ireland and Wall[16] state that anatomic differences, including a wide pelvis, increased femoral anteversion, a greater Q-angle, and increased tibial vara, increase forces on the ACL and create a greater risk of injury.

The dimensions of the intercondylar notch as defined by a smaller notch width index correlate significantly with ACL tears. La Prade and Burnett[17] and Souryal and Freeman[18] concluded that there were no gender differences in this association. It is well known that individuals with ACL deficiency and pathologic laxity have a greater potential for further injury and degenerative osteoarthritis.[19] Identification of the athlete with anterolateral rotatory instability is essential to limit participation in high school, collegiate, and professional sports. Anterolateral rotatory instability is not to be confused with hyperlaxity, which commonly is present in the female athlete and has not been correlated with a greater risk. In contradistinction, Nicholas[20] believed that there was a strong correlation to injury. Most recently, it has been suggested that the increased elasticity may come from a direct estrogen relaxin response. Liu and associates[21] found that estrogen and progesterone inhibit fibroblast proliferation. The question that remains is what is the relationship between normal cyclical hormonal changes and the connective tissue's normal and pathologic response to adaptive changes of sports participation.

During sports participation, the athlete physically depends on neuromuscular balance, proprioception, reflexes, and reaction time for athletic performance. Proprioception is defined as having three components: (1) sensory modality of the joint, (2) kinesia or movement of the joint, and (3) position of the joint. Most recently, proprioception of the knee can be measured with a Fastex (Cybex Brand, by Lumex, Inc, Ronkonkoma, NY), which can measure balance, coordination, reaction time, and single stance stability. Perhaps proprioception is at the center of etiology for ACL injuries including (1) the normal athlete who is at risk for injuring the ACL; (2) the athlete whose ACL has been partially or completely torn; and (3) the athlete whose ligament has been torn and reconstructed, and who has been rehabilitated back to sports. The question in each of these athletic groups is how optimally to restore proprioceptive function. Barrack and associates[22] noted that with ACL injury there was a "partial deafferentiation" of the knee. This theory corroborated that a diminished hamstring reflex results in less stabilization; this was confirmed by two studies.[23,24] Clearly, the function of the ACL is to protect from anterolateral subluxation of the tibia with ground reactive forces. This is most optimally measured in physical examination using the Lachman, anterior drawer, and pivot shift tests. Videotape analysis has shown that athletes with ACL deficiency use a body position and kinetics that are significantly different in comparison to athletes who have intact ACLs. It is well accepted that ACL reconstruction followed by an accelerated and a comprehensive rehabilitation program will restore proprioceptive function.[25]

Extrinsic risk factors include the field, synthetic or otherwise, and grass turf in which there may be holes or uneven surfaces.[26] Some authors believe that even a hard dry surface may be a cause. Shoes have also been theorized to have a role in ACL tears. Lambson and associates[27] demonstrated that football cleats with an edge design have a significant correlation to ACL tears. Finally, it is well known that foul play rule violations have a greater potential for knee injury but result in contact-induced knee injury.[28,29]

Overall, a consensus has been reached in evaluating all extrinsic and intrinsic risk factors. Neuromuscular control deficits seem to be the major factor that causes the ACL injury. The explosion of female soccer participants has resulted in a greater number of knee injuries, specifically ACL injuries.[3] However, the exact mechanism of injury remains obscure. Both intrinsic and extrinsic variables may have a multifactorial relationship in causation that includes notch width dimensions, a muscle imbalance, neuromuscular loss of proprioception and, perhaps, a collagen catabolism resulting in a "stress" fracture of the ACL. Because all these factors work in concert, any one can be an important variable at one time or another. It is imperative to design a preventive strategy program that identifies risk factors by evaluating epidemiologic patterns of incidence and prevalence. Once a program is developed, it can be communicated to athletes, parents, coaches, athletic trainers, and physicians.

Meniscus Injuries

In the athlete with an ACL injury, there is a 60% to 75% incidence of associated meniscus tears. The role of the meniscus in normal function is to distribute load and provide stability for knee kinematics. Roos and associates[30] report the incidence of meniscus tears in Sweden is 6 per 10,000 inhabitants. Young athletes tear the menisci traumatically, and in middle age, degenerative tears are much more common. Athletes in general have a higher incidence of meniscus tears. Of former soccer players, 14% had arthroscopic surgery for meniscus tears versus only 2% of a control group.[30]

Articular and Osteochondral Lesions

The incidence of articular cartilage injuries in the general population remains obscure. Curl and associates[31] evaluated 35,000 arthroscopic procedures and found the incidence of articular cartilage defects to be 2%. In the ACL-injured patient, there appears to be a close relationship between ligament injury and articular cartilage degeneration, or chondropenia. In addition, ACL injuries have been found to cause a consistent rapid elevation of the metalloproteinase enzyme stromelysin and other cytokines that cleave articular cartilage.[32,33] Subchondral bone bruises, most commonly in the lateral compartment, are present in 80% of the ACL injuries evaluated with magnetic resonance imaging (MRI).[34,35] This injury combination is more common in soccer and basketball and less common in skiing in which the mechanism is more distraction without axial compression. These studies, therefore, illuminate the biochemical and mechanical complexities with respect to the etiology and the long-term natural history of these entities with respect to articular cartilage injury and potential degeneration. This is most evident in a 9-year data registry of an ACL-injured population, of whom 1.9% have an incidence of articular cartilage defects with acute ACL injury but a 19% incidence over the 9-year period (Johnson RJ, personal communication, unreferenced database). These and other studies suggest that acute ACL injury with disruption of the osteochondral "functional unit" and an unstable ligamentous environment unleashes a destructive biochemical process that may result in injury and a progressive deterioration of articular cartilage.[34,35]

In summary, the female athlete, by virtue of a greater incidence of knee and ACL injuries, undergoes a greater mechanical and biochemical injury to the menisci and the functional articular and load-bearing unit.

Contemporary Management of Knee Injuries

The goals of the sports medicine orthopaedic surgeon are injury care, injury prevention, and performance maximization. In the situation of an ACL injury and associated internal derangements, the major goals will be to restore stability and performance and minimize the probability of joint degeneration.

To accomplish these goals, it is imperative to make an efficient diagnosis leading to an effective treatment. The method used to arrive at a diagnosis includes obtaining a history, physical examination, and radiographic evaluation. Radiographs and MRI examinations determine the severity and the consequent injury to articular cartilage, bone, ligament, and menisci. Using the arthroscope as an interventive tool, the orthopaedic surgeon can refine the characterization of the injury and effectively treat the process systematically.

Meniscus Injuries

Meniscus injuries are among the most common knee injuries. The meniscus has many important functions, including load transmission, lubrication, shock absorption, and passive stabilization. The medial meniscus is most commonly injured in the stable and chronic ACL-deficient knee. The lateral meniscus is most commonly injured with an acute ACL tear. The primary function of the meniscus is to distribute loads transmitted across the knee joint. Early in the 1900s, the meniscus was thought of as an expendable structure, and complete removal of the meniscus was common. In 1948, Fairbank[36] suggested that the meniscus had an important load-bearing function when he showed loss of articular cartilage, flattening of the femoral condyles, and osteophyte formation in patients who had undergone total meniscectomy. The effects of partial meniscectomy demonstrate increasing contact stresses with removing larger portions of the meniscus. In one study, after removing the inner one third of the meniscus, the contact area was decreased by 10%, and the contact stresses increased by 65%.[37] The load-sharing property of the meniscus is so crucial that orthopaedic surgeons must compromise between removing the torn cartilage and preserving as much cartilage as possible. In addition to its load-sharing properties, the meniscus also provides significant stability to the knee, especially in an ACL-deficient knee.

Diagnostic studies should include MRI and standard knee radiographs to exclude fractures. In a large study examining 1,014 patients, the accuracy of MRI ranged from 64% to 95% in detecting medial meniscus lesions, from 83% to 94% for lateral meniscus lesions, and from 78% to 97% for an ACL injury.[38] Treatment of meniscus tears includes a wide spectrum of options including conservative treatment, partial meniscectomy, or meniscus repair. Several factors need to be considered when deciding on treatment, including patient's age, activity level, chronicity of symptoms, the type of meniscus tear, and associated ligamentous pathology. The overriding rule based on the biochemical and biomechanical principles is restoration and preservation at all times. Since the advent of arthroscopy, many studies have shown that arthroscopic partial meniscectomy results in decreased morbidity and allows earlier return to function than previous open menisectomy. Excellent or good short-term results can be expected in 80% to 95% of the patients. In a long-term study, 82% of the patients had satisfactory knee function at a minimum 5-year follow-up after partial meniscectomy.[39] Although functional results did not correlate with radiographic findings, significant radiographic changes can occur with partial meniscectomy. The most favorable results following partial meniscectomy were seen in the patients younger than 40 years of age, in a single fragment tear (bucket-handle, flap, or radial tears), and with minimal arthritic changes present. The long-term outcome of meniscus tears in young people increases the probability of osteoarthritis.

The understanding of the load-sharing properties and the importance of preserving the meniscus has led to the development of a spectrum of techniques for meniscus repair. Excellent results have been reported in selected tears regardless of technique used. A ligamentously stable knee is important for successful meniscus repair and healing. Meniscus repairs are successful up to

90% to 100% when associated with concomitant ACL reconstruction. In contrast, a success rate of 30% to 70% has been reported in unstable knees. The long-term effect of meniscus repair on decreasing degenerative changes of the knee is unknown. Human meniscus allograft transplantation is currently limited to certain study groups and investigational protocols but is performed with the rationale to improve load sharing. Long-term follow-up is limited, and meniscus transplantation therefore requires further investigation to assess its effectiveness in restoring normal meniscus function and preventing arthritis.

ACL Reconstruction and Rehabilitation

In recent years, accelerated rehabilitation following arthroscopic ACL reconstruction using patellar and quadriceps tendon or hamstrings has been the focus of many investigators. Application of these techniques when performed isometrically and with stable fixation allows optimal restoration of joint stability and performance. Noyes and associates,[40] Shelbourne and associates,[41] and Mandelbaum (Mandelbaum BR, unpublished data, 1998) have been instrumental in the advancement of postoperative rehabilitation protocols following ACL reconstruction. These programs now advocate early weight bearing, immediate active "safety zone" exercise, and sport-specific progressions, leading to return to sports. Outcome studies demonstrate that with these protocols excellent functional results are achieved without compromise of graft integity. There appear to be no gender differences in the functional outcome after ACL reconstruction in athletes, although there are no available studies.

Management of Articular Cartilage Defects

The contemporary orthopaedic surgeon must understand the complexities of articular cartilage biochemistry, biomechanics, physiology, and the natural course of the lesion. This comprehensive interpretation then can be applied to the specific lesion and the particular dilemmas of the problem. In addition, several important principles are essential: (1) When the knee is injured there is a release of intra-articular degradative enzymes such as stromelysin[32] and other cytokines[33] that may contribute to degradation rather than reparation. (2) Partial-thickness lesions do not heal; they remain static because there are no biologic mechanisms to create a reparative cascade. (3) Full-thickness lesions heal with fibrous type I fibrocartilage that lacks organization and composition to provide wear characteristics and integrity for the long term. (4) Defects < 2 cm^2 that are well contained or shouldered may be asymptomatic and nondegenerative for a long unspecified amount of time, thus having the best potential prognosis. (5) Defects > 2 cm^2 that are poorly contained or shouldered have a lower probability of regenerative success, which translates into lower levels of function with increased pain and swelling. (6) Malalignments and ligament instabilities must be identified and treated simultaneously or in sequence with the articular procedure of choice. (7) Once a comprehensive history, physical examination, and all survey and secondary diagnostic tests are completed, the clinician has completed the necessary evaluation that will lead to a treatment plan.

Once the efficacy and safety objectives are understood it is appropriate to develop a practical algorithm that divides protocols into femoral condyle groups < 2 cm^2 and > 2 cm^2, patellar, and tibial defects. Defects in the femoral condyle < 2 cm^2 group have the best potential prognosis. If the defect is contained, it is appropriate to consider the primary mesenchymal stimulation options of drilling, debridement, or the pick procedure with the expectation of being successful in the short term of 3 to 5 years without progression to degenerative joint disease.[42] Hubbard[43] has stated that in the low-demand patient the small focal and contained defect has a probability of success of 50% for up to 5 years. In this group, clinical failure may be treated with autologous chondrocyte implantation (ACI) as a secondary option, a procedure with a success rate of 90% for return to sports and activities of daily life. Mosaicplasty can be offered as another option. It will convert a chondral defect to a osteochondral repair at a low cost with a minimally invasive arthroscopic option.[44]

For femoral condyle defects > 2 cm^2, the probability of degenerative joint disease is higher because the repaired fibrocartilage tissue will be unable to contain or shoulder the defect. In the individual with low athletic demands, the mesenchymal stimulation procedures are acceptable as a primary approach, and if this fails, ACI remains the secondary option. In the patient with higher athletic demands, ACI can be considered as the primary approach in view of its > 85% success rate. Failure of ACI can be revised with ACI secondarily or with an osteochondral allograft.

In the femoral osteochondritis group, initial approaches should include bioabsorbable fixation of the fragment if possible.[34] If the fragment cannot be repaired and is lost, primary techniques in lesions < 2 cm^2 include drilling or the microfracture procedure or mosaicplasty. If the lesion is > 2 cm^2 or quite deep and cystic, ACI should be considered as a primary technique, and if the lesion is particularly deep it may require staging with initial bone graft, followed by ACI 4 to 12 months later.

The Increased Risk of Osteoarthritis

Gender Differences

There are some gender differences in anatomy, biomechanics, and physiology of the knee joint. The woman's knee joint is smaller and is aligned differently than in men. The pelvis is wider, there is a greater degree of femoral anteversion, the Q-angle is greater, and there is more tibial vara in women. The resultant differential in anatomic alignment creates a differential response to similar stresses, loads, and positions. The consequence of these differences is a greater incidence of patellofemoral and other disorders yet to be characterized by this association.

The principal function of articular cartilage as a viscoelastic material is variable load bearing through a range of motion and functional activities. This function depends on the specific composition and organization of this composite structure. Functional stress reduction on subchondral bone and minimization of friction is essential. Normal articular cartilage is composed of matrix, chondrocytes, and water that is contiguous with and overlies the subchondral bone. The matrix principally is made up of type II collagen fibers, but type V, VI, IX, X, and XI collagens are present in smaller amounts. Sulfated proteoglycans are linked to hyaluronate. It is this lattice framework in conjunction with the collagen fibrils that is responsible for its structural properties, including its tensile strength and resiliency. It is the resilience of the functional load-bearing unit that is essential in the normal athlete.[42]

There are few preliminary animal and clinical studies that address gender differences in joint anatomy and physiology. Larbre and associates[45] found lower levels of proteoglycan and collagen and a higher glycosaminoglycan loss in female rats. Moreover, in vitro assays in cartilage from female rats had higher rates of proteoglycan synthesis. In addition, female cartilage was more sensitive to interleukin-1 inhibition of proteoglycan synthesis.

Cova and associates[46] and Cicuttini and associates[47] independently demonstrated with MRI that men had a significantly greater cartilage thickness and volume than age-matched women at all measurement sites. In addition, there was an inverse relationship between age and cartilage thickness. Manicourt and associates[48] found that serum levels of stromelysin increased with age and were two times higher in men than in women. Levels of stromelysin were also elevated in patients with osteoarthritis. These results demonstrate that there are gender differences in cartilage anatomy, biochemistry, metabolism, and susceptibility to inflammatory mediators. These differences may have important consequences for sports-related articular injury and the rationale for potentially creative therapies and strategies.

Biochemical Response to Knee Injury and the Pathogenesis of Osteoarthritis

Lohmander and associates[33] observed that the synovial fluid of ACL- and/or meniscus-injured patients had greater concentrations of aggrecan fragments, which are markers of increased matrix turnover. In addition, cartilage oligomeric matrix protein, C-propeptide of type II collagen, bone sialoprotein, and matrix metalloproteinases 1 and 3 (stromelysin and tissue inhibitor of metalloproteinase 1) were elevated. These also provide direct evidence of cartilage catabolism and turnover. It appears that these biochemical responses are the initial steps in articular cartilage injury, which lead to the progressive and natural course leading to chondropenia (the loss of articular cartilage) and the ultimate consequence of osteoarthritis. There are several issues about the female athlete that need to be further elucidated in this progression and mechanism. There is a greater spectrum of knee injuries that occur at a younger age in the female athlete. This gender difference creates a larger population with significant injury and the resultant catabolic response to articular cartilage. Studies suggest that acute ACL injury with disruption of the osteochondral "functional unit" and an unstable ligamentous environment unleashes a destructive biochemical process that may result in a progressive deterioration of articular cartilage.[32,33]

To date there are no controlled studies that reveal gender differences in osteoarthritis progression with nonsurgical or surgical intervention. Andersson and associates[49] found that after ACL reconstruction there is a decreased risk of meniscus injury. Moreover, most patients return to their sports at the highest level. Daniel and associates,[50] in a prospective uncontrolled outcome study, found that ACL-injured and reconstructed patients had a higher incidence of radiographic osteoarthritis. The limitation of this study is that patients with the more severe injuries were selected for surgery, and thus it was skewed. In addition, reconstructed athletes returned to their previous levels of sports without modification of the duration, intensity, and frequency of training or competition.[50] Several studies show that after meniscal surgery including partial or total meniscectomy, there is a significant risk of osteoarthritis.[51,52] Meniscus preservation and repair have theoretical benefits. Sommerlath[53] found that meniscus repair has a decreased potential for osteoarthritis. Gillquist and Messner[54] found that there is difficulty in conducting randomized studies because most meniscus tears have a preexisting degenerative component. Roos and associates[52] demonstrated a 50% incidence of radiographic degenerative changes 10 to 15 years after ACL tear and reconstruction. Other variables, such as changed gait pattern and/or loss of proprioception or motor control, may contribute to the development of osteoarthritis. There is no conclusive evidence that meniscus or ACL surgery decreases the potential for osteoarthritis. Therefore, knee injury involving the ACL or meniscus in combination with articular and subchondral injury (with or without surgical intervention) is associated with chondropenia with progression to osteoarthritis. As a consequence, these findings highlight the prevention of knee injury as the most important and effective intervention.

Dose-Response Issues

A working hypothesis and "dose-response model" of mechanisms for joint adaptation and maladaptation have been developed to practically apply and evaluate these concepts. On the Y-axis is the dose of activity, which includes the duration, intensity, and frequency. On the X-axis the articular cartilage response of adaptation to activity is featured. Conceptually, there is a positive linear relationship until a threshold is reached for the normal male and female athletes. At this threshold, every unit increase in dose results in a negative response or "injury zone" chondropenia and perhaps osteoarthritis in the long term. In animal study corellates, Kiviranta and associates[55,56] found that moderate running of 4 km/day increased stiffness and matrix content of proteoglycan in normal female beagle dogs, whereas 20 km/day decreased proteoglycan content. Arokoski and associates[57] found that long-term running in the dog model demonstrated a loss of proteoglycan and softening of articular cartilage as the adaptive response. In a human study, Felson and associates[58] demonstrated that women whose occupations involve increased loading with bending and lifting, such as firefighting, coal mining, labor, farming, and construction work, have a greater risk of osteoarthritis of the knee. In addition, in this model, the normal female athlete is placed lower on the dose curve to account for her qualitative focus on less impact and more proprioception, pliometrics, and other preventive strategies. Therefore, in the first group of high-demand participation by occupation and sport, any increase in activity and loading beyond this threshold may result in an overuse response and the negative adaptive consequences of injury to articular cartilage, chondropenia, and an increased risk of osteoarthritis.

The second population includes athletes involved in sports such as soccer and basketball who have sustained a significant ACL, meniscus, and articular injury. In this group, by virtue of these injuries occurring at a younger age, there is a potentially accelerated pathogenesis and progression toward osteoarthritis. It is this group that returns to sports after injury, surgery, and rehabilitation that may be at greatest risk. The pathogenesis of osteoarthritis is a multivariant phenomenon, such that there are negative and positive modulators. Important negative risk factors and modulators of this maladaptive response include sports participation, chronic ligamentous instability, patellofemoral or varus/valgus malalignment, hormonal and estrogen defiencies, and obesity.

Roos and associates[52] have stated that the longer the time after an ACL tear, the higher the risk of radiologic signs of osteoarthritis. Therefore, an ACL injury will put the 20- to 40-year-old athlete at greatest risk for early osteoarthritis. Roos and associates[59] also found that soccer as a independent variable places the athlete at risk for osteoarthritis. After selecting out knee-injured athletes, the occurrence of osteoarthritis was 11% in former players versus 4% in nonsoccer players who served as controls. Among elite soccer players, risk of osteoarthritis is 2.3 to 3.7 times greater in the hip and 4.4 to 5.2 times greater in the knee. In former elite soccer players (mean age 63 years) the prevalence of osteoarthritis was 15% versus 4% for the control population. This was not the case in players at lower levels of competition.[59] In former female soccer players (13 years of participation), mean age 43 years, osteoarthritis of the hip was comparable, but osteoarthritis of the knee was greater (17% versus 0% in controls). In soccer players there is an increased prevalence of knee and hip osteoarthritis.[60,61] Spector and associates[62] corroborated in female soccer and tennis players an increased prevalence of knee osteoarthritis and lower hip osteoarthritis in comparison to male players. In addition they found a greater incidence of patellofemoral arthritis in runners.

Kujala and associates[63] noted a prevalence of 29% of osteoarthritis in soccer and weightlifting and none in shooters and runners. In general, long-distance running has not been correlated with increased risk of or with acceleration of the progression of already present osteoarthritis.[63,64] Konradsen and associates[65] found that that there may be a greater incidence of hip osteoarthritis when comparing runners to bobsled controls. Therefore, athletes, by virtue of higher injury rates in conjunction with years of participation in sports, undergo a chondropenic evolution that results in a higher incidence of osteoarthritis.

In comparison, the female athlete has a higher rate of osteoarthritis of the knee and the male athlete of the hip. Women who have estrogen deficiencies suffer direct consequences on cartilage thickness, resulting in chondropenia with a greater potential for osteoarthritis. Turner and associates[66] evaluated ovariectomized sheep and found that estrogen deficiency was responsible for a decreased cartilage thickness and intrinsic material properties that could be ameliorated by replacement. Interestingly, women with osteoarthritis of the knee have a greater bone mineral density of the hip and lumbar sacral spine than those without arthritis. Dennison and associates,[67] studying women scheduled for hip replacement, found a significantly increased risk of osteoarthritis after oophorectomy. This risk could be decreased by 40% after hormone replacement therapy. Therefore, estrogen has direct effects on cartilage as deficiencies are correlated with a chondropenia and osteoarthritis that can be ameliorated with estrogen replacement strategies.

Furthermore, along with the aging process, the consequent loss of muscle (sarcopenia) and bone mass (osteopenia) and the escalation of body fat percent and obesity are directly correlated with cartilage loss (chondropenia) and osteoarthritis as an independent variable. Manninen and associates[68] evaluated Finnish farmers over a 10-year period and found that obesity in women is a strong risk factor for disabling knee osteoarthritis. Hart and associates[69] also demonstrated that obesity and aging are risk factors for development of osteoarthritis. Moreover, Cerhan and associates,[70] using Cox regression analysis, found a correlation between increased numbers of joints affected with osteoarthritis and decreased survival. Therefore, the deleterious consequences of severe polyarticular arthritis are both increased morbidity and mortality. The socioeconomic impact and consequences may be significant, considering the increasing longevity of the US population.

Conclusion

As knowledge grows regarding the female athlete's knee, several conclusions can be reached: (1) The female knee joint is anatomically, biomechanically, and biochemically different from the knee joint of the male and responds differently to inflammatory mediators. (2) Moderate to high intensity exercise may cause biochemical, material property, and morphology changes to the articular cartilage and load-bearing unit. (3) There are gender differences with respect to early age, incidence, and prevalence of knee, ACL, meniscal, and articular injury. The major etiologic and risk factor appears to be an instantaneous loss of compensatory neuromuscular control in the female athlete. (4) The injured knee, especially when injured early in life, is at greater risk of osteoarthritis whether treated with surgery or not. (5) There are populations at risk for osteoarthritis, such as soccer players, ballet dancers, and manual workers. There is also a dose-response relationship with respect to duration (years of participation and competition), intensity (elite>>>amateur), and frequency of sports. (6) A woman is at higher risk for osteoarthritis of the knee, especially if she is estrogen deficient and obese.

Prevention Strategies

Ekstrand and associates[71] have demonstrated that implementation of a multilevel approach to soccer in the male athlete can diminish injuries by 75%. The elements of a prevention program for the female athlete should consist of:

(1) correction of training problems; in the female athlete it is essential to recognize that more is not better and that quality should be considered over quantity at all times; (2) provision of optimum equipment including shin guards and shoes, and maintenance of good quality fields; (3) prophylactic ankle taping or bracing with proprioceptive ankle taping; (4) controlled rehabilitation and identification of those athletes who have not adequately healed or been rehabilitated; (5) exclusion of players with marked knee ligament instability and optimal conditioning and rehabilitation for those athletes who have normal knees and those whose knees have been reconstructed; (6) education about the importance of disciplined play and the significance of the increased risk of injury from foul play (a Fédération Internationale de Football Association study [Dvorak and associates, unpublished data] demonstrates that fair play is an important factor in limiting injuries in male elite soccer players); (7) supervision of games by doctor(s) and athletic trainer(s); (8) identification and treatment of athletes with eating disorders, with supplementation of calcium, iron, and calories and other components when appropriate; (9) identification and treatment of menstrual abnormalities; and (10) establishment of a systematic preseason and regular season motor control enhancement and proprioceptive training program to minimize the probability of knee injury.[72–75]

Overall, there are complex factors that differentiate the female athlete from her male counterpart with respect to performance and injury. These facts in conjunction with the rapid expansion of girls' and women's participation in soccer in the United States and worldwide necessitate a heightened level of awareness of these issues. Physiologically, the female athlete performs with less power, strength, and agility and levels of aerobic capacity. Three populations must be considered with respect to strategies for prevention: (1) the uninjured and seemingly normal athlete; (2) the knee-injured athlete; and (3) the individual with knee osteoarthritis.

References

1. Schnitzer PG, Runyan CW: Injuries to women in the United States: An overview. *Womens Health* 1995;23:9–27.
2. Möller-Nielsen J, Hammar M: Women's soccer injuries in relation to the menstrual cycle and oral contraceptive use. *Med Sci Sports Exerc* 1989;21:126–129.
3. Arendt E, Dick R: Knee injury patterns among men and women in collegiate basketball and soccer: NCAA data and review of literature. *Am J Sports Med* 1995;23:694–701.
4. Lindenfeld TN, Schmitt DJ, Hendy MP, Mangine RE, Noyes FR: Incidence of injury in indoor soccer. *Am J Sports Med* 1994;22:364–371.
5. Sullivan JA, Gross RH, Grana WA, Garcia-Moral CA: Evaluation of injuries in youth soccer. *Am J Sports Med* 1980;8:325–327.
6. Engström B, Johansson C, Törnkvist H: Soccer injuries among elite female players. *Am J Sports Med* 1991;19:372–375.
7. Noyes FR, Mooar PA, Matthews DS, Butler DL: The symptomatic anterior cruciate-deficient knee: Part I: The long-term functional disability in athletically active individuals. *J Bone Joint Surg* 1983;65A:154–162.

8. Ekstrand J, Gillquist J: Soccer injuries and their mechanisms: A prospective study. *Med Sci Sports Exerc* 1983;15:267–270.
9. Boden B, Dean G, Feagin J, Garrett WE Jr: Mechanisms of anterior cruciate ligament injury. *Orthopedics* 2000;23:573–578.
10. Shoemaker SC, Adams D, Daniel DM, Woo SL: Quadriceps/anterior cruciate graft interaction: An in vitro study of joint kinematics and anterior cruciate ligament graft tension. *Clin Orthop* 1993;294:379–390.
11. Arms SW, Pope MH, Johnson RJ, Fischer RA, Arvidsson I, Eriksson E: The biomechanics of anterior cruciate ligament rehabilitation and reconstruction. *Am J Sports Med* 1984;12:8–18.
12. Berchuck M, Andriacchi TP, Bach BR, Reider B: Gait adaptations by patients who have a deficient anterior cruciate ligament. *J Bone Joint Surg* 1990;72A:871–877.
13. Huston LJ, Wojtys EM: Neuromuscular performance characteristics in elite female athletes. *Am J Sports Med* 1996;24:427–436.
14. Garrick JG, Requa RK: Football cleat design and its effect on anterior cruciate ligament injuries. *Am J Sports Med* 1996;24:705–706.
15. Gray J, Taunton JE, McDenzie DC, Clement DB, McConkey JP, Davidson RG: A survey of injuries to the ACL of the knee in female basketball players. *Int J sports Med* 1985;6:314–316.
16. Ireland ML, Wall C: Abstract: Epidemiology and comparison of knee injuries in elite male and female United States basketball athletes. *Med Sci Sports Exer* 1980;(suppl 22):S82.
17. La Prade RF, Burnett QM II: Femoral intercondylar notch stenosis and correlation to anterior cruciate ligament injuries: A prospective study. *Am J Sports Med* 1994;22:198–203.
18. Souryal TO, Freeman TR: Intercondylar notch size and anterior cruciate ligament injuries in athletes: A prospective study. *Am J Sports Med* 1993;21:535–539.
19. Sherman MF, Warren RF, Marshall JL, Savatsky GJ: A clinical and radiographical analysis of 127 anterior cruciate insufficient knees. *Clin Orthop* 1988;227:229–237.
20. Nicholas J: Mechanisms of injury, in Nicholas J, Herschman E (eds): *The Lower Extremity and Spine in Sports Medicine.* Philadelphia, PA, Mosby, 1995, p 3.
21. Liu SH, Al-Shaikh RA, Panossian V, Finerman GA, Lane JM: Estrogen affects the cellular metabolism of the anterior cruciate ligament: A potential explanation for female athletic injury. *Am J Sports Med* 1997;25:704–709.
22. Barrack RL, Skinner HB, Buckley SL: Proprioception in the anterior cruciate deficient knee. *Am J Sports Med* 1989;17:1–6.
23. Beard DJ, Kyberd PJ, O'Connor JJ, Fergusson CM, Dodd CA: Reflex hamstring contraction latency in anterior cruciate ligament deficiency. *J Orthop Res* 1994;12:219–228.
24. Solomonow M, Baratta R, Zhou BH, et al: The synergistic action of the anterior cruciate ligament and thigh muscles in maintaining joint stability. *Am J Sports Med* 1987;15:207–213.
25. Borsa PA, Lephart SM, Irrgang JJ, Safran MR, Fu FH: The effects of joint position and direction of joint motion on proprioceptive sensibility in anterior cruciate ligament-deficient athletes. *Am J Sports Med* 1997;25:336–340.
26. Ekstrand J, Nigg BM: Surface-related injuries in soccer. *Sports Med* 1989;8:52–62.
27. Lambson RB, Barnhill BS, Higgins RW: Football cleat design and its effect on anterior cruciate ligament injuries: A three-year prospective study. *Am J Sports Med* 1996;24:155–159.

28. Ekstrand J, Gillquist J: Soccer injuries and their mechanisms: A prospective study. *Med Sci Sports Exerc* 1983;15:267–270.

29. Ekstrand J, Gillquist J: The avoidability of soccer injuries. *Int J Sports Med* 1983;4:124–128.

30. Roos H, Lindberg H, Gärdsell P, Lohmander LS, Wingstrand H: The prevalence of gonarthrosis and its relation to meniscectomy in former soccer players. *Am J Sports Med* 1994;22:219–222.

31. Curl WW, Krome J, Gordon ES, Rushing J, Smith BP, Poehling GG: Cartilage injuries: A review of 31,516 arthroscopies. *Arthroscopy* 1997;13:456–460.

32. Cameron ML, Fu FH, Paessler HH, Schneider M, Evans CH: Synovial fluid cytokine concentrations as possible prognostic indicators in the ACL-deficient knee. *Knee Surg Sports Traumatol Arthrosc* 1994;2:38–44.

33. Lohmander LS, Roos H, Dahlberg L, Hoerrner LA, Lark MW: Temporal patterns of stromelysin, tissue inhibitor and proteoglycan fragments in synovial fluid after injury to knee cruciate ligament or meniscus. *J Orthop Res* 1994;12:21–28.

34. Mink JH, Deutsch A: Occult cartilage and bone injuries of the knee: Detection, classification, and assessment with MR imaging. *Radiology* 1989;170:823–829.

35. Rosen MA, Jackson DW, Berger PE: Occult lesions documented by magnetic resonance imaging associated with anterior cruciate ligament ruptures. *Arthroscopy* 1991;7:45–51.

36. Fairbank TJ: Knee joint changes after meniscectomy. *J Bone Joint Surg* 1948;30B:664–670.

37. Radin EL, de Lamotte F, Maquet P: Role of the menisci in the distribution of stress in the knee. *Clin Orthop* 1984;185:290–294.

38. Mink JH, Levy T, Crues JV: Tears of the anterior cruciate ligament and menisci of the knee: MR imaging evaluation. *Radiology* 1988;167;769–774.

39. Newman AP, Daniels AU, Burks RT: Principles and decision making in meniscal surgery. *Arthroscopy* 1993;9:33–51.

40. Noyes FR, Mangine RE, Barber S: Early knee motion after open and arthroscopic anterior cruciate ligament reconstruction. *Am J Sports Med* 1987;15:149–160.

41. Shelbourne KD, Klootwyk TE, Wilckens JH, De Carlo MS: Ligament stability two to six years after anterior cruciate ligament reconstruction with autogenous patellar tendon graft and participation in accelerated rehabilitation program. *Am J Sports Med* 1995;23:575–579.

42. Mandelbaum BR, Browne JE, Fu F, et al: Articular cartilage lesions of the knee. *Am J Sports Med* 1998;26:853–861.

43. Hubbard MJ: Articular debridement versus washout for degeneration of the medial femoral condyle: A five-year study. *J Bone Joint Surg* 1996;78B:217–219.

44. Bobic V: Arthroscopic osteochondral autograft in anterior cruciate ligament reconstruction: A preliminary clinical study. *Arthroscopy* 1996;3:262–264.

45. Larbre JP, Da Silva JA, Moore AR, James IT, Scott DL, Willoughby DA: Cartilage contribution to gender differences in joint disease progression: A study with rat articular cartilage. *Clin Exp Rheumatol* 1994;12:401–408.

46. Cova M, Freza F, Shariat-Razavi I, Ukmar M, Mucelli RS, Dalla Palma L: Magnetic resonance assessment of knee joint hyaline cartilage according to age, sex, and body weight. *Radiol Medi* 1996:92:171–179.

47. Cicuttini F, Forbes A, Morris K, Darling S, Bailey M, Stuckey S: Gender differences in knee cartilage volume as measured by magnetic resonance imaging. *Osteoarthritis and Cartilage* 1999;7:265–271.

48. Manicourt DH, Fujimoto N, Obata K, Thomar EJ: Serum levels of collagenase, stomelysis-1: Age- and sex-related differences in normal subjects and relationship

to the extent of the joint involvement and serum levels of antigenic keratan sulfate in patients with osteoarthritis. *Arthritis Rheum* 1994;37:1774–1783.

49. Andersson C, Odensten M, Good L, Gillquist J: Surgical or non-surgical treatment of acute rupture of the anterior cruciate ligament: A randomized study with long-term follow-up. *J Bone Joint Surg* 1989;71A:965–974.
50. Daniel DM, Stone ML, Dobson BE, Fithian DC, Rossman DJ, Kaufman KRl: Fate of the ACL injured patient: A prospective outcome study. *Am J Sports Med* 1996;22:632–644.
51. Hede A, Jensen DB, Blyme P, Sonne-Holm S: Epidemiology of meniscal lesions in the knee: 1,215 open operations in Copenhagen 1982-84. *Acta Orthop Scand* 1990;61:435–437.
52. Roos H, Adalberth T, Dahlberg L, Lohmander LS: Osteoarthritis of the knee after injury to the anterior cruciate ligament or meniscus: The influence of time and age. *Osteoarthritis Cartilage* 1995;3:261–267.
53. Sommerlath KG: Results of meniscal repair and partial meniscectomy in stable knees. *Int Orthop* 1991;15:347–350.
54. Gillquist J, Messner K: Long-term results of meniscal repair. *Sports Med Arthroscopic Rev* 1993;1:159–163.
55. Kiviranta I, Tammi M, Jurvelin J, Arokoski J, Saamanen AM, Helminen HJ: Articular cartilage thickness and glycosaminoglycan distribution in the canine knee joint after strenuous running exercise. *Clin Orthop* 1992;283:302–308.
56. Kiviranta I, Tammi M, Jurvelin J, Saamanen AM, Helminen HJ: Moderate running exercise augments glycosaminoglycans and thickness of articular cartilage in the knee joint of young beagle dogs. *J Orthop Res* 1988;6:188–195.
57. Arokoski J, Kiviranta I, Jurvelin J, Tammi M, Helminen HJ: Long-distance running causes site-dependent decrease of cartilage glycosaminoglycan content in the knee joints of beagle dogs. *Arthritis Rheum* 1993;36:1451–1459.
58. Felson DT, Hannan MT, Naimark A, Berkeley J, Gordon G, Wilson PW, et al: Occupational physical demands, knee bending, and knee osteoarthritis: Results from the Framingham study. *J Rheumatol* 1991;18:1587–1592.
59. Roos H, Ornell M, Gardsell P, Lohmander LS, Lindstrand A: Soccer after anterior cruciate ligament injury–an incompatible combination? A national survey of incidence and risk factors and a 7-year follow-up of 310 players. *Acta Orthop Scand* 1995;66:107–112.
60. Chantraine A: Knee joint in soccer players: Osteoarthritis and axis deviation. *Med Sci Sports Exerc* 1985;17:434–439.
61. Klünder K, Rud B, Hansen J: Osteoarthritis of the hip and knee joint in retired football players. *Acta Orthop Scand* 1980;51:925–927.
62. Spector TD, Harris PA, Hart DJ, et al: Risk of osteoarthritis associated with long term weight-bearing sports: A radiologic survey of the hips and knees in female ex-athletes and population controls. *Arthritis Rheum* 1996;39:988–995.
63. Kujala UM, Kettunen J, Paananen H, et al: Knee osteoarthritis in former runners, soccer players, weight lifters, and shooters. *Arthritis Rheum* 1995;38:539–546.
64. Kohatsu ND, Schurman DJ: Risk factors for the development of osteoarthrosis of the knee. *Clin Orthop* 1990;261:242–246.
65. Konradsen L, Berg Hansen E-M, Söndergaard L: Long distance running and osteoarthrosis. *Am J Sports Med* 1990;18:379–381.
66. Turner AS, Athanasiou KA, Zhu CF, Alvis MR, Bryant HU: Biochemical effects of estrogen on articular cartilage in ovariectomized sheep. *Osteoarthritis Cartilage* 1997;5:63–39.

67. Dennison EM, Arden NK, Kellingray S, Croft P, Coggon D, Cooper C: Hormone replacement therapy, other reproductive variables and symptomatic hip osteoarthritis in elderly white women: A case-control study. *Br J Rheumatol* 1998;37:1198–1202.

68. Manninen P, Piihimaki H, Heliovaara M, Makela P: Overweight, gender, and knee osteoarthritis. *Int J Obes Relat Metab Disord* 1996;20:595–597.

69. Hart DJ, Doyle DV, Spector TD: Incidence and risk factors for radiographic knee osteoarthraitis in middle-aged women: The Chingford Study. *Arthritis Rheum* 1999;42:17–24.

70. Cerhan JR, Wallace RB, el-Khoury GY, Moore TE, Long CR: Decreased survival with increasing prevalence of full-body, radiographically defined osteoarthritis in women. *Am J Epidemiol* 1995;141:225–234.

71. Ekstrand J, Gillquist J, Liljedahl SO: Prevention of soccer injuries: Supervision by doctor and physiotherapist. *Am J Sports Med* 1983;11:116–120.

72. Caraffa A, Cerulli G, Projetti M, Aisa G, Rizo A: Prevention of anterior cruciate ligament injuries in soccer: A prospective controlled study of proprioceptive training. *Knee Surg Sports Traumatol Arthrosc* 1996;4:19–21.

73. Ettlinger CF, Johnson RJ, Shealy JE: A method to help reduce the risk of serious knee sprains incurred in alpine skiing. *Am J Sports Med* 1995;23:531–537.

74. Henning CE, Griffis ND, Vequist SW, et al: Sport-specific knee injuries, in Renström P (ed): *Sports Injury Prevention and Care V of the Encyclopaedia of Sports Medicine*. Portland, OR, IOC Medical Commission, 1994, pp 164–178.

75. Hewett TE: The effect of neuromuscular training on the incidence of knee injury in female athletes: A prospective study. *Am J Sports Med* 1999;27:699–706.

Chapter 10
Patellofemoral Disorders

Elizabeth A. Arendt, MD

The patellofemoral (PF) joint is composed of two osseous components, the patella and the femoral trochlear surface, with a shared articulating surface. It is different from most other joints in that the patella is enclosed within the confines of the extensor mechanism of the lower limb, that is, the quadriceps muscle and its associated soft-tissue attachments. Therefore, its function is intimately associated with the dynamic muscle activity of the lower extremity.

Any discussion of a topic depends on dividing the larger topic into smaller components. However, the first problem with understanding PF joint disorders is that there is no consensus in the literature on their classification.

Classification Systems

Radin,[1] in 1979, recognized four categories of PF pain, including traumatic lesions of the patella, osteoarthritis of the PF joint, synovial fringe entrapment syndrome, and patellar malalignment/subluxation. Insall[2] defined eight categories based on the presence or absence of damage to the articular surface of the PF joint. Carson[3] divided extensor mechanism disorders into three basic categories: (1) abnormalities of the PF articulation; (2) abnormalities of the supporting muscles, tendons, ligaments, and retinaculum; and (3) malalignment of the extremity causing altered knee mechanics. Yates and Grana,[4] in 1986, divided PF disorders into four major categories, with the category of patellar tracking disorders being further subdivided into four subcategories including PF malalignment, PF compression syndrome, recurrent subluxation, and recurrent dislocation. Fulkerson and Shea[5] categorized anterior knee pain into three categories: inflammatory, mechanical, and miscellaneous.

More recently, Merchant,[6] recognizing the need for a uniform classification system, proposed a classification of PF disorders based on etiologies rather than symptoms. He recognized that treatment protocols and outcome studies depend on a comparative classification system. His classification system has seven major categories and 15 minor categories. The seven major categories are: acute trauma, repetitive trauma, PF dysplasia, idiopathic chondromalacia patella, osteochondritis dissecans, synovial plicae syndromes, and iatrogenic disorders. Many of his categories relate to orthopaedic ICD-9-CM expanded diagnostic codes.

There is little commonality between these systems, perhaps because there is much confusion and disagreement as to the etiology of the disease process that creates clinical symptoms. A brief historical review of the development of the knowledge base of PF disorders may help to explain why the confusion exists.

Historical Review

Chondromalacia Patellae

Before the advent of modern imaging, classification of PF disorders was based largely on clinical presentation (anterior knee pain) or surgical findings (chondromalacia patellae). Büdinger[7] was the first to describe cartilaginous changes on the inferior patellar surface. The term chondromalacia patellae was introduced into the literature by Aleman[8] in 1928. He described a degeneration of patellar articular cartilage, which he termed "chondromalacia posttraumatica patellae," that he had observed in one third of 220 knees at the time of surgery. As the years advanced, chondromalacia patellae was used alone as a diagnosis without reference to etiology and became equated with anterior knee pain.

There is debate as to the clinical pathologic significance of chondromalacia or cartilage softening and breakdown of the articular patellar surface. Moreover, there is little evidence to suggest that chondromalacia patellae is a precursor to osteoarthritis.[9–11] Many consider chondromalacia of the patella as a normal part of aging that is found in the knees of most people older than 30 years.[12]

Chondromalacia patellae is frequently observed along the medial odd facet and increases with advancing age.[13–16] Owre[17] described pathologic changes, including a significant percentage of cartilaginous lesions in young people, at random autopsy in 106 cadavers. It has been noted from observations in the hip and elbow that chondromalacia frequently was found in the nonweightbearing part of articular cartilage.[18,19] Therefore, habitual disuse of that area of the cartilage was believed to be an important etiologic factor in the development of chondromalacia patellae.

Patellar Malalignment

In the late 1970s and early 1980s, clinicians began to discuss the association between pain in the anterior aspect of the knee and patellar malalignment. Merchant and associates[20] were among the first to separate chondromalacia patellae into two types, that with normal alignment and that with abnormal alignment. They suggested the use of a specific 30° radiograph of the patella to distinguish between the two types. Other forms of axial radiographic imaging have suggested schemes for radiographic malalignment categorization.[11,21,22] Insall[23] stated that most young people with patellar pain have a malalignment syndrome, and it is this malalignment syndrome rather than abnormalities of articular cartilage that is responsible for the pain.

With advancing use of axial radiographic imaging, a category of PF disorders was described by Ficat and Hungerford.[24] Lateral patellar compression syndrome ("Syndrome d'hyperpression esterne de la totule") was believed to be functional lateralization of the patella created by increased lateral forces, decreased medial forces, or both, which can lead to increased cartilage wear and pain. Ficat and Hungerford described chondromalacia patellae at the median ridge and the lateral facet, a different area than the previously described medial or odd facet. This finding was believed to represent overload of the articular cartilage and was associated with radiographic evidence of overload, including subchondral sclerosis and lateralization of the patella trabeculae. It gave further support to the malalignment theory of PF disorders.

Computed tomography[21,25–27] has improved the ability to evaluate the relationship of the patella to the trochlear groove. Schutzer and associates[25] gave specific computed tomographic criteria for normal patellar alignment based on precise midpatella transverse cuts at 0°, 20°, and 30° of flexion. This was based on a population of 20 clinically symptomatic patients and 10 control subjects. They described four categories: type I was subluxation alone, type II was subluxation and tilt, type III was tilt without subluxation, and type IV was no malalignment. Although others have published series with slightly larger numbers,[28,29] there continues to be little understanding of the correlation of imaging findings and clinical symptoms, and the distribution of "normal" within populations.

The malalignment theory of the extensor mechanism pain assumes that malalignment could be associated with an increase in PF contact force, a decrease in PF contact area, or both. This resulting increased PF contact pressure could be the mechanical stimulus triggering damage to the cartilage.[30,31] PF contact forces have been investigated in numerous biomechanical studies. Most of these are in vitro cadaver studies and are well delineated elsewhere.[32] There are inherent limitations of the cadaver model, most important of which is the inability to duplicate the in vivo actions of the quadriceps and its associated dynamic complex. However, collectively, in vitro studies have demonstrated that alterations in the biomechanics of the PF joint can lead to changes in magnitude, distribution, and pattern of PF contact pressures.

The relationship of PF contact pressure to clinically symptomatic PF disorders is less clear. There is a suggestion that pain results from increased subjacent bone plate being subject to increased pressure variations from which they are normally defended by the energy-absorbing function of cartilage.[33]

Tissue Overload/Rotational Variances

Another theory is that PF pain is due to overload of the soft tissues and articular structures. This tissue overload is more powerful than any faulty mechanics and is the dominant factor in the genesis of anterior knee pain.[34] The relationship of the patellar tracking mechanism within the trochlear groove would be important to understand in relationship to a potential overload syndrome because maltracking may be a continuum of normal alignment, with tissue overload occurring faster along the continuum, commensurate with degrees of maltracking. This malalignment depends on coronal and rotational plane alignments about the knee. Coronal plane deformities about the knee (varus and valgus at the tibiofemoral joint) are recognized as capable of producing pathologic change in the joint. Coronal plane deformities involving the PF joint (lateral tibial tubercle displacement, patellar tilt, patellar subluxation) are better imaged and visualized but continue to be less well-understood compared to coronal plane deformities of the tibiofemoral joint. These coronal plane abnormalities likely vary with the dynamic action of the quadriceps muscle complex, as well as the dynamic rotational relationship of lower limb components. Coronal plane relationships of the PF joint frequently address the rotational relationships of the limb, specifically the rotational orientation of the tibia to the femur, and the femur to the pelvis. In children, rotational deformities such as femoral anteversion and tibial torsion (both physiologic and pathologic) are better understood. However, there is little effort to relate these findings to adult pathology, particularly to those disorders of a PF nature.

The term miserable malalignment[35] has been used by clinicians to describe a malalignment syndrome that frequently presents clinically as PF or anterior knee pain. This syndrome originally was described as a rotational malalignment of the extensor mechanism produced by a combination of internal femoral torsion and compensatory external torsion. It can be seen in combination with genu recurvatum, genu valgum, tibial varum, foot pronation, and/or axial tilt on radiographs. More recently, this miserable malalignment syndrome has focused further up the kinetic chain where it can be associated with an anteriorly rotated pelvis with obligate internal rotation of the femur.[36] Although these rotational variances can be associated with patellar malalignment, Merchant[6] ascribes rotational variances as a type of developmental abnormality and refers to them as rotational dysplasias. True dysplasias should be constitutional features of a person's body habitus and not subject to change through postural muscle control. Recently, physical examination measurements of limb malrotation and radiographic axial malalignment of the patella were improved with the use of an exercise program and Protonics brace.[36] These data cast further confusion on the role of rotation of the femur and patella position in the trochlear groove (patellar tilt/subluxation) in the pathogenesis of PF pain.

Although miserable malalignment has been associated with anterior knee pain, the determination of which components may play a role in associated PF problems is inconclusive. The Q angle or quadriceps angle is an angular measurement of the vector from the anterosuperior iliac spine to the midpatella, bisecting the vector from the midpatella to the tibial tubercle's insertion of the patellar tendon. The underlying assumption is that the larger the Q angle, the larger will be the lateral moment on the patella. Q angle measurements are widely used, but no direct correlation with the incidence of PF disorders has been established by scientific criteria.

According to a cadaver study, an increase or decrease in Q angle is associated with abnormal patterns of cartilage loading and increased peak PF pressure.[37] Increased Q angle has been associated with patellar chondropathy in several studies.[38–40] The range of normal values established by multiple studies is wide. Although some authors have used Q angles as one of the criteria to determine alignment strategies, approaches are empirical. Although it is a traditional part of PF discussions, actual clinical utility of the Q-angle measurement itself is uncertain despite extensive study.[41,42] More recently, the International Patellofemoral Study Club had a majority consensus that the clinical utility of a Q-angle measurement is minimal, given the knowledge to date.

The condition of an inwardly pointed knee so often is associated with chronic anterior knee pain that it typically is ascribed to femoral anterversion.[43,44] Femoral deformities have been noted in relationship to chondromalacia patellae.[35,45] Smillie[46] and others[47–49] have noted the prevalence of abnormal torsion in panarticular osteoarthritis of the knee.

More recently, external tibial torsion was believed to be the primary pathologic limb feature in people with chronic anterior knee pain and abnormal torsion of the limb. However, this was not associated with concomitant femoral anterversion.[50,51] External torsion of the tibia and the tibial tubercle brings the plane of the patellar tendon laterally and posterior to the plane of the patella. This torsion can create increased contact forces in the trochlear groove. Knee flexion obligates internal rotation of the tibia. It was found that there is less derotation of the tibia in flexion in patients with PF pain;[24,52] however, this finding did not hold up with additional study.[53,54] Foot pronation has been associated with a chondropathy.[55–58]

Tissue Overload/Tissue Homeostasis

With the advent of arthroscopy, clinicians have a tool to directly examine the articular surface of the kneecap. It was hoped that this could lead to better understanding of the relationship of articular lesions and clinical symptoms. However, many have noted patients with anterior knee pain who have completely normal patellar articular cartilage at the time of the arthroscopy.[59–61] In addition, articular cartilage changes were found in several patients without any preoperative physical examination findings.[62]

Few studies relate physical examination and/or imaging studies to clinical symptoms and/or treatment results. This lack of correlation between current physical examination measurements, imaging studies, and clinical symptoms with PF pain has led several clinicians to rethink the etiology of PF pain. Dye and associates[63–65] have advanced the theory that PF pain reflects the loss of tissue homeostasis, frequently arising from biologic tissue about the PF joint exceeding tissue load acceptance capacity. This problem can result in a microfailure of a variety of anatomic components that can induce a biologic cascade of excessive cytokine production, resulting in not only nerve irritation and perceived pain, but also decreased structural strength. They believe that structural malalignment and/or the presence of cartilage damage in itself is not a reason for PF pain. It is not until a person steps outside his or her own envelope of tissue acceptance that the person has clinical pain and dysfunction.

Natural History/Predictive Factors

Few longitudinal natural history studies are available for review. Nimon and associates[66] followed a consecutive series of 63 girls (average age 15.5 years), initially seen by Sandow and Goodfellow[67] at Nuffield Orthopaedic Centre in Oxford, England, between 1974 and 1980. Treatment consisted of reassurance, and in some cases physical therapy and cast immobilization. All patients were told that the condition was benign and would go away in time. Fifty-four of the 63 original patients responded to a questionnaire at an average of 3.8 years of follow-up. Fifty percent improved during the first 4 years of the study. Forty-nine of these patients responded to the 1994 survey (an average follow-up of

16 years). The 1994 study showed that an additional 23% improved during the subsequent 12 years, for a total of 73% improvement in the original follow-up group of 63. Nimon and associates[66] also performed a statistical analysis of radiographic measurements, quadriceps wasting, joint effusion, and various physical examination signs. They could not identify any factor on which to predict the patients who made up the 27% failure group. In this group, those with PF pain who did not improve still had no evidence of significant structural disease.[67]

When analyzing potential predictive factors with a prospective study design, one group of investigators looked at a variety of constitutional features, including sex, age, body composition, athletic activity, and duration of symptoms. They also measured 10 physical examination features and radiographic indices. They showed that 70% of their patient population improved with conservative rehabilitation consisting of strengthening activities, nonsteroidal anti-inflammatory drugs, and reduction of the aggravating activity. Age was the only factor that showed significant predictive value; the younger the age the more likely a favorable outcome.[68]

Exercise Intervention for PF Pain

Exercise interventions for patients with PF pain already have been investigated individually; the literature is most abundant in this area. Variations on exercise themes surface on a regular basis. Questions remain with regard to the following issues: (1) the core neuromuscular control strategies used by the central nervous system to control knee joint musculature and stability; (2) changes to these strategies that may occur in the presence of pain, particularly PF pain, and the relationship of these strategies to the onset, duration of, and recovery from PF pain; and (3) the relationship between changes in the control strategies and patellar function. From where does the pain come? Is it centrally or locally controlled? What is the relationship between pain and PF forces and pressures? How does muscular strengthening change this relationship?

Neuromotor control is assumed to be disturbed in the presence of PF pain, thus leading to quadriceps inhibition (and knee dysfunction). The restoration of normal neuromuscular control is one of the primary goals of conservative treatment, at least implicitly. Conservative treatment has been reported to be successful in 63% to 90% of patients.[69–71]

Summary of PF Pain

The etiology of PF pain is unclear and likely varied. This lack of fundamental knowledge on the pathogenesis of PF disorders has hindered progress in communicating what is already known. Progress would be aided by: (1) consensus on a classification system; (2) consistency in the terminology used; (3) improvement in knowledge of common physical examination measurements of the PF joint and their relationship to clinical symptoms; (4) clearer representation of the normal variations in PF physical examination measurements and imaging results in the population; (5) understanding the relationship between cartilage damage and clinical pain; (6) outcome studies using similar terminology and tests to define the prevalence of PF disorders in the population at various age groups and longitudinal studies concerning PF pain and its expression over time; and (7) understanding the relationship between improving the neuromuscular control of the PF joint and improvement of symptoms.

Patellofemoral Instability

Patellar instability is described for the purpose of this chapter as the traumatic disruption of normal or previously uninjured tracking relationship of the patella to the femoral groove. It merits separate consideration on some discussion points. However, PF pain can coexist with PF instability.

PF instability has been associated with a variety of anatomic factors including trochlear dysplasia, patellar tilt, tibial tubercle lateralization (high Q angle) and patellar height. The most consistent physical examination feature associated with patellar instability has been patella alta.[41,72–75] Torsional deformities have been noted in relationship to PF instability, including increased external tibial torsion[24,48,76,77] and femoral torsion deformities.[5,46]

Q angles have not been found to be greater in a group of patients with patellar subluxation than in control subjects.[78] However, when measurement is rigorously controlled for locating the patella in the center of the trochlear groove, Q angles were higher in patients with a history of patellar subluxation.[79] This was true in both the injured knee and the contralateral knee, with the uninvolved knee having a higher Q angle compared to the normal population of 94 control subjects.

Nonsurgical treatment of patellar dislocations followed over time noted that dislocations became less frequent with advancing age, and there was little evidence of osteoarthritis.[80] However, no studies are recent or included articular cartilage damage and/or soft-tissue damage that might be evaluated through the use of magnetic resonance imaging and/or arthroscopy.

Surgical procedures aimed at stabilizing the patella are often successful in eliminating instability, but frequently the patient is left with symptomatic pain.[81,82] Despite a low recurrence rate, neither surgical nor conservative treatment of PF dislocations address the issue of persistent symptoms of anterior knee pain.

More than 100 operations have been described for treatment of PF disorders. These surgical procedures are directed primarily at treating PF instability. Treatment of PF pain using instability principles is based primarily in the malalignment theory of the etiology of PF pain. Treatment of PF problems is based on the clinician's belief concerning the etiology of the underlying pathophysiology. Nowhere is this more apparent than in the surgical management of PF disorders.

Surgical procedures can be divided into seven principal categories: (1) arthroscopic debridement of localized synovitis and/or debridement of frayed cartilage, (2) proximal soft-tissue balancing procedures, including release or lengthening of the lateral retinaculum, imbrication, tightening, or reconstruction of passive medial structures, and vastus medialis obliquus (VMO) advancement consisting of moving the VMO muscle with variable midline and/or distal advancement; (3) distal bony procedures including medialization of the patellar tendon insertion into the tibial tubercle anterior displacement; (4) proximal bony procedures involving changing the configuration of the trochlear groove; (5) combined soft-tissue and bony procedures; (6) patellectomies with or without realignment of the extensor mechanism; and (7) derotation osteotomies of the lower limb (femur and/or tibia).

Schematic indications for the various surgical procedures are discussed elsewhere.[83] However, most lack uniformity in preoperative measurements, consistency in imaging methodology, and validated outcome scales.

Scoring System/Outcome Studies

Few outcome questionnaires have been designed specifically for the PF joint; the most popular is Kujala and associates.[84] The International Patellofemoral Study Club and a subgroup of the International Knee Documentation Society are working on a validated outcome measure specifically for PF disorders.

General Variables

Clinicians have anecdotally agreed for years that PF disorders are more common in women. Given the difficulty in classifying patient groups, literature support for this supposition is meager. However, the following physical examination features are worthy of mention: (1) Investigators have agreed that female subjects generally have a greater Q angle. (2) Because of the broader pelvis in women, the lower extremities assume a more valgus position at the knee, which can have subsequent accommodation with increased pronation of the foot. (3) In women, there is a higher prevalence of increased femoral anteversion, which in turn affects the biomechanics of the PF joint. Increased femoral anteversion and a wide pelvis are associated with increased quadriceps angle.[85,86] (4) Patella alta is more common in women.[87] Patella alta is associated with PF osteoarthritis[87] and PF instability.[41,72–74]

Gender Differences in Injury Incidence

DeHaven and Lintner[69] reported that among patients with knee disorders presenting over a 7-year period, disorders in 18.1% of men and 33.2% of women were associated with PF pain.

In an epidemiologic study of acute knee injuries in a Danish hospital over a 1-year period, the rate of dislocations of the PF joint were equal to the rate of ACL injuries. Patellar dislocation and PF overuse were both more common in women.[82,88]

Historically, patellar dislocation and subluxation have been considered primarily disorders of women.[89,90] Cash and Hughston, however, found that of 60 patients studied, 72% of the athletes and 42% of the entire group were men.[91] Others report a nearly 1:1 ratio.[92] Studies on acute patellar dislocations, although few are current, continue to show male preponderance.[82,93,94] A few studies,[95,96] supported by many physicians' personal impressions, report that recurrent patellar dislocations occur more frequently in women. It is difficult to interpret these findings because most studies reporting acute dislocations in men are not prevalent studies and date from a time when men constituted most of the athletes. However, a collective review of the studies does suggest that women have a higher incidence of recurrent patellar dislocation.

This information suggests that acute patellar dislocations occur more in men, whereas women experience more recurrent dislocations. Further study in this area, documenting the degree of soft-tissue and cartilage damage, physical examination features, bony morphology, and treatment rendered, would be necessary to determine whether gender is a factor for recurrent patellar dislocations.

References

1. Radin EL: A rational approach to the treatment of patellofemoral pain. *Clin Orthop* 1979;144:107–109.
2. Insall J: Patellar pain. *J Bone Joint Surg* 1982;64A:147–152.
3. Carson WG Jr: Diagnosis of extensor mechanism disorders. *Clin Sports Med* 1985;4:231–246.
4. Yates C, Grana WA: Patellofemoral pain: A prospective study. *Orthopedics* 1986;9:663–667.
5. Fulkerson JP, Shea KP: Disorders of patellofemoral alignment. *J Bone Joint Surg* 1990;72A:1424–1429.
6. Merchant AC: Clinical classifications of patellofemoral disorders. *Sports Med Arthrosc Rev* 1994;2:211–219.
7. Büdinger K: Über Traumatische Knorpelrisse im Kniegelenk. *Deutsch Z Chir* 1908;92:510–536.
8. Aleman O: Chondromalacia posttraumatica patellae. *Acta Chir Scand* 1928;63:149–190.
9. Goodfellow J, Hungerford DS, Woods C: Patellofemoral joint mechanics and pathology: 2. *J Bone Joint Surg* 1976;58B:291-299.
10. Bentley G: Articular cartilage changes in chondromalacia patellae. *J Bone Joint Surg* 1985;67B:769–774.
11. Karlson S: Chondromalacia patellae. *Acta Chir Scand* 1940;83:347–381.
12. Bennett GA, Waine H, Bauer W (eds): *Changes in the Knee Joint at Various Ages: With Particular Reference to the Nature and Development of Degenerative Joint Disease*. New York, NY, Commonwealth Fund, 1942.
13. Outerbridge RE: The etiology of chondromalacia patellae. *J Bone Joint Surg* 1961;43B:752–757.
14. Emery IH, Meachim G: Surface morphology and topography of patello-femoral cartilage fibrillation in Liverpool necropsies. *J Anat* 1973;116:103–120.

15. Casscells SW: The place of arthroscopy in the diagnosis and treatment of internal derangement of the knee: An analysis of 1000 cases. *Clin Orthop* 1980;151:135–142.

16. Casscells SW: Gross pathological changes in the knee joint of the aged individual: A study of 300 cases. *Clin Orthop* 1978;132:225–232.

17. Owre A: Chondromalacia patellae. *Acta Chir Scand* 1936;41(suppl):7–156.

18. Goodfellow JW, Bullough PG: The pattern of ageing of the articular cartilage of the elbow joint. *J Bone Joint Surg* 1967;49B:175–181.

19. Harrison MHM, Schajowicz F, Trueta J: Osteoarthritis of the hip: A study of the nature and evolution of the disease. *J Bone Joint Surg* 1953:35B:598–626.

20. Merchant AC, Mercer RL, Jacobsen RH, Cool CR: Roentgenographic analysis of patellofemoral congruence. *J Bone Joint Surg* 1974;56A:1391–1396.

21. Malghem J, Maldauge B: Patellofemoral joint: 30 degrees axial radiograph with lateral rotation of the leg. *Radiology* 1989;170:566–567.

22. Laurin CA, Lèvesque HP, Dussault R, Labelle H, Peides JP: The abnormal lateral patellofemoral angle: A diagnostic roentgenographic sign of recurrent patellar subluxation. *J Bone Joint Surg* 1978;60A:55–60.

23. Insall J: "Chondromalacia patellae": Patellar malalignment syndrome. *Orthop Clin North Am* 1979;10:117–127.

24. Ficat RP, Hungerford DS (eds): *Disorders of the Patello-Femoral Joint*. Paris, France, Masson, 1977, p 117.

25. Schutzer SF, Ramsby GR, Fulkerson JP: Computed tomographic classification of patellofemoral pain patients. *Orthop Clin North Am* 1986;17:235–248.

26. Schutzer SF, Ramsby GR, Fulkerson JP: The evaluation of patellofemoral pain using computerized tomography: A preliminary study. *Clin Orthop* 1986;204:286–293.

27. Shellock FG, Mink JH, Fox JM: Patellofemoral joint: Kinematic MR imaging to assess tracking abnormalities. *Radiology* 1988;168:551–553.

28. Inoue M, Shino K, Hirose H, Horibe S, Ono K: Subluxation of the patella: Computed tomography analysis of patellofemoral congruence. *J Bone Joint Surg* 1988;70A:1331–1337.

29. Reikerås O, Høiseth A: Patellofemoral relationships in normal subjects determined by computed tomography. *Skeletal Radiol* 1990;19:591–592.

30. Fulkerson JP, Hungerford DS (eds): *Disorders of the Patellofemoral Joint*, ed 2. Baltimore, MD, Williams & Wilkins, 1990, p 98.

31. Outerbridge RE, Dunlop JA: The problem of chondromalacia patellae. *Clin Orthop* 1975;110:177–196.

32. Grabiner MD, Koh TJ, Draganich LF: Neuromechanics of the patellofemoral joint. *Med Sci Sports Exerc* 1994;26:10–21.

33. Goodfellow J, Hungerford DS, Woods C: Patello-femoral joint mechanics and pathology: 2. Chondromalacia patellae. *J Bone Joint Surg* 1976;58B:291–299.

34. Fairbank JC, Pynsent PB, van Poortvliet JA, Phillips H: Mechanical factors in the incidence of knee pain in adolescents and young adults. *J Bone Joint Surg* 1984;66B:685–693.

35. James SL: Chondromalacia of the patella in the adolescent, in Kennedy JC, Fowler PJ (eds): *The Injured Adolescent Knee*. Baltimore, MD, Williams & Wilkins, 1979, pp 205–251.

36. Jansa S: Femoralpatellar dysfunction: A new description of an old problem. *Adv Phys Ther Phys Ther Assts* 1999;35:47.

37. Huberti HH, Hayes WC: Patellofemoral contact pressures: The influence of Q-angle and tendofemoral contact. *J Bone Joint Surg* 1984;66A:715–724.

38. Aglietti P, Cerulli G: Chondromalacia and recurrent subluxation of the patella: A study of malalignment, with some indications for radiography. *Ital J Orthop Traumatol* 1979;5:187–201.

39. Insall J, Falvo KA, Wise DW: Chondromalacia patellae: A prospective study. *J Bone Joint Surg* 1976;58A:1–8.

40. Reider B, Marshall JL, Warren RF: Clinical characteristics of patellar disorders in young athletes. *Am J Sports Med* 1981;9:270–274.

41. Insall J, Goldberg V, Salvati E: Recurrent dislocation and the high-riding patella. *Clin Orthop* 1972;88:67–69.

42. Kujala UM, Österman K, Kormano M, Nelimarkka O, Hurme M, Taimela S: Patellofemoral relationships in recurrent patellar dislocation. *J Bone Joint Surg* 1989;71B:788–792.

43. Engel GM, Staheli LT: The natural history of torsion and other factors influencing gait in childhood: A study of the angle of gait, tibial torsion, knee angle, hip rotation, and development of the arch in normal children. *Clin Orthop* 1974;99:12–17.

44. Fabry G, MacEwen GD, Shands AR Jr: Torsion of the femur: A follow-up study in normal and abnormal conditions. *J Bone Joint Surg* 1973;55A:1726–1738.

45. Bandi W: Trauma-induced chondromalacia patellae, in Hungerford DS (ed): *Leg Length Discrepancy: The Injured Knee*. Berlin, Germany, Springer-Verlag, 1977, pp 131–141.

46. Smillie IS: *The Biomechanical Basis of Osteoarthritis of the Knee in Total Knee Replacement*. London, England, Mechanical Engineering Publications, 1974, p 8.

47. Eckhoff DG, Johnston RJ, Stamm ER, Kilcoyne RF, Wiedel JD: Version of the osteoarthritic knee. *J Arthroplasty* 1994;9:73–79.

48. Turner MS, Smillie IS: The effect of tibial torsion on the pathology of the knee. *J Bone Joint Surg* 1981;63B:396–398.

49. Weber U: Malrotation of distal femur. *Z Orthop Ihre Grenzgeb* 1977;115:707–715.

50. Cooke TD, Price N, Fisher B, Hedden D: The inwardly pointing knee: An unrecognized problem of external rotational malalignment. *Clin Orthop* 1990;260:56–60.

51. Reikerås O: Is there a relationship between femoral anteversion and leg torsion? *Skeletal Radiol* 199;20:409–411.

52. Simmons E Jr, Cameron JC: Patella alta and recurrent dislocation of the patella. *Clin Orthop* 1992;274:265–269.

53. Sargent JR, Teipner WA: Abstract: Medial patellar retinacular repair for acute and recurrent dislocation of the patella: A preliminary report. *J Bone Joint Surg* 1971;53A:386.

54. Kujala UM, Kvist M, Österman K, Friberg O, Aalto T: Factors predisposing Army conscripts to knee exertion injuries incurred in a physical training program. *Clin Orthop* 1986;210:203–212.

55. Buchbinder MR, Napora NJ, Biggs EW: The relationship of abnormal pronation to chondromalacia of the patella in distance runners. *J Am Podiatry Assoc* 1979;69:159–162.

56. Jernick MS, Heifizt NM: An investigation into the relationship of foot pronation to chondromalacia patellae. *Arch Podiatr Med Foot Surg* 1980;62B:346.

57. Lutter LD: Foot-related knee problems in the long distance runner. *Foot Ankle* 1980;1:112–116.

58. Subotnick SI: A biomechanical approach to running injuries. *Ann NY Acad Sci* 1977;301:888–899.

59. McGinty JB, McCarthy JC: Endoscopic lateral retinacular release: A preliminary report. *Clin Orthop* 1981;158:120–125.
60. Metcalf RW: An arthroscopic method for lateral release of subluxating or dislocating patella. *Clin Orthop* 1982;167:9–18.
61. Bentley G, Dowd G: Current concepts of etiology and treatment of chondromalacia patellae. *Clin Orthop* 1984;189:209–228.
62. Stougard J: Chondromalacia of the patella: Physical signs in relation to operative findings. *Acta Orthop Scand* 1975;46:685–694.
63. Dye SF, Chew MH: The use of scintigraphy to detect increased osseous metabolic activity about the knee. *J Bone Joint Surg* 1993;75A:1388–1406.
64. Dye SF, Stäubli HU, Biedert RM, Vaupel GL: The mosaic of pathophysiology causing patellofemoral pain: Therapeutic implications. *Oper Tech Sports Med* 1999;7:46–54.
65. Dye SF, Vaupel GL: The pathophysiology of patellofemoral pain. *Sports Med Arthrosc Rev* 1994;2:203–210.
66. Nimon G, Murray D, Sandow M, Goodfellow J: Natural history of anterior knee pain: A 14-20 year follow-up of nonoperative management. *J Ped Orthop* 1998;18:118-122.
67. Sandow MJ, Goodfellow JW: The natural history of anterior knee pain in adolescents. *J Bone Joint Surg* 1985;67B:36–38.
68. Kannus P, Niittymäki S: Which factors predict outcome in the nonoperative treatment of patellofemoral pain syndrome? A prospective follow-up study. *Med Sci Sports Exerc* 1994;26:289–296.
69. DeHaven KE, Lintner DM: Athletic injuries: Comparison by age, sport, and gender. *Am J Sports Med* 1986;14:218–224.
70. Bentley G: Chondromalacia patellae. *J Bone Joint Surg* 1970;52A:221–232.
71. O'Neill DB, Micheli LJ, Warner JP: Patellofemoral stress: A prospective analysis of exercise treatment in adolescents and adults. *Am J Sports Med* 1992;20:151–156.
72. Aglietti P, Insall JN, Cerulli G: Patellar pain and incongruence: Part 1. Measurements of incongruence. *Clin Orthop* 1983;176:217–224.
73. Blackburne JS, Peel TE: A new method of measuring patellar height. *J Bone Joint Surg* 1977;59B:241–242.
74. Lancourt JE, Cristini JA: Patella alta and patella infera: Their etiological role in patellar dislocation, chondromalacia, and apophysitis of the tibial tubercle. *J Bone Joint Surg* 1975;57A:1112–1115.
75. Nagamine R, Otani T, White SE, McCarthy DS, Whiteside LA: Patellar tracking measurement in the normal knee. *J Orthop Res* 1995;13:115–122.
76. Fox TA: Dysplasia of the quadriceps mechanism: Hypoplasia of the vastus medialis muscle as related to the hypermobile patella syndrome. *Surg Clin North Am* 1975;55:199–226.
77. Eckhoff DG, Brown AW, Kilcoyne RF, Stamm ER: Knee version associated with anterior knee pain. *Clin Orthop* 1997;339:152–155.
78. Koskinen SK, Kujala UM: Patellofemoral relationships and distal insertion of the vastus medialis muscle: A magnetic resonance imaging study in nonsymptomatic subjects and in patients with patellar dislocation. *Arthroscopy* 1992;8:465–468.
79. Rorabeck CH, Bobechko WP: Acute dislocation of the patella with osteochondral fracture: A review of eighteen cases. *J Bone Joint Surg* 1976;58B:237–240.
80. Crosby EB, Insall J: Recurrent dislocation of the patella: Relation of treatment to osteoarthritis. *J Bone Joint Surg* 1976;58A:9–13.

81. Sallay PI, Poggi J, Speer KP, Garrett WE: Acute dislocation of the patella: A correlative pathoanatomic study. *Am J Sports Med* 1996;24:52–60.

82. Hawkins RJ, Bell RH, Anisette G: Acute patellar dislocations: The natural history. *Am J Sports Med* 1986;14:117–120.

83. Papagelopoulos PJ, Sim FH: Patellofemoral pain syndrome: Diagnosis and management. *Orthopedics* 1997;20:148–157.

84. Kujala UM, Jaakkola LH, Koskinen SK, Taimela S, Hurme M, Nelimarkka O: Scoring of patellofemoral disorders. *Arthroscopy* 1993;9:159–163.

85. Staheli LT: Rotational problems of the lower extremities. *Orthop Clin North Am* 1987;18:503–512.

86. Hvid I, Andersen LI: The quadriceps angle and its relation to femoral torsion. *Acta Orthop Scand* 1982;53:577–579.

87. Ahlbäck S, Mattsson S: Patella alta and gonarthrosis. *Acta Radiol Diagn (Stockh)* 1978;19:578–584.

88. McNab I: Recurrent dislocation of the patella. *J Bone Joint Surg Am* 1952;34:957–976.

89. Hughston JC: Subluxation of the patella. *J Bone Joint Surg Am* 1968;50:1003–1026.

90. Kettlecamp DB: Current concepts review: Management of the patellar malalignment. *J Bone Joint Surg Am* 1981;63:1344–1348.

91. Cash JD, Hughston JC: Treatment of acute patella dislocation. *Am J Sports Med* 1988;16:244–249.

92. Henry JH, Crosland JW: Conservative treatment of patellofemoral subluxation. *Am J Sports Med* 1979;7:12–14.

93. Coffield RH, Bryan RS: Acute dislocation of the patella: Result of conservative treatment. *Trauma* 1977;17:526–531.

94. Vanioppa S, Laasonon E, Silvennionen T, Vasenius J, Rokkanen P: Acute dislocation of the patella: A prospective review of operative treatment. *J Bone Joint Surg Am* 1990;72:365–369.

95. Halbrecht JL, Jackson DW: Acute dislocation of the patella, in Fox JM, Del Pizzo (eds): *The Patellofemoral Joint*. New York, NY, McGraw Hill, 1993, pp 123–156.

96. Larsen E, Lauriden F: Conservative treatment of patellar dislocations: Influence of evident factors on the tendency to redislocation and the therapeutic results. *Clin Orthop* 1982;171:131–136.

Chapter 11

Noncontact Anterior Cruciate Ligament Injuries in Women: New Insights Into Prevention Strategies

Letha Y. Griffin, MD, PhD

Introduction

Over the last two decades there has been a marked rise in the number of women participating in recreational and competitive sports. For example, only 96 women competed for the United States in the 1972 Olympics, whereas in 1996, 280 US women competed, making an extremely strong showing in multiple sports. Colleges are seeking to provide women with scholarship opportunities equal to those for men, and the number of high school female athletes rose from approximately 300,000 in 1971 to almost 2 million in 1990. Moreover, women now represent more than 33% of college athletes and 37% of US Olympic athletes.[1] As the numbers of female athletes have grown, several injuries that occur more commonly in female athletes have received increasing recognition.

Knee injuries, especially injuries to the knee's central ligament, the anterior cruciate ligament (ACL), are one such group of injuries. Because this ligament is a key stabilizer of the knee joint, injuring it can predispose the knee joint to recurrent injury and subsequent arthritis. During the last decade, great strides have been made to improve the understanding of the complexities of the many risk factors associated with this injury. The ultimate goal is to use this knowledge to develop effective prevention strategies. This chapter, after briefly reviewing the epidemiology of ACL injuries, will examine common risk factors associated with noncontact ACL injuries and the relationship of these factors to prevention strategies.

Epidemiology

ACL injuries occur at an alarming rate in competitive and recreational athletes. In college football, Hewson and associates[2] reported 42 ACL injuries per 1,000 players at risk per year. This would extrapolate to a 16% chance of ACL injury in a 4-year collegiate career and a hundredfold increase in injury compared with the general population. Feagin and associates[3] reported an average of one ACL injury per day at a large ski area, which represented an average of 1.2 ACL injuries per 1,000 skiers a day. If the incidence of injury is similar at the other US ski slopes, this would equate to more than 100,000 ACL injuries per year from skiing alone. The rate of ACL injuries as reported in the Kaiser Permanente population over a 3-year period was 0.38 per 1,000 members per year, of which 61% were sports related.[4] In a report from Denmark,[5] 76 ACL injuries were found in more than 250,000 inhabitants for a rate of 0.30 ACL injuries per thousand inhabitants per year, 27% of which were sports related. The incidence in female athletes in National Collegiate Athletic Association (NCAA) schools has been estimated at 10,000 injuries annually and in high school, it has been estimated that 25,000 ACL injuries will occur each year in female athletes.[6] Moreover, Garrick and Requa[7] have reported that over half of all ACL injuries occur in individuals from the ages of 15 to 25 years. Sports that require frequent jumping, twisting, and cutting movements, such as volleyball, soccer, skiing, and basketball, account for the majority of the sports-related injuries.

Not only does it appear that younger athletes in certain sports are more at risk for ACL injuries, but women participating in these sports appear to be more likely than men to sustain an ACL injury. A study done by Arendt and Dick[8] on the incidence of ACL injuries in collegiate soccer and basketball players, using the NCAA Injury Surveillance System data from 1989 to 1993[7] and recently updated by Arendt and associates[9] with data from 1994 to 1998, confirmed previous reports[10,11] that ACL injuries were more common in women, approximately two to three times as frequent in women playing soccer than in men and three times as frequent for female basketball players when compared with male players. Moreover, the mechanism of injury in an overwhelming number of ACL injuries was "no apparent contact" (Table 1).

Further substantiation of the prevalence of noncontact ACL injuries in women can be found throughout the literature published in the 1980s and 1990s. In 1982, Zelisko and associates[12] compared men's and women's professional basketball injuries and found women were 1.6 times more likely to be injured than men, with the knee being the most commonly injured site in women. Hunter and Torgan[13] in 1983 expressed concern over the high rate of ACL injuries in female gymnasts. No comparison was made with the incidence of ACL injuries in male gymnasts, although in reality, the apparatuses used by each sex in this sport differ significantly.

In 1985, Gray and associates[14] reported a retrospective study of female basketball injuries presenting to a single orthopaedic clinic over a 30-month period. Seventy-six injuries occurred in women, of which 55 (72%) involved

Table 1 Mechanisms of injury

	Contact		Noncontact	
	Women	**Men**	**Women**	**Men**
Soccer	31	34	53	32
Basketball	34	16	137	30

(Adapted with permission from Arendt E, Dick R: Knee injury patterns among men and women in collegiate basketball and soccer. *Am J Sports Med* 1995;23:694–701.)

the knee; of these, 19 (35%) were ACL injuries. Over the same time period, 151 injuries occurred in men, of which four involved the ACL. The average age of the women injured was 17 years and most of those injured had at least 2 years of playing experience.

DeHaven and Lintner,[15] in a 1986 survey of injuries in high school, intramural, professional, intercollegiate, and recreational athletic participants seen over 7 years in the sports medicine department of the University of Rochester, reported an increase in the number of knee injuries in female athletes when compared with male athletes. In basketball, ACL injuries were 8.5% of all injuries for men, but 20.7% of all injuries for women.

One Norwegian study reported a higher rate of ACL injuries in female team handball players compared with male players,[16] while an Italian study reported a higher rate of ACL injuries occurring in female volleyball players as compared with male players.[17]

Recently the lay press has given significant publicity to the incidence of ACL injuries in women. *Sports Illustrated* highlighted noncontact ACL injuries in female athletes in the February 1995 issue.[18] The ACL injury statistics for collegiate basketball players as quoted in this article demonstrates the prevalence of this injury in female players (Table 2). The September 1998 *New York Times Magazine* featured one woman's personal account of her experience with multiple reconstructions of her injured ACL.[19] Frequently over the last 5 years local newspapers have published accounts of injured star athletes in the community.[20–22]

Risk Factors for Injury

Several authors of ACL injury surveys in women have speculated on the mechanism of ACL injury. Strand and associates[23] believed that the mechanism of injury in the Norwegian handball players surveyed was decelerating and pivoting. Ferretti and associates[17] surveyed injuries in volleyball and reported altered balance on landing as a primary mechanism of injury, and Hunter and Torgan[13] blamed awkward landings from difficult dismounts done when the gymnast was fatigued at the end of a routine. Gray and associates'[14] findings agree with those of Strand and associates[23] and

Table 2 ACL Injuries in collegiate basketball players

Conference	Number of Players	
	Women	**Men**
ACC	20	4
Big East	9	4
SEC	15	5
Big Ten	15	7
Big 8	10	1
Pac-10	14	5

(Adapted with permission from McCallum J: Out of joint. *Sports Illustrated* Feb. 13, 1995, pp 44–53.)

Ferretti and associates[17]—that is, that landing from a jump and pivoting appear to be the two most frequent injury mechanisms.

It has been speculated that ACL injuries result from out of control play, such as taking off and landing one-footed and spinning in the air,[18] or occur because women are not exposed to motor learning skills at critical periods of their early development, which results in their having "impaired neuromuscular coordination."[18]

Arendt and Dick[8] speculated that the cause for the increased incidence of ACL injuries in female athletes is multifactorial, consisting of both intrinsic and extrinsic factors. Intrinsic factors include joint laxity, limb alignment, femoral notch dimension, ligament size, and hormonal influences. Extrinsic factors include muscular strength, neuromuscular control, body movement, skill level, and shoe/surface interface.

Joint Laxity

Hypermobility was first introduced as the cause of musculoskeletal symptoms in 1964 by Carter and Wilkinson,[24] who proposed five tests for hypermobility: (1) hyperextension of the fingers so that they lie parallel to the forearm; (2) abduction of the thumb so that it touches the forearm; (3) hyperextension of the elbow of more than 10°; (4) hyperextension of the knee of more than 10°; and (5) dorsiflexion of the ankle of more than 45°.

Using these criteria or the various modifications of them, the incidence of hypermobility in the general population has been found to be between 4% to 7%.[17,25,26] Joint hypermobility appears to be a genetically inherited trait, but musculotendinous flexibility can be increased through conditioning. Laxity is the combination of joint hypermobility and musculotendinous flexibility. A question that has been posed is: Do women have greater knee joint laxity and, if so, does this laxity predispose them to knee ligament injuries?

Studies have documented that laxity is more prevalent among women than men,[27] but more specifically it has been found that collegiate female athletes have greater knee laxity than collegiate men.[28,29] The relationship of hypermobility or laxity to injury is not as well defined. Nicholas,[30] using a modification of the Carter-Wilkinson criteria (Table 3), examined 37 professional football players who sustained knee ligament injuries over a 5-year period and found 28 had at least three indices of hypermobility. Of the total of 139 players studied, 39 had three indices of looseness. Twenty-eight of these 39 loose players ruptured their knee ligaments (72%). Of the remaining 100 players with two or fewer indices, only 9% ruptured their ligaments. Hence, he concluded that there was an increased likelihood of knee ligament rupture when a person had joint hypermobility as measured by his modification of the Carter-Wilkinson criteria. This finding has not been duplicated in other studies. In 1982, Moretz and associates[31] found no correlation between laxity test scores and knee ligament injuries in collegiate football players. Godshall[32] found no correlation between knee and ankle ligament injuries and laxity classification in high school players. Kalenak and Morehouse[33] evaluated 401 college football players and found no

Table 3 Nicholas' hypermobility criteria

1. The ability to flex the spine so that the palms can touch the floor with the knees fully extended.
2. The presence of recurvatum of the knee of 20° or more.
3. With knees flexed to 15° to 30° and with the hips, knees, and ankles turned out to the maximum external rotation, the feet can turn from a straight angle of 180° heel to heel with the toes out.
4. The ability to lie or sit flat on the floor with the knees or ankles parallel to the floor.
5. The presence of upper extremity laxity as noted by hypersupination of the forearm to position the hypothenar eminence including cephalad in a vertical plane with the elbows extended and the forearms supinated. This demonstrates shoulder flexion, elbow hyperextension, and hypersupination of the forearm.

(Adapted with permission from Grahame R: Joint hypermobility: Clinical aspects. *Proc R Soc Med* 1971;64:692–694.)

relationship between joint laxity tests and knee ligament injuries. However, Acasuso Diaz and associates[34] published a study of 675 17-year-old male soldiers and found that those who were classified as lax on the hypermobility test did have more musculoligamentous lesions. Hence, it would appear that the relationship between hypermobility and knee ligament injuries is still unresolved.

Forster and associates[35] reported that the uninjured knee in ACL-injured patients had greater laxity than the average knee laxity in normal subjects; that is, individuals who tear their ACL may not have generalized joint laxity, but perhaps their knee joints are looser than those of the average person. These data have not been verified by others.

Studies have also shown a mild increase in anterior and posterior knee laxity (18% to 20%) in certain sports (basketball and jogging) performed for longer than 30 minutes.[36] This laxity returned to normal after 60 minutes. Power lifters doing squats did not demonstrate a significant increase in laxity. Such data raise the issue of whether there could be an association between increased laxity associated with exercise, which is most likely a normal physiologic response to exercise, and potential for ligamentous injury.

Limb Alignment

The woman's lower extremity alignment has been implicated as a potential causative factor in a variety of lower-leg overuse injuries. Recently it has been blamed for an increased susceptibility to ACL injuries. Some feel the woman's increased hip varus, knee valgus, and foot pronation may contribute to increased forces on the ACL during functional activity.[37] Meister and associates[38] reported on a difference with respect to thigh-foot angle in a group of 51 ACL-injured female athletes compared with a matched cohort of 65 uninjured female athletes. Their report suggested that an increase in thigh-foot angle may play a predisposing role in noncontact ACL injuries in the female athlete. They found no difference with respect to femoral anteversion in the two groups studied.

Femoral Notch

Arendt[39] has summarized much of the available information on the relationship of the width of the femoral intercondylar notch to the incidence of ACL injuries. Shelbourne and associates[40] published data demonstrating that patients with narrow notches (< 15 mm as measured radiographically as well as intraoperatively at the time of their ACL reconstruction) had a higher incidence of tearing their contralateral ACL (23 of 388 patients versus four of 326 patients whose notches were > 15 mm). Furthermore, their data showed that with height and weight as covariates, women had statistically significantly narrower notches compared with men. The study population consisted of 336 patients with acute ACL tears and 378 patients with chronic tears.

Although much has been written regarding the relationship of small notches to ACL injury (Table 4), the great variability in techniques used to measure the notch results in difficulties with reproducibility of data. At present, the relationship of small athletes, small femurs, small notches, and small ACLs to ACL injuries remains inconclusive.

Hormonal Influences

Estrogen's effect on collagen metabolism and neuromuscular performance has been appreciated for a number of years,[49,50] but it was not until Liu and associates'[51] award-winning paper identifying, through immunohistochemical localization, estrogen and progesterone receptors in 17 specimens of human ACLs obtained at surgery from 13 women and four men that the interest in estrogen as a potential causative factor of ligamentous injuries intensified. Hormonal receptor sites have also been identified in the synovial lining of the knee joint, in the fibroblasts present in the ACL stroma, and in cells within the vessel walls of the ligament.

Wojtys and associates[52] reported an increased susceptibility to ACL injuries in women during the ovulatory phase of the menstrual cycle (days 10 to 14) when estrogen levels are high (Fig. 1). However, Thomas and associates, examining normal knee laxity of 31 collegiate athletes during the three phases of the menstrual cycle, identified the premenstrual phase (days 21 to 28) as the time of greatest laxity (unpublished data, 1998). They felt that this normal cyclic increase in ligamentous laxity might contribute to a decrease in proprioceptive awareness. In a study of 87 athletes in NCAA schools sustaining an ACL injury during the 1996 to 1999 academic years, the majority of athletes appeared to be injured during the early part of their cycle, not during the ovulatory phase (E Arendt, unpublished data, 2000). Mirzayan and associates (unpublished data, 1999) studied the effects of estradiol on the biomechanical properties of the ACL in rabbits and found that the force to failure of the ACLs from oophorectomized rabbits was similar to that of male rabbits. The addition of estradiol to the diet of female rabbits before sacrifice decreased the time to ACL failure.

Because all gender differences ultimately are hormonally rooted, the role of sex hormones as a major factor in the increased risks to women of noncontact ACL injuries is intriguing. However, present studies are conflicting, and no firm causal relationships can be drawn. Use of urine or serum measurements of hormonal status rather than estimates based on self-reported onset of menses may help to resolve these differences.

Table 4 Intercondylar notch size versus anterior cruciate ligament injury

References	Population	Measurement Technique	Conclusion	Comments
Anderson et al[41]	Patients with bilateral ACL injury, unilateral injury, and no known knee injury Retrospective study	Computed tomography scan	An association exists between anterior outlet stenosis of the ICN and ACL rupture	
Houseworth et al[42]	Patients with acute ACL injury and no known injury Retrospective study	Computer graphic study	A narrow posterior notch may predispose to ACL failure	
Souryal et al[43]	Patients with bilateral ACL injury, acute ACL injury, and normal knees Retrospective study	Notch radiographic view; NWI defined as ratio of width of ICN to width of femoral condyle, using radiographic landmarks	NWI bilateral ACL injury < NWI acute ACL injury and normal knees; NWI acute injuries = NWI normal knees	No gender difference, though population largely male
Good et al[44]	Patients with acute and chronic unilateral ACL injury (Normal measured from cadaver knees) Retrospective study	Direct measurement of anterior notch opening using a caliper technique	Normal notch width 18.1 mm to 20.4 mm; acute ACL injury had narrower notch measurements	
Souryal and Freeman[45]	902 high school athletes Prospective study	Notch radiographic view, measuring NWI	Athletes with no contact ACL injury have smaller notches	NWI in females < NWI in males
Schickendantz and Weicker[46]	Patients with unilateral and bilateral ACL injury, and normal knees Retrospective study	Used 8 different mathematical measurements from notch radiographic view	ICN measurements from radiographs may not be reliable predictors of ACL injury	
Lund-Hanssen et al[47]	Female Norwegian national team handball players Retrospective study	Notch radiographic view, direct measurement of notch width	Notch width < 17 mm are at high risk of injury	Only females studied

Continued on next page

Table 4 *continued*

References	Population	Measurement Technique	Conclusion	Comments
LaPrade and Burnett[48]	213 Division I athletes Prospective study	Notch radiographic view, measured NWI	Athletes playing certain sports with stenotic notches are at high risk for ACL injury	No significant difference between sex and average NWI or rate of ACL tears

(Adapted with permission from Arendt EA: Relationship between notch width index and risk of noncontact ACL injury, in *Prevention of Noncontact ACL Injuries*. Rosemont, IL, American Academy of Orthopaedic Surgeons, 2001.)
ACL = anterior cruciate ligament; NWI = notch width index; ICN = intercondylar notch

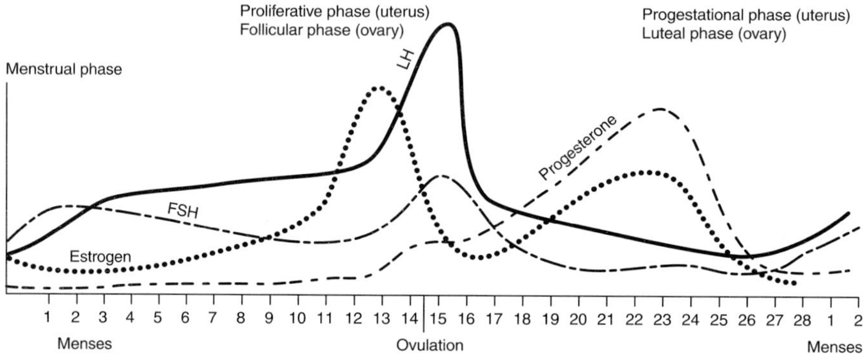

Fig. 1 Hormonal fluctuations during the menstrual cycle.

Muscle Strength and Neuromuscular Control

It has been well established that women have less muscle mass per total body weight than men (approximately 36.0% versus 44.8%).[53] Huston and Wojtys[28] in their evaluation of 40 Division I female athletes, 60 Division I male football players, and 60 control athletes (average age 23.5 years) found not only were female athletes statistically weaker, with less endurance in both quadriceps and hamstrings when compared with either male athletes or controls, but they generated maximal torque in the quadriceps before hamstrings in response to anterior tibial translation.

Boden and associates[54] have speculated that an ACL injury could occur secondary to the development of a strong eccentric quadriceps contraction simultaneously with a varus or valgus force on the knee in or near full extension. They have theorized that the quadriceps is preactivated to stop the knee's forward progress at heel strike, but then an unplanned event occurs (a slip or sudden change in direction), resulting in an "unbalanced" maximal quadriceps contraction while the foot is planted. Research by his group has shown that when the knee is minimally flexed, the force generated by a maximal quadriceps contraction exceeds the tensile strength of the ACL. This study is consistent with prior theories of Griffis and associates,[55] who describe what they call the "quad-cruciate interaction," that is, the ability of a maximum quadriceps contraction to tear the ACL when the knee is at near or full extension. The quad-cruciate interaction was also stressed by Markolf and associates,[56] who used cadaver specimens to evaluate the effects of knee angle on ACL loads. They advised limiting active extension of the quadriceps against resistance in the range of 0° to 45° if a person wished to limit forces on the ACL or ligament graft.

Mechanoreceptors have been found in human ACL,[29,57–59] leading to speculation that ligament stress may initiate muscular contraction or alteration in tone to stabilize the joint in a reflexive manner[60] (Fig. 2). A fatigued muscle may be unable to respond adequately to such signals from an ACL. Moreover, research by Lephart and Fu[59] and DeMont and Lephart[60] suggests that altered afferent feedback mechanisms reflecting proprioceptor deficits can result in a decrease in neuromuscular control and an increased risk of ACL injury.

Body Movement

Investigations are underway for evaluating the differences in body movement between men and women. Ireland (unpublished data, 1999) has analyzed videos of female and male basketball players performing jump shots, rebounds, and pivots. She reported differences in body mechanics. Recently, Malinzak and associates[61] studied 11 male and 9 female recreational athletes and found the women performed running, cross cutting, and side cutting maneuvers with significantly less knee flexion, more knee valgus, and less hip flexion than the men. Huston (unpublished data, 1999) reported significant

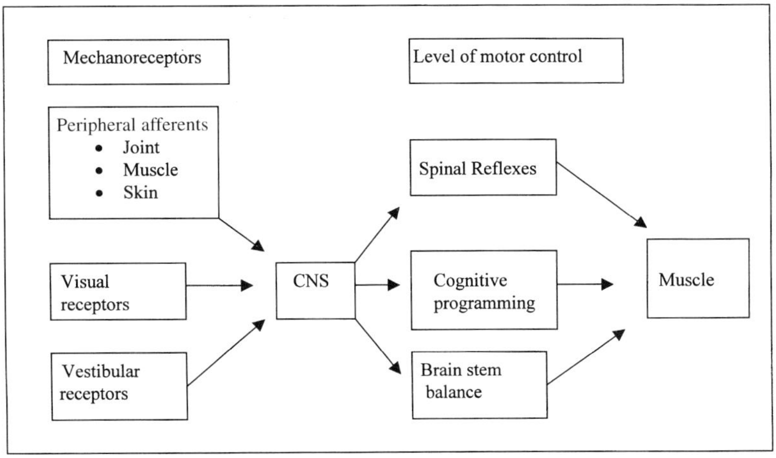

Fig. 2 Neuromuscular control pathways; CNS = Central nervous system. (Reproduced with permission from DeMont R, Lephart S: Repetition drives neuromuscular recovery after ACL injury. Biomechanics *1998;April:31–36.)*

gender differences in knee flexion angles at ground impact on landing from a drop landing, with women landing with less knee flexion than men. Subjects performed three unconstrained jumps from three different vertical heights (20, 40, and 60 cm) onto a concrete floor. The largest gender differences in knee angle occurred when landing from the lowest height of 20 cm, and there were no significant gender differences when landing from the 60 cm height.

Shoe/Surface Interface

Studies of team handball athletes in Norway[16] have shown an increased incidence of ACL injuries in players wearing shoes with a high coefficient of friction. No differences between men and women were identified, but total body size compared to shoe size was theorized as a potential influencing factor. In high school football, shoe cleat design has been found to influence the rate of ACL injuries,[62] and Scranton and associates,[63] in a retrospective review of noncontact ACL injuries in National Football League games over a 5-year period, found that there were approximately twice as many noncontact ACL injuries on natural grass than on artificial turf (40 to 21), and more injuries occurred on dry than wet grass. Dr. Bill Youmans has been quoted as saying, "There is no question the incidence of torn cruciates would go down— if I could get the young ladies and men to wear a fairly slick surface shoe that did not have much traction."[18]

Economic and Emotional Impact of ACL Injuries

The economic and emotional impact of ACL injuries on the injured athlete, the athlete's family, and society as a whole is great. If one estimates 250,000 ACL injuries each year[64] and a cost of $17,000 for surgical repair and rehabilitation of this injury,[65,66] the annual economic impact if only one half of the ACL-injured athletes are surgically reconstructed would be over $2 billion. This figure does not account for the costs incurred in the nonsurgical care of the remainder of the injured athletes.

Prevention Strategies

The ultimate goal of identifying injury risk factors is to use such information to formulate prevention strategies to decrease the injury rate. Previously published neuromuscular training prevention programs include that of Griffis and associates,[55] Caraffa and associates,[67] Ettlinger and associates,[68] and Hewett and associates.[64,69] Henning's program as reported by Griffis and associates[55] in 1989 was based on a 10-year review of ACL injuries in Division I female basketball players; the conclusion was that most ACL injuries were noncontact (75%) and that the most common mechanisms of injury were planting and cutting on a straight knee (29%), landing from a jump with a straight knee (28%), and a one-step stop with the knee extended (26%). Interestingly, 10 years later (1999), an NCAA survey of 69 ACL-injured female athletes[70] found the most commonly reported mechanism of injury was planting and pivoting and the second most common was decelerating and jumping. Henning's prevention program consisted of practice drills in which athletes were taught to change the plant-and-cut maneuver to an accelerated rounded turn, landing from a jump with a straight knee to landing from a jump with a bent knee, and modifying the one-step stop with a straight knee or hyperextended knee to a three-step stop with the knee flexed. He instituted his program in two Division I basketball programs in the Wichita, Kansas, area and found an 89% decrease in the rate of ACL injuries. Despite this early success, Henning's untimely death shortly after institution of the program unfortunately resulted in its abandonment.

In 1996, Caraffa and associates[67] reported on a prospective controlled study of proprioceptive training in 600 soccer players (300 controls and 300 test subjects) using balance board training and found a tenfold decrease in injury rates in athletes who participated in the balance board training program.

Hewett and associates'[71] neuromuscular training program consisting of a three-part program of stretching, weight training, and plyometrics has been shown to decrease impact forces on landing, improve neuromuscular control, improve hamstring muscle power, improve hamstring to quadriceps muscle peak torque ratios, and increase vertical jump. Three hundred sixty-six female high school volleyball and basketball athletes who underwent the 6-week preseason program demonstrated a significant decrease in the rate of ACL injury with the incidence of injury (injuries per 1,000 exposures) in untrained female athletes reported as 0.432 compared with 0.116 in the trained female athletes.[47]

Ettlinger and associates[68] reported on the Vermont ski safety program, a program developed in 1993 after the analysis of more than 1,400 ACL injuries sustained in Alpine skiing over a 22-year period. The program is based on a technique they call "guided discovery," a process in which skiers view videos of skiers sustaining ACL injuries with instructions to try to recognize potentially dangerous situations and to strategize how they would respond quickly and effectively if these situations were encountered. The participants were also encouraged to avoid high-risk behavior. In the 1993–1994 ski season, the on-slope staff (4,700 instructors and ski patrollers) from 20 ski areas participated in the program, resulting in a 69% decrease in serious knee sprains.

In June of 1999, an ACL Consensus Conference was organized in Hunt Valley, Maryland, on the day preceding the NIH-AAOS Symposium on "Women's Health in Sports and Exercise" to evaluate prevention strategies for noncontact ACL injuries in female athletes. Twenty participants representing orthopaedic surgeons, biomechanists, and athletic trainers attended the conference funded by the Orthopaedic Research and Education Foundation; the American Orthopaedic Society for Sports Medicine; the National Athletic Trainers Association Research and Education Foundation; and the NCAA. Because of overlapping areas that occur when risk factors are categorized into intrinsic and extrinsic groups, this conference used the Wojtys scheme of dividing risk factors into subcategories of environmental, anatomic, hormonal, and biomechanical risk factors. Participants, after carefully reviewing available data in each of these risk categories, formulated consensus statements on prevention strategies for each category. The following is a summary of those statements.

Environmental Risk Factors

The participants examined data on knee brace and shoe/surface interactions. They believe that at present there is no evidence that knee braces prevent ACL injuries. It was thought that increasing the shoe/surface coefficient of friction may improve performance, but also may increase the risk of injury to the ACL. Because shoe/surface interaction is modifiable, the participants thought this area of prevention research merits further investigation.

Anatomic Risk Factors

Although there is much literature on the role of the femoral notch size and ACL injuries, the group felt that because of the difficulty in achieving valid and reliable measurements, no consensus on the notch's role in the ACL injury is reachable at this time. Moreover, at present there are insufficient data on ACL size (absolute or proportional) to support that ligament size is related to the risk of injury. In addition to notch and ACL size, other lower extremity anatomic features have been implicated as causative factors in female ACL injury. At present, there is insufficient data to relate any lower extremity anatomic feature to ACL injury, but the group felt further studies in this area need to be done.

Hormonal Risk Factors

No consensus exists at present in the scientific community that sex-specific hormones play a role in the increased incidence of ACL injury in female athletes. The consensus participants did not recommend modification of activity or restriction of sport for women at any time during the menstrual cycle, but they did recommend continued investigation of hormonal influences on ACL injury.

Biomechanical Risk Factors

The group reemphasized that the knee is one part of a kinetic chain and anatomic sites other than the knee including the trunk, hip, and ankle may contribute to ACL injuries. Common biomechanical factors involved with many (not all) injuries include impact on the whole foot rather than on the toes (forefoot only) during landing or changing directions, awkward dynamic body movements, and perturbation prior to the injury. The common at-risk situations for noncontact ACL injuries appear to be deceleration, cutting or changing directions, and landing from a jump. The group believed that neuromuscular factors are significant in the increased risk of ACL injuries in women. Furthermore, at the present time, neuromuscular factors appear to be the most important reason for the differing ACL injury rates between male and female athletes. A strong quadriceps activation during eccentric contraction was believed to be a major factor in injury to the ACL.

After reviewing the existing neuromuscular training prevention programs, participants agreed on the following statements regarding prevention strategies. First, early data show that specific training programs that enhance body control reduce ACL injury rates in female athletes and may enhance athletic performance. Training and conditioning programs for male and female athletes in the same sport may need to be different. Those involved in the care of athletes should identify sports-specific at-risk motions and positions and encourage athletes to avoid these at-risk situations when possible. Strategies for activating protective neuromuscular responses when at-risk situations are encountered should also be identified.

With regard to future research direction in the area of biomechanical risk factors, the consensus group emphasized the need to continue to define the specific neuromuscular, proprioreceptive, and motor control factors associated with injury. However, until specific predictive and protective factors are definitively identified, training and prevention programs should continue to be implemented, assessed, and improved. The group believed that there is a pressing need to improve public and participant awareness of the risk of ACL injury and the possibilities of prevention.

Summary

In sports involving pivoting and deceleration, noncontact ACL injuries are more common in women than in men. Although research and the knowledge base on this topic have grown, the cause for this increased incidence is still unknown. The cause is likely multifactorial, consisting of environmental, anatomic, hormonal, and biomechanical risk factors. Neuromuscular risk factors appear at present to be the major factors in the development of noncontact ACL injuries. While continuing to further define risk factors for injury, it does appear appropriate to begin instituting available neuromuscular training programs for "at-risk" athletes.

References

1. CDC recommendations for previous exercise related injuries in women. *Women's Health, Orthopedic Edition* 2000;3:90-92.
2. Hewson GF Jr, Mendini RA, Wang JB: Prophylactic knee bracing in college football. *Am J Sports Med* 1986;14:262–266.
3. Feagin JA Jr, Lambert KL, Cunningham RR, Anderson LM, Riegel JR, King PH, VanGenderen L: Consideration of the anterior cruciate ligament injury in skiing. *Clin Orthop* 1987;216:13–18.
4. Miyasaka KC, Daniel DM, Stone ML, Hirshman P: The incidence of knee ligament injuries in the general population. *Am J Knee Surg* 1991;4:3–8.

5. Nielsen AB, Yde J: Epidemiology of acute knee injuries: A prospective hospital investigation. *J Trauma* 1991;31:1644–1648.
6. Huston LJ, Greenfield ML, Wojtys EM: ACL injuries in the female athlete: Potential risk factors. *Clin Orthop*. 2000;372:50-73.
7. Garrick J, Requa R: Anterior cruciate ligament injuries in men and women: How common are they? in *Prevention of Noncontact ACL Injuries*. Rosemont, IL, American Academy of Orthopaedic Surgeons, 2001.
8. Arendt E, Dick R: Knee injury patterns among men and women in collegiate basketball and soccer. *Am J Sports Med* 1995;23:694–701.
9. Arendt EA, Agel J, Dick RW: Anterior cruciate ligament injury patterns among collegiate men and women. *J Athletic Train* 1999;34:86–92.
10. Hutchinson MR, Ireland ML: Knee injuries in female athletes. *Sports Med* 1995;19:288–302.
11. Ireland ML, Wall C: Abstract: Epidemiology and comparison of knee injuries in elite male and female United States basketball athletes. *Med Sci Sports Exerc* 1990;22(suppl):491.
12. Zelisko JA, Noble HB, Porter M: A comparison of men's and women's professional basketball injuries. *Am J Sports Med* 1982;10:297–299.
13. Hunter LY, Torgan C: Dismounts in gymnastics: Should scoring be reevaluated? *Am J Sports Med* 1983;11:208–210.
14. Gray J, Taunton JE, McKenzie DC, Clement DB, McConkey JP, Davidson RG: A survey of injuries to the anterior cruciate ligament of the knee in female basketball players. *Int J Sports Med* 1985;6:314–316.
15. DeHaven KE, Lintner DM: Athletic injuries: Comparison by age, sport, and gender. *Am J Sports Med* 1986;14:218–224.
16. Myklebust G, Engebretsen L, Nilsson S, Hegermann C, Strand T, Maehlum S: Abstract: Registration of ACL injuries in the 3 upper divisions in Norwegian team handball: A prospective study. *Med Sci Sports Exerc* 1993;25:S50.
17. Ferretti A, Papandrea P, Conteduca F, Mariani PP: Knee ligament injuries in volleyball players. *Am J Sports Med* 1992;20:203–207.
18. McCallum J: Out of joint. *Sports Illustrated* Feb. 13,1995;44–53.
19. Gorney C: How the knee became the back. *New York Times Magazine* Sept. 6, 1998; section 6:42–47.
20. Curtright G: Anchor of a fan. *Atlanta Journal Constitution* Jan. 31, 1999.
21. Dorr V Jr: Knee deep in injuries. *Richmond Times Dispatch* Feb. 27, 1996.
22. Parker W: ACL injuries are taking a toll on the country's top teams *Atlanta Journal Constitution* March 13, 1998.
23. Strand T, Tvedte R, Engebretsen L, Tegnander A: Anterior cruciate ligament injuries in handball playing: Mechanisms and incidence of injuries. *Tidsskr Nor Laegeforen* 1990;110:2222–2225.
24. Carter C, Wilkinson J: Persistent joint laxity and congenital dislocation of the hip. *J Bone Joint Surg* 1964;46B:40–45.
25. Grahame R: Joint hypermobility: Clinical aspects. *Proc Roy Soc Med* 1971;64:692–694.
26. Jessee EF, Owen DS Jr, Sagar KB: The benign hypermobile joint syndrome. *Arthritis Rheum* 1980;23:1053–1056.
27. Grana WA, Moretz JA: Ligamentous laxity in secondary school athletes. *JAMA* 1978;240:1975–1976.
28. Huston LJ, Wojtys EM: Neuromuscular performance characteristics in elite female athletes. *Am J Sports Med* 1996;24:427–436.

29. Rozzi SL, Lephart SM, Gear WS, Fu FH: Knee joint laxity and neuromuscular characteristics of male and female soccer and basketball players. *Am J Sports Med* 1999;27:312–319.

30. Nicholas JA: Injuries to knee ligaments: Relationship to looseness and tightness in football players. *JAMA* 1970;212:2236–2239.

31. Moretz JA, Walters R, Smith L: Flexibility as a predictor of knee injuries in college football players. *Phys Sportsmed* 1982;10(suppl 7):93–97.

32. Godshall RW: The predictability of athletic injuries: An eight-year study. *J Sports Med* 1975;3:50–54.

33. Kalenak A, Morehouse CA: Knee stability and knee ligament injuries. *JAMA* 1975;234:1143–1145.

34. Acasuso Diaz M, Collantes Estevez E, Sanchez Guijo P: Joint hyperlaxity and musculoligamentous lesions: Study of a population of homogeneous age, sex and physical exertion. *Br J Rheumatol* 1993;32:120–122.

35. Forster IW, Warren-Smith CD, Tew M: Is the KT1000 knee ligament arthrometer reliable? *J Bone Joint Surg* 1989;71B:843–847.

36. Steiner ME, Grana WA, Chillag K, Schelberg-Karnes E: The effect of exercise on anterior-posterior knee laxity. *Am J Sports Med* 1986;14:24–29.

37. Ireland ML: Special concerns of the female athlete, in Fu FH, Stone DA (eds): *Sports Injuries: Mechanisms, Prevention and Treatment*. Baltimore, MD, Williams & Wilkins, 1994, pp 153–187.

38. Meister K, Huegel MO, Rolle GA, Indelicato PA, Horodyski MB: Abstract: The influence of rotational alignment of the lower extremity on noncontact injuries to the anterior cruciate ligament on the female athlete. Proceedings of the American Academy of Orthopaedic Surgeons 65th Annual Meeting, New Orleans, LA. Rosemont, IL, American Academy of Orthopaedic Surgeons, 1998, p 79.

39. Arendt EA: Relationship between notch width index and risk of noncontact ACL injury, in *Prevention of Noncontact ACL Injuries*. Rosemont, IL, American Academy of Orthopaedic Surgeons, 2001.

40. Shelbourne KD, Davis TJ, Klootwyk TE: The relationship between intercondylar notch width of the femur and the incidence of anterior cruciate ligament tears: A prospective study. *Am J Sports Med* 1998;26:402–408.

41. Anderson AF, Lipscomb AB, Liudahl KJ, Addlestone RB: Analysis of the intercondylar notch by computed tomography. *Am J Sports Med* 1987;15:547–552.

42. Houseworth SW, Mauro VJ, Mellon BA, Kieffer DA: The intercondylar notch in acute tears of the anterior cruciate ligament: A computer graphics study. *Am J Sports Med* 1987;15:221–224.

43. Souryal TO, Moore HA, Evans JP: Bilaterality in anterior cruciate ligament injuries: Associated intercondylar notch stenosis. *Am J Sports Med* 1988;16:449–454.

44. Good L, Odensten M, Gillquist J: Intercondylar notch measurements with special reference to anterior cruciate ligament surgery. *Clin Orthop* 1991;263:185–189.

45. Souryal TO, Freeman TR: Intercondylar notch size and anterior cruciate ligament injuries in athletes: A prospective study. *Am J Sports Med* 1993;21:535–539.

46. Schickendantz MS, Weiker GG: The predictive value of radiographs in the evaluation of unilateral and bilateral anterior cruciate ligament injuries. *Am J Sports Med* 1993;21:110–113.

47. Lund-Hanssen H, Gannon J, Engebretsen L, Holen KJ, Anda S, Vatten L: Intercondylar notch width and the risk for anterior cruciate ligament rupture: A case-control study in 46 female handball players. *Acta Orthop Scand* 1994;65:529–532.

48. LaPrade RF, Burnett QM II: Femoral intercondylar notch stenosis and correlation to anterior cruciate ligament injuries: A prospective study. *Am J Sports Med* 1994;22:198–203.
49. Fischer GM: Comparison of collagen dynamics in different tissues under the influence of estradiol. *Endocrinology* 1973;93:1216–1218.
50. Fischer GM, Swain ML: Effect of sex hormones on blood pressure and vascular connective tissue in castrated and noncastrated male rats. *Am J Physiol* 1977;232:H617–H621.
51. Liu SH, Al-Shaikh R, Panossian V, et al: Primary immunolocalization of estrogen and progesterone target cells in the human anterior cruciate ligament. *J Orthop Res* 1996;14:526–533.
52. Wojtys EM, Huston LJ, Lindenfeld TN, Hewett TE, Greenfield ML: Association between the menstrual cycle and anterior cruciate ligament injuries in female athletes. *Am J Sports Med* 1998;26:614-619.
53. Wells CL: Physical differences and similarities, in *Women: Sport and Performance: A Physiological Perspective*. Champaign, IL, Human Kinetics, 1985.
54. Boden BP, Griffin LY, Garrett WE: Etiology and prevention of noncontact ACL injury. *Physician Sportsmed* 2000;28:53–60.
55. Griffis ND, Vequist SW, Yearout KM, Henning CE, Lynch MA: Injury prevention of the anterior cruciate ligament. *Orthop Trans* 1990;14:239.
56. Markolf KL, Gorek JF, Kabo JM, Shapiro MS: Direct measurement of resultant forces in the anterior cruciate ligament: An in vitro study performed with a new experimental technique. *J Bone Joint Surg* 1990;72A:557–567.
57. Barrack RL, Skinner HB, Buckley SL: Proprioception in the anterior cruciate deficient knee. *Am J Sports Med* 1989;17:1–6.
58. Kennedy JC, Alexander IJ, Hayes KC: Nerve supply of the human knee and its functional importance. *Am J Sports Med* 1982;10:329–335.
59. Lephart SM, Fu FH: The role of proprioception in the treatment of sports injuries. *Sports Exercise Injury* 1995;1:96–102.
60. DeMont R, Lephart S: Repetition drives neuromuscular recovery after ACL injury. *Biomech* 1998;5:31–37.
61. Malinzak RA, Colby SM, Kirkendall DT, Garrett WE Jr: Abstract: Electromyographic and 3-dimensional kinematic analysis of cutting maneuvers in men and women: Implications for anterior cruciate ligament injury. Proceedings of the American Academy of Orthopaedic Surgeons 66th Annual Meeting, Anaheim, CA. Rosemont, IL, American Academy of Orthopaedic Surgeons, 1999, p 74.
62. Lambson RB, Barnhill BS, Higgins RW: Football cleat design and its effect on anterior cruciate ligament injuries: A three-year prospective study. *Am J Sports Med* 1996;24:155–159.
63. Scranton PE Jr, Whitesel JP, Powell JW, et al: A review of selected noncontact anterior cruciate ligament injuries in the National Football League. *Foot Ankle Int* 1997;18:772–776.
64. Hewett T, Murazzi D: Videotape: Cincinnati Sportsmetrics: *A Jump Training Program Designed for the Prevention of Knee Injuries*. Cincinnati, Ohio, Cincinnati Sportsmedicine Research and Education Foundation, 1997.
65. Kao JT, Giangarra CE, Singer G, Martin S: A comparison of outpatient and inpatient anterior cruciate ligament reconstruction surgery. *Arthroscopy* 1995;11:151–156.
66. Malek MM, DeLuca JV, Kunkle KL, Knable KR: Outpatient ACL surgery: A review of safety, practicality, and economy, in Pritchard DJ (ed): *Instructional Course Lectures 45*. Rosemont, IL, American Academy of Orthopaedic Surgeons, 1996, pp 281–286.

67. Caraffa A, Cerulli G, Projetti M, Aisa G, Rizzo A: Prevention of anterior cruciate ligament injuries in soccer: A prospective controlled study of proprioceptive training. *Knee Surg Sports Traumatol Arthrosc* 1996;4:19–21.

68. Ettlinger CF, Johnson RJ, Shealy JE: A method to help reduce the risk of serious knee sprains incurred in alpine skiing. *Am J Sports Med* 1995;23:531–537.

69. Hewett TE, Riccobene JV, Lindenfeld TN: The effect of neuromuscular training on the incidence of knee injury in female athletes. A prospective study. *Am J Sports Med* 1999;27:699-706.

70. Arendt E, Agel J, Dick R: Profile of the noncontact ACL-injured athlete, in *Prevention of Noncontact ACL Injuries*. Rosemont, IL, American Academy of Orthopaedic Surgeons, 2001.

71. Hewett TE, Stroupe AL, Nance TA, Noyes FR: Plyometric training in female athletes: Decreased impact forces and increased hamstring torques. *Am J Sports Med* 1996;24:765–773.

Chapter 12

Stress Fractures in the Female Athlete

Lisa R. Callahan, MD

Introduction

Stress fractures were first described approximately 150 years ago as "march fractures" in military personnel. In the decades since, they have been recognized as overuse injuries of bone that are common in athletes as well as military populations. Traditionally, variables such as training errors, anatomic and biomechanical differences, road surface, and footwear were blamed for this injury, which occurs when repetitive stress applied to the skeleton exceeds the bone's reparative capability. Recently, it has become clear that this injury is even more common in women than in men, generating a great amount of interest in other possible contributing factors, such as underlying bone health, menstrual irregularities, and dietary restrictions.

This chapter will review the current understanding of stress fracture etiology and treatment with special attention to the variables that make stress fractures a particular concern for female athletes.

Epidemiology and Risk Factors

With the growth in popularity of both recreational and competitive athletics, and the ready availability of sophisticated imaging techniques, stress fractures have become a frequently diagnosed overuse injury. They have been reported in practically all sports,[1–7] with the greatest reported incidence in running, accounting for 4.4% to 15.6% of all injuries to runners.[4,8]

Numerous investigators have reported increased numbers of stress fractures in women, with reported relative risk ranging from 1.5 to 12 times greater in women than in men.[1,6,8–11] However, much of the oft-quoted epidemiologic data is from military experience. When these data are excluded, and only athletes are considered, the increased risk to female athletes is generally reported as no more than 3.5 to 4 times that of male athletes.[1,5,12–15] In fact, a recent study by Bennell and associates[2] showed no significant difference between elite male and female runners. This raises the possibility that when equally highly trained, female and male athletes may experience similar rates of stress fractures.

The lower extremity is the most frequent site of stress fractures in both women and men, with most stress fractures reported in the tibia regardless of gender.[4,5,12] The femur, pelvis, and metatarsals are more common locations of stress fractures in women than in men, while the fibula is more commonly a site of stress fracture in men.[1,2,10,12,16]

Traditionally, stress fractures have been labeled as either fatigue fractures or insufficiency fractures. The former occurs when an abnormal amount of stress is placed on a normal bone, whereas the latter results from a normal stress applied to an abnormal bone. This labeling suggests that fatigue-type fractures should be seen in athletes, while insufficiency fractures occur in sufferers of osteoporosis. It fails to account for the unique but not uncommon development of stress fracture resulting from abnormal stress applied to an abnormal bone, as appears to occur in the female athlete triad. (The female athlete triad, consisting of disordered eating, amenorrhea, and osteoporosis, is discussed in detail in Chapter 32.) It is unknown how many of the stress fractures sustained by female athletes belong to this third category.

Bone size and density, anatomy and biomechanics, conditioning, nutrition, and hormonal state are elements receiving attention as possible contributors to the increased risk of stress fractures in women. Much of the current literature, although compelling, is anecdotal; rigorous, prospective studies are needed to establish which factors are causative and which are merely associative.

Bone Size and Density

The independent roles of bone size and density in stress fracture development are unclear. A frequent assumption is that stress fractures occur more frequently in women simply because their bones are smaller than men's bones. Narrowness of the tibia has been associated positively with an increased risk for stress fracture, independent of gender.[4,14] Ballet dancers have been found to have cortical hypertrophy in the tibia as well as the other bones of the lower extremity, which has been postulated to be a protective response to repetitive load,[15] occurring most consistently in female dancers.

It has been known for quite some time that decreased bone mineral density (BMD) is positively correlated with increased risk for insufficiency fractures; whether or not a similar decrease is associated with stress fractures in female athletes is currently an area of intense investigation. Myburgh and associates[17] found a significantly lower BMD in athletes with stress fractures, although male athletes were also included in this study. Bennell and associates[12] found that mean BMD was somewhat lower in female track and field athletes with stress fractures than in those without stress fractures, but the difference was not great enough to be statistically significant. Cline and associates[18] found no difference in BMD in female US Army recruits with and without stress fractures. Race was not evaluated as a possible confounding variable in this study, which included black, white, and Hispanic women, although previous military studies have shown whites are at greater risk of stress fractures than blacks. It has been postulated that this is secondary to a protective effect provided by higher BMD.[1] Unpublished data from a retrospective study at the Women's Sports Medicine Center at the Hospital for Special Surgery in New York City concluded that female athletes with stress fractures of cancellous bone had significantly lower BMD, whereas those with stress fractures of cortical bone did not. A larger prospective study is in process to explore this finding.

Currently, there is no consensus recommendation for obtaining BMD measurements in the female athlete with a stress fracture. A large, carefully controlled study is needed to investigate BMD as an independent risk factor for stress fracture in female athletes.

Hormonal Influence

The relationship between menstrual dysfunction and stress injury to bone is another area of great interest in the female athlete. Adequate quantities of estrogen are required for development of optimal peak bone mass. Amenorrhea and oligomenorrhea may result in loss of 2% of bone mass per year at a time when a young woman should be gaining 2% to 4% bone mass per year,[19] resulting in decreased vertebral and peripheral BMD in amenorrheic female athletes.[20–24] To date, studies indicate that such loss is not reversible even when normal menses are restored.[14,21,22,25,26]

There appears to be a strong association between menstrual abnormalities and stress fracture occurrence. The study by Bennell and associates,[12] which did not show statistically significant decreases in BMD, did find that stress fractures were more common in athletes with a history of menstrual dysfunction. A study of female Marines also found a positive association between stress fracture and menstrual dysfunction.[27] Yet another study reported that stress fractures occurred in 49% of women runners with a history of very irregular menses and 29% of those with a history of regular menses.[28]

Several reports of an inverse association between oral contraceptive use and stress fractures[12,14,24,28,29] have led physicians who work with female athletes to recommend hormone replacement therapy in the setting of amenorrhea. One survey of sports medicine physicians showed that 92% had prescribed replacement hormone therapy for amenorrheic female athletes. While it has been assumed that this therapy reduces the incidence of stress fractures by improving bone density or at least reducing bone loss, no controlled study to date has confirmed this popular belief.[30]

Nutritional Factors

The role of nutrition is one of the most poorly understood but frequently suspected risk factors for stress fracture development. There are very few controlled studies that include evaluation of nutritional factors, although it is known that many female athletes practice disordered eating behaviors including bingeing, purging, use of diet pills and laxatives, and aggressive restriction of fat, protein, or total caloric intake. Bennell and associates[12] found that female track and field athletes with stress fractures scored higher on the EAT-40 test (a validated, 40 question eating attitudes test) and had a higher incidence of restrictive eating habits, increasing their risk of stress fracture eightfold. It has been postulated that inadequate total caloric intake causes an energy deficit state[14,31–33] that contributes to bone loss, but it is unclear exactly how this relates to stress fracture incidence. Disordered eating, amenorrhea, and low BMD resulting in osteoporosis in the young woman with vigorous exercise habits has become well-recognized as the female athlete triad. It is critical that physicians recognize that not all female athletes with stress fractures are at risk for the female athlete triad, an error that could negatively impact the tremendous gains that women have made in the world of athletics. However, some studies suggest that osteoporosis associated with the female athlete triad is not reversible, even with calcium supplementation and estrogen replacement therapy or resumption of menses.[14,26,31] Therefore, it is imperative that physicians working with female athletes evaluate risk factors for the triad, especially in the setting of stress injury to bone.

Other Risk Factors

Many other factors have been implicated in the development of stress fractures, including training patterns and surface, footwear, biomechanical and anatomic variations, and conditioning. It is not clear whether any of these variables are of more concern in women than in men. Some suspect that the amount of muscle mass in the leg is inversely related to the development of lower extremity stress fracture,[4] which would increase relative risk of injury in women with less muscle mass. Controlled studies of strength training programs would be helpful in evaluating this possible structural variable. Additionally, some investigators have reported an increased incidence of stress fractures in female military recruits who were less physically fit prior to entering a specific training program.[18,27] Similarly, controlled studies of conditioning programs and training patterns would help to delineate such factors.

Diagnosis and Treatment

Clinical presentation, imaging, and treatment of stress fractures is not known to vary with gender. However, in the female athlete with a stress fracture, it is prudent to record nutritional and menstrual histories. Because the exact role of nutrition in stress fracture etiology is unknown, it may be wise to also query young men with stress fractures about their dietary habits. Although eating disorders and disordered eating are reported much more frequently in women than in men, male athletes have been known to suffer from such behaviors as well. If nutritional status is an independent risk factor for stress fracture, male athletes with disordered eating may also be at increased risk.

Most stress fractures are uncomplicated and can be treated successfully with conservative intervention, regardless of gender. It is imperative that the athlete stop the causative activity for healing to occur; it is equally important for the treating physician to recognize that doing so may be especially anxiety provoking for women with body image concerns. By encouraging an appropriate alternative activity such as stationary biking or exercise in a pool, the treating physician can decrease any anxiety associated with cessation of the original activity, possibly improving compliance with the treatment protocol while preventing loss of aerobic conditioning. As muscle mass has been inversely correlated with stress fracture occurrence,[4] a strength training program may be helpful in prevention of recurrence, as well as providing another alternate activity while healing occurs. It is not known whether such a program would be more beneficial in women than in men.

Although most stress fractures do respond to conservative treatment, it is important to note that some stress fractures require a more aggressive management strategy, with immobilization, strict avoidance of weightbearing, and consideration of surgical fixation. The femoral neck is one such site; femoral neck stress fractures have been seen predominately in women. Two recent case reports of femoral neck stress fractures were in amenorrheic female athletes, both of whom had fractures requiring surgical repair.[34,35] It is unknown if the presence of any of the aforementioned risk factors, including amenorrhea and low BMD, have predictive value for need for surgical intervention.

References

1. Bennell KL, Brukner PD: Epidemiology and site specificity of stress fractures. *Clin Sports Med* 1997;16:179–196.
2. Bennell KL, Malcolm SA, Thomas SA, Wark JD, Brukner PD: The incidence and distribution of stress fractures in competitive track and field athletes: A twelve-month prospective study. *Am J Sports Med* 1996;24:211–217.
3. Karlson KA: Rib stress fractures in elite rowers: A case series and proposed mechanism. *Am J Sports Med* 1998;26:516–519.
4. Leach RE, Zecher SB: Stress fractures, in Guten GN (ed): *Running Injuries.* Philadelphia, PA, WB Saunders, 1997, pp 30–42.
5. Matheson GO, Clement DB, McKenzie DC, Taunton JE, Lloyd-Smith DR, MacIntyre JG: Stress fractures in athletes: A study of 320 cases. *Am J Sports Med* 1987;15:46–58.
6. Reeder MT, Dick BH, Atkins JK, Pribis AB, Martinez JM: Stress fractures: Current concepts of diagnosis and treatment. *Sports Med* 1996;22:198–212.
7. Taimela S, Kujala UM, Orava S: Two consecutive rib stress fractures in a female competitive swimmer. *Clin J Sport Med* 1995;5:254–257.
8. Burr DB: Bone, exercise, and stress fractures. *Exerc Sport Sci Rev* 1997;25:171–194.
9. Greaney RB, Gerber FH, Laughlin RL, et al: Distribution and natural history of stress fractures in US Marine recruits. *Radiology* 1983;146:339–346.
10. Hulkko A, Orava S: Stress fractures in athletes. *Int J Sports Med* 1987;8:221–226.
11. Milgrom C, Giladi M, Stein M, et al: Stress fractures in military recruits: A prospective study showing an unusually high incidence. *J Bone Joint Surg* 1985;67B:732–735.
12. Bennell KL, Malcolm SA, Thomas SA, et al: Risk factors for stress fractures in female track- and field-athletes: A retrospective analysis. *Clin J Sport Med* 1995;5:229–235.
13. Kadel NJ, Teitz CC, Kronmal RA: Stress fractures in ballet dancers. *Am J Sports Med* 1992;20:445–449.
14. Nattiv A, Armsey TD Jr: Stress injury to bone in the female athlete. *Clin Sports Med* 1997;16:197–224.
15. Schneider HJ, King AY, Bronson JL, Miller EH: Stress injuries and developmental change of lower extremities in ballet dancers. *Radiology* 1974;113:627–632.

16. Coady CM, Micheli LJ: Stress fractures in the pediatric athlete. *Clin Sports Med* 1997;16:225–238.
17. Myburgh KH, Hutchins J, Fataar AB, Hough SF, Noakes TD: Low bone density is an etiologic factor for stress fractures in athletes. *Ann Intern Med* 1990;113:754–759.
18. Cline AD, Jansen GR, Melby CL: Stress fractures in female army recruits: Implications of bone density, calcium intake, and exercise. J *Am Coll Nutr* 1998;17:128–135.
19. Lane JM, Riley EH, Wirganowicz PZ: Osteoporosis: Diagnosis and treatment. *J Bone Joint Surg* 1996;78A:618–632.
20. Cann CE, Martin MC, Genant HK, Jaffe RB: Decreased spinal mineral content in amenorrheic women. *JAMA* 1984;251:626–629.
21. Drinkwater BL, Bruemner B, Chesnut CH III: Menstrual history as a determinant of current bone density in young athletes. *JAMA* 1990;263:545–548.
22. Drinkwater BL, Nilson K, Chesnut CH III, Bremner WJ, Shainholtz S, Southworth MB: Bone mineral content of amenorrheic and eumenorrheic athletes. *N Engl J Med* 1984;311:277–281.
23. Lindberg JS, Fears WB, Hunt MM, Powell MR, Boll D, Wade CE: Exercise-induced amenorrhea and bone density. *Ann Intern Med* 1984;101:647–648.
24. Marcus R, Cann C, Madvig P, et al: Menstrual function and bone mass in elite women distance runners: Endocrine and metabolic features. *Ann Intern Med* 1985;102:158–163.
25. Lindberg JS, Powell MR, Hunt MM, Ducey DE, Wade CE: Increased vertebral bone mineral in response to reduced exercise in amenorrheic runners. *West J Med* 1987;146:39–42.
26. Wirganowicz PZ, Lane JM: Postmenopausal osteoporosis: An update for the clinician. *J Musculoskel Med* 1996;13:29–38.
27. Winfield AC, Moore J, Bracker M, Johnson CW: Risk factors associated with stress reactions in female Marines. *Mil Med* 1997;162:698–702.
28. Barrow GW, Saha S: Menstrual irregularity and stress fractures in collegiate female distance runners. *Am J Sports Med* 1988;16:209–216.
29. Loucks AB, Horvath SM: Athletic amenorrhea: A review. *Med Sci Sports Exerc* 1985;17:56–72.
30. Haberland CA, Seddick D, Marcus R, Bachrach LK: A physician survey of therapy for exercise-associated amenorrhea: A brief report. *Clin J Sport Med* 1995;5:246–250.
31. Nattiv A, Agostini R, Drinkwater B, Yeager KK: The female athlete triad: The inter-relatedness of disordered eating, amenorrhea, and osteoporosis. *Clin Sports Med* 1994;13:405–418.
32. Putukian M: The female triad: Eating disorders, amenorrhea, and osteoporosis. *Med Clin North Am* 1994;78:345–356.
33. Shangold MM: Menstruation and menstrual disorders, in Shangold MM, Mirkin G (eds): *Women and Exercise: Physiology and Sports Medicine*, ed 2. Philadelphia, PA, FA Davis, 1994, pp 152–171.
34. Haddad FS, Bann S, Hill RA, Jones DH: Displaced stress fracture of the femoral neck in an active amenorrhoeic adolescent. *Br J Sports Med* 1997;31:70–72.
35. Voss L, DaSilva M, Trafton PG: Bilateral femoral neck stress fractures in an amenorrheic athlete. *Am J Orthop* 1997;26:789–792.

Chapter 13

The Role of Physical Activity and Injury in Knee and Hip Osteoarthritis

Leena Sharma, MD

Introduction

As the most common form of arthritis, osteoarthritis (OA) is associated with substantial individual and societal cost. OA is a leading cause of chronic disability at older ages. Disability resulting from OA is in large part caused by knee and hip involvement. Knee OA alone is as often associated with disability as heart and chronic obstructive lung diseases.1 Over 13% of US residents aged 55 to 64 years and over 17% aged 65 to 74 years have pain and functional limitation related to knee OA alone.2 The societal burden of OA relates to its pervasiveness. It is estimated that 12.1% of Americans (or 21 million in 1990) between ages 25 and 75 years have clinical signs and symptoms of OA.3 The increase in the prevalence of symptomatic OA with age, coupled with the inadequacy of symptom-relieving or disease-modifying treatment, contributes to the overall burden of OA.

Epidemiologic studies have demonstrated that gender influences the risk of OA at certain sites. The mechanism of the effect of gender is not well understood. Gender effects are likely complex and may be mediated through multiple, diverse routes that possibly include hormonal influences on cartilage and/or bone metabolism and gender differences in the mechanical environment of the joint. Within the last several years, there has been an increase in sports and exercise participation by women in all age groups. With this has come a concern about the possibility of an increase in the development of OA either as a direct consequence of certain physical activities or via injury. However, certain effects of sports and exercise may well protect against the development of OA and/or the disability with which it is associated. Whether the positive or negative effects of physical activity on OA risk differ between men and women is unclear.

The purpose of this chapter is to review, for hip and knee OA, gender differences in OA incidence and prevalence; the epidemiologic evidence of relationships between physical activity and OA and between injury and OA; whether there is any evidence that physical activity or injury may be a more potent risk factor for OA in women than in men; and potential effects of sports and exercise on pain and disability in OA.

The Definition of OA

The 20th century has witnessed an evolution in the definition of OA from hypertrophic arthritis at the outset of the century to the current consensus definition:[4]

> OA diseases are a result of both mechanical and biologic events that destabilize the normal coupling of degradation and synthesis of articular cartilage chondrocytes and extracellular matrix, and subchondral bone. Although they may be initiated by multiple factors, including genetic, developmental, metabolic, and traumatic, OA diseases involve all of the tissues of the diarthrodial joint. Ultimately, OA diseases are manifested by morphologic, biochemical, molecular, and biomechanical changes of both cells and matrix which lead to a softening, fibrillation, ulceration, loss of articular cartilage, sclerosis and eburnation of subchondral bone, osteophytes, and subchondral cysts. When clinically evident, OA diseases are characterized by joint pain, tenderness, limitation of movement, crepitus, occasional effusion, and variable degrees of inflammation without systemic effects.

OA usually is classified as primary (idiopathic) or secondary (secondary to metabolic conditions, anatomic abnormalities, trauma, or inflammatory arthritis).[5] The proportion of idiopathic OA that is attributable to overuse or injury is unclear.

Knee OA

Both the incidence and prevalence of knee OA are greater in women than in men. Oliveria and associates[6] evaluated the incidence of symptomatic, radiographic knee OA in a large health maintenance organization (HMO) in central Massachusetts; they found higher rates in women and an increase in incidence with age until age 80 years, after which there was a leveling off or decline in the for all joints.[6] The overall age- and sex-standardized incidence for knee OA was 240/100,000 person-years (95% confidence interval [CI], 218 to 262). Among women, the incidence rates for knee OA ranged from a low of 0/100,000 person-years among those ages 20 to 29 years to a high of 1,082/100,000 person-years for those ages 70 to 79 years. Among men, the incidence rates for knee OA ranged from a low of 5/100,000 person-years among those ages 20 to 29 years to a high of 839 among those ages 70 to 79 years. In a Framingham study of subjects with a mean age of 70.8 years (range, 63 to 91) and no knee OA at baseline, in women, 2%/yr developed radiographic knee OA, and about 1%/yr developed symptomatic, radiographic knee OA, as compared with 1.4% and 0.7% of men, respectively.[7] In a population-based study in Holland with participants aged 46 to 66 years at baseline followed for 12 years, 25% of women (about 2%/yr) and 10% of men (about 0.8%/yr) developed radiographic knee OA.[8]

There is a striking increase in the prevalence of radiographic knee OA with age in women, from 1% to 4% in those aged 24 to 45 years to 53% to 55% in those 80 years and older.[9–11] Framingham data suggest about one third of older women with radiographic OA are symptomatic.[10] In men, the prevalence rises from 1% to 6% in those 45 years and younger to 22% to 33% in those 80 years and older.[9–11]

Gender, Physical Activity, and Injury in the Development of Knee OA

Gender and Hormonal Factors

Gender influences the risk of knee OA. Available data suggest that the effect of gender in knee OA is independent of physical activity and injury. In a longitudinal study of the Framingham cohort (mean age 70.5 years), in analyses adjusted for age, body mass index (BMI), smoking, injury, chondrocalcinosis, hand OA, and physical activity, women had a greater risk than men (odds ratio [OR], 1.8; 95% CI, 1.1 to 3.1) of developing OA over an 8-year period.[12]

Several cross-sectional studies support a role for gender in the development of knee OA. Analyses of National Health and Nutrition Examination Survey (NHANES) I data revealed that in those aged 45 to 74 years, bilateral knee OA was twice as prevalent in women as in men.[13] No gender difference was seen in the prevalence of unilateral OA. Anderson and Felson[14] found that, among NHANES I subjects aged 35 to 74 years, radiographic OA increased with age in both sexes, and beginning in those aged 45 to 54 years was greater in women than in men.[14] In the Zoetermeer survey,[11] knee OA was more prevalent in women at all ages. Though mild radiographic OA was more prevalent in women, severe radiographic OA was much more prevalent in women.

A significant gender difference in the incidence and prevalence of knee OA first becomes apparent during the menopausal years,[6,14] suggesting a role for hormonal factors. Estrogen may have direct effects on articular cartilage or may influence OA development via its effects on bone. Postmenopausal estrogen replacement therapy (ERT) may provide some protection against the development of knee OA. Although in many studies the relationship is not statistically significant, the consistency of both the direction and magnitude of the findings is notable, as is the fact that there appears to be a gradient of protection (that is, greater protection conferred with current ERT use versus past use). In a longitudinal Framingham study, the OR for past ERT use versus never use was 0.8 (95% CI, 0.5 to 1.4) and for current use versus never use, 0.4 (95% CI, 0.1 to 3.0), adjusting for age, BMI, femoral neck bone mineral density, physical activity, weight change, knee injury, smoking, and baseline knee OA severity.[15] Similarly, a nonsignificant protective effect for incident knee osteophytes was seen with current ERT in the longitudinal Chingford study (OR, 0.41; 95% CI, 0.12 to 1.42), adjusted for hysterectomy, smoking, physical activity, knee pain, and social class.[16]

Physical Activity

It is believed that abnormal joint anatomy, malalignment, previous injury, surgery, joint laxity, obesity, disturbed innervation, or muscle weakness may increase the physical activity-associated risk of knee OA.[17] The interaction of these factors with physical activity has not been examined as yet.

Occupational Activity The relationship between occupational physical activity and knee OA is better understood in men than in women, in large part because previous studies have predominantly assessed paid labor, giving less attention to homemaking or child-rearing tasks. In a longitudinal study of the Framingham cohort, in men, risk of later radiographic knee OA was highest in those whose jobs, ascertained 20 years earlier, had at least medium physical demands and involved knee bending (OR, 2.2; 95% CI, 1.4 to 3.6) versus a job with sedentary demands and no knee bending.18 Analyses were adjusted for age, BMI, history of knee injury, education, and smoking. Analyses of NHANES I data revealed that radiographic knee OA was more common in men and women (aged 55 to 64 years) whose current job by title included much knee bending versus some knee bending (OR, 2.45; 95% CI, 1.2 to 4.9 for men and OR, 3.49; 95% CI, 1.2 to 10.5 for women), after adjusting for race, education level, and BMI.14 In women, but not in men, jobs with high versus moderate strength demands were associated with knee OA (OR, 3.1; 95% CI, 1.1 to 9.4). Kivimaki and associates19 directly measured duration of knee bending activities in male carpenters, floor layers, and painters and also found an association between knee bending and knee OA.19

In a case-control study, an increased risk of knee OA was found in those whose main job entailed > 30 min/day squatting or kneeling, or climbing more than 10 flights of stairs, adjusting for BMI and the presence of Heberden's nodes.[20] Regularly lifting > 25 kg, as well as kneeling, squatting, or climbing stairs was associated with a fivefold increase in risk of knee OA, versus no exposure to these activities. No association was found between knee OA and prolonged walking, standing, sitting, or driving. Men and women were not analyzed separately. Other studies have suggested an increased knee OA in male miners[21] and dock workers.[22]

Nonoccupational Physical Activity Although a link between elite athletics and knee OA has been demonstrated in men and women, there is currently no evidence that recreational running or leisure activities are associated with knee OA.

A comparison of 81 female former elite athletes including 67 runners and 14 tennis players to age-matched women revealed that ex-athletes had greater rates of tibiofemoral OA (OR, 3.57; 95% CI, 1.89 to 6.71) and patellofemoral OA (OR, 3.50; 95% CI, 1.80 to 6.81) than did controls after adjusting for height and weight differences.[23] Results were not affected by further adjustment for injury, smoking, menopause, hysterectomy, BMI, age, or weight. In another study involving male ex-elite athletes, soccer players had the highest prevalence of tibiofemoral OA (26%) and weight lifters the highest prevalence of patellofemoral OA (28%).[24] Previous knee injury, higher BMI at age 20, and hours of participation in team sports predicted tibiofemoral OA, and previous knee injury, higher BMI at age 20, years spent in heavy work and work involving kneeling or squatting predicted patellofemoral OA. Of note, unlike the general population,[25] elevations in BMI well within the nonobese range were linked to knee OA in these athletes, suggesting that the pathogenetic role of excess weight in knee OA may be modified by the nature and intensity of physical activity.

Although elite runners may have an increased risk of knee OA, this does not appear to be the case for recreational runners. In a prospective comparison of rates of knee OA development over a 5-year period between runners and controls matched for age, sex, education, and occupation, Lane and associates[26] found that, of 73 subjects, nine developed knee OA by American College of Rheumatology (ACR) criteria: five were controls (4 men and 1 woman), and 4 were runners (3 men and 1 woman). All subjects were between the ages of 50 and 72 years. The women runners averaged 282 min of exercise/wk (225 min running) at baseline and 335 min of exercise/wk (196 min of running) at 5-year follow-up. Running did not accelerate the development of radiographic or clinical knee OA in women or in men. Panush and associates[27] similarly found no difference in rate of OA development between 17 male runners (53% marathon runners) and age- and weight-matched controls.

A link between leisure activities and knee OA in older subjects has not been detected. In a case-control study, there was no association in men or in women aged 55 years and older between knee OA and lifetime leisure activities including walking (> 1 hr/day), cycling (> 2 hrs/wk), gardening (> once/wk), dancing (> 1 hr/wk), and outdoor sports (> once/wk).[28]

In a study of subjects 79 years of age, Bagge and associates[29] found no association between leisure physical activity (light, moderate, or heavy, accounting for number of years) and knee OA in all subjects considered together or in men and women considered separately; as noted by the authors, ability to detect a relationship may have been limited by the small number of subjects in the heavy-activity group.

Composite Physical Activity Available data raise the possibility that the physical activity-associated risk of OA may differ on the basis of age. There is currently no evidence that the relationship between physical activity and knee OA differs between men and women. A Framingham study found that habitual physical activity (a weighted and summed measure of hours/day at various activities), assessed at two previous examinations (1954 to 1957 and 1971 to 1973), did not predict the presence of radiographic knee OA in 1983 to 1985, in unadjusted analyses or after adjusting for age, BMI, injury, smoking, and education.[30] The mean age of the subjects was 73 years (range, 63 to 93). In the highest quartile of habitual physical activity compared with the least active, the adjusted OR for men was 1.34 (95% CI, 0.66 to 2.74) and for women was 1.09 (95% CI, 0.63 to 1.90).

Longitudinal studies have had conflicting results. In the Chingford population (1,000 women aged 45 to 64 years, mean 54), physical activity was not linked to incident OA in the uninvolved knee in those with unilateral knee OA,[31] nor was it linked to incident OA in the full cohort;[16] as the authors note, these studies may have lacked sufficient power.

Longitudinal Framingham studies involving an older cohort have detected a link between current physical activity and knee OA.[12,32] In participants with a mean age of 70.1 years at baseline (including 295 women and 178 men), the odds of developing knee OA between two examinations about 8 years apart were increased by heavy physical activity assessed by a questionnaire at midpoint in the study, adjusting for age, gender, BMI, weight loss, injury, health status, calorie intake, and smoking. OR steadily rose between 2, 3, and 4 hours of heavy activity per day. For > 4 hrs/day, OR was 7.2 (95% CI, 2.5 to 20) for radiographic OA and 5.3 (95% CI, 1.2 to 24) for symptomatic OA.[32] Risk was greatest in those subjects in the highest tertile of BMI. No relationship was detected between radiographic or symptomatic knee OA and moderate or light physical activity, number of blocks walked, or number of flights of stairs climbed daily. Findings were similar in men and women.

Injury

Several cross-sectional studies have demonstrated a link between knee injury and knee OA.[13,28,33] There is currently no epidemiologic evidence that injury is more likely to lead to knee OA in women. Although linked to both unilateral and bilateral knee OA, knee injury was more closely associated with unilateral OA in analyses of NHANES I data.[13] Knee injury (OR, 16.3; 95% CI, 6.50 to 40.89) was a stronger predictor than obesity (OR, 3.4; 95% CI, 1.55 to 7.29) of unilateral knee OA. More men (4%) than women (3%) reported at least one of the three categories of knee injury (severe knee twisting, fracture, other injury). Although bilateral knee OA was more common in women, there was no difference between men and women in the prevalence of unilateral knee OA.

In a case-control study, a history of knee injury was associated with symptomatic knee OA (OR, 3.4; 95% CI, 1.7 to 6.7) adjusting for BMI, family history of knee arthritis, and Heberden's nodes. Also, injury increased the risk of OA at both tibiofemoral and patellofemoral sites.[28] Analyses were not performed separately for men and women.

In the Michigan Bone Health Study involving 573 white women aged 24 to 45 years, 478 women reported no previous knee injury.[33] In these subjects there was radiographic evidence of knee OA in eight right knees and 13 left knees. Of the 95 women who reported a history of knee injury, radiographic evidence of OA was present in six right knees and six left knees.

The link between knee injury and OA has not been confirmed in longitudinal studies of the Framingham or Chingford populations.[12,16] This likely reflects insufficient power, or, as described by Felson and associates,[12] in the older Framingham cohort, those with past knee injury may have developed knee OA before the baseline examination and would therefore have been ineligible for the current study, which included only those free of disease at baseline. However, there remains a possibility that recall bias has contributed to the association detected in cross-sectional studies.

Risk Factors for Knee OA Influenced by Sports and Exercise

Weight

Epidemiologic studies have strongly demonstrated that obesity is linked to the development of knee OA. In the Framingham cohort, baseline weight predicted the presence of knee OA 36 years later;[34] a decrease in BMI of 2 units or more over the previous 10 years decreased the odds of knee OA;[25] and both baseline BMI and weight change were linked to the risk of incident knee OA in an 8-year study of subjects free of radiographic OA at baseline.[12] Findings were consistent in a 4-year study of the Chingford population.[16] Also, in Chingford subjects with unilateral knee OA, BMI predicted development of OA in the uninvolved knee.[31] By preventing weight gain or contributing to weight loss in overweight subjects, appropriate sports and exercise may protect against the development of knee OA.

Muscle Weakness and Proprioception

Quadriceps weakness may be a risk factor and not only a consequence of knee OA. In a community-based study of subjects 65 years or older, among women with tibiofemoral OA, extensor weakness was present in those without significant knee pain or muscle atrophy.[35] After adjusting for body weight, age, and sex, quadriceps weakness remained predictive of radiographic knee OA. In women after adjusting for body weight, knee extensor strength was 18% lower at baseline among those who developed incident knee OA than among controls.[36] Reduced quadriceps strength relative to body weight may be a risk factor for knee OA. Also, there is some evidence that knee proprioception declines with age[37] and that varus-valgus laxity increases with age.[38] Exercise may preserve periarticular muscle strength, improve proprioceptive accuracy, and by increasing strength, compensate for soft-tissue changes that occur with aging. By enhancing neuromuscular joint protection through such routes, exercise may reduce the risk of knee OA.

Progression of Knee OA

Several studies involving cohorts of subjects with established knee OA to determine risk factors for disease progression have not revealed a relationship between gender and OA progression assessed using a variety of approaches to assess progression.[7,38–43] Single studies have not found a relationship between occupational factors[39] or physical activity[31] and knee OA progression. Gender differences in the potency of physical activity or injury as risk factors for disease progression have not been examined.

Hip OA

Oliveria and associates[6] report an overall age- and sex-standardized incidence for symptomatic, radiographic hip OA of 88/100,000 person-years (95% CI, 75 to 101).[6] The incidence rates for women ranged from a low of 0/100,000 person-years among those ages 20 to 29 years and 40 to 49 years to a high of 583/100,000 person-years among those ages 70 to 79 years. For men the incidence rates ranged from a low of 0/100,000 person-years among those ages 20 to 29 years to a high of 445/100,000 person-years among those ages 70 to 79 years.

Over an 8-year period, Nevitt and associates[44] found that 3.5% to 11.9% (depending on how hip OA was defined) of women aged 65 years and over developed incident radiographic changes of hip OA.

Lawrence and associates[9] found radiographic hip OA in 6.2% of women and 16.5% of men older than 55 years. Danielsson and associates[45] found that the prevalence of radiographic hip OA rose from 0.4% in women between 40 and 54 years of age to 10% in women aged 85 to 89 years, and from 0% in men aged 40 to 44 years to 11.5% in men aged 80 to 84 years.[45] Van Saase and associates[11] found hip OA prevalence rose from 2.6% in women aged 45 to 49 years to 26% in women 80 years or older, and from 2.8% in men aged 45 to 49 years to 11.1% in men 80 years or older.

Gender, Physical Activity, and Injury in the Development of Hip OA

Gender

Available information suggests that the female preponderance of knee and hand OA is not seen with hip OA, although there is some evidence that hip OA is more common in women than in men at older ages. Danielsson and associates[45] found no difference in the prevalence of hip OA between men and women. Jorring,[46] however, found an overall female-to-male ratio of 3:2. For mild hip OA, there was no gender difference. In those older than 60 years, severe hip OA was more common in women. In the Zoetermeer survey, between ages 55 and 64 years, hip OA appeared to be more common in men; in those aged 65 years and older, hip OA was more common in women.[11] Analyses of the NHANES I data revealed no association between hip OA and gender, in univariate or multivariate analyses.[47] Parity, age at menarche, and age at menopause were not linked to the presence of hip OA.

Consistent with results of studies involving women with knee OA, in a cross-sectional study of over 4,000 white women ≥ 65 years from the Study of Osteoporotic Fractures, current users of ERT had a significantly reduced risk of any hip OA (OR, 0.62; 95% CI, 0.49 to 0.86), and of moderate to severe hip OA.[48] Current users for ≥ 10 years had a greater reduction in risk of any hip OA versus users < 10 years. Current use for ≥ 10 years was associated with a nonsignificant trend for a reduced risk of moderate to severe symptomatic hip OA.

Physical Activity

Occupational Activity Reports are not available concerning the relationship between occupational activity (either outside or in the home) and hip OA in women. As summarized by Maetzel and associates,[49] a consistently positive though weak relationship between work-related exposure (farming in particular) and hip OA in men has been reported. Farming for ≥ 10 years versus < 1 year was associated with hip OA (OR, 2.0; 95% CI, 0.9 to 4.4) adjusting for age, height, and weight.[50,51]

There is evidence that high workloads predispose to hip OA. Veterans Administration clinic patients with primary hip OA and controls were surveyed about lifetime occupational and recreational activities and categorized based on estimates of joint compression forces produced.[52] Subjects in the intermediate work category had 2.0 times (95% CI, 1.0 to 3.8) and those in the heavy work category had 2.4 times (95% CI, 1.3 to 4.3) the odds of having hip OA. The results for heavy work were minimally affected by adjusting for obesity, history of cancer, or football participation or running.

Nonoccupational Physical Activity There is some evidence linking high levels of nonoccupational physical activity to hip OA in men; data are not available for women. A case-control study of men up to age 49 years with total hip replacements versus men from the general population revealed that high exposure to sports of all kinds (in hours, based on subject report) increased the risk of hip OA (relative risk 3.5 to 4.5, depending on number of years of exposure), adjusted for age, BMI, smoking, and occupational physical activity.[53] Track and field sports and racket sports appeared to be associated with the highest risk, although small numbers for individual sports make conclusions difficult.

Puranen and associates[54] found that hip OA prevalence was no greater in male former Finnish champion distance runners (4%) than in controls who were not runners or different from population-based prevalence figures. Marti and associates,[55] however, found, in a study including baseline assessments of intensity of activity, that radiographic changes of hip OA were more prevalent in male former national team long-distance runners than in bobsled competitors or controls. Age and mileage run in 1973 predicted radiographic hip OA in 1988. These findings suggest that high-intensity, high-mileage running in elite athletes may be a risk factor for hip OA in men.

Injury

In analyses of NHANES I data, hip trauma was associated with hip OA (OR, 7.84; 95% CI, 2.11 to 29.10) adjusted for sex, age, race, and education.[47] When men and women were examined separately, injury was more strongly associated with hip OA in men (OR, 24.2; 95% CI, 3.84 to 153.10) than in women (adjusted OR, 4.17; 95% CI, 0.50 to 34.71) adjusting for age, race, and education. Hip trauma was significantly associated with unilateral hip OA (adjusted OR, 13.74; 95% CI, 3.69 to 51.13); no hip trauma was reported among those with bilateral hip OA.

Risk Factors for Hip OA Influenced by Sports and Exercise

Of risk factors for hip OA potentially influenced by sports and exercise, information is available only for body weight. In contrast to the knee, a more modest association between measures of body weight and hip OA has been found. In analyses of NHANES I data, obesity and fat distribution were not associated with hip OA when both men and women were considered together or when each gender was considered separately.[47] Being overweight was, however, more closely associated with bilateral hip OA (OR, 2.0; 95% CI, 0.97 to 4.15) than unilateral hip OA (OR, 0.54; 95% CI, 0.26 to 1.16), adjusting for gender, age, race, and education. In the Zoetermeer survey, obesity was linked to OA in the right but not the left hip in men, and was not linked to OA presence in women.[56] In another study involving men, in which farming was associated with an increased risk of hip OA, the risk was highest in the tallest and heaviest members of the sample, although the association with weight, height, or BMI did not achieve significance.[50]

Potential Effect of Sports and Exercise on Pain and Disability in OA

More information is available for radiographic disease, as outlined in preceding sections, than for symptoms or patient function. Risk factor profiles differ for each of the three domains—structural disease, pain, and disability—although there may be some overlap. Current knowledge of determinants of pain and disability is based upon a number of cross-sectional studies. Determinants of pain in knee OA that are positively influenced by exercise include psychological factors and strength. Among subjects with knee and/or hip OA, an association has been reported between joint pain and poor psychological well-being,[57] "feeling in low spirits,"[58] depression, anxiety, or coping style,[59–61] and hypochondriasis.[62] Quadriceps weakness and pain have also been associated.[61,63]

Determinants of physical function in knee OA that may be positively influenced by exercise include pain coping,[64] psychological well-being,[64] self-efficacy,[65] depression, and/or anxiety.[59–61,66] In a study concurrently examining psychosocial and physiologic factors, Rejeski and associates[65] found that pain and self-efficacy independently predicted physical function, explaining a significant portion of the variance in both self-assessed physical function and task performance even after controlling for aerobic capacity and strength in patients with knee OA.[65] Finally, several studies have linked quadriceps strength and function in knee OA.[63–65,67,68]

Given the myriad positive effects on both psychological (including self-efficacy) and physiological (including strength and aerobic capacity) factors, appropriate sports and exercise have the potential to significantly improve the symptoms and disability associated with lower extremity OA. Used correctly, sports and exercise may have dramatic effects on the preservation of functional independence and the prevention of aging-associated frailty in women and men.

Summary

The incidence and prevalence of knee OA are greater in women, especially after menopause, suggesting that hormonal factors play a role. ERT may protect against the development of knee OA. For physical activity in general, very little information is available to compare the effect of activity between men and women. Occupations requiring at least medium physical demands and knee bending are associated with an increased risk of knee OA in men and probably also in women. Homemaking or child-rearing tasks have been minimally considered in previous studies. Squatting, kneeling, or stair climbing may also be associated with an increased risk of knee OA. A small number of studies suggest an increased risk of OA in elite athletes. Recreational running was not linked with development or progression of knee OA in older subjects. A small number of studies suggest that leisure activity does not increase the risk of OA in elderly subjects, although these studies are limited by the small number of subjects involved in heavy activity. Among studies of composite physical activity, one longitudinal study found the risk of OA to be increased in those participating in heavy physical activity. Although injury and knee OA have been linked in several cross-sectional studies, the association remains to be confirmed in a longitudinal study. At present, there is no evidence that men and women differ with respect to the effect of physical activity or injury on the risk of knee OA.

Less information is available for hip OA. The female preponderance of knee OA is not seen with hip OA although there is some evidence that hip OA is more common in women than men at older ages. ERT may reduce the risk of hip OA. There is no information available concerning physical activity and the risk of hip OA for women. In men, a relationship between work-related exposure (farming, high workload) and hip OA has been reported. Based on a small number of studies, sports exposure and elite running in particular may increase the risk of hip OA in men. Hip injury was more closely associated with hip OA in men than in women.

Though it is believed that risk factors for OA may differ between men and women, little specific information to support this notion is available.

References

1. Guccione AA, Felson DT, Anderson JJ, et al: The effects of specific medical conditions on the functional limitations of elders in the Framingham Study. *Am J Public Health* 1994;84:351–358.
2. Maurer K (ed): *Basic Data On Arthritis: Knee, Hip, and Sacroiliac Joints In Adults Aged 25–74 Years: United States, 1971–1975*. Hyattsville, MD, US Department of Health, Education and Welfare, 1979 [PHS] 79–1661.
3. Lawrence RC, Helmick CG, Arnett FC, et al: Estimates of the prevalence of arthritis and selected musculoskeletal disorders in the United States. *Arthritis Rheum 1998;41:778–799.*
4. Kuettner KE, Goldberg VM: Introduction, in Kuettner KE, Goldberg VM (eds): *Osteoarthritic Disorders*. Rosemont, IL, American Academy of Orthopaedic Surgeons 1995, pp xxi–xxv.
5. Altman R, Asch E, Bloch D, et al: Development of criteria for the classification and reporting of osteoarthritis: Classification of osteoarthritis of the knee. Diagnostic and Therapeutic Criteria Committee of the American Rheumatism Association. *Arthritis Rheum* 1986;29:1039–1049.
6. Oliveria SA, Felson DT, Reed JI, Cirillo PA, Walker AM: Incidence of symptomatic hand, hip, and knee osteoarthritis among patients in a health maintenance organization. *Arthritis Rheum* 1995;38:1134–1141.
7. Felson DT, Zhang Y, Hannan MT, et al: The incidence and natural history of knee osteoarthritis in the elderly: The Framingham Osteoarthritis Study. *Arthritis Rheum* 1995;38:1500–1505.
8. Schouten JSAG: *A 12-Year Follow-Up Study on Osteoarthritis of the Knee in the General Population: An Epidemiological Study of Classification Criteria, Risk Factors and Prognostic Factors*. Rotterdam, The Netherlands, Erasmus University Medical School, 1991. Dissertation.
9. Lawrence JS, Bremner JM, Bier F: Osteo-arthrosis: Prevalence in the population and relationship between symptoms and x-ray changes. *Ann Rheum Dis* 1966;25:1–24.
10. Felson DT, Naimark A, Anderson J, Kazis L, Castelli W, Meenan RF: The prevalence of knee osteoarthritis in the elderly: The Framingham Osteoarthritis Study. *Arthritis Rheum* 1987;30:914–918.
11. van Saase JL, van Romunde LK, Cats A, Vandenbroucke JP, Valkenburg HA: Epidemiology of osteoarthritis: Zoetermeer survey. Comparison of radiological osteoarthritis in a Dutch population with that in 10 other populations. *Ann Rheum Dis* 1989;48:271–280.

12. Felson DT, Zhang Y, Hannan MT, et al: Risk factors for incident radiographic knee osteoarthritis in the elderly: The Framingham Study. *Arthritis Rheum* 1997;40:728–733.
13. Davis MA, Ettinger WH, Neuhaus JM, Cho SA, Hauck WW: The association of knee injury and obesity with unilateral and bilateral osteoarthritis of the knee. *Am J Epidemiol* 1989;130:278–288.
14. Anderson JJ, Felson DT: Factors associated with osteoarthritis of the knee in the first National Health and Nutrition Examination Survey (HANES I): Evidence for an association with overweight, race, and physical demands of work. *Am J Epidemiol* 1988;128:179–189.
15. Zhang Y, McAlindon TE, Hannan MT, et al: Estrogen replacement therapy and worsening of radiographic knee osteoarthritis: The Framingham Study. *Arthritis Rheum* 1998;41:1867–1873.
16. Hart DJ, Doyle DV, Spector TD: Incidence and risk factors for radiographic knee osteoarthritis in middle-aged women: The Chingford Study. *Arthritis Rheum* 1999;42:17–24.
17. Buckwalter JA, Lane NE: Athletics and osteoarthritis. *Am J Sports Med* 1997;25:873–881.
18. Felson DT, Hannan MT, Naimark A, et al: Occupational physical demands, knee bending, and knee osteoarthritis: Results from the Framingham study. *J Rheumatol* 1991;18:1587–1592.
19. Kivimaki J, Riihimaki H, Hanninen K: Knee disorders in carpet and floor layers and painters. *Scand J Work Environ Health* 1992;18:310–316.
20. Cooper C, McAlindon T, Coggon D, Egger P, Dieppe P: Occupational activity and osteoarthritis of the knee. *Ann Rheum Dis* 1994;53:90–93.
21. Kellgren JH, Lawrence JS: Rheumatism in miners: Part II. X-ray study. *Br J Industr Med* 1952;9:197–207.
22. Partridge RE, Duthie JJ: Rheumatism in dockers and civil servants: A comparison of heavy manual and sedentary workers. *Ann Rheum Dis* 1968;27:559–568.
23. Spector TD, Harris PA, Hart DJ, et al: Risk of osteoarthritis associated with long-term weight-bearing sports: A radiologic survey of the hips and knees in female ex-athletes and population controls. *Arthritis Rheum* 1996;39:988–995.
24. Kujala UM, Kettunen J, Paananen H, et al: Knee osteoarthritis in former runners, soccer players, weight lifters, and shooters. *Arthritis Rheum* 1995;38:539–546.
25. Felson DT, Zhang Y, Anthony JM, Naimark A, Anderson JJ: Weight loss reduces the risk for symptomatic knee osteoarthritis in women: The Framingham study. *Ann Intern Med* 1992;116:535–539.
26. Lane NE, Michel B, Bjorkengren A, et al: The risk of osteoarthritis with running and aging: A 5-year longitudinal study. *J Rheumatol* 1993;20:461–468.
27. Panush RS, Hanson CS, Caldwell JR, et al: Is running associated with osteoarthritis? An eight-year follow-up study. *J Clin Rheumatol* Preview: October 1994.
28. Cooper C, McAlindon T, Snow S, et al: Mechanical and constitutional risk factors for symptomatic knee osteoarthritis: Differences between medial tibiofemoral and patellofemoral disease. *J Rheumatol* 1994;21:307–313.
29. Bagge E, Bjelle A, Eden S, Svanborg A: Factors associated with radiographic osteoarthritis: Results from the population study of 70-year-old people in Goteborg. *J Rheumatol* 1991;18:1218–1222.
30. Hannan MT, Felson DT, Anderson JJ, Naimark A: Habitual physical activity is not associated with knee osteoarthritis: The Framingham Study. *J Rheumatol* 1993;20:704–709.

31. Spector TD, Hart DJ, Doyle DV: Incidence and progression of osteoarthritis in women with unilateral knee disease in the general population: The effect of obesity. *Ann Rheum Dis* 1994;53:565–568.

32. McAlindon TE, Wilson PW, Aliabadi P, Weissman B, Felson DT: Level of physical activity and the risk of radiographic and symptomatic knee osteoarthritis in the elderly: The Framingham Study. *Am J Med* 1999;106:151–157.

33. Sowers MF, Hochberg M, Crabbe JP, Muhich A, Crutchfield M, Updike S: Association of bone mineral density and sex hormone levels with osteoarthritis of the hand and knee in premenopausal women. *Am J Epidemiol* 1996;143:38–47.

34. Felson DT, Anderson JJ, Naimark A, Walker AM, Meenan RF: Obesity and knee osteoarthritis: The Framingham study. *Ann Intern Med* 1988;109:18–24.

35. Slemenda C, Brandt KD, Heilman DK, et al: Quadriceps weakness and osteoarthritis of the knee. *Ann Intern Med* 1997;127:97–104.

36. Slemenda C, Heilman DK, Brandt KD, et al: Reduced quadriceps strength relative to body weight: A risk factor for knee osteoarthritis in women? *Arthritis Rheum* 1998;41:1951–1959.

37. Sharma L: Proprioceptive impairment in knee osteoarthritis. *Rheum Dis Clin North Am* 1999;25:299–314.

38. Sharma L, Lou C, Felson DT, et al: Laxity in healthy and osteoarthritic knees. *Arthritis Rheum* 1999;42:861–870.

39. Schouten JS, van den Ouweland FA, Valkenburg HA: A 12 year follow up study in the general population on prognostic factors of cartilage loss in osteoarthritis of the knee. *Ann Rheum Dis* 1992;51:932–937.

40. Dougados M, Gueguen A, Nguyen M, et al: Longitudinal radiologic evaluation of osteoarthritis of the knee. *J Rheumatol* 1992;19:378–384.

41. Spector TD, Dacre JE, Harris PA, Huskisson EC: Radiological progression of osteoarthritis: An 11 year follow up study of the knee. *Ann Rheum Dis* 1992;51:1107–1110.

42. Dieppe P, Cushnaghan J, Young P, Kirwan J: Prediction of the progression of joint space narrowing in osteoarthritis of the knee by bone scintigraphy. *Ann Rheum Dis* 1993;52:557–563.

43. Sharif M, George E, Shepstone L, et al: Serum hyaluronic acid level as a predictor of disease progression in osteoarthritis of the knee. *Arthritis Rheum* 1995;38:760–767.

44. Nevitt MC, Arden NK, Lane NE, Gore LR, Hochberg MC: Abstract: Incidence of radiographic changes of hip OA in elderly white women? *Arthritis Rheum* 1998;41(suppl):S181.

45. Danielsson L, Lindberg H, Nilsson B: Prevalence of coxarthrosis. *Clin Orthop* 1984;191:110–115.

46. Jorring K: Osteoarthritis of the hip: Epidemiology and clinical role. *Acta Orthop Scand* 1980;51:523–530.

47. Tepper S, Hochberg MC: Factors associated with hip osteoarthritis: Data from the First National Health and Nutrition Examination Survey (NHANES-I). *Am J Epidemiol* 1993;137:1081–1088.

48. Nevitt MC, Cummings SR, Lane NE, et al: Association of estrogen replacement therapy with the risk of osteoarthritis of the hip in elderly white women: Study of Osteoporotic Fractures Research Group. *Arch Intern Med* 1996;156:2073–2080.

49. Maetzel A, Makela M, Hawker G, Bombardier C: Osteoarthritis of the hip and knee and mechanical occupational exposure: A systematic overview of the evidence. *J Rheumatol* 1997;24:1599–1607.

50. Croft P, Coggon D, Cruddas M, Cooper C: Osteoarthritis of the hip: An occupational disease in farmers. *BMJ* 1992;304:1269–1272.

51. Croft P, Cooper C, Wickham C, Coggon D: Osteoarthritis of the hip and occupational activity. *Scand J Work Environ Health* 1992;18:59–63.

52. Roach KE, Persky V, Miles T, Budiman-Mak E: Biomechanical aspects of occupation and osteoarthritis of the hip: A case-control study. *J Rheumatol* 1994;21:2334–2340.

53. Vingard E, Alfredsson L, Goldie I, Hogstedt C: Sports and osteoarthrosis of the hip: An epidemiologic study. *Am J Sports Med* 1993;21:195–200.

54. Puranen J, Ala-Ketola L, Peltokallio P, Saarela J: Running and primary osteoarthritis of the hip. *Br Med J* 1975;2:424–425.

55. Marti B, Knobloch M, Tschopp A, Jucker A, Howald H: Is excessive running predictive of degenerative hip disease? Controlled study of former elite athletes. *BMJ* 1989;299:91–93.

56. van Saase JL, Vandenbroucke JP, van Romunde LK, Valkenburg HA: Osteoarthritis and obesity in the general population: A relationship calling for an explanation. *J Rheumatol* 1988;15:1152–1158.

57. Davis MA, Ettinger WH, Neuhaus JM, Barclay JD, Segal MR: Correlates of knee pain among US adults with and without radiographic knee osteoarthritis. *J Rheumatol* 1992;19:1943–1949.

58. Hochberg MC, Lawrence RC, Everett DF, Cornoni-Huntley J: Epidemiologic associations of pain in osteoarthritis of the knee: Data from the National Health and Nutrition Examination Survey and the National Health and Nutrition Examination–I Epidemiologic Follow-up Survey. *Semin Arthritis Rheum* 1989;18(suppl 2):4–9.

59. Summers MN, Haley WE, Reveille JD, Alarcon GS: Radiographic assessment and psychologic variables as predictors of pain and functional impairment in osteoarthritis of the knee or hip. *Arthritis Rheum* 1988;31:204–209.

60. Lunghi ME, Miller PM, McQuillan WM: Psycho-social factors in osteoarthritis of the hip. *J Psychosom Res* 1978;22:57–63.

61. O'Reilly SC, Jones A, Muir KR, Doherty M: Quadriceps weakness in knee osteoarthritis: The effect on pain and disability. *Ann Rheum Dis* 1998;57:588–594.

62. Lichtenberg PA, Skehan MW, Swensen CH: The role of personality, recent life stress and arthritic severity in predicting pain. *J Psychosom Res* 1984;28:231–236.

63. Lankhorst GJ, Van de Stadt RJ, Van der Korst JK: The relationships of functional capacity, pain, and isometric and isokinetic torque in osteoarthrosis of the knee. *Scand J Rehabil Med* 1985;17:167–172.

64. van Baar ME, Dekker J, Lemmens JA, Oostendorp RA, Bijlsma JW: Pain and disability in patients with osteoarthritis of hip or knee: The relationship with articular, kinesiological, and psychological characteristics. *J Rheumatol* 1998;25:125–133.

65. Rejeski WJ, Craven T, Ettinger WH Jr, McFarlane M, Shumaker S: Self-efficacy and pain in disability with osteoarthritis of the knee. *J Gerontol B Psychol Sci Soc* 1996;51:P24–P29.

66. Salaffi F, Cavalieri F, Nolli M, Ferraccioli G: Analysis of disability in knee osteoarthritis: Relationship with age and psychological variables but not with radiographic score. *J Rheumatol* 1991;18:1581–1586.

67. McAlindon TE, Cooper C, Kirwan JR, Dieppe PA: Determinants of disability in osteoarthritis of the knee. *Ann Rheum Dis* 1993;52:258–262.

68. Fisher NM, Pendergast DR, Gresham GE, Calkins E: Muscle rehabilitation: Its effect on muscular and functional performance of patients with knee osteoarthritis. *Arch Phys Med Rehabil* 1991;72:367–374.

Directions for Future Research

Identify risk factors for common musculoskeletal injuries.

Prevention of an injury is predicated on knowing risk factors and modifying them when possible. Risk factors link exposures with outcomes, in this case, injury. Unfortunately, very few risk factors for sports injuries have stood up to scientific scrutiny. If a modifiable risk factor is identified, intervention programs aimed at modifying the risk factor can have a very positive effect on injury outcome. Catastrophic injury outcome has been reduced successfully by this approach in several cases, most notably reduction of serious neck injuries by modifying tackling technique in football and increasing water depth at dive entry in swimming. Such strategies need to be extended to common musculoskeletal injuries such as ankle sprains because they have a profound effect on society in terms of health care costs and time lost from work.

Identify and characterize motor control strategies/movement patterns and relate them to risks of acute and chronic injuries.

Understanding a pattern of injury mechanism in the creation of joint damage and dysfunction is fundamental to the development of interventional prevention programs. There is increasing evidence that some acute musculoskeletal injuries, such as the noncontact anterior cruciate ligament (ACL) injury, have their etiology in disordered motor patterns. Early evidence suggests a gender difference in neuromuscular function and/or motor patterns, and these patterns correlate with injuries that are more prevalent in girls and women. Data supporting decreases in joint injuries as a result of improvement in motor/muscle patterns are limited. This is a fruitful area of research because it is likely a modifiable factor that can lead to injury reduction.

Investigate whether joint injury leads to osteoarthritis.

Injury is a potential risk of exercise and sport. Musculoskeletal injury, in particular joint injury, can lead to chronic dysfunction that reduces overall quality of life. Joint trauma can result from acute injury or chronic overload. Sometimes, joint trauma can be occult, with the sequelae of an acute injury leading to dysfunction at a time remote from the injury. Effects of macro- and microtrauma to the joint are currently difficult to characterize and quantify. Little is known about the relationship between acute joint trauma or chronic overuse joint injury and the development of joint osteoarthritis. More information is needed regarding the natural history of joint injury and subsequent degenerative joint disease, and if treatment strategies alter these results.

Better characterize bone remodeling and its role in different load states and at different stages in life.

Tissue markers for bone remodeling (resorption and formation) have been identified and characterized in the postmenopausal woman. Bone remodeling as characterized in the postmenopausal woman may not be applicable in growing bone. There is a need to better characterize bone remodeling in different life cycles, under different load conditions (jumping, walking), and with repetitive loading. In addition to load, muscle strength and muscle fatigue play an important role in transference of joint load. Better characterization of bone remodeling would aid in the understanding and treatment of stress fractures and maintenance of bone health.

Design prospective studies that relate prevention strategies to modifiable risk factors or modifiable injury mechanisms.

Injury prevention programs ideally target at-risk populations, modifying a risk factor or known injury mechanism, resulting in injury reduction. There is early evidence that noncontact ACL injuries can be reduced in high school girls when a specified training program is used. Studies such as these need to be further developed to identify the factor(s) that were modified by such a program. Variables such as strength, body size, previous sport experience, and proprioception all may be confounding factors in the etiology of this injury.

Investigate neuromuscular control strategies used by the central nervous system to control joint musculature and stability in the normal and injured states.

There are several musculoskeletal conditions with a primary symptom of pain that clinically improve with rehabilitation, including a strengthening program. Among these are patellofemoral overuse syndrome, shoulder impingement syndrome, and lateral elbow epicondylitis. Implicitly, it appears that pain is related to loss of normal joint neuromuscular control. Regaining strength and/or neuromuscular control of the joint improves the clinical symptoms, ie, pain and dysfunction. What strategies are used by the body to restore normal neuromuscular control? Are these strategies similar for men and women? Understanding this neuromuscular relationship with joint control would greatly advance the treatment of many musculoskeletal conditions.

Encourage scientific journals and their editorial review boards to require gender/race stratification of their data reporting.

Review of current musculoskeletal literature reveals few studies that stratify data reporting by gender and race. This is particularly true for literature on rehabilitation issues and postoperative results. With the ever-growing body of knowledge concerning a difference in outcomes based on gender, it is essential to stratify data in statistical reporting to further clarify this issue. Little is known about race in regard to potential outcomes differences.

Encourage musculoskeletal organizations to develop consensus regarding uniform classification systems, imaging techniques, outcome measures, and parameters to measure/record physical examination (anatomic) features.

Lack of a uniform language hampers progress in clarifying etiology and treatment of an injury or disease. Perhaps this is best exemplified in patellofemoral disorders. There is currently a paucity of studies linking physical examination and/or imaging techniques to clinical symptoms and/or treatment results. Physical examination measurements are inexact with high intra- and intervariability. No uniform imaging system and classification system exists. Yet treatment strategies, including surgery, are often based on these physical examinations and imaging measurements. A uniform process by which data are recorded will greatly aid in communicating injury and disease states in a reproducible manner and allow for collective and comparative research investigations.

Section Three

Sport-Specific Injuries

Section Editor:
Letha Y. Griffin, MD, PhD

W. Benjamin Kibler, MD
Mary Lloyd Ireland, MD
Bert R. Mandelbaum, MD
Jill L. McNitt-Gray, PhD
Margot Putukian, MD, FACSM
Carol C. Teitz, MD

Overview

When analyzing musculoskeletal injuries in specific sports, it is necessary to appreciate that it is the interaction of the sport's demands and the individual athlete that determines performance and risk of injury. Each sport has unique requirements of body movements, power, strength, and endurance, as well as proprioception, flexibility, agility, and size and shape of the athlete. Although many sports have movements in common, e.g., running, jumping, or pivoting, others require highly specific movements such as tumbling, swinging from one bar to another, skating, and spinning on one leg. Athletes may have an easy or difficult time learning these movements, depending on their individual attributes.

Strength and the ability to use it rapidly, ie, power, are useful in all sports. Yet certain sports demand more strength in the upper extremity than others. Trunk strength is especially critical for athletes in throwing and racquet sports.

Endurance is required in aerobic activities such as running, dance, and basketball, but it also may prevent injuries secondary to fatigue in anaerobic sports. Proprioception is known to be critical for gymnasts and may also be important for good body control in all sports.

Flexibility is required in dance, gymnastics, and hurdling, but too much flexibility (ie, hyperelasticity) may be detrimental. Agility is critical for athletes who have to change direction frequently, such as soccer or basketball players.

The size and shape of the athlete may affect her ability to be competitive (or participate) in various sports. For example, it may be advantageous for a gymnast to be short, ie, have a low center of gravity. On the other hand, track and field athletes who must generate momentum in order to put the shot or throw the discus require a larger, heavier frame.

Although the ability to meet the above requirements determines to a point an individual's ability to be successful in a given sport, additional nonphysiologic demands of the sport also may affect performance and injury risk and must be met by the athlete. For example, equipment, such as footwear, braces, or pads must fit the female athlete in order to protect her adequately and allow her to perform optimally. Environmental demands are also important. Women with exercise-induced bronchospasm do better in an aqueous environment. The ability to tolerate heat and altitude are related to conditioning. Protection from the sun may be more important for fair-skinned athletes.

Ideally the athlete should match her individual attributes to the demands of a given sport. These attributes can be divided into a number of areas, many of which are genetically influenced.

Within the musculoskeletal system, there are individual variations in static anatomic features such as leg length, as well as in dynamic features such as strength, flexibility, and patterns of muscle recruitment. An individual's distribution of various muscle fiber types (ie, anaerobic and aerobic) as well as her cardiopulmonary capabilities (eg, anaerobic threshold) also influence her chances of success in specific sports.

The athlete's own psychosocial environment, including support (or lack thereof) from parents, friends, and coaches, influences sports performance and risk. Coaches, in addition to their psychological influence, are critical in establishing an athlete's sport technique and in educating her about the history and rules of the sport.

Nutrition plays a major role in athletic performance and risk of injury. Evidence suggests that an athlete needs to have sufficient caloric input to meet demands and that the lack thereof may lead to osteoporosis and endocrinologic disorders. Adequate iron is needed for maximum oxygen-carrying capacity by the red blood cells. Physiologic differences in premenarchal, pregnant, and postmenopausal female athletes may affect their performance and risk of injury. Furthermore, comorbid conditions of athletes, such as diabetes, exercise-induced bronchospasm, or abnormal thyroid status, must not be overlooked.

In summary, any analyses of sport-specific injuries and sport-specific performance must recognize the unique contributions of the athlete and the sport.

LETHA Y. GRIFFIN, MD, PHD

Chapter 14
Soccer

Margot Putukian, MD, FACSM
Bert R. Mandelbaum, MD

Introduction

Soccer is the world's most common sport, with 200 million players participating and growth continuing. The interest and involvement of women in soccer is increasing exponentially, and nowhere has this been more apparent than in the United States. It has not always been acceptable for women to participate, and they were banned from participation by the European Football Association from 1921 until 1971. With the passage of Title IX in 1972, the opportunities for women in the United States to participate increased. The growth of National Collegiate Athletic Association (NCAA) women's soccer programs has increased dramatically, from 230 programs in 1986 to 746 in 1998–1999. The United States won the first Women's World Cup, held in China in 1991, and the Olympics held in Atlanta in 1998. Of the players in the United States, 43% are girls and women, whereas 22% of worldwide players are female. The future for women's soccer is extremely bright; as the United States hosted the Women's World Cup in 1999, the spotlight showed the women's athleticism, talent, and enthusiasm for the sport.

The overall picture for women's participation in soccer is exciting and positive, with the growth of the sport in the United States paralleling an increasing understanding of and love for the game. There are certain medical considerations that should be emphasized in that they either occur more commonly in soccer or are conditions that represent serious concerns for the overall health and well being of the female athlete participating in soccer. The primary areas of concern in the musculoskeletal system include the increased incidence of knee and in particular anterior cruciate ligament (ACL) injuries, stress fractures and other overuse injuries, and ankle injuries. Nutrition and hydration issues are important as are the elements of the female athlete triad (menstrual dysfunction, disordered eating patterns and their association with bone loss stress fractures, and premature osteoporosis). Finally, the incidence of concussions and concern for brain injury due to repetitive blows to the head from heading also raise particular concerns in soccer. This chapter will focus on what is known about these issues, with an emphasis on exploring areas where future research can be directed.

Physiology of the Female Player

Soccer is a sport that requires a combination of endurance training and discontinuous sprinting. The sport-specific skills demand the ability to turn quickly, pivot, jump in the air, and run both forward and backward. All body surfaces are used except for the hands and arms, which are used only by field players for throw-ins, and by the goalkeeper. Because so many of the sport-specific skills require balancing on one leg, there is high emphasis on lower extremity and trunk strength as well as balance and proprioception.

The female athlete runs approximately 8,471 m in a game, sprinting roughly 100 times an average distance of 14.9 m. The average percent body fat for a female player is between 19% and 22%, and the average maximal oxygen uptake (Vo_{2max}) is between 47 and 56 ml/kg/min.[1] These numbers represent data from European players in 1986 and may not reflect the physiologic characteristics of the current day soccer player. It might be expected that the body fat percentage of athletes in the United States now would be slightly lower, and the Vo_{2max} would be higher.

There are significant health benefits of participation for the female athlete, some of which transcend sport. These include a lower teen pregnancy rate, lower drug and alcohol use, higher graduation rates, improved self-esteem and body image, less depression, and improved teamwork and goal setting abilities.[2] There are also health benefits from exercise, such as reduction of heart disease, obesity, and diabetes, that affect long-term health. These benefits must be weighed against some of the potential risks of participation.

Fluids and Nutrition

Proper nutrition and hydration are essential given the physiologic demands that soccer play places on the athlete. Maintaining and restoring these energy demands are even more important when ambient temperatures are high, or when multiple games are played in succession. There are also special nutritional needs to consider in the female athlete that may affect performance.[3] These nutritional needs should be discussed with the athletes to optimize their training and performance.

Female soccer players, similar to other female athletes, are often deficient in their total caloric intake as well as their quality of intake. They are often deficient in iron and calcium intake, and may also struggle with trying to attain body composition or weight goals that are not appropriate. In an attempt to reach weight goals that may or may not be appropriate, these athletes may try "whatever works" to reach the goals they are unable to obtain. This may lead to experimentation with pathologic weight control behaviors, or true eating disorders. How eating disorders and menstrual dysfunction affect bone health is described later in this chapter.

The most important nutritional deficiency seen in the female athlete is iron deficiency, which can negatively affect performance. This most often occurs as a result of poor dietary intake along with the blood loss that normally occurs with menses. Asking questions at the beginning of the season that pertain to nutritional practices can help screen for athletes at risk. A determination of their hemoglobin (Hgb) along with ferritin can assess iron stores and the presence or absence of iron deficiency, with additional studies indicated if either of these is abnormal.

Fatigue on the soccer field generally is due to depletion of carbohydrate reserves. Dehydration is another concern for the soccer player, and this is more important when exercising in a warm environment. Some studies have demonstrated a decrease in exercise performance when an athlete is 2% dehydrated. The exercising athletes will not experience thirst until they are already 3% dehydrated, and generally will not drink enough on their own to replace their losses. Work capacity can diminish by 30% once an athlete loses 5% of his or her body weight.[4] Soccer-specific studies[5] have demonstrated that voluntary intake of fluids is often not sufficient and that athletes may benefit from hyperhydration.

Heat illness and heat exhaustion are the most serious side effects of dehydration and result from an inability to dissipate heat. In a youth soccer tournament in Minnesota, the incidence of heat-related illness over the several days of the tournament was decreased by modifications made by the medical staff covering the tournament.[6] Several factors can increase the risk for the development of heat illness including preexisting medical disease (cardiovascular disease, diabetes, alcoholism, hyperthyroidism), prepubertal or elderly age, poor conditioning, inadequate acclimatization, dehydration, obesity, fatigue, prior heat injury, current or recent febrile illness, and certain medications.

Fluid ingestion during activity can satisfy both fluid and carbohydrate needs and enhance performance. The optimal timing and content of the fluid used should be individualized to meet the demands of the exercise, the environmental conditions, and the preferences of the athlete. Muscle glycogen depletion and maintenance of hydration during soccer activity can be delayed by adding carbohydrate to fluids.[7] With either 90 to 180 minutes of exercise at 60% to 80% Vo_{2max} or 15 to 30 minutes of exercise at 90% to 130% Vo_{2max} performed in 1 to 5 min intervals, depletion of muscle glycogen occurs.[8,9] Ingesting carbohydrates is beneficial because it spares muscle glycogen stores, enhances performance, and increases work output and the time to exhaustion.[10–13] Ingesting carbohydrates as soon after exercise as possible has also been demonstrated to maximize the replacement of muscle glycogen energy stores in preparation for the next exercise session.[14]

Leatt and Jacobs[15] prospectively examined the effects of carbohydrate and fluid ingestion in soccer performance. Muscle biopsies were performed before and after a game in players who ingested glucose polymer before and during a soccer match. In players who ingested glucose, the muscle glycogen content was 31% higher than in those players given a placebo. A similar study assessed the effects of glucose polymer ingestion between two successive indoor matches. The study was single-blind, crossover design in which each player served as his or her own control. From film analysis, the amount of time each player spent walking, sprinting, or cruising was measured in both halves of both games. The players spent the same amount of time walking in the first and second halves and the same cruising or sprinting in the first half. However, the athletes given glucose polymer spent 40% more time sprinting and cruising in the second half, and covered 20% more distance overall than the athletes given a placebo.[16] Recent studies[17] assessing the use of low and high carbohydrate intake before soccer activity demonstrate that the increase in performance seen with high-carbohydrate diets tends to be in physiologic parameters (pre-game muscle glycogen, higher intensity work volume), not technical variables (passing skills).

It is clear from these studies that proper fluid and carbohydrate ingestion can not only prevent dehydration and thermoregulatory complications, but also may play a role in enhancing performance. The American College of Sports Medicine (ACSM) has useful recommendations for fluid and carbohydrate replacement. They recommend 30 to 60 g of carbohydrate per hour to maintain glucose levels and spare muscle glycogen, with the fluid needed based on the environmental conditions present. Athletes should be reminded to drink early and often during an exercise, and remember not to rely on their thirst as a gage for dehydration. When exercising in the heat, fluid intake is more important than substrate, and adding sodium may be useful in maintaining the osmotic drive to drink, enabling the kidney to hold onto sodium, and making fluids more palatable.[18]

Injury Patterns

The overall injury incidence in soccer is favorable, with considerably fewer injuries than in American football. In soccer players younger than 10 years of age, the injury incidence is extremely low.[19–21] At the high school level, injuries increase tenfold.[19,22] In the younger age levels, girls have a higher incidence of injury than boys. One study noted an injury incidence in women of 12 per 1,000 player hours compared with 5 per 1,000 player hours for men,[23] and another study found an incidence of 17.6 versus 7.4 per 1,000 player hours for girls and boys, respectively.[24] In young Danish players, the injury incidence for various levels of play was 11.9 to 18.5 per 1,000 hours, with 84% of injuries occurring in the lower extremity and 34% due to overuse injuries. Ankle sprains were the most common injury (36%) and occurred equally at all levels of play.[25] It is often difficult to compare injury studies because of differences in injury definition and settings evaluated. Some of these results are summarized in Table 1.

At the collegiate level, the disparity between injury incidence in men and women becomes less striking. The Injury Surveillance System (ISS) of the NCAA is a well-designed injury tracking system that uses time loss as definition for injury. There are disadvantages to this system in that mild injuries

Table 1 Injuries in soccer: Boys versus girls

Injuries (per 1,000 Player Hours) in Boys Versus Girls		
Study	**Girls**	**Boys**
Engstrom et al[23]*	12	5
Nilsson and Roass[26]	32	14
Maehlum[27]	17.6	8.9
Schmidt-Olsen et al[24]	17.6	7.4

*Denotes study using time loss from practice/play as definition of injury

that do not result in time loss may be missed. However, despite these limitations, because the injury incidence provides a denominator (number of athlete exposures) the data are very useful in comparing sports and genders as well as determining the specific types of injuries that occur.

Using the NCAA data through 1995–1996 (Table 2), women's soccer incurs a game injury rate of 17.3 per 1,000 athlete exposures (A-E) and a practice injury rate of 5.8 per 1,000 A-E, compared with 20.2 and 4.8, respectively, for men's soccer. This incidence ranks sixth in all sports followed by the NCAA, behind football, wrestling, women's gymnastics, spring football, and men's soccer. However, the injuries that occur are generally mild, with 72% of injuries resulting in time loss less than 7 days. This places women's soccer 12th in the 16 sports in terms of greatest severity. According to the data regarding practice and game injuries in fall and spring soccer in 1997, the practice rates were 5.8 and 5.6 per 1,000 A-E, respectively, and the game rates were 19.7 and 23.4 per 1,000 A-E, respectively. The spring data have only recently been examined.

Using the NCAA data from 1998–1999, injuries to the ankle, knee, and head accounted for 57% of all the injuries that occur during women's games. In assessing the body parts injured from 1986 to 1998, the knee, ankle, and upper leg account for the top three throughout, and account for an average of 55% of all injures that occur during both games and practices. Excluding the spine, 76% of the game injuries occur in the lower extremity. Concussions accounted for an injury rate of 2.09 per 1,000 A-E (11% of all injuries), with grade I concussions accounting for 89% of these.

Table 2 Injury data from NCAA injury surveillance system, through 1995–1996

Sport	Practice Injury Rate per 1,000 A-E*	Game Injury Rate per 1,000 A-E
Football	4.1	36.1
Wrestling	7.2	30.6
Women's gymnastics	8.1	21.4
Spring football	9.4	20.8
Men's soccer	4.8	20.2
Women's soccer	5.8	17.3
Ice hockey	2.3	16.9
Men's gymnastics	4.7	15.7
Men's lacrosse	3.8	15.7
Men's basketball	4.6	10.1
Women's basketball	4.4	9.4
Field hockey	4.2	9.4
Women's lacrosse	3.5	7.2
Baseball	2.2	6.2
Women's volleyball	4.6	5.2
Women's softball	3.3	4.9

(Reproduced with permission from Dick R: NCAA data 1995 to 1996. Overland Park, KS, NCAA.)
*A-E = athlete exposures

In elite female players from Sweden, the incidence of injuries during games was 24 per 1,000 player hours and 7 per 1,000 hours for practices. Of these, 88% were lower extremity injuries and 49% were in the ankle or knee; 49% also were considered minor, and 58% of the major injuries were knee ligament or meniscal injuries. This study reported 28% of the injuries as being overuse injuries.[23] These data compare to data for elite male players from Finland, where the incidence was 14.2 and 11.3 for injured and noninjured players, respectively, during games and 2.3 and 1.8, respectively, for practices. The authors of this study also reported that most injuries (76%) occurred in the lower extremities. They reported thigh injuries as the most frequent (22%) and overuse injuries rarely (6%). In this study, 18% of players required surgery, and most of these (58%) were due to knee injuries.[28]

The knee injury rates at the NCAA level from 1989 to 1993 were 1.6 and 1.3 per 1,000 A-E for women and men, respectively, with an ACL injury rate of 0.31 and 0.13 per 1,000 A-E for women and men, respectively.[29] These data have recently been re-addressed, and the ACL injury rates for women and men from 1994 to 1998 were 0.33 and 0.12 per 1,000 A-E, respectively.[30] These data confirm the increased rate of knee and specifically ACL injuries in female soccer players and are discussed in greater detail later in this chapter.

Indoor Soccer

In indoor soccer the injury data are sparse with only 2 studies that have included women.[31] In 1 study of indoor league play, the injury incidence for men and women was similar; 5.04 and 5.03 injuries per 100 player hours, respectively. The authors' injury definition was broad, including anything for which a player requested medical attention or for which play was stopped. An increased incidence of ACL injuries was found in women compared to men.

In a 3-day indoor tournament injury study, the rates of injury per 100 player hours were 5.79 and 4.74 in men and women, respectively.[32] This study used a time-loss definition of injury, with mild, moderate, and severe injuries corresponding to time loss of less than 1 week, more than 1 week but less than 1 month, and more than 1 month, respectively. Of the injuries, 65.8% were mild, 15.8% were moderate, and 18.4% were severe. The difference between the incidence of injuries in men and women was insignificant, and there was no difference in knee injuries. Injuries that were severe were more likely to have a noncontact mechanism. As in the outdoor game, 71.4% of the injuries incurred were in the lower extremity. The amount of injury information available for the indoor game is sparse, and more research is needed.

The types of injuries that occur in soccer are similar in the outdoor and indoor games, especially if a stricter time-loss definition is used. Because it is almost exclusively played on an artificial surface and often inside a hockey rink, the number of abrasions and contusions are greater in the indoor game, but generally these injuries do not lead to significant time loss. The 1996–1997 NCAA data demonstrate that the injury incidence is significantly greater on artificial surface versus natural grass; 15.4 versus 10.3 per 1,000 A-E, respectively. Examining injury epidemiology is useful in determining where injuries occur commonly and potentially identifying ways in which these can be prevented. More injury data are needed in the women's game, especially as the level of play has become more competitive.

Specific Injury Patterns

When considering musculoskeletal injuries in the female soccer player, it is important to emphasize knee injuries, specifically ACL injuries; stress fractures; ankle injuries; and ankle impingement syndromes. There are several skills that are unique to the sport of soccer. For example, kicking the ball with various surfaces of the foot—the inside, outside, and instep—can be associated with different injury patterns. An additional area of increasing concern is head injuries and the possibility of injury related to repetitive heading in soccer. Heading the ball, a skill unique to soccer, requires jumping, striking the ball with the head, and landing. Figures 1 through 4 illustrate some of the sport-specific skills used in soccer. These issues will be discussed in greater detail below, and help raise additional areas where more research is needed.

Knee Injuries

At the collegiate level, knee injuries account for 15% to 24% of the injuries that occur in practices and games.[29] As mentioned earlier, the NCAA data

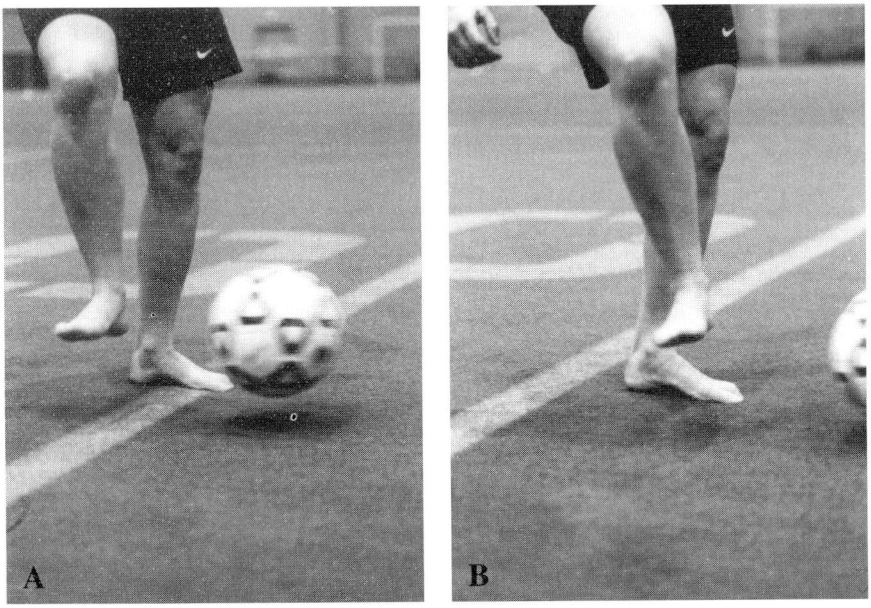

***Fig. 1** Inside-of-foot pass. **A**, The foot is in dorsiflexion and the hip is externally rotated. **B**, The medial aspect of the ankle is used to strike the ball. (Photos courtesy of University Photographics, S. Manuel.)*

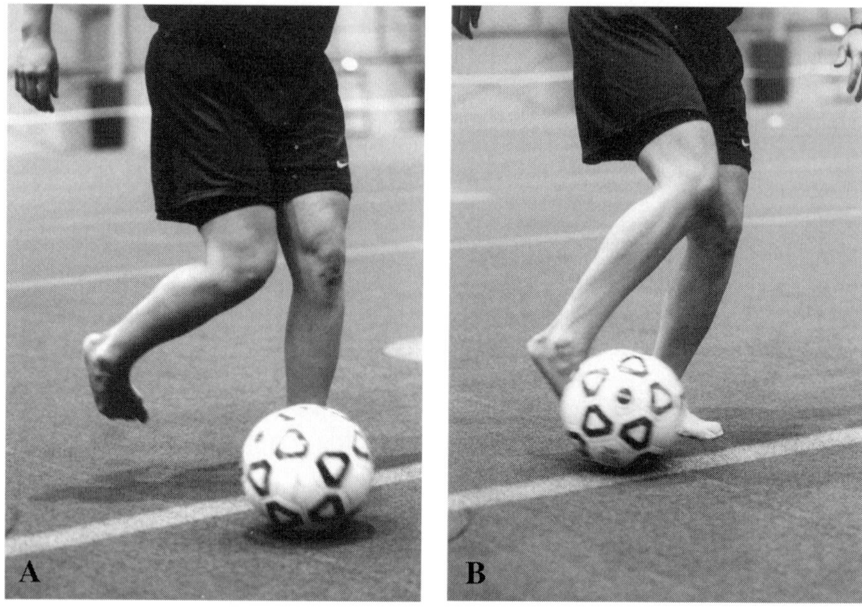

Fig. 2 *Outside-of-foot pass.* ***A****, The hip is internally rotated and the foot is inverted and plantarflexed.* ***B****, The lateral aspect of the foot/ankle is used to strike the ball. (Photos courtesy of University Photographics, S. Manuel.)*

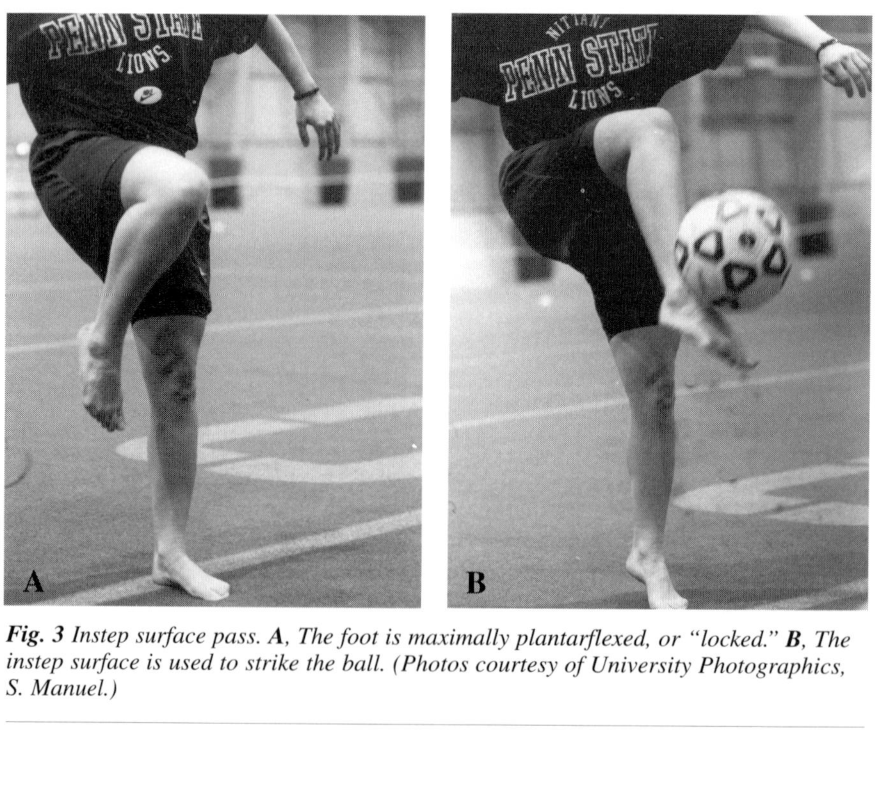

Fig. 3 *Instep surface pass.* ***A****, The foot is maximally plantarflexed, or "locked."* ***B****, The instep surface is used to strike the ball. (Photos courtesy of University Photographics, S. Manuel.)*

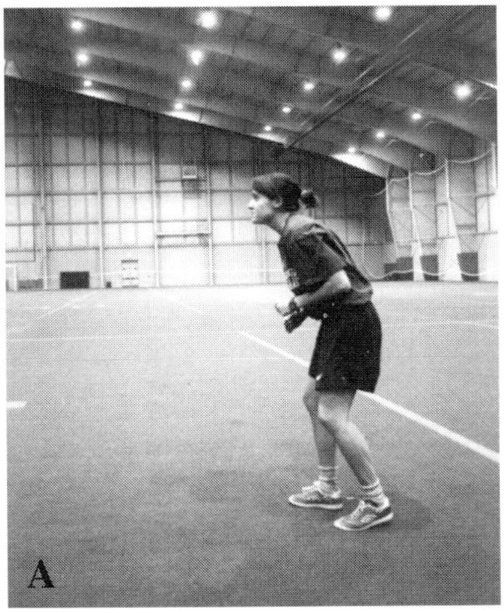

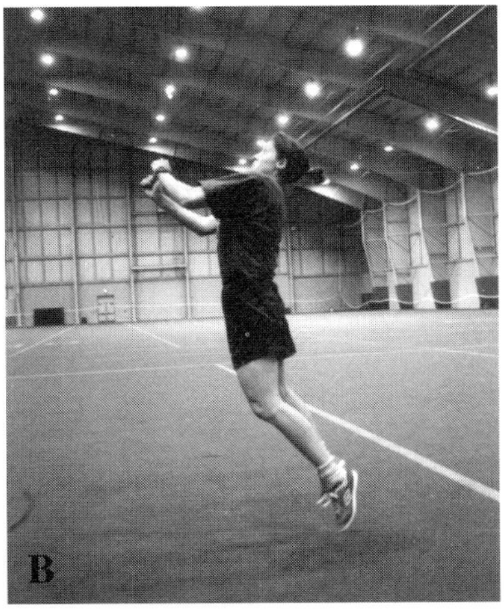

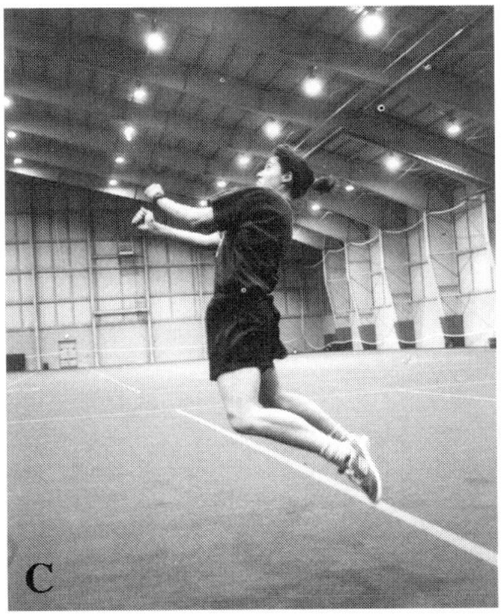

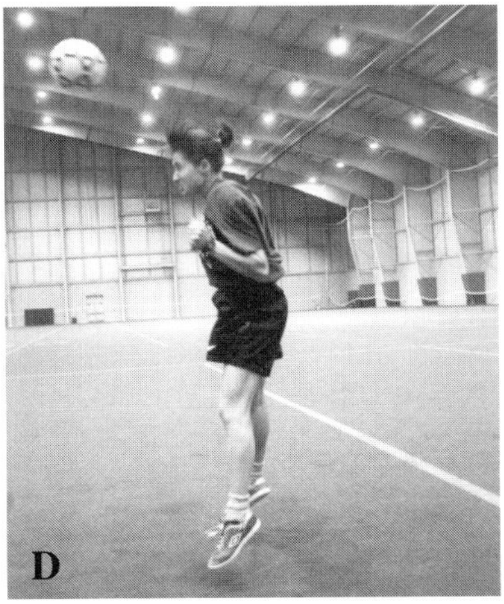

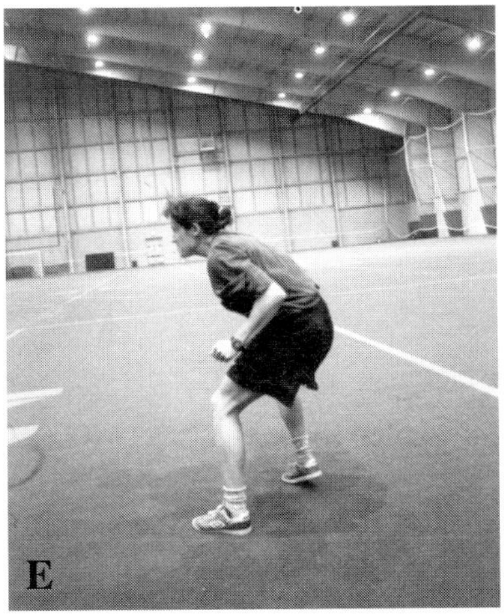

***Fig. 4* A** *through* **E,** *Jumping header. These photographs show the series of techniques involved in the jumping header. The ball is struck when the player is at the maximal height of the jump, with the player's eyes open. Impact with the ball is made at the forehead/hairline, with the head striking forward, through the ball. (Photos courtesy of University Photographics, S. Manuel.)*

from 1989 to 1993 demonstrated an increased incidence of total knee and ACL injuries in women, with the latter representing a 40% greater risk in the female player.[29] This increased ACL injury rate in female soccer players was also demonstrated in Norwegian players.[33] This increase in knee injuries, and specifically ACL tears in women compared to their male counterparts, is seen in all sports tracked by the NCAA, although the difference in soccer in particular is very striking. The other knee structures injured in soccer in both men and women are shown in Table 3, and along with ACL injuries, there is also an increase in meniscal injuries seen in women compared to men. The reasons for the increased incidence of ACL injuries in women is certainly a paramount question warranting further research.

A majority of ACL injuries occur secondary to a noncontact mechanism.[29,34–36] In the study by Arendt and Dick,[29] noncontact was the mechanism for 63% of the ACL injuries in women, whereas in the men, the noncontact mechanism was reported in only 48%. However, in these data, men also experienced a greater incidence of medial collateral ligament injuries. In the study by Noyes and associates,[34,35] 78% of ACL injuries were noncontact. Bjordal and associates[33] found that 46% of ACL injuries in men and women were contact injuries from tackling. When the mechanism is contact, it generally entails an illegal tackle from behind.[37]

The mechanism for noncontact ACL injury has been reported by Noyes and associates[34,35] to be on landing from a jump, while cutting, or with sudden deceleration. In a study assessing 85 athletes with ACL tears, 72% were due to a noncontact mechanism during deceleration in which the knee was flexed an average of 23°. The injury occurred during a pivot (23%), during a varus moment (19%), with hyperextension (13%), valgus (6%), and contact varus (2%).[38] In the NCAA data from 1996–1998, the most common mechanisms of ACL injury were landing from a jump (12.2%), planting or pivoting (57.1%), deceleration (12.2%), and hyperextension (12.2%).[30]

In a prospective study of female basketball players competing at the Division I level, the mechanisms of ACL injury were again planting and cutting (29%), landing on a straight knee (28%), and a 1-step land on a hyperextended knee (26%).[39] These researchers then instituted a modified training program that

Table 3 Knee structures injured in soccer (1989–1993)

Men's Soccer			Women's Soccer		
No.	**Rate***		**No.**	**Rate***	***P*†**
316	0.51	Collateral	192	0.62	0.02
119	0.19	Torn meniscus	105	0.34	0.00
130	0.21	Patella/P tendon	92	0.30	0.01
81	0.13	Anteroir cruciate	97	0.31	0.00
22	0.04	Posterior cruciate	12	0.04	
626,223		Athlete exposures	308,748		

(Reproduced with premission from Arendt EA, Dick R: Collegiate soccer injuries, in Garrett WE, Kirkendall DT, Contiguglia SR (eds): *U.S. Soccer Sports Medicine*. Baltimore, MD, Williams & Williams, 1996, p 454.)
*per 100,000
†Variance

emphasized landing with a bent knee, making pivots round instead of sharp, and a 3-step stop with a flexed knee. They reported an 89% reduction in ACL injury over 2 subsequent years. The idea of modifying biomechanical techniques to reduce injury is an area in which further research certainly is needed.

Several risk factors have been put forth to explain the increased risk for ACL injury. These have been divided into intrinsic and extrinsic factors.[29] Intrinsic factors include quadriceps/hamstring strength and firing patterns, fitness, limb alignment, dimensions of the intracondylar notch, hormonal influences, and proprioception. Extrinsic factors include shoe type, field surface, and rules of the game and their enforcement. More research is needed to assess ACL risk factors.

The hamstring muscles augment the action of the ACL, whereas the quadriceps is the major antagonist of ACL action. Wojtys and associates[40] demonstrated less quadriceps and hamstring strength in women and a reversal of the firing pattern of both muscles, with the quadriceps firing before the hamstrings in women versus the reverse pattern in men. Aerobic and anaerobic fitness has also been suggested as a risk factor for ACL injury, with poor fitness in women increasing the possibility of an ACL tear. Quadriceps/hamstring strength imbalances have also been associated with increased incidence of knee injuries in female athletes.[41]

The importance of general limb alignment has been controversial in regard to risk for ACL injury. No correlation was found between Q angle, femoral-tibial alignment, and ACL injury by Gray and associates,[42] whereas Ireland and Wall[43] have reported that a wider pelvis, increased femoral anteversion, a greater Q angle, and increased tibial vara predispose to ACL injury. A small intercondylar notch has been correlated with an increased incidence of ACL injury.[44] These biomechanical factors and their correlation with an increased risk for ACL injury remain an interesting area for future research.

There has been recent interest in the possibility that hormonal influences may be risk factors for ACL injury and help explain the increase in female athletes. There may be increased elasticity secondary to an estrogen effect on the ACL, and changes may be related to estrogen and progesterone effects on fibroblast proliferation.[45] What remains unanswered is the exact effect of hormonal changes on connective tissue, and whether this effect has any impact on the physiologic or pathologic responses to loads on these structures. Moller-Nielsen and Hammar[46] demonstrated in a study assessing the timing of injuries in soccer relative to the menstrual cycle that players were more susceptible to traumatic injuries during the premenstrual and menstrual phases of the cycle. This same study also demonstrated that women on an oral contraceptive pill (OCP) were less likely to sustain injury than those not on an OCP.

Proprioception, neuromuscular balance, and reaction time are important factors that may play a role in preventing ACL injuries. Loading of the ACL occurs after landing,[47] and at the high school level in basketball, proprioceptive training may reduce the incidence of ACL injury.[48] It is important to consider proprioception in various situations; the normal, uninjured athlete, the ACL-deficient athlete, and the athlete after ACL reconstruction. Changes that occur after an ACL tear may affect the risk for further injury. "Partial deafferentation" of the knee has been demonstrated after ACL injury.[49] This theory was substantiated by Solomonow and associates[50] in demonstrating that the balance of quadriceps and hamstring firing is important as stabilizers and that in the ACL-deficient knee, the hamstrings work to stabilize the joint. The kinetics of body position and muscle firing patterns in the ACL-competent and ACL-deficient knee are clearly different, and certainly an important goal of ACL reconstruction and rehabilitation is to restore proprioceptive function.[51] The exact role of proprioceptive training in all types of patients (ACL-deficient, ACL-reconstructed, uninjured athlete) is an area for future research.

Extrinsic factors felt to contribute to the incidence of ACL injuries include the field, cleats, and rules of the game and their enforcement. Lambson and associates[51] demonstrated that certain types of cleats may be associated with an increased incidence of ACL tears. In handball players, a higher friction rate of certain shoes on certain materials correlated with a higher incidence of ACL injury.[52] How this might relate to the soccer player given different shoe surfaces is unclear. In addition, artificial surfaces or fields that are uneven may play a role in ACL injuries[53] (R Dick, personal communication).

A primary area for future research in soccer is a better understanding of the ACL injury, especially in the female player. A better understanding of the biomechanical factors and kinesiology of soccer-specific skills and how these may relate to injury is needed. Understanding the role of motor recruitment and muscle imbalance in injury and the potential role of flexibility and strength training in preventing injury is also important. Continued research assessing the role of proprioception and proprioceptive training in injury and injury prevention is needed. Finally, a better understanding of the effects of hormonal influences on ACL integrity and injury is also needed. These intrinsic factors as well as the extrinsic factors specific to the sport of soccer are areas where future research should be emphasized.

Meniscal injuries are also common in soccer, due to the same sport-specific skills that put the athlete at risk for ACL injuries. A person needs only to watch a soccer player pivot and cut back and forth, change direction while decelerating, take a cross with a half-volley, or cross the ball from one side of the field to another to understand why soccer players may be at an increased risk for knee pathology. In the setting of ACL deficiency, the impact of concomitant meniscal injury is more dramatic.

In a retrospective study of 77 soccer players with both meniscal and ACL injuries, Neyret and associates[54] followed patients after rim-preserving menisectomy. Five years after menisectomy, it was demonstrated that those patients with ACL deficiency were less likely to be playing soccer (52% versus 75%), less happy with their knees (74% versus 97%), and more likely to have radiographic evidence for osteoarthritis (77% versus 24%). The ACL-deficient athlete is at an increased risk for chondromalacia of the tibia, femur, and patella, as well as degenerative meniscal tears.[55,56] The coexistence of injuries to the menisci and ligamentous injuries to the knee should not be underestimated when addressing the soccer player. These injuries in isolation may not prohibit activity, whereas in combination, they may make it difficult to return to high-level soccer performance.

Medial collateral ligament (MCL) injuries also occur frequently in the soccer player, although as with meniscal injury, no clear gender-specific concerns are present. The sport-specific skills of passing the ball with the inside of the foot, redirecting the ball onto goal, and block tackling put the athlete at risk for MCL injuries because of the direct valgus force that is incurred. If an athlete is not prepared going into a tackle for the ball against another stronger player, the MCL can be injured. In addition, because of these sport-specific skills, rehabilitation and return to play issues are often more complicated. The importance of proper skill techniques (keeping body weight over the ball) and lower extremity strengthening should be emphasized, especially in the young player.

Stress Fractures

Another common problem in women's soccer is overuse injuries and, specifically, stress fractures. Because of the physiologic demands of the sport and the training regimen that most high-level players participate in, overuse injuries and stress-related injuries occur and can result in significant time loss from play. Several factors that put the female athlete at a higher risk for stress fractures should be considered. These factors include playing surface, cleat and indoor shoe requirements, changes in training regimens and intensity, and hormonal and/or nutritional influences.

Most overuse injuries and stress fractures in the soccer player occur in the lower extremity. The incidence of stress fractures in soccer would be expected to be similar to that in other sports that emphasize running activities. In a study of bone scan positive stress fractures in athletes, Matheson and associates[57] reported them to occur most commonly in the tibia (49.1%), tarsals (25.3%), metatarsals (8.8%), femur (7.2%), fibula (6.6%), pelvis (1.6%), sesamoids (0.9%), and spine (0.6%). Given the high demand for running in soccer, these injuries can be devastating to a season or career, and prevention and detection of risk factors is an area that should be emphasized early on.

It is important to differentiate stress fractures from insufficiency fractures. In stress fractures, repetitive submaximal forces overwhelm the reparative process, but the bone itself is initially normal. In insufficiency fractures, normal stresses on a bone that has a decreased resistance to fracture because of an underlying condition, such as osteoporosis, lead to fracture.

Factors that predispose to the development of stress fractures include training and equipment errors as well as biomechanical abnormalities. Matheson and associates[57] found that training errors accounted for 22.4% of the stress fractures. The training and equipment errors identified in another study[58] included an abrupt change in playing surface; an abrupt change in the training schedule, including increased distance, intensity, or speed of activity; or insufficient recovery time between sessions. Inappropriate shoes may be causative in the development of stress fractures, and this may be particularly important in soccer players because many of the soccer cleats worn are often poor in controlling rearfoot and forefoot motion. Biomechanical issues include leg-length discrepancies, foot pronation, femoral anteversion, or increased knee valgus.[58] These factors should be considered in the preparticipation physical examination as well as in athletes who present with overuse injuries.

Although many of these factors are well studied, more research is needed specifically in the female player as to the effect of biomechanical influences and shoe/surface issues. More importantly, addressing the possibility of hormonal or nutritional deficiencies in respect to stress fractures is paramount in the overall health and morbidity of the soccer player. Disordered eating, menstrual dysfunction, and abnormalities in bone mineral density (BMD) have become known together as "the female athlete triad."[59–61] Though the entities of the female athlete triad have commonly been associated with sports that emphasize leanness (cross-country running, swimming) or subjective scoring (gymnastics, skating), they occur in all sports including soccer.

Drinkwater and associates[62] demonstrated that runners with amenorrhea had lower BMD than eumenorrheic runners, and subsequently have shown that there is a linear relationship between menstrual cycle history, both past and present, and BMD.[63] Athletes with stress fractures were found to have low BMD, a low calcium intake, negative calcium balance, and a higher incidence of menstrual irregularities and oral contraceptive use.[64] Myburgh and associates[65] have subsequently demonstrated that amenorrheic athletes have lower BMD at both axial and appendicular sites measured by dual energy x-ray absorptiometry (DEXA) scan. These and other studies[66,67] have demonstrated that menstrual dysfunction, especially amenorrhea, is associated with decreased BMD in both trabecular and cortical bone, which subsequently increases the risk for both stress fractures and premature osteoporosis.

Disordered eating patterns are also important to address in the female athlete, and unfortunately are seen in a variety of sports, including soccer. In one study of collegiate athletes, 32% practiced at least one form of pathogenic eating behavior; 16% used laxatives, 20% binged, 20% purged, and 25% used diet pills or diuretics.[68] It has also been demonstrated that athletes start experimenting with these methods of weight control in their early teens.[69] Eating disorders, anorexia nervosa and bulimia nervosa, are psychological problems that have at their core a disordered body image; the person believes he or she is fat when indeed she or he is too thin. For a variety of reasons, eating disorders are more common in athletes than their nonathletic counterparts.[70,71] There are several complications of eating disorders including infertility, thermoregulatory disturbances, depression, immune dysfunction, poor healing, low BMD, and consequently an increased risk for stress fractures.[72–74]

A dose-response curve that describes the balance between bone response to changes in physical training and the intensity, frequency, and duration of activity has been suggested by Knapp and Mandelbaum.[75] This hypothesis assumes a normal cyclic response of connective tissue and bone adaptations to an increased physical stress. If an individual is weightless (astronaut) or immobilized, the reverse occurs with a negative response. If an athlete trains in a progressive manner, he or she remains healthy and on the performance side of the curve. If a significant aberrancy in the athlete's training occurs, or if the athlete has a concomitant eating disorder or abnormality in menstrual function, she can fall into the injury zone with resultant overuse injury and stress fracture. This dose-response curve can be useful in educating the athlete with regard to the multiple factors that contribute to bone injury and the importance of optimizing nutrition, training, and normal hormonal balances to optimize performance.

Ankle Injuries and Impingement Syndrome

Ankle sprains account for a majority of injuries that occur in soccer, and given the sport-specific skills of soccer, these usually mild injuries are very important to detect and treat appropriately.[71,76] The usual mechanism is an inversion plantar flexion injury. One of the skills used in soccer is the outside-of-foot pass, in which the foot is in this position and the ball is struck (Fig 2). This technique is used because it is particularly deceptive during passing, and when a player is running at full speed where it is easier to strike the ball using this surface as part of the normal running stride. Ankle injuries are not uncommon, with the use of the outside-of-foot pass adding an additional mechanism to consider in the sport of soccer.

Ankle injuries are generally mild with little time lost from practice or play. The immediate treatment of these injuries is no different in the soccer player, but the injuries may be very debilitating if not addressed aggressively with early treatment and rehabilitation. Ankle sprains can sometimes be more complicated and involve the lateral ligaments as well as additional structures such as the articular cartilage and bone. Because soccer players rely on their mobility and "touch" on the ball, the challenge often lies in returning athletes to 100% functional activity.

The most common complications associated with ankle injuries to consider include fractures of the talar dome or fifth metatarsal, chronic instability, synovitis, sinus tarsi syndrome, and posterior, anterior, and anterolateral impingement syndromes with meniscoid lesions. The tibial diaphyseal fracture that occurs in soccer has been called the "footballer's fracture" and generally occurs from the impact of a tackle.[77] Syndesmotic injuries, or fractures of the lateral process of the talus, anterior process of the calcaneus, or tibial plafond occur less commonly. It is important to consider all of these complications and associated injuries in those athletes that do not respond appropriately to adequate treatment. Rehabilitation after ankle injury, especially if it involves the syndesmosis or involves additional structures, is essential and its importance should not be trivialized. In addition, if significant ankle laxity is detected during the preparticipation physical examination, a strengthening and proprioceptive program should be initiated and consideration of prophylactic taping or bracing should be discussed.

There is a subgroup of athletes with ankle sprains that continue to experience pain and disability after injury, and this group of "ankle impingement" syndromes are often difficult to treat in the soccer player. In the setting of anterolateral pain, no instability, and history of prior ankle sprains, impingement syndromes should be considered. Athletes often complain of pain while trying to pivot or push off of one foot, as well as difficulty and pain while shooting the ball with the instep. Impingement syndrome occurs as a result of hypertrophic scar formation, synovium, and fibrocartilage in the anterolateral tibiotalar space extending from the anterior capsule posteriorly into the lateral gutter. McCarroll and associates[78] have described these as "meniscoid" lesions in soccer players after inversion ankle sprains. Stress radiographs generally do not reveal significant ligamentous laxity, though anterior spurring of the tibia may be present and increase the soft-tissue impingement.

Knapp and Mandelbaum[79] have recommended an ankle impingement syndrome classification that describes 4 grades: I, normal radiographs, anterolateral capsular thickening seen on magnetic resonance imaging (MRI) and verified arthroscopically; II, extra-articular or intra-articular osteophytes with articular surface surfaces entirely normal; III, bony abnormalities involving articular surface (osteochondritis dissecans); and IV, previous intraarticular fracture. If aggressive physical therapy and rehabilitation does not provide resolution of impingement problems, these lesions often respond well to arthroscopic debridement.

An impingement syndrome can also occur posteriorly, especially if an os trigonum is present. Other entities to consider in the posterior ankle include achilles tendonitis, retrocalcaneal bursitis, Haglund's deformity, posterior tibialis tendonitis, and tarsal tunnel syndrome. These entities can usually be detected by careful history and physical examination, occasionally supplemented with additional testing.

Head Injuries

Heading the ball is the most unique sport-specific skill in soccer (Fig. 4). It has been estimated that approximately 300 games are played and 200 blows to the head are sustained in a typical male professional player's career.[80] The head is used to clear the ball defensively, pass to a teammate, and strike the ball toward the goal in attempt to score. When a ball is kicked, it travels at an approximate average speed of 114 km/hr and from 10 m away, strikes with an impact of 116 kpm.[81] The ball stays in contact with the head from 1/63 to 1/128 s.

There has been some concern that repetitive heading may lead to chronic changes similar to those seen in the "punch drunk" syndrome in boxing. Early European studies reported central cerebral atrophy on computed tomography (CT) scanning, electroencephalogram changes, and neuropsychological changes as a result of soccer activity.[80,82,83] These studies have methodologic problems in that they lacked good control groups, did not screen for alcohol use or previous history of head injury, and did not separate acute head injuries. In a study of US National Team players, no statistical differences were seen between track athletes and soccer players using MRI scans.[84]

The head injuries that occur in soccer are most often concussions, or mild traumatic brain injury, which generally occur as a result of impact with another player, the ground, or the goal posts. Head injuries account for 1.2% to 8% of injuries in soccer, depending on the study. In 1996–1997, there were 0.46 injuries per 1,000 A-E in women's NCAA soccer, accounting for 4.4% of the total injuries seen. In a study of collegiate players, Delfico and Garrett[38] found an incidence of concussion in men and women over two seasons to be 0.6 and 0.4 per 1,000 A-E, respectively. Most of these injuries were due to contact with an opponent (48%), the ground or surrounding surface (13%), the ball (24%), or a combination of objects. None of these injuries were the result of intentional heading.

In a prospective, cross-over study of collegiate male and female soccer players, a battery of neuropsychological tests was used before and after a training session where 20 out of 90 minutes were secured for heading exercises. Athletes were matched with another player and either participated in the heading or not; 2 days later the practice was repeated with the roles reversed (those not heading on day 1 now participated and vice versa). No deficits were seen in cognitive function as assessed by the neuropscyhological tests, although all groups demonstrated a practice effect. There was also some difference in performance based on gender, and the need for baseline testing was confirmed.[2] Additional prospective research focusing on the impact of heading over the course of a season and college career is under way. Further research is needed to differentiate the effects of multiple or severe head injuries from those caused by repetitive heading.

The management and assessment of mild traumatic brain injuries remain difficult and controversial. Athletes should be closely assessed for abnormalities in cognitive function and evidence of underlying intracranial abnormalities and cervical spine injury, and not allowed to return to play if they are symptomatic. Several concussion classification systems and return to play guidelines exist in the literature and are not discussed further here.[85–87] This is an area where exciting new research is ongoing.

There has been recent interest in the use of neuropsychological testing in the assessment and return to play decisions in the head-injured athlete.[88–91] Neuropsychological tests provide a reliable assessment and quantification of brain functioning by examining brain-behavior relationships. These measurements assess memory recall, attention and concentration, problem solving abilities, visual tracking, reaction time, and speed of information processing as well as other measures of cognitive function. There are a variety of different tests available, many of which are well validated. There has been research using neuropsychological testing specifically with an athletic population.[82,92,93]

If a battery of neuropsychological tests is performed before the season is under way, a "baseline" of function in these various realms of cognitive function is obtained. If the athlete subsequently sustains a head injury, additional testing can be obtained and then compared with the baseline studies. Limitations currently include the time and cost of testing, as well as the normal "learning curve" that occurs with repetitive testing. In addition, it is important currently that these tests be interpreted correctly with the help of qualified neuropsychologists, which may limit their application. This type of research is ongoing with college athletes, with exciting information being gained.[91] Despite the limitations mentioned above, neuropsychological testing remains useful in detecting mild head injuries[82,88–90,92–96] and in assessing acute and chronic effects, and may be more sensitive than classical testing in assessing cognitive function.[32,92] As the research in this area evolves, the way head injuries are treated and return to play decisions are made, may change.

Prevention of Injuries

Though the frequency and severity of injuries in soccer are generally mild, preventing these injuries can only manage to make the game safer and more enjoyable. Ekstrand and Gillquist[97] demonstrated in male soccer players that certain preventative measures decreased injury. Measures that should be implemented in the women's game are listed in Outline 1.

Outline 1 Measures that should be implemented to decrease injury in women's soccer

1. Assessing and correcting training errors, especially overtraining
2. Use of proper equipment (shin guards, shoes, field maintenance)
3. Use of prophylactic ankle taping if laxity is present
4. Rehabilitation for injuries that have not adequately healed or have been inappropriately rehabilitated
5. Exclusion of athletes with significant pathological knee ligamentous laxity (laxity that is asymmetric and/or symptomatic)
6. Aggressive strengthening and conditioning of the lower extremities, especially if after knee reconstruction
7. Education about association of injury to foul play
8. Appropriate medical care for practices and games
9. Nutritional education, including both energy and fluid intake
10. Education, early identification, and treatment of athletes with eating disorders
11. Education, early identification, and treatment of menstrual dysfunction
12. Emphasis on proper technique, especially during tackling and heading
13. Emphasis on strengthening of the lumbar and cervical spine musculature in response to heading

Conclusion

Soccer is a tremendous team sport that enjoys a relatively low injury rate, a reliance on both endurance and sprinting conditioning, strength, and sport-specific skills. The most common injury is the ankle sprain, which generally is mild and minimally affects the athlete's performance, although if impingement syndromes occur, it can be more complicated. Additional research assessing the effectiveness of prophylactic taping, bracing, and proprioceptive training is needed. By far the most serious injury, which occurs at an alarming rate, is the ACL injury; this injury occurs at a greater incidence in the female player than in male players. Further research is clearly needed to understand both of these injuries, along with their risk factors, ideal treatment, and rehabilitation and prevention.

Head injuries desperately warrant further research energy. It is important to differentiate concussions from the potential injuries sustained by repetitive heading. Early recognition of concussion in soccer is important, and new methods of assessing these injuries and making return to play decisions are currently being researched. Additional research is needed in addressing the biomechanical forces associated with heading, especially in the women's game. This research may impact on safety issues and/or preventative measures that may minimize the occurrence of these injuries. Gender differences for both concussion and potential injury from heading should be examined.

Finally, the incidence of overuse injuries, including stress fractures, needs to be assessed in further detail, with identification of risk factors specific to the soccer player. This will undoubtedly include physiological profiling of the elite and college-level athlete and assessment for nutritional intake optimal for peak soccer performance. Understanding the importance of educating athletes and coaches regarding the entities of the female athlete triad and initiating treatment as soon as these problems are recognized is essential. With additional research in the women's game, all of these important questions can undoubtedly be answered.

References

1. Ekblom B (ed): *Football (Soccer): Handbook of Sports Medicine and Science.* Oxford, England, Blackwell Scientific Publications, 1994.
2. Putukian M, Echemendia RJ, Mackin S: The acute neuropsychological effects of heading in soccer: A pilot study. *Clin J Sport Med* 2000;10:104–109.
3. Brewer J: Nutritional aspects of women's soccer. *J Sports Sci* 1994;12:S35–S38.
4. Saltin B, Costill D: Fluid and electrolyte balance during prolonged exercise, in Horton ES, Terjung RL (eds): *Exercise, Nutrition, and Energy Metabolism.* New York, NY, MacMillan, 1988, pp 150–158.
5. Rico-Sanz J, Frontera WR, Rivera MA, Rivera-Brown A, Mole PA, Meredith CN: Effects of hyperhydration on total body water, temperature regulation and performance of elite young soccer players in a warm climate. *Int J Sports Med* 1996;17:85–91.
6. Elias SR, Roberts WO, Thorson DC: Team sports in hot weather: Guidelines for modifying youth soccer. *Phys Sportsmed* 1991;19:67–80.
7. Coyle EF, Montain SJ: Carbohydrate and fluid ingestion during exercise: Are there trade-offs? *Med Sci Sports Exerc* 1992;24:671–678.
8. Coggan AR, Coyle EF: Carbohydrate ingestion during prolonged exercise: Effects on metabolism and performance. *Exerc Sport Sci Rev* 1991;19:1–40.
9. Keizer HA, Kuipers H, van Kranenburg G, Geurten P: Influence of liquid and solid meals on muscle glycogen resynthesis, plasma fuel hormone response, and maximal physical working capacity. *Int J Sports Med* 1987;8:99–104.
10. Coyle EF, Coggan AR, Hemmert MK, Ivy JL: Muscle glycogen utilization during prolonged strenuous exercise when fed carbohydrate. *J Appl Physiol* 1986;61:165–172.
11. Hargreaves M, Costill DL, Coggan A, Fink WJ, Nishibata I: Effect of carbohydrate feedings on muscle glycogen utilization and exercise performance. *Med Sci Sports Exerc* 1984;16:219–222.
12. Ivy JL, Miller W, Dover V, et al: Endurance improved by ingestion of a glucose polymer supplement. *Med Sci Sports Exerc* 1983;15:466–471.
13. Murray R, Eddy DE, Murray TW, Seifert JG, Paul GL, Halaby GA: The effect of fluid and carbohydrate feedings during intermittent cycling exercise. *Med Sci Sports Exerc* 1987;19:597–604.

14. Ivy JL, Katz AL, Cutler CL, Sherman WM, Coyle EF: Muscle glycogen synthesis after exercise: Effect of time of carbohydrate ingestion. *J Appl Physiol* 1988;64:1480–1485.

15. Leatt PB, Jacobs I: Effect of glucose polymer ingestion on glycogen depletion during a soccer match. *Can J Sport Sci* 1989;14:112–116.

16. Foster C, Thompson NN, Dean J, Kirkendall DT: Abstract: Carbohydrate supplementation and performance in soccer players. *Med Sci Sports Exerc* 1986;18(suppl):S12.

17. Balsom PD, Wood K, Olsson P, Ekblom B: Carbohydrate intake and multiple sprint sports: With special reference to football (soccer). *Int J Sports Med* 1999;20:48–52.

18. Convertino VA, Armstrong LE, Coyle EF, et al: American College of Sports Medicine position stand: Exercise and fluid replacement. *Med Sci Sports Exerc* 1996;28:i–vii.

19. Hoff GL, Martin TA: Outdoor and indoor soccer: Injuries among youth players. *Am J Sports Med* 1986;14:231–233.

20. Keller CS, Noyes FR, Buncher CR: The medical aspects of soccer injury epidemiology. *Am J Sports Med* 1987;15:230–237.

21. Backous DD, Friedl KE, Smith NJ, Parr TJ, Carpine WD Jr: Soccer injuries and their relation to physical maturity. *Am J Dis Child* 1988;142:839–842.

22. Sullivan JA, Gross RH, Grana WA , Garcia-Moral CA: Evaluation of injuries in youth soccer. *Am J Sports Med* 1980;8:325–327.

23. Engstrom B, Johansson C, Tornkvist H: Soccer injuries among elite female players. *Am J Sports Med* 1991;19:372–375.

24. Schmidt-Olsen S, Jorgensen U, Kaalund S, Sorensen J: Injuries among young soccer players. *Am J Sports Med* 1991;19:273–275.

25. Nielsen AB, Yde J: Epidemiology and traumatology of injuries in soccer. *Am J Sports Med* 1989;17:803–807.

26. Nilsson S, Roass A: Soccer injuries in adolescents. *Am J Sports Med* 1978;6:358–361.

27. Maehlum S: Frequency of injuries in a youth soccer tournament. *Phys Sportsmed* 1984;12:114–117.

28. Luthje P, Nurmi I, Kataja M, et al: Epidemiology and traumatology of injuries in elite soccer: A prospective study in Finland. *Scand J Med Sci Sports* 1996;6:180–185.

29. Arendt E, Dick R: Knee injury patterns among men and women in collegiate basketball and soccer: NCAA data and review of literature. *Am J Sports Med* 1995;23:694–701.

30. Arendt EA, Agel J, Dick R: Anterior cruciate ligament injury patterns among collegiate men and women. *J Athletic Training Assoc* 1999;34:86–92.

31. Lindenfeld TN, Schmitt DJ, Hendy MP, Mangine RE, Noyes FR: Incidence of injury in indoor soccer. *Am J Sports Med* 1994;22:364–371.

32. Putukian M, Knowles WK, Swere S, Castle NG: Injuries in indoor soccer: The Lake Placid Dawn to Dark Soccer Tournament. *Am J Sports Med* 1996;24:317–322.

33. Bjordal JM, Arnly F, Hannestad B, Strand T: Epidemiology of anterior cruciate ligament injuries in soccer. *Am J Sports Med* 1997;25:341–345.

34. Noyes FR, Mooar PA, Matthews DS, Butler DL: The symptomatic anterior cruciate-deficient knee: Part I. The long-term functional disability in athletically active individuals. *J Bone Joint Surg* 1983;65A:154–162.

35. Noyes FR, Matthews DS, Mooar PA, Grood ES: The symptomatic anterior cruciate-deficient knee: Part II. The results of rehabilitation, activity modification, and counseling on functional disability. *J Bone Joint Surg* 1983;65A:163–174.

36. Strand T, Tvedte R, Engebretsen L, Tegnander A: Anterior cruciate ligament injuries in handball playing: Mechanisms and incidence of injuries. *Tidsskr Nor Laegeforen* 1990;110:2222–2225.

37. Ekstrand J, Gillquist J: Soccer injuries and their mechanisms: A prospective study. *Med Sci Sports Exerc* 1983;15:267–270.

38. Delfico AJ, Garrett WE Jr: Mechanisms of injuries of the anterior cruciate ligament in soccer players. *Clin Sports Med* 1998;17:779–785.

39. Griffis ND, Vequist SW, Yearout KM, Henning CE, Lynch MA: Abstract: Injury prevention of the anterior cruciate ligament, in *American Orthopaedic Society for Sports Medicine: Meeting Abstracts, Symposia, and Instructional Courses, 15th Annual Meeting*. Chicago, IL, American Orthopaedic Society for Sports Medicine, 1989.

40. Wojtys EM, Wylie BB, Huston LJ: The effects of muscular fatigue on neuromuscular function and anterior tibial translation in healthy knees. *Am J Sports Med* 1996;24:615–621.

41. Knapik JJ, Bauman CL, Jones BH, Harris JM, Vaughan L: Preseason strength and flexibility imbalances associated with athletic injuries in female collegiate athletes. *Am J Sports Med* 1991;19:76–81.

42. Gray J, Taunton JE, McKenzie DC, Clement DB, McConkey JP, Davidson RG: A survey of injuries to the anterior cruciate ligament of the knee in female basketball players. *Int J Sports Med* 1985;6:314–316.

43. Ireland ML, Wall C: Abstract: Epidemiology and comparison of knee injuries in elite male and female United States basketball athletes. *Med Sci Sports Exerc* 1990;22(suppl):S82.

44. Souryal TO, Freeman TR: Intercondylar notch size and anterior cruciate ligament injuries in athletes: A prospective study. *Am J Sports Med* 1993;21:535–539.

45. Yu WD, Liu SH, Hatch JD, Panossian V, Finerman GA: Effect of estrogen on cellular metabolism of the human anterior cruciate ligament. *Clin Orthop* 1999;366:229–238.

46. Moller-Nielsen J, Hammar M: Women's soccer injuries in relation to the menstrual cycle and oral contraceptive use. *Med Sci Sports Exerc* 1989;21:126–129.

47. Caraffa A, Cerulli G, Projetti M, Aisa G, Rizzo A: Prevention of anterior cruciate ligament injuries in soccer: A prospective controlled study of proprioceptive training. Knee *Surg Sports Traumatol Arthrosc* 1996;4:19–21.

48. Henning CE, Griffis ND, Vequist SW, et al: Sport-specific knee injuries, in Renström FH (ed): *The Encyclopedia of Sports Medicine*. Oxford, England, Blackwell Scientific, 1994, vol 5, pp 164–178.

49. Barrack RL, Skinner HB, Buckley SL: Proprioception in the anterior cruciate deficient knee. *Am J Sports Med* 1989;17:1–6.

50. Solomonow M, Baratta R, Zhou BH, et el: The synergistic action of the anterior cruciate ligament and thigh muscles in maintaining joint stability. *Am J Sports Med* 1987;15:207–213.

51. Lambson RB, Barnhill BS, Higgins RW: Football cleat design and its effect on anterior cruciate ligament injuries: A three-year prospective study. *Am J Sports Med* 1996;24:155–159.

52. Myklebust G, Maehlum S, Engebretsen L, Strand T, Solheim E: Registration of cruciate ligament injuries in Norwegian top level team handball: A prospective study covering two seasons. *Scand J Med Sci Sports* 1997;7:289–292.

53. Ekstrand J, Nigg BM: Surface-related injuries in soccer. *Sports Med* 1989;8:56–62.

54. Neyret P, Donell ST, DeJour D, DeJour H: Partial meniscectomy and anterior cruciate ligament rupture in soccer players: A study with a minimum 20-year followup. *Am J Sports Med* 1993;21:455–460.

55. Menke W, Schneider T, Schmitz B, Michiels I: Results of follow-up of untreated anterior cruciate ligament rupture. *Sportverletz Sportschaden* 1990;4:169–174.

56. Kohn D: Arthroscopy in acute injuries of anterior cruciate-deficient knees: Fresh and old intraarticular lesions. *Arthroscopy* 1986;2:98–102.

57. Matheson GO, Clement DB, McKenzie DC, Taunton JE, Lloyd-Smith DR, MacIntyre JG: Stress fractures in athletes: A study of 320 cases. *Am J Sports Med* 1987;15:46–58.

58. Reeder MT, Dick BH, Atkins JK, Pribis AB, Martinez JM: Stress fractures: Current concepts of diagnosis and treatment. *Sports Med* 1996;22:198–212.

59. Yeager KK, Agostini R, Nattiv A, Drinkwater B: The female athlete triad: Disordered eating, amenorrhea, osteoporosis. *Med Sci Sports Exerc* 1993;25:775–777.

60. Putukian M: The female althlete triad. *Clin Sports Med* 1998;17:679–696.

61. Putukian M: The female athlete triad: Eating disorders, amenorrhea and osteoporosis. *Med Clin NA* 1994;78:345–356.

62. Drinkwater BL, Nilson K, Chesnut CH III, Bremner WJ, Shainholtz S, Southworth MB: Bone mineral content of amenorrheic and eumenorrheic athletes. *N Engl J Med* 1984;311:277–281.

63. Drinkwater BL, Bruemner B, Chesnut CH III: Menstrual history as a determinant of current bone density in young athletes. *JAMA* 1990;263:545–548.

64. Myburgh KH, Hutchins J, Fataar AB, Hough SF, Noakes TD: Low bone density is an etiologic factor for stress fractures in athletes. *Ann Intern Med* 1990;113:754–759.

65. Myburgh KH, Bachrach LK, Lewis B, Kent K, Marcus R: Low bone mineral density at axial and appendicular sites in amenorrheic athletes. *Med Sci Sports Exerc* 1993;25:1197–1202.

66. Prior JC, Vigna YM, Schechter MT, Burgess AE: Spinal bone loss and ovulatory disturbances. *N Engl J Med* 1990;323:1221–1227.

67. Rencken ML, Chesnut CH III, Drinkwater BL: Bone density at multiple skeletal sites in amenorrheic athletes. *JAMA* 1996;276:238–240.

68. Rosen LW, McKeag DB, Hough DO, Curley V: Pathogenic weight-control behavior in female athletes. *Phys Sportsmed* 1986;14:79–86.

69. Dummer GM, Rosen LW, Heusner WW, Roberts PJ, Counsilman JE: Pathogenic weight-control behaviors of young competitive swimmers. *Phys Sportsmed* 1987;15:75–86.

70. Sundgot-Borgen J: Risk and trigger factors for the development of eating disorders in female elite athletes. *Med Sci Sports Exerc* 1994;26:414–419.

71. Putukian M: The female athlete triad: Eating disorders, amenorrhea, and osteoporosis. *Med Clin North Am* 1994;78:345–356.

72. Otis CL, Drinkwater B, Johnson M, Loucks A, Wilmore J: American College of Sports Medicine position stand: The female athlete triad. *Med Sci Sports Exerc* 1997;29:i–ix.

73. Palla B, Litt IF: Medical complications of eating disorders in adolescents. *Pediatrics* 1988;81:613–623.

74. Pomeroy C, Mitchell JE: Medical issues in the eating disorders, in Brownell KD, Rodin J, Wilmore JH (eds): *Eating, Body Weight, and Performance in Athletes: Disorders of Modern Society*. Philadelphia, PA, Lea & Febiger, 1992, pp 202–221.

75. Knapp TP, Mandelbaum BR: Stress fractures, in Garrett WE Jr, Kirkendall DT, Contiguglia SR (eds): *The U.S. Soccer Sports Medicine Book*. Baltimore, MD, Williams & Wilkins, 1996, pp 326–345.

76. Ekstrand J, Tropp H: The incidence of ankle sprains in soccer. *Foot Ankle* 1990;11:41–44.

77. Cattermole HR, Hardy JR, Gregg PJ: The footballer's fracture. *Br J Sports Med* 1996;30:171–175.

78. McCarroll JR, Schrader JW, Shelbourne KD, Rettig AC, Bisesi MA: Meniscoid lesions of the ankle in soccer players. *Am J Sports Med* 1987;15:255–257.

79. Knapp TP, Mandelbaum BR: Ankle sprains and impingement syndromes, Garrett WE Jr, Kirkendall DT, Contiguglia SR (eds): *The U.S. Soccer Sports Medicine Book*. Baltimore, MD, Williams & Wilkins, 1996, pp 360–368.

80. Tysvaer AT, Storli OV, Bachen NI: Soccer injuries to the brain: A neurologic and electroencephalographic study of former players. *Acta Neurol Scand* 1989;80:151–156.

81. Smodlaka VN: Medical aspects of heading the ball in soccer. *Phys Sportsmed* 1984;12:127–131.

82. Tysvaer AT, Lochen EA: Soccer injuries to the brain: a neuropsychologic study of former soccer players. *Am J Sports Med* 1991;19:56–60.

83. Sortland O, Tysvaer AT, Storli OV: Changes in the cervical spine in association football players. *Br J Sports Med* 1982;16:80–84.

84. Jordan SE, Green GA, Galanty HL, Mandelbaum BR, Jabour BA: Acute and chronic brain injury in United States National Team soccer players. *Am J Sports Med* 1996;24:205–210.

85. *Guidelines for the Management of Concussion in Sports*. Denver, CO, Colorado Medical Society, 1991.

86. Cantu RC: Return to play guidelines after a head injury. *Clin Sports Med* 1998;17:45–60.

87. Report of the Quality Standards Subcommittee, American Academy of Neurology: Practice parameter: The management of concussion in sports (summary statement). *Neurology* 1997;48:581–585.

88. Abreau F, Templer DI, Schuyler BA, et al: Neuropsychological assessment of soccer players. *Neuropsychology* 1990;4:175–181.

89. Rimel RW, Giordani B, Barth JT, Boll TJ, Jane JA: Disability caused by minor head injury. *Neurosurgery* 1981;9:221–228.

90. Rimel RW, Giordani B, Barth JT, Jane JA: Moderate head injury: Completing the clinical spectrum of brain trauma. *Neurosurgery* 1982;11:344–351.

91. Echemendia RJ, Putukian M, Mackin S, et al: Neuropsychological test performance prior to and following sports-related mild traumatic brain injury. *Clin J Sports Med*, in press.

92. Alves WM, Rimel RW, Nelson WE: University of Virginia prospective study of football-induced minor head injury: Status report. *Clin Sports Med* 1987;6:211–218.

93. Levin HS, Williams D, Crofford MJ, et al: Relationship of depth of brain lesions to consciousness and outcome after closed head injury. *J Neurosurg* 1988;69:861–866.

94. Levin HS, Amparo E, Eisenberg HM, et al: Magnetic resonance imaging and computerized tomography in relation to the neurobehavioral sequelae of mild and moderate head injuries. *J Neurosurg* 1987;66:706–713.

95. Porter MD, Fricker PA: Controlled prospective neuropsychological assessment of active experienced amateur boxers. *Clin J Sport Med* 1996;6:90–96.

96. McLatchie G, Brooks N, Galbraith S, et al: Clinical neurological examination, neuropsychology, electroencephalography and computed tomographic head scanning in active amateur boxers. *J Neurol Neurosurg Psychiatry* 1987;50:96–99.

97. Ekstrand J, Gillquist J: The avoidability of soccer injuries. *Int J Sports Med* 1983;4:124–128.

Chapter 15
Gymnastics

Jill L. McNitt-Gray, PhD

The Problem: Control of Reaction Forces Using Effective Load Distribution Strategies

In gymnastics, large reaction forces are applied to the musculoskeletal system during hand or foot interaction with the apparatus. Large forces and moments need to be generated by muscle-tendon units to counteract or control the translation and rotation effects of these large reaction forces[1] (Fig. 1). If the muscle-tendon units are unable to effectively control the forces and moments created by the reaction forces imposed on the system, ligaments, bone, and other soft tissues may experience an increase in load. The ability of muscle-tendon units to generate force may be compromised by an inability of the gymnast to anticipate impending load, weakness at a specific muscle-tendon unit length or velocity, inadequate coordination of muscle activation and/or segment motion, pathology, or neuromuscular fatigue.

The high incidence of injury to the extremities of competitive gymnasts, which has been reported in the literature, indicates mechanical loading of the musculoskeletal system is out of balance with the ability of the body to positively adapt to the loads experienced. A causal relationship between load and injury, however, has been difficult to establish because of the inability to directly measure forces experienced by individual components of the musculoskeletal system.[2,3] Another limitation is the result of current methods of determining load exposure and tissue response in relation to the hormonal and nutritional environment of growing gymnasts.

This chapter aims to define what is and is not known regarding the dynamic imbalance between mechanical loading encountered during gymnastics participation and the response of the musculoskeletal system to these loads. The context in which loading is applied is discussed first by providing an overview of the sport of gymnastics. Second, factors contributing to musculoskeletal loading are summarized and related to injuries reported in the literature. Third, research results specific to load distribution and tissue response to load are discussed in light of reported injuries. Gender specific issues are highlighted throughout as they arise.

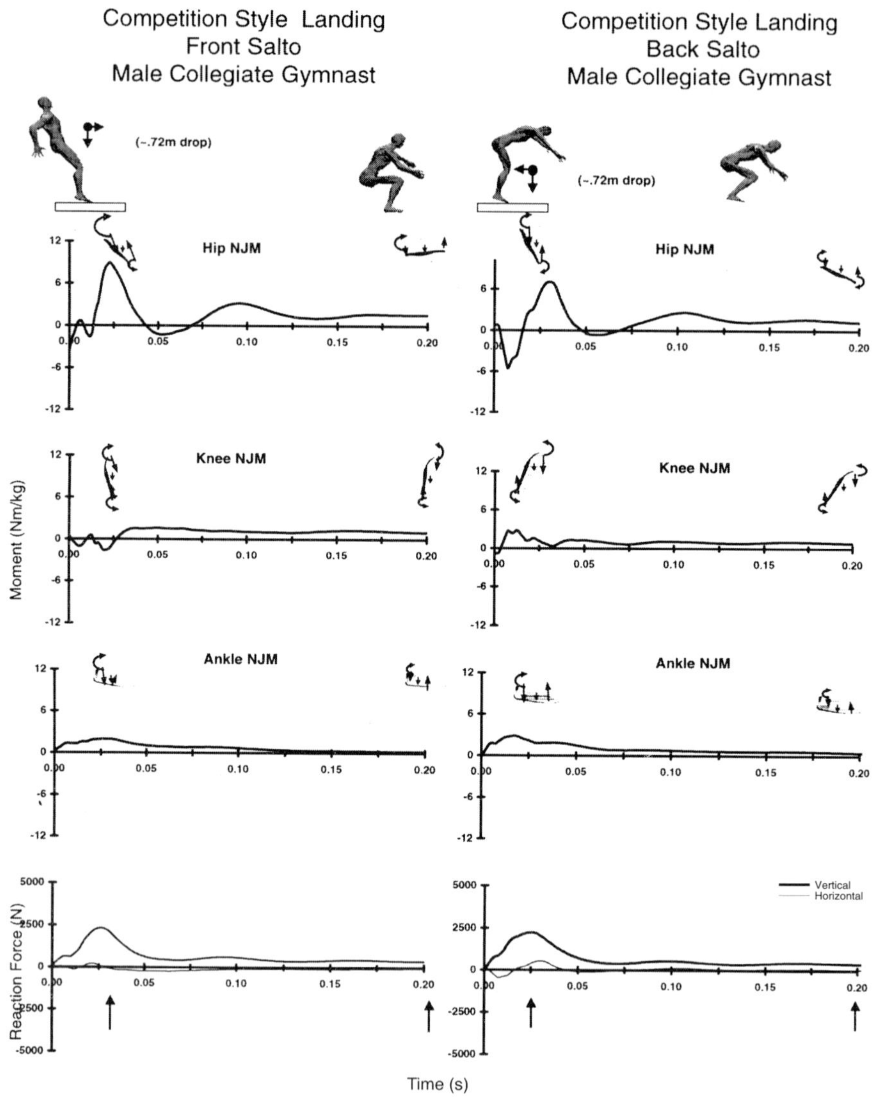

Fig. 1 During interaction with the apparatus and landing surfaces, gymnasts experience large external reaction forces. These forces are progressively attenuated as they are transmitted through the musculoskeletal system. If the forces act at an angle relative to the segment, the forces will also cause moments that must be controlled by muscle-tendon units and soft tissue. These free body diagrams illustrate how the magnitude and direction of the lower extremity net joint moments are influenced by the angle of the proximal and distal net joint forces (NJF) relative to the segment angle as well as the adjacent joint net joint moment (NJM). Note the differences in knee and hip NJM demand between the landing tasks. These data were acquired for male collegiate gymnasts during the landing of front and back saltos onto regulation landing mats supported by force plates from a platform 0.72 m above the landing surface.[1] Although these joint kinetics are based on data acquired for male gymnasts, the difference in mechanical demand imposed on the knee and hip between tasks is likely to be similar for female gymnasts. The free body diagrams are drawn at the times indicated by the arrows along the x axis. Time zero is the time of first contact with the landing surface.

Gymnastics Overview

Historical Perspective

Sport

Gymnastics is often considered fundamental for all sports. Participants develop skills critical to the performance of many movements including balance, agility, flexibility, strength, biomechanical coordination, and self-discipline. Gymnastics has existed for over 2,000 years.[4] In the 1930 World Championships in Luxembourg, the competition included the pole vault, the broad jump, shot put, rope climb, and a 100-m sprint. In the 1928 Olympic Games, the team combined exercise was introduced as the first women's event. Today, the Internationale Federation de Gymnastique (FIG) governs five forms of gymnastic expression: Men's Artistic Gymnastics, Women's Artistic Gymnastics, Rhythmic Sports Gymnastics, General Gymnastics, and Sports Aerobics. According to the 1995 census, more than 25 million people are affiliated with gymnastics worldwide.[4] Today, more than 71,000 athletes are registered in competitive gymnastics programs within the United States and compete in 3,000 competitions sanctioned by USA Gymnastics.

Age of Participants

The mean age of gymnasts participating in official international competitions has declined. For example, during the period between the 1968 Olympic Games in Mexico and the 1988 Olympic Games in Seoul, the mean age of the top six men's teams decreased by 3.5 years (25 to 21.5 years), whereas the mean age of the women's teams decreased by 6.5 years (24 to 17.5 years).[5] During the Tokyo Olympic Games in 1964, the mean chronologic age of female gymnasts (N = 102) was 22.7 years, whereas during the World Championships at Rotterdam, The Netherlands, in 1987, the mean age (N = 201) was 16.5 years.[6]

The age of the gymnast at the initiation of gymnastics training has also decreased. For example, in 1948 boys began training at 16 years of age and girls began training at 13 years of age. In contrast, in 1991 boys initiate gymnastics training at 6 to 7 years of age and girls begin at 5 to 6 years of age.

The number and duration of annual competitions has also increased (from 5 to 6 per year to 15 to 16 per year), as has the number and duration of training sessions.[5] The increase in training corresponds to the increasing value due to more difficult movements as defined by the current Code of Points.[5]

Performance Evaluation

During competition, the performance of the gymnast is evaluated by a panel of judges according to the Code of Points. The Code of Points is a working document that evolves with the sport. Artistic presentation; routine composition; and skill amplitude, originality, and difficulty are heavily weighted in the evaluation process. To remain competitive, gymnasts must master more difficult skills. As skill amplitude and difficulty increase, the total body center of mass (TBCM) velocity at contact and the magnitude of the reaction force experienced during contact with the apparatus also increase. Therefore, as gymnasts advance in skill level they must master these tasks without injuring themselves during interaction with the apparatus and landing surface.

Athlete Preparation Process

As part of their participation in gymnastics, gymnasts develop strength, power, and flexibility through a range of angles and velocities. In addition, gymnasts learn to anticipate and control large reaction forces applied to the body in a variety of directions during hand and foot interaction with the mats and apparatus. Gymnasts also learn to stabilize joints effectively as a means of resisting external forces and/or limiting body segmentation in order to improve movement aesthetics. Gymnasts also tend to be stronger relative to their body mass than age matched norms.[7] Gymnasts tend to weigh less and be shorter than age matched controls; however, segment lengths relative to the stature were observed to be similar.[7] Gymnasts tend to be less endomorphic and more mesomorphic than controls.[7] Their capacity to generate muscle force and consistently control multijoint movement enables them to use effective compensatory responses when the body is perturbed.

Many questions remain regarding effective methods for balancing musculoskeletal loading with the repetition needed for consistent skill performance, particularly when training individuals with immature musculoskeletal systems. Gymnasts have been observed to exhibit a delay in skeletal maturity of about 1.5 years compared to reference subjects. Late maturation may contribute to the desire of an individual to continue gymnastics participation.[8] For those who had attained menarche, mean age at menarche was 15.1 ± 1.3 years.

USA Gymnastics has addressed the needs of their 50,000 registered female athletes, most of them adolescents, by creating a wellness program. The mission of the wellness program is to create a positive environment for gymnasts to acquire the physical and mental tools needed to pursue their goals, secure their well being, and enjoy the sport of gymnastics. Wellness Program recommendations for gymnasts include: participation in a national team mentoring system to further develop self-esteem, encourage communication about challenges and fears, and decrease the sense of isolation. As part of this program, gymnasts are also encouraged to discuss concerns regarding nutrition and psychology with professionals and to learn how to address their coach and parents regarding their concerns and experiences. This goal is being achieved by establishing educational opportunities and a referral network under the direction of a former Olympic gymnast.[9]

Factors Contributing to Musculoskeletal Loading Experienced During Gymnastics Skills

Apparatus

Gender Issues

Female gymnasts compete in four events: balance beam, uneven bars, vaulting horse, and floor exercise. Male gymnasts compete in 6 events: high bar, parallel bars, pommel horse, vaulting horse, rings, and floor exercise. In all events, with the exception of the floor exercise event, the height, shape, and mechanical properties of the apparatus will vary between events. For example, the height and orientation of the vaulting horse is different in the male and female events. The bar materials, suspension system, bar shape, and height are different in male and female bar events. The thickness of landing surfaces used also varies between male and female events. Therefore, analysis of gender differences in injury patterns needs to consider the geometric constraints and the mechanical properties of the specific apparatus when characterizing the stress imposed on the gymnast by the environment.

Although a male and a female gymnast may execute the same skill, the differences in the apparatus often pose unique challenges from a mechanical loading perspective. For example, skills performed by male gymnasts often require more upper extremity control of large reaction forces applied to the hands by the apparatus (eg, on rings, parallel bars, pommel horse) than skills typically performed by female gymnasts. In the uneven bar event, the presence of the low bar reduces the time and limits the distance the female gymnast can position her TBCM away from the bar during the downswing of a giant circle performed on the high bar. In contrast, a male gymnast performing a giant swing on the high bar is unrestricted during the downswing of a giant swing. The consequence of this mechanical disadvantage to the female gymnast presented during the downswing may result in the need to decrease the distance of her TBCM relative to the bar during the upswing. One means of reorienting the TBCM relative to the bar is to hyperextend the back. Recent modifications of the uneven bar apparatus have been effective in reducing the mechanical disadvantage imposed by the low bar by allowing the bars to be placed farther apart. This modification enables the gymnast to position her TBCM farther from the high bar for a longer period of time and thus reduces the need for compensatory responses during the upswing phase of the giant swing. Even with these apparatus modifications, however, female gymnasts do not have the same relative mechanical advantage as male gymnasts during the downswing phase of the giant swing.

In the vaulting event, female gymnasts need to initiate hand contact with the horse oriented perpendicular to the runway, whereas the length of the horse is oriented parallel to the runway in men's vaulting. The perpendicular orientation of the horse creates a much narrower margin for error in the direction of the run than in the parallel orientation. Initiation of hand first contact with the horse is further complicated during round-off entry vaults during which the gymnast dives backward towards the horse from a springboard. In the floor-exercise event, the construction and properties of the sprung floor, made up of layers of springs, wood, foam, and carpet, is the same for the 80-lb female gymnast and the 160-lb male gymnast.

Competition Issues

Effective interaction between the athlete and equipment is critical for maximizing performance. Successful performance of advanced skills depends on the ability of the gymnast to use features of the apparatus. Before the competition, gymnasts have limited exposure to landing surfaces and apparatus placed on podiums. During competition, gymnasts have only one opportunity to demonstrate mastery of the apparatus. As skills increase in difficulty, the solution space for accomplishing the task narrows.[10]

Mechanical Properties

Although gymnastics equipment used in international competition must fall within guidelines established by the FIG governing body, these standards are broad and allow for great variations in equipment between venues. The purpose of these standards has been to ensure justice in competition by establishing uniformity of equipment used during sanctioned gymnastics competitions. Although standardization of apparatus in advance of the competition is critical to ensure gymnasts can adequately prepare for specific competition conditions, the standard has not been specifically designed to promote effective interaction between the gymnast and the surface. While rigid body tests provide repeatable results in characterizing the impact between inanimate objects, they fail to assess the internal loading implications of strategies gymnasts use to interact with different surfaces.[3,11,12]

Mechanical Loading Issues

The response characteristics of the apparatus in relation to the movement of the gymnast will influence both the mechanical effectiveness of the interaction and the musculoskeletal loading experienced during each hand and/or foot contact. Effective interaction with the apparatus during hand and foot contact often must occur in less than 0.025 s. Therefore, even small differences in the mechanical response characteristics of the apparatus between venues may significantly change the parameters of the skill and, thus, require the gymnast to modify his or her technique just before or during the performance. For example, every hand and foot contact with the apparatus gives the gymnast the opportunity to generate or lose momentum. Because total body momentum is progressively generated by performing a series of skills, a negative interaction during one hand or foot contact in the series may have a detrimental effect on the final skill of the series.

Gymnasts performing skills on an apparatus unlike the apparatus they have trained on for years will most likely experience significant changes in musculoskeletal loading patterns. For example, suspension of the rings using leather or nylon materials will change the mechanical response of the rings in relation to the gymnast's movements. While the response of the ring suspension system may have little effect on static strength moves (eg, cross), the more dynamic nature of current skills (eg, double back) tends to amplify the differences in response characteristics. An unanticipated experience of external load applied to the hands may mechanically overload components of the upper extremity. Similarly, if the floor exercise surface recoils more quickly than anticipated, the orientation of the joint and segment at the time of recoil may be different than usual. As gymnasts adapt their movement patterns to mechanical response characteristics of the apparatus, they are reported to experience more jerky movements than normal in unusual segment and/or joint positions. These observations suggest the lack of coordinated muscles or insufficient activation of muscles needed to control moments induced by the external force experienced at the hands or feet. In addition, muscle-tendon units throughout the body may be at unusual lengths or velocities and, therefore, may be unable to generate the same magnitude of force. If the neuromuscular and skeletal systems are unprepared for changes in loading (eg, contact time, loading rate, and force magnitude) induced by a change in the mechanical characteristics of the board, excessive mechanical loading of the system may occur.

The need to adapt to variations in apparatus occurs in all ten events. For example, the vaulting board used during competition may be a Reuther (slower recoil) or spring (faster recoil) type board. The response characteristics of each board will also vary with the vaulting skill performed (eg, round-off entry versus handspring). Wood bars and fiberglass bars used in the uneven and parallel bar events have different mechanical response characteristics. The parallel bar event may be further complicated because of differences in response characteristics between bars. If the covers on the vaulting horse or balance beam are too firm, the gymnast may experience higher loads or opt to flex the joints to dissipate the load. If the covers are too soft, the gymnast may experience a potentially detrimental increase in wrist extension during periods of high loading.

Given this potential for apparatus modifications between venues, gymnasts need to be trained in a manner that enables them to effectively control reaction forces under a variety of conditions and to quickly and effectively adapt to changes in the mechanical properties of their apparatus and landing surfaces. If the gymnast is unable to adapt quickly to apparatus modifications, the repetition required to master multiple skills under a variety of apparatus and landing surface conditions would significantly add to mechanical loading that the body must endure to remain competitive. In addition, the use of compensatory actions to control the changes in reaction forces may result in detrimental load distribution patterns.

Relating Mechanical Loading to Reported Injuries

To avoid injury, musculoskeletal load experienced by the gymnast needs to be kept in balance with the ability of musculoskeletal structures to respond to stress induced by loading.[13] A positive training regime ensures that the exposure to load is balanced with sufficient recovery time, the hormonal environment provides a cyclical estrogen cycle, and the nutritional environment ensures that the rate of replenishment exceeds use. The interplay between load exposure and blood levels of reproductive hormones (estrogen, progesterone) and calcium can be of great significance in the development of bone mineral density (BMD).[7] Because BMD has been reported to account for 80% to 90% of the variance in bone compressive strength, the interaction between load exposure and the hormonal and nutritional environment plays an important role in skeletal adaptations to load.[14]

In a negative training regime, the exposure to load exceeds recovery, there is an absence of an estrogen cycle, and the rate of use of nutritional resources exceeds replenishment. Adolescent females with menstrual dysfunction, such as delayed menarche and/or missed menses, typically exhibit lower BMD and lower bone cortical thickness than healthy age-matched controls. Although participation in gymnastics appears to protect adolescent girls against excessive bone loss as compared to age matched controls,[13,15,16] we do not know whether this response is sufficient for the musculoskeletal system to withstand the extraordinary large forces experienced during take-offs and landings from gymnastics apparatus.

One excessive load may result in acute injury (eg, fracture, sprain) or may lead to chronic injury (eg, cartilage damage). Repetitive loading may produce positive effects such as increased critical limits of musculoskeletal components or negative effects such as fatigue fracture, muscle soreness, or chronic pain. The cumulative effect of hand and foot interactions with the apparatus adds to the complexity of determining injury mechanisms. Although ineffective interaction with the apparatus may have a limited effect on the mechanics of a single hand or foot contact phase, successful performance of complex skills depends on the outcome of a series of skills performed before the complex skill. Therefore, a series of negative interactions with the apparatus may lead to insufficient generation of linear and/or angular momentum at take-off. Inadequate linear and angular momentum at take-off leads to insufficient time or rotation to complete the aerial skill and prepare for a high velocity landing on the floor. Repeated miscues experienced by the gymnast during the equipment adaptation period most likely lead to a cumulative overloading of the musculoskeletal system. Whereas load exposure is necessary to improve skill levels and competitive performance, positive adaptations in the musculoskeletal and neurologic systems in response to the mechanical forces experienced by gymnasts can be achieved only in a healthy hormonal and nutritional environment.

Interpretation of Epidemiology Literature

The injuries reported in the literature reflect an inability to control the forces and moments created by large reaction forces applied during contact with the apparatus. In general, structures located closest to the point of force application tend to experience the highest incidence of injury. Care must be taken when interpreting injury data reported in the literature. First, musculoskeletal loading experienced by an individual gymnast may vary greatly between gymnasts due to the unique mechanical demands imposed by the numerous skills gymnasts may elect to perform (> 3,000 skills). For example, a gymnast competing in all four events will experience compressive, tensile, and torsional loads at multiple musculoskeletal sites. Therefore, it is difficult to establish a causal relationship between load and injury. In contrast, establishing an associative relationship between pain and the performance of a particular skill is relatively easy. Second, the incidence of injury reported for patient populations may be significantly different than that for the population of gymnasts participating in the sport who are not patients. Third, interpretation of injury rates and disordered eating needs to consider the prevalence of the problem in like populations that are not participating in gymnastics. For example, self-esteem of all preadolescent females tends to plummet by as much as 30%. Because most recreational, competitive, and elite female gymnasts are in middle and high school, the design of experiments needs to differentiate between gymnasts and age-matched controls with similar activity levels. Fourth, quantitative assessment of musculoskeletal loading using biomechanical methods is labor and technologically intensive. Therefore, hypotheses are tested using data obtained from relatively few gymnasts who often compete and train as a gymnastics team. Finally, few studies assess the many benefits of gymnastics participation if kept in balance. For example, the female athlete triad, defined as the interrelatedness of disordered eating, amenorrhea, and osteoporosis, has been identified as an area of concern for all female athletes. Recent studies on BMD, however, indicate gymnasts tend to have higher BMD than age-matched controls.

Reported Injuries

Published literature on gymnastics ranges from single case studies[17,18] to prospective studies.[19,20] From these studies, the location and type of injury experienced has been documented. However, none, due to methodologic challenges, have been able to report the status of the musculoskeletal system and define the mechanical load experienced and the resulting injury. Suggestions for establishing injury patterns and risk characteristics include large-scale prospective studies.[21] To be effective in elucidating causal relationships between load and injury, a means to characterize and assess load exposure in relation to the current state of the musculoskeletal system is needed. In addition, the experimental design will need to control for the effect of coaching and medical personnel skills, mechanical properties of the apparatus, and landing surfaces on load exposure.[21]

Gymnasts experience large diverse repetitive loads that are skill, surface, and gymnast dependent.[22–24] These loads produce positive and negative adaptations in the musculoskeletal system. The response of the musculoskeletal system to stress induced by gymnastics participation has potentially long-lasting effects on the health of the individual (eg, BMD, growth plate, arthritis). For example, of 21 patients with stress injury of the distal radial growth plate, 11 patients also exhibited other osteochondritides including Osgood-Schlatter disease, Scheuermann disease, Sever disease, and Sinding-Larsen disease.[25] These observations suggest the gymnasts' musculoskeletal system was not able to withstand forces at multiple sites. The growth plate is particularly vulnerable when at its thickest during the growth spurt or when widened as a result of repetitive trauma.[25]

One way to prevent injuries is to identify effective load distribution mechanisms and define load exposure cycles that permit adequate recovery time for tissues to adapt to induced stress. In general, the epidemiology literature has consistently arrived at a similar distribution of injuries across body parts. The lower extremities account for 50% to 66% of the reported injuries.[7,19,20,26–31] Ankle and knee injuries account for 28% to 37% of the reported injuries, whereas the low back accounts for approximately 10% to 20% of the injuries reported for female gymnasts.[21,27,29] Floor exercise and the uneven bars account for close to 60% of the reported injuries for female gymnasts. Male gymnasts also exhibit similar percent of ankle and low back injuries with less knee and more shoulder and wrist injuries as compared to the female gymnasts.[27,31] The observed difference in shoulder injuries has been associated with the additional upper extremity loading associated with the men's events (pommel horse, rings, and parallel bars). In a retrospective study of 116 elite artistic gymnasts at the Australian Institute of Sport training an average of 36 to 40 hours per week over a 10-year period, no catastrophic injuries were reported.[27] Acute injuries accounted for 60% of injuries for both male and female gymnasts, whereas, chronic injuries accounted for 40% of injuries for both male and female gymnasts.[27]

The number of injuries appears to be proportional to the skill level.[19,32–34] Injury rates tend to increase as gymnasts transition between performance of individual skills and routines.[29] This observation points toward a decrease in the ability of the gymnast to control the external forces applied to the system, as well as a potential change in the force-time characteristics experienced by the gymnasts when landing on less-forgiving surfaces. Strains, sprains, and tendinitis account for approximately 50% of the reported injuries to female college gymnasts.[27,31] Related issues also include the inability to maintain momentum when transitioning between skills, thereby requiring the gymnast to create greater reaction forces to increase momentum or initiate compensatory technique modifications to accommodate for less momentum available before the initiation of the skill. Either way, unusual loads are experienced that may overload a component of the musculoskeletal system. The influence of neuromuscular control or anatomic alignment, however, has not been elucidated.

Bones closest to the point of force application may experience contusions during inadvertent collisions with the apparatus (eg, kick by mistake, land on bar teeth first) or may experience a fracture of a bone. Most bone adapts to stress through remodeling. However, stress fractures have been observed in bone close to the point of external reaction forces. Joints closest to the application of the reaction force, wrist and ankle, experience pain during forced dorsiflexion and wrist extension and, in some cases, impingement.[35,36] Sprains may be medial or lateral and, from a mechanical perspective, are most likely linked to the moment induced by the reaction force.

Swinging on bars and hand first landings on a variety of surfaces, including a spring floor, balance beam, vaulting runway, and the vaulting horse, load the wrist and hand in a variety of ways. During the course of a practice, a gymnast may experience load during interaction under all of these conditions. Therefore, without more information regarding the load exposure scenario associated with the injury, a causal relationship cannot be established. The hand and wrist are the structures closest to the point of force application during interaction with the apparatus, and therefore, they are likely to experience high loads. Distal radial growth plate injury has been associated with gymnastics participation;[7,17,25,37–43] this may lead to slowed, interrupted, or retarded skeletal development.[44] Ulnar variance associated with gymnastics participation, however, may be overstated in the literature.[7] Recent research with age-matched controls, however, indicates 80% of the gymnasts studied fell within the 95% confidence interval for normal ulnar variance parameters.[7] Other wrist injuries include scaphoid/lunate impaction syndrome, scaphoid stress fracture, ulnar impaction, and carpal chondromalacia.[45] Soft-tissue injuries include capsulitis, impingement, wrist splints, fibrocartilage tears, ganglia, instability, De Quervain tendinitis, Squeakers syndrome, contusions, and sprains.[43,45] Wrist injuries tend to be aggravated during dorsiflexion involving hand-first impact and rotation[25] and may be related to dowel grip use.[41]

As with the hand and wrist, the foot and ankle are the structures closest to the point of force application during foot-first contact with the apparatus and, therefore, they experience high loads. As the force is transmitted through the musculoskeletal system, the forces created by muscles controlling the moments induced by the reaction force will add to the load experienced by the gymnast. If muscles are unable to control these moments induced by the reaction forces, injuries may result. For example, ankle injuries include Achilles tendinitis, bursitis, inversion, and capsular sprain/inpingement. The different regions of ankle injuries likely are due to the interaction between the foot position, the point of force application of the reaction force, and the ability of the gymnast to control the moment induced by the reaction force. For example, if a gymnast lands using a toe-heel pattern, and the plantar flexors are unable to control the large, rapid dorsiflexor moment induced by the reaction force, the Achilles tendon and plantar flexor muscle group are likely to experience a large rapid increase in tensile load. Similarly, if the gymnast lands on the side of her foot and is unable to control the inversion or eversion moment created by the reaction force, structures opposing the moment created by the reaction force are likely to experience a large rapid increase in tensile load. As force is transmitted through the lower extremity, intersegmental forces are created. If the moments created by these transmitted forces about the shaft of the long bones are unopposed by muscular forces, bending moments may be induced that lead to bone fracture. For example, a tibia fracture[46] was reported during a landing on a springboard.

During foot-first interaction with the landing surface or apparatus, the knee flexes. The degree of knee flexion may differ depending on the goal of the task or the mechanical properties of the landing surface. Reported knee injuries include capsular sprain, meniscal tears, patellofemoral dislocation, synovitis, tendinitis,[36] ligament rupture, anterior cruciate ligament (ACL) injury with and without meniscal or ligamentous damage, patellofemoral pain, Osgood-Schlatter disease, Sinding-Larsen-Johansson disease, and muscle strains.[21,27] Injuries of the ACL have been associated with a twist at landing or hyperextension. These injuries reflect the diverse role the knee plays in either transmitting force by maintaining the knee angle or attenuating the force by allowing controlled flexion of the knee.

In contrast to the knee, the role of the elbow tends to be to transmit force applied at the hand to the shoulder complex. The reported elbow injuries, including arthrosis, nodules,[47] dislocation,[27] and olecranon fracture,[26] reflect the role of the elbow as a force transmitter.

During the flight phase, the trunk plays an active role in controlling the resistance of the body to rotation (moment of inertia). If gymnasts need to rotate faster in a layout position, the spine is placed in a hyperextended position so that the distribution of the body mass is closer to the TBCM. During interaction with the landing surfaces and apparatus, the structures of the trunk, pelvis, and shoulder complex experience whatever force has not been attenuated through the extremities. Therefore, the pelvis and spine need to be aligned in an advantageous position to handle them when they experience these transmitted forces. The trunk injuries reported to be in the lumbosacral spine reflect this mechanical demand during foot-first landings. Trunk injuries include spondylolysis related disorders,[48] stress fracture of the pars interarticularis at the level of L5,[49–52] stress fracture, disc degeneration, and structural abnormalities, particularly in older gymnasts.[53–55] Trunk injuries tend to be aggravated by activities involving control of large forces, rotation, or hyperextension,[51,54,56] apophyseal injury, and spinal flexion at T12 after a landing. Back pain during gymnastics is not suggestive of disk degeneration; however, evidence of disk degeneration may appear in retired gymnasts.[53]

Research Regarding Musculoskeletal Loading Experienced by Gymnasts

While current technology limits the ability to directly measure forces experienced by individual components of the musculoskeletal system in vivo, joint kinetics, kinematics, and electromyographic techniques have been successful in providing insight regarding load distribution strategies used by gymnasts. For example, the examination of work done by net joint moments provides an "index of softness" that can be used to categorize landings that favor loading of muscle or bone.[57] Examination of load distribution strategies used during the landings of complex gymnastics skills performed under realistic circumstances have also enabled assessment of internal loading implications of the strategies gymnasts use to interact with different surfaces. Continued biomechanical analyses of these types of data will contribute to the development of improved training methods and of surfaces that facilitate successful performance and minimize the potential for injury. Musculoskeletal modeling may assist in inferring internal loads experienced by gymnastics during the performance of gymnastics skills. Accurate estimates, however, require adequate representations of the individual's physical plant (musculoskeletal system) and control strategies (muscle activation patterns). Extrapolation of results obtained from mechanical tests of specimens in vitro to in vivo performance requires caution. Loading of in vitro specimens also requires knowledge regarding the load-exposure profiles observed in vivo.

Landing Preparation

Musculoskeletal loading during hand- and foot-first landing is influenced by the strategies a gymnast uses to prepare for the impending collision and to distribute load during the landing. Because the musculoskeletal system experiences large loads immediately following contact, strategies used to attenuate and control the reaction force must be initiated before contact.[58] The ability of a gymnast to prepare for contact may be compromised by the preparation time, segment kinematics, and visual conditions before contact.[59–62] The inability to prepare for effective interaction with the landing surface may result in serious injury. For example, 76% of trampoline related injuries occurred when someone else was on the trampoline, thereby changing the anticipated response characteristics of the landing surface.[63]

The landing preparation time during the flight phase preceding touchdown influences the ability of the athlete to prepare for contact. Preparation for contact may include placement of segments in an advantageous position at touchdown, adjustment of lower extremity segment velocity before contact, and/or activation of the muscles responsible for controlling the reaction force. For example, gymnasts attempting to land more softly than normal will reduce the reaction force magnitude experienced after contact by pulling up the lower extremity (decrease downward velocity) just before contact. Therefore, skills performed preceding the landing task must be performed in a way that ensures adequate preparation time is available before touchdown. During the flight phase of simple drop landings, joints of the lower extremity approach full extension and then flex just before touchdown.[58,64,65] Landings of more complex tasks from relatively low apparatus, however, may limit the time a gymnast has to prepare for contact.

Compensatory kinematics associated with reductions in landing preparation time were also observed in a within-subject comparison of dismount landings performed by gymnasts during the 1996 Olympic Games. In general, dismounts with longer flight times provided the gymnast with more time to complete the required rotations and to extend the joints in preparation for contact, whereas dismounts with shorter flight times provided the gymnast with less time to complete both the rotation and preparation for foot-first contact. For example, greater hip angles at touchdown and greater flight times were observed for landings of backward rotating dismounts performed from the high bar than for those from the parallel bars.[66] The longer flight times observed for the high bar dismounts were associated with the higher height of the apparatus and the greater TBCM vertical velocity at the time of release from the high bar as compared to the height and velocity observed at time of release from the parallel bars. Differences in the hip angle at touchdown between tasks influences the musculoskeletal loading characteristics by requiring hip muscles to generate moments at different muscle lengths.

Landing preparation time may also be compromised by decreases in time to view the landing surface. For example, the success rate of forward rotating handspring vaults performed by male gymnasts during the 1992 Olympic compulsory competition was less than 15% of those performed.[67] In addition, male and female gymnasts apparently chose to avoid landings of forward rotating skills when choreographing their optional routines for the 1992 Olympic Gymnastics Competition.[67] The avoidance of forward rotating tasks may also reflect difficulty in preparing for and controlling large forces and moments after touchdown.

Reaction Forces During Landing

The amplitude, direction, and loading rate of reaction force experienced during take-off and landings of gymnastics skills have been found to vary with linear and angular velocity at contact, surface properties, direction of rotation,[61,68–73] and athlete skill level. For example, male gymnasts competing at the Junior National level experience large vertical reaction forces during take-off and landings of tumbling skills (eg, feet first: 10 to 14 times body weight [BW];[70,71,74] hand first: 1.5 to 2.5 BW).[23,24,75] These large compressive forces create the need for bones to increase their resistance to large multidirectional load. Positive adaptations in bone will result in greater resistance to the forces applied. Therefore, greater than normal BMD observed in athletes experiencing high reaction forces during impact activities is consistent with current theories regarding bone remodeling. Load exposure characteristics unique to gymnastics also include the magnitude and direction of horizontal reaction forces experienced by both the hands and feet (eg, 3 to 5 BW versus running at 0.75 BW)[23,24,75,76] and the generation and reduction of total body angular momentum during take-offs and landings of gymnastics skills. Both hand- and foot-first interactions with the apparatus and landing surfaces are characterized by high frequency force after contact followed by a second lower frequency force.[23,24,72]

Landing Kinematics

Comparison of minimum knee and hip angles observed during gymnastics landings performed from progressively higher heights with and without landing mats indicates that landing on a mat may reduce the need for knee and hip flexion.[72] Accomplishing the landing task with less lower extremity joint flexion may allow the gymnast to generate the net joint moments needed to control the large reaction force at more advantageous muscle lengths. If less joint flexion were required to perform a landing, then more knee and hip range of motion would become available to compensate for instability and/or unexpected events.[65]

Landing Kinetics

Within-subject comparison of force-time characteristics observed during gymnastics landings performed with and without mats indicates the time to peak reaction force tends to be delayed when landing on a mat.[77] Time to peak force may also be delayed when gymnasts voluntarily attempt to reduce the peak reaction force experienced during landing by slowing the downward velocity of the lower extremity before contact and initiating contact with a more vertical foot position.[10,78] The more vertical foot position appears to provide the gymnast with more time to reduce the velocity of the heel before contact with the landing surface.[78] The ability to control the foot during contact, however, may be compromised when the muscles are fatigued.[79]

During landings of front and back saltos, the horizontal component of the reaction forces changes direction multiple times (Fig. 1). The initial direction of the horizontal component appears to act to reduce the angular momentum at contact. However, the direction of the net horizontal impulse during the landing phase acts to reduce the horizontal momentum of the TBCM at contact.

Joint kinetics during gymnastics landings and load distribution between joints appear to be influenced by task, momentum, skill level, and surface.[72] These observed differences in load are associated with differences in segment kinematics and reaction forces between landing conditions. For example, the differences in kinematics and reaction forces at contact between front and back salto landings contributed to the need for different knee net joint moments between tasks (Fig. 1).

Task differences in load distribution were also observed between front and back salto landings performed by the same gymnast[1] (Fig. 1). The negative work by the ankle net joint movement made up a greater percent of the total negative work during the back salto landings than during the front salto landings. In contrast, work done by the hip net joint movement was a greater percent of the total negative work during the front salto landings than during the back salto landings.

Landing Practice

The intensity of training regimes needs to accommodate potential changes in musculoskeletal loading when athletes make transitions between landing surfaces. For example, when gymnasts learn new skills they often land the aerial skill in a deep foam pit. Reaction forces experienced during the take-off phase of tumbling skills, however, are similar in magnitude to those experienced during landings of aerial skills (10 to 14 times body weight[80]). Although the internal loading consequences of these reaction forces during the take-off and landing phase tumbling skills may be different because of the differences in body position and mechanical objectives between tasks, the loading is significant.

As an intermediate step during skill development, gymnasts may perform the landing of an aerial skill onto 0.2-m crash pads placed on top of the spring floor. Although the mat thickness provides the gymnast with additional time to reduce body momentum, the deformation pattern of the surface around the foot may increase the potential for foot, subtalar, and ankle instability. Because less energy is being absorbed by the surface, the athlete must absorb more energy. Therefore, training regimes need to be adjusted to accommodate changes in musculoskeletal loading associated with different surfaces.

In summary, gymnasts need to practice take-offs and landings under a variety of velocity, rotation, surface, and preparation conditions using a training regime that balances load exposure with recovery time. Uncontrolled landings reduce team score and may result in excessive loading of the musculoskeletal system. Training regimes need to consider modifications in musculoskeletal loading when athletes make transitions between landing surfaces.

Acknowledgments

This research was funded in part by USA Gymnastics; the US and International Olympic Committees; American Athletics, Inc; Speith; and Carolina Gym Supply. In addition, I would like to thank the coaches and athletes who have volunteered as subjects in these studies, as well as the administrators actively involved in the governance of the sport at the International and National levels. I would also like to thank the graduate and undergraduate research assistants at the University of Southern California who have contributed to the data collection and analysis portions of these projects.

References

1. McNitt-Gray JL, Irvine DME, Eagle J: Relative work of net joint moments during landings of front and back saltos, in *Proceedings of the XIXth American Society of Biomechanics (ASB) Meeting*. Stanford, CA, American Society of Biomechanics, 1995, pp 132–133.
2. Nigg B, Denoth, Neukomm: Quatifying the load on the human body: Problems and some possible solutions. *Biomechanics* 1981;8:88–98.
3. Nigg BM, Bobbert M: On the potential of various approaches in load analysis to reduce the frequency of sports injuries. *J Biomech* 1990;23:3–12.
4. USAGymnastics: http://www.usa-gymnastics.org.
5. Hadjiev N: Gymnastics chronic trauma: Methodological aspects, in *Proceedings of the 1991 World Gymnastics Championships FIG Scientific/Medical Symposium*. Indianapolis, IN, Internationale Federation de Gymnastique, 1991, pp 64–68.
6. Claessens AL, Lefevre J: Morphological and performance characteristics as drop-out indicators in female gymnasts. *J Sports Med Phys Fitness* 1998;38:305–309.
7. Claessens AL, Lefevre J, Beunen G, De Smet L, Veer AM: Physique as a risk factor for ulnar variance in elite female gymnasts. *Med Sci Sports Exerc* 1996;28:560–569.
8. Baxter Jones AD, et al: Menarche in intensively trained gymnasts, swimmers and tennis players. *Ann Hum Biol* 1994;21:407–415.
9. Marshall NT (ed): *The Athlete Wellness Book*. Indianapolis, IN, USA Gymnastics, 1999.
10. McNitt-Gray JL, Koff SR, Hall BL: The influence of dance training and foot position on landing mechanics. *Med Probl Perform Artists* 1992;7:87–91.
11. Nigg BM: The validity and relevance of test used for the assessment of sports surfaces. *Med Sci Sports Exerc* 1990;22:131–139.
12. Nigg BM, Yeadon MR: Biomechanical aspects of playing surfaces. *J Sports Sci* 1987;5:117–145.
13. Bass S, Pearce G, Bradney M, et al: Exercise before puberty may confer residual benefits in bone density in adulthood: Studies in active prepubertal and retired female gymnasts. *J Bone Miner Res* 1998;13:500–507.
14. Benardot D: Working with young athletes: Views of a nutritionist on the sports medicine team. *Int J Sport Nutr* 1996;6:110–120.

15. Hinton JDN, DiMarco NM, Sanborn CF: Effect of retirement from women's gymnastics on bone mineral density, diet, and body composition. *Med Sci Sports Exerc* 1998;30:47.

16. Fuchs RKS: Longitudinal case study of an amenorheic gymnast: High impact loading activity in amenorheic women athletes. *Med Sci Sports Exerc* 1998;30:292.

17. Albanese SA, Palmer AK, Kerr DR, Carpenter CW, Lisi D, Levinsohn EM: Wrist pain and distal growth plate closure of the radius in gymnasts. *J Pediatr Orthop* 1989;9:23–28.

18. Sward L, et al: Acute injury of the vertebral ring. Apophysis & IVD in adolescent gymnasts. *Spine* 1990;15:144–148.

19. Garrick JG, Requa RK: Epidemiology of women's gymanstics injuries. *Am J Sports Med* 1980;8:261–264.

20. Pettrone FA, Ricciardelli E: Gymnastic injuries: The Virginia experience. *Am J Sports Med* 1987;15:59–62.

21. McAuley E, Hudash G, Shields K, et al: Injuries in women's gymnastics. *Am J Sports Med* 1987;15:558–565.

22. McNitt-Gray JL, Yokoi T: The influence of surface characteristics on the impulse characteristics of drop landings, in *Proceedings of the XIIIth American Society of Biomechanics (ASB) Meeting*, Stanford, CA, American Society of Biomechanics, 1989, pp 92–93.

23. Koh TJ, Grabiner MD, Weiker GG: Technique and ground reaction forces in the back handspring. *Am J Sports Med* 1992;20:61–66.

24. Markolf KL, et al: Wrist loading patterns during pommel horse exercises. *J Biomech* 1990;23:1001–1011.

25. Carter SR, Aldridge MJ: Stress injury of the distal radial growth plate. *J Bone Joint Surg* 1988;70B:834–836.

26. Mattuli N, Chan D, Aldridge MJ: Overuse injuries of the olecranon in young gymnasts. *J Bone Joint Surg* 1992;74B:305–308.

27. Dixon M, Fricker P: Injuries to elite gymnasts over 10 years. *Med Sci Sports Exerc* 1993;25:1322–1329.

28. Kirby RL, Simms FC, Symington VJ, Garner JB: Flexibility and musculoskeletal symptomatology in female gymnasts and age-matched controls. *Am J Sports Med* 1981;9:160–164.

29. Sands WA, Shultz BB, Newman AP: Women's gymnastics injuries: A 5-year study. *Am J Sports Med* 1993;21:271–276.

30. Snook GA: Injuries in women's gymnastics: A 5-year study. *Am J Sports Med* 1979;7:242–244.

31. NCAA, *Men's & Women's Gymnastics*. Injury Surveillance System. Mission, KS, NCAA, 1997–1998.

32. Lowry CB, Leveau BF: A retrospective study of gymnastics injuries to competitors and non-competitors in private clubs. *Am J Sports Med* 1982;10:237–239.

33. Weiker GG: Club gymnastics. *Clin Sports Med* 1985;4:39–43.

34. Weiker GG: Injuries in club gymnastics. *Phys Sportsmed* 1985;13:63–66.

35. Barron JL, Yocum LA: Recognized achilles tendon rupture associated with ipsilateral medial malleolar fracture. *Am J Sports Med* 1993;21:629–631.

36. Wadley GH, Albright JP: Women's intercollegiate gymnastics: Injury patterns and permanent medical disability. *Am J Sports Med* 1993;21:314–320.

37. Caine D, Howe W, Ross W, Bergman G: Does repetitive physical loading inhibit radial growth in female gymnasts? *Clin J Sport Med* 1997;7:302–308.

38. DiFiori JP, Mandelbaum BR: Wrist pain in a young gymnast: Unusual radiographic findings and MRI evidence of growth plate injury. *Med Sci Sports Exerc* 1996;28:1453–1458.

39. Liebling MS, Berdon WE, Ruzal-Shapiro C, Levin TL, Roye D Jr, Wilkinson R: Gymnast's wrist (pseudorickets growth plate abnormality) in adolescent athletes: Findings on plain films and MR imaging. *Am J Radiology* 1995;164:157–159.

40. Roy SD, Caine D, Singer KM: Stress changes of the distal radial epiphysis in young gymnasts. *Am J Sports Med* 1985;13:301–308.

41. Ruggles DL, Peterson HA, Scott SG: Radial growth plate injury in female gymnasts. *Med Sci Sports Exerc* 1991;23:393–396.

42. Yung-Hing K, Wedge JH, Bowen CVA: Chronic injury to distal ulnar and radial growth plates in an adolescent gymnast: A case report. *J Bone Joint Surg* 1988;70A:1087–1089.

43. Weiker GG: Hand and wrist problems in the gymnast. *Clin Sports Med* 1992;11:189–202.

44. Howe HB: Wrist pain: Gymnastics. *Med Sci Sports Exerc* 1997;29:151.

45. Dobyns JH, Gabel GT: Gymnast's wrists. *Hand Clinics* 1990;6:493–505.

46. Burks RT, Lock TR, Negendank WG: Occult tibial fracture in a gymnast: Diagnosis by magnetic resonance imaging. *Am J Sports Med* 1992;20:88–91.

47. Nocini S, Silvy S: Clinical and radiological aspects of gymnast's elbow: Note 2. *J Sports Med* 1982;22:54–59.

48. Wiltse LL, Widell EH, Jackson DW: Fatigue fracture: The basic lesion in isthmic spondylolisthesis. *J Bone Joint Surg* 1975;57A:17–22.

49. Jackson DW, Wiltse LL, Cirincione RJ: Spondylolysis in the female gymnast. *Clin Orthop* 1985;117:68–73.

50. Ciullo JV, Jackson DW: Pars interarticularis stress reaction, spondylolysis, and spondylolysthesis in gymnasts. *Clin Sports Med* 1985;4:95–108.

51. Weber MD, Woodall WR: Spondylogenic disorders in gymnasts. *J Orthop Sports Phys Ther* 1991;14:6–13.

52. Dubousset J: Treatment of spondylolysis and spondylolisthesis in children and adolescents. *Clin Orthop* 1997:77–85.

53. Tertti M, Paajanen H, Kujala UM, Alanen A, Salmi TT, Kormano M: Disc degeneration in young gymnasts: An MRI study. *Am J Sports Med* 1990;18:206–208.

54. Goldstein JD, Berger PE, Windler GE, Jackson DW: Spine injuries in gymnasts and swimmers. An epidemiological investigation. *Am J Sports Med* 1991;19:463–468.

55. Tsai L, Wredmark T: Spinal posture, sagittal mobility, and subjective rating of back problems in former female elite gymnasts. *Spine* 1993;18:872–875.

56. Micheli LJ, Wood R: Back pain in young athletes: Significant differences from adults in causes and patterns. *Arch Pediatr Adolesc Med* 1995;149:15–18.

57. Zatsiorsky VM, Prilusky BI: Soft and stiff landing, in Jonsson B (ed): *Biomechanics X-B*. Champaign, IL, Human Kinetics, 1987, pp 739–743.

58. McKinley P, Pedotti A: Motor strategies in landing from a jump: The role of skill in task execution. *Exp Brain Res* 1992;90:427–440.

59. Nigg BM: Biomechanics, load analysis and sport injuries in the lower extremities. *Sports Med* 1985;2:367–379.

60. McNitt-Gray JL, Nelson RC: Abstract: Segment and joint kinematics of Olympic vault landings. *Med Sci Sport Exerc* 1988;20(suppl):S48.

61. McNitt-Gray JL: The influence of impact speed on joint kinematics and impulse characteristics of drop landings, in *Proceedings of the XIIth International Congress of Biomechanics (ISB) Meeting*. UCLA, Los Angeles, CA, International Congress of Biomechanics, 1989, pp 159–160.
62. Sidaway B, McNitt-Gray JL, Davis G: Visual timing of muscle preactivation in preparation for landing. *Ecol Psychol* 1989;1:253–264.
63. Smith GA, Shields BJ: Trampoline-related injuries to children. *Arch Pediatr Adolesc Med* 1998;152:694–699.
64. Munkasy BA, McNitt-Gray JL: Segment velocity prior to contact in normal and softer than normal landings, in *Proceedings of the Second North American Congress on Biomechanics (NACOB II)*, Chicago, IL, NACOB, 1992, pp 257–258.
65. McNitt-Gray JL, Yokoi T, Millward C: Landing strategy adjustments made by female gymnasts in response to drop height and mat composition. *J Appl Biomech* 1993;9:173–190.
66. McNitt-Gray JL, et al: Invariant features of multijoint control strategies used by gymnasts during landings performed in Olympic competition, in *Proceedings of the Third North American Congress on Biomechanics*. Waterloo, Canada, 1998, pp 441–442.
67. McNitt-Gray JL: Biomechanical factors contributing to successful landings: We need to stick in '96! *USGF Sports Sci Pub* 1992;9:19–25.
68. Ozguven, Berme: An experimental and analytical study of impact forces during human jumping. *J Biomech* 1988;21:1061–1066.
69. Hyoku C: Effect of dropping height on a buffer action in landing, in *Proceedings of the Japanese Society of Biomechanics*. Nagoya, Japan, Japanese Society of Biomechanics, 1984.
70. Panzer VP: *Lower Extremity Loads in Landing of Elite Gymnasts*. University of Oregon, 1987. Dissertation.
71. Bruggemann P: Biomechanics in gymnastics. *Med Sport Sci* 1987;25:142–176.
72. McNitt-Gray JL, Yokoi T, Millward C: Landing strategy adjustments made by female gymnasts in response to drop height and mat composition. *J Appl Biomech* 1993;9:173–190.
73. McNitt-Gray JL, et al: The effect of landing surface on muscle activity in preparation for landing, in *Proceedings in the XVth American Society of Biomechanics (ASB) Meeting*. Stanford, CA, American Society of Biomechanics, 1991, pp 230–231.
74. McNitt-Gray JL: Kinetics of the lower extremities during drop landings from three heights. *J Biomech* 1993;25:1037–1046.
75. McNitt-Gray JL, Munkasy B, Welch M: External reaction forces experienced by gymnasts during the take-off and landing of tumbling skills. *Technique* 1994;14:10–16.
76. McNitt-Gray JL, et al: Differences in reaction forces experienced by gymnasts during landings in front and back saltos, in *Proceedings of the XVth American Society of Biomechanics (ASB) Meeting*. Stanford, CA, American Society of Biomechanics, 1991, pp 228–229.
77. McNitt-Gray JL, Yokoi T, Millward C: Landing strategies used by gymnasts on different landing surfaces. *J Appl Biomech* 1994;10:237–252.
78. Irvine DME, et al: Muscle activity and kinetics during landings with reduced vertical reaction forces, in *Proceedings of the Second North American Congress on Biomechanics (NACOB II)*. Chicago, IL, NACOB, 1992, pp 547–548.

79. McNitt-Gray JL, et al: Modifications in joint kinetics during stop and go landing movements under fatigued and non-fatigued conditions, in *Proceedings of the XXth American Society of Biomechanics (ASB) Meeting*. Atlanta, GA, American Society of Biomechanics,1996, pp 47–48.

80. Munkasy B, McNitt-Gray JL, Welch M: Reaction forces and impulses experienced during the take-off and landing of tumbling skills, in *Proceedings of the XVIIIth American Society of Biomechanics (ASB) Meeting*. Stanford, CA, American Society of Biomechanics, 1994, pp 97–98.

Chapter 16
Basketball

Mary Lloyd Ireland, MD

Introduction

Over the last three decades, the game of women's basketball has changed drastically. Many girls start playing at a very young age and have older role models who are making a living playing professional basketball. Women now play the sport very similarly to men; it is a fast-paced, highly competitive game. Thirty years ago, the game was played by 6 players: 2 rovers crossed the center court, and 2 players stayed on each side of the court.

Basketball is the number one sport in which girls and women participate at the high school and collegiate levels. According to the National Collegiate Athletic Association (NCAA),[1] during the 1997–1998 season 13,750 women and 15,029 men played basketball at the college level. During the 1997–1998 high school year, 454,000 girls participated in basketball compared to 544,463 boys. These high and still increasing numbers of participants have resulted in trends of injury that are of concern. Noncontact anterior cruciate ligament (ACL) tears are 3 to 4 times higher in female players than in male players. In the 1997–1998 season, among 11% of member institutions surveyed, there were 10 ACL injuries in male players and 30 ACL injuries in female players. If these numbers were extrapolated to all member institutions, there would be 273 ACL-injured female players and 91 male players. Extrapolating the cost estimates at $17,000 for an ACL reconstruction, which would include $10,000 for hospitalization, $3,600 for physician, $600 for anesthesia, and $2,800 in rehabilitation, estimates can be made of the financial impact of these injuries. The cost of ACL reconstruction would be $4,641,000 for the female players and $1,547,000 for the male players. The NCAA extrapolated injury rates from the 1997–1998 NCAA surveillance rates (male:female ratios) for ACL tears (3), finger injuries (2.75), meniscus tears (2.2), stress fractures (1.88), collateral ligament (1.85), concussion (1.73), low back (1.06), wrist (0.54), and eye (0.50).[1]

History

Senda Berenson, the director of physical education at Smith College in Northampton, Massachusetts, started basketball for women in the 1890s and has been called "The Mother of Women's Basketball."[2] Berenson studied with James Naismith at Springfield College, where men's basketball began. The 6-girl game was born with 2 players assigned to each of 3 areas of the court and no one allowed to run its full length. Dribbling was limited to 3 lady-like bounces. The women's basket was not open-bottomed. A chain had to be pulled to release the hatch. It was believed that this would slow down the game, lest the participants become infertile.

In the 1930s, the Red Heads, created by promotor and coach Orwell Moore, were the Harlem Globetrotters of the women's game.[2] They played men's rules against male semiprofessional and military teams. The requirements were to be an excellent basketball player and to dye one's hair red. Ninety-five percent of the time, according to Mickey Childress, they won. The Flying Queens played women's basketball at Wayland Baptist in Plainview, Texas, in the 1960s.[2] Coach Harley Redin's record was 431 wins and 66 losses. They traveled in planes. Nera White was believed to be the greatest female player ever. She played for Wayland Baptist's biggest rival, the Nashville Business College, and led the United States to a world title in 1957.

In 1999–2000, the Women's National Basketball Association (WNBA) has just completed its third year. Many of the players have been on Olympic teams and played internationally. It is encouraging for aspiring basketball players that they can continue to play professionally in this country instead of overseas as in the past. There are 12 teams with 132 women participating, and expansion occurs every year.

Participation

The National Federation of State High School Associations has been keeping track of the number of boys and girls participating in programs for the last 9 years.[3] The number of boys and girls participating in high school sports continues to increase. For all sports in the 1997-1998 survey, girls numbered 2,570,333, an increase of 98,290 from the previous year. Boys' participation numbered 3,763,120, an increase of 56,895. Of the high school athletes, 59% were boys and 41% were girls. The most popular sport among girls was basketball, with 454,000 participants. The number of boys in basketball was 544,463. The largest gain in girl participants was in competitive spirit squads, which were up 23,584 from the previous year. The number of students participating in basketball in the top 10 states is given in Table 1.

Table 1 1998 high school basketball participation: Top 10 states, number of schools, and number of participants

	Females		Males	
State	**Schools**	**Participants**	**Schools**	**Participants**
Texas	1,163	70,365	1,165	70,558
California	1,098	30,979	1,144	39,846
Michigan	698	19,948	710	24,718
Pennsylvania	634	19,020	636	19,080
Ohio	786	18,448	785	24,975
Illinois	588	17,148	651	24,702
New York	702	17,039	718	21,610
Missouri	532	12,631	558	15,476
Iowa	397	12,588	400	14,721
Indiana	380	12,466	381	13,883

(Data taken from National Federation of State High School Associations.)

Epidemiology

High School

According to the National Federation of State High Schools Association Handbook, there are 6,000,000 high school youths from 20,000 high schools participating in sports. Estimates are that these young high school athletes account for 2,000,000 injuries, 500,000 doctor visits, and 30,000 hospitalizations.[4,5]

NCAA Information

Since the 1988–1989 season, the NCAA has kept injury statistics. The rates of injury are reported as number of injuries per 1,000 athlete exposures (A-Es). Surveys of 11% to 15% of member institutions are reported in the NCAA Injury Surveillance System (ISS). Unfortunately, the rates of ACL injuries have not changed despite players playing earlier, improvements in the coaching, and gradual improvement in skill and talent level of the basketball athletes. In 1997–1998, the rate of ACL tears in female athletes compared to male athletes was five times greater in games and two times greater in practice.[1] In comparing overall injury rates occurring in practices and games per 1,000 A-Es, the injury rate is 5.37 in women and 4.42 in men.

The types of basketball injuries incurred by men and women in practice and during games[1] are given in Table 2. Compared to men, women have fewer contusions and more tendinitis, complete ligament sprains, muscle strains, stress fractures, and concussions. Certain injuries occur at a significantly greater rate in women during a game. These injuries include complete tear of a ligament, partial dislocation, stress fractures, and concussions. The category for type of injuries is general without specific mention of time loss. Further gender comparison needs to be done regarding injury types.

Table 2 Basketball injuries per 1,000 A-Es by type 1997–1998[1]

	Practices			Games			Overall
	Males	Females	Ratio F/M	Males	Females	Ratio F/M	F/M
Laceration	0.11	0.05	0.45	0.51	0.14	0.27	0.36
Ligament sprain (incomplete tear)	1.02	1.23	1.21	2.63	2.86	1.09	1.15
Ligament sprain (complete tear)	0.10	0.10	1.00	0.11	0.65	5.91*	3.45*
Muscle-tendon strain (incomplete tear)	0.64	1.03	1.61	0.72	0.71	0.99	1.30
Muscle-tendon strain (complete tear)	0.02	0.02	1.00	0.07	0.03	0.43	0.71
Dislocation (partial)	0.09	0.08	1.00	0.18	0.37	2.06*	1.53
Dislocation (complete)	0.04	0.06	1.50	0.18	0.10	0.56	1.03
Fracture	0.23	0.22	0.96	0.97	0.75	0.77	0.86
Stress fracture	0.14	0.28	2.00*	0.04	0.17	4.25*	3.13*
Concussion	0.13	0.22	1.69	0.22	0.51	2.32*	2.01*

*Injury rate ratio (F:M) greater than 2

Types of Injuries

Concussion

Concussion rates are greater in women (0.51) than in men (0.22) during games, for a ratio of 2.3 times greater in women. In practices, rates are more similar, 0.22 in women and 0.13 in men, for a ratio of 1.7[1] (Fig. 1). In general, injuries are more common in games than in practices.

Eye Injuries

At the collegiate level, eye injury rates per 1,000 A-Es are 0.04 in practice for both genders and 0.18 in games for men and 0.03 in games for women.[1] Up to 10% of all basketball injuries involve the face or scalp.[6] Eye injuries are very common. In a report of eye injuries evaluated by a single ophthalmologist, 30% were sustained while playing basketball. Six percent required surgery and 3% resulted in permanent visual loss.[7] The most common type of eye injury is corneal abrasion. Frank tears, hyphema, lens injury, and posterior segment injury (0.51 per 1,000 A-Es in women and 0.22 per 1,000 A-Es in men during games, 0.22/1,000 A-Es for women and 0.13 for men in practice) occur less frequently. Information regarding protective eyewear in patients who have undergone laser keratotomy should be gathered up to 10 years from the procedure. Persistent corneal weakness and risk of critical injury can occur following the procedure.[8] Use of commercially available eye protectors is recommended if there has been previous serious eye injury or previous surgery such as laser keratotomy.

In a case study, there were two cases of traumatic ruptures of the cornea along the keratotomic incisions at 4 years and 5 months after athletic and

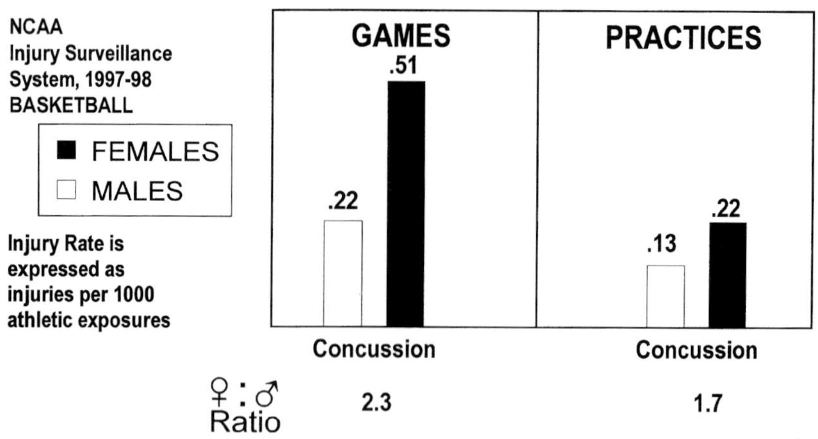

Fig. 1 Concussion injury rates.[1]

occupational injuries.[9] Polycarbonate lenses should be used during athletic activities, particularly in such sports as basketball where there is significant risk of eye injury.[10] Vinger[10] believed that radial keratotomy should not be recommended to athletes who will participate in contact sports.

Musculoskeletal Injuries

Women sustained more lower leg, foot, ankle, and knee injuries than did men. Injuries to the lower back, pelvis, and groin are similar in both genders. Neck injuries were more common in the female athlete, particularly in games, although they were relatively rare (0.1 per 1,000 A-Es for women and 0.04 for men). The rates for the 1997–1998 season are given in Table 3. Rates that are more than double for women include the knee, ACL, meniscus, collateral ligaments, lower leg, fingers, and neck. Injury rates increase in games as compared to practices for the ACL, collateral ligaments, and neck. The patellar reports include patella and patellar tendon and are relatively equal in men and women. A specific patellar diagnosis is not confirmed; there is no category for patellar subluxation, plica syndrome, patellar tendinitis. Therefore, the patellar diagnosis does not correspond with my experience of patellofemoral disorders being more common in the female athlete, particularly at the high school level (Kentucky Sports Medicine, unpublished data).

The most common joint injured in basketball is the ankle, with increased rates during games. Similar rates are seen in men and women (Table 3). The next most commonly injured joint is the knee. The ACL injury rate is significantly higher in women during games (0.68) than in men (0.14). In practices, the rates are double in the female players. Progress is being made in revising and improving the ISS (R Dick, NCAA, Overland Park, Kansas, personal communication).

Upper Extremity Injuries

Upper extremity injuries are not that common in basketball. However, upper extremity injuries are unusual in practices, but the rates of shoulder injuries increase in games for both male (0.54) and female (0.48) athletes[1] (Table 3). Other rates that increase in games and are greater in the female athlete are injuries to the fingers.

The most common upper extremity injury in basketball is an anterior glenohumeral subluxation. The typical mechanism of injury is as the player dives for a ball, blocks a shot, and gets his or her arm in an abducted externally rotated position. From personal experience, I have treated an anterior glenohumeral dislocation in a collegiate athlete who was 4 weeks postpartum. She had increased laxity of all joints. She responded to a rehabilitation program and did not have any recurrence.

Documentation with the precise diagnosis in shoulder injuries is very important. In the younger athletes, physiologic laxity, which in some cases is multidirectional, is very common. Secondary involvement of the rotator cuff with weakness occurs in the event of subluxation episodes. With the advances in arthroscopic treatment of the shoulder, including arthroscopic devices for labral reattachment and thermal capsular modification to shrink the capsular

Table 3 Basketball injuries per 1,000 A-Es by body part 1997–1998[1]

	Practices			Games			Overall
	Males	Females	Ratio F/M	Males	Females	Ratio F/M	F/M
Lower Extremity							
Upper leg	0.26	0.31	1.19	0.47	0.17	0.36	0.66
Knee	0.35	0.78	2.23*	0.76	1.56	2.05*	2.11*
ACL	0.05	0.10	2.00*	0.14	0.68	4.86*	4.11*
Meniscus	0.08	0.23	2.88*	0.29	0.54	1.86	2.08*
Collateral ligament	0.07	0.10	1.43	0.22	0.54	2.45*	2.21*
Patella	0.10	0.18	1.80	0.18	0.17	0.94	1.25
Lower leg	0.13	0.42	3.23*	0.14	0.34	2.43*	2.81*
Ankle	0.91	0.95	1.04	1.99	2.38	1.20	1.15
Heel/Achilles	0.05	0.09	1.80	0.04	0.03	0.75	1.33
Foot	0.24	0.35	1.46	0.32	0.34	1.06	1.23
Upper Extremity							
Shoulder	0.16	0.09	0.56	0.54	0.48	0.89	0.81
Clavicle	0.00	0.01	—	0.11	0.00	0.00	0.09
Acromioclavicular separation	0.02	0.00	0.00	0.04	0.07	1.75	1.17
Elbow	0.04	0.03	0.75	0.11	0.10	0.91	0.87
Forearm	0.02	0.00	0.00	0.11	0.03	0.27	0.23
Wrist	0.03	0.04	1.33	0.32	0.10	0.31	0.40
Hand	0.10	0.04	0.40	0.11	0.03	0.27	0.33
Finger(s)	0.04	0.14	3.50*	0.11	0.24	2.18*	2.53*
Thumb(s)	0.06	0.05	0.83	0.14	0.10	0.71	0.75
Other							
Head	0.18	0.23	1.28	0.32	0.61	1.91	1.68
Eye	0.04	0.04	1.00	0.18	0.03	0.17	0.32
Neck	0.00	0.03	—	0.04	0.10	2.50*	3.25*
Lower back	0.18	0.29	1.61	0.47	0.20	0.43	0.75
Pelvis, groin, hip	0.25	0.21	0.84	0.40	0.14	0.35	0.54

*Injury rate ratio (F:M) greater than 2

tissues, it is even more important to document the rates of shoulder injuries in the female athlete. Many arthroscopic procedures are being performed on the female athlete's shoulder, most notably thermal capsular modification. Exact diagnosis preoperatively and follow-up based on the type of procedure are very important and must be documented.

Lower Extremity Injuries

Ankle injuries are the most common injury in basketball. Rates are similar in male and female players and are greater in games than in practices. The exact diagnosis is not available. Injuries involving the ankle are reported, but sprain versus fractures and time off are not reported[1,11] (Table 3). The rate of injury essentially doubles in games compared to practice. If these rates are extrapolated, the number of ankle injuries is 1,545 in female athletes and 1,481 in male athletes. At the high school level, the ankle was the joint injured in 32% of boys and 31% of girls. The difference of ankle injuries is not significant. However, a statistically significant higher injury rate was found involving the knee, 10% (53/543) in boys and 20% (86/436) in girls ($p = 0.0001$). Boys had a higher incidence of facial injuries—11% (58/543) in boys and 5% (21/436) in girls ($p = 0.023$). Fortunately, with the nature of ankle sprains, protective equipment, such as ankle braces, taping, and a proprioceptive rehabilitation program, is quite successful. It is unusual for ankle surgery to be required following an ankle sprain.

Lower leg injuries are more common in the female athlete during practices than in the male athlete and remain more common in games. Stress fractures are more common in the female basketball player than in the male player, with a two times greater rate documented in practices and a 4.25 greater rate documented in games (Table 2). Specific reasons for the increased rate of stress fractures include hormonal imbalance, disordered eating, improperly fitting shoes, and reduced strength. The shoes for female players have, in the past, been a reduced model of those for male players. There is progress in the development of an athletic shoe contoured to the female athlete, with a true women's last and a reduced heel width.

Knee Injuries

Many articles have been written regarding the nature and location of injury patterns in boys and girls.[12–16] Specific sports have also been looked at.[17–20] Comparison studies also have been done.[21–24]

The joint of greatest cause for concern is the knee. A continued two- to four-time greater rate of ACL injuries in women compared to men is of great concern (see chapter 11). Patellofemoral disorders are more common in the female athlete, specifically patellofemoral stress syndrome, patellar instability, and plica syndrome.[24]

Professional Level Injury Patterns

In a study published in 1982 comparing men's and women's professional basketball injuries over two seasons, women were injured 1.6 times more than men.[19] The ankle was the most frequently injured body part for both sexes. Men had more muscle spasms, while women had more knee and thigh injuries and sprains, strains, and contusions. No ACL injury rates were included in the study. Injury data for the WNBA are being recorded but are not yet available.

Olympic Level Knee Injuries

In 1988, at the US Olympic basketball trials for men and women, where the coaches picked the elite male and female players in the country, detailed surveys were completed by the participants.[25,26] Of the 64 female basketball players at the Olympic trials, 20 underwent 25 surgeries, with the diagnosis of ACL tear in 13. Of the 80 male participants, 6 required 6 surgeries, with 3 ACL tears diagnosed. Eight of the 13 females and all of the three males underwent ACL reconstruction[25,26] (Table 4). Many of these national level female players are still playing professional basketball in the WNBA.

Table 4 Injuries sustained during 1988 Olympic basketball trials

Parameter	Males	Females	Total
Number of participants	80	64	144
Athletes with knee injuries	11*	34	45
ACL injuries	3	13	16
Number of athletes requiring surgery	6†	20	26
Number of procedures	6	25	31
Type of procedure			
Arthroscopy	3	17	20
ACL Reconstruction	3	8	11

ACL = anterior cruciate ligament
, † indicate a statistically significant difference between male and female athletes (= $p < 0.0001$; † = $p < 0.0007$)
(Reproduced with permission from Hutchinson MR, Ireland ML: Knee injuries in female athletes. *Sports Med* 1995;19:288–302.)

High School Injury Patterns

In a study over a 3-year period, information was gathered on 3,200 team seasons and 75,000 player seasons, 4.4 A-Es, and 2,500 reportable injuries.[5] In girls' basketball, there were 395 team seasons, 6,083 player seasons, and 394,143 A-Es. In boys' basketball, there were 406 team seasons, 6,831 player seasons, and 444,338 A-Es. Only football has more A-Es at 1,300,446. Sprains were the most common type of injury, accounting for 44.8% of the boys' injuries and 45.2% of the girls' injuries. The highest rate of reinjury was in girls' basketball, at 13.6%. The injury rates per 1,000 A-Es were greater in basketball games than in practice. Similar incidences were seen for boys' basketball. The percentage of injuries was greater in practice than games (53.2% in practice and 42.8% in games) in girls' basketball. In boys' basketball, the percentage was 58% in practice and 42% in games. In girls' basketball and girls' soccer, the players sustained a higher proportion of knee injuries than boys. The need for knee surgery in girls' basketball was one case per eight team seasons compared to one case per 18 team seasons for boys' basketball. This greater rate of knee injuries requiring surgery in girls' basketball continues to be observed and is not dropping over time.

A 2-year injury surveillance study was performed by athletic trainers in Iowa for 121 schools.[27] It was estimated in 1990 by the National Athletic Trainers' Association that 714,000 students play basketball at 19,000 high schools. Of these, 47% are girls and 53% boys. There is a total of approximately 1.3 million injuries per year. Based on time loss, girls have a slightly higher percentage of moderate and major injuries than boys. Over 2 years, the girls had 67% minor, 19% moderate, and 14% major injuries, while the boys had 73% minor, 17% moderate, and 11% major injuries. Games produced twice the injury rate as practice in both genders. The girls sustained a higher rate of major injuries per game than did the boys: 1.17% injuries per 1,000 A-Es for girls and 0.72% injuries per 1,000 A-Es for boys. The injured body parts in the girls were ankle (31%), knee (14%), and fingers (7%), and in the boys the injured body parts were ankle (38%), knee (8%), and thigh

(5%). Statistically, significantly more major knee injuries occurred in the girls (44%) than in the boys (23%). Although details of the surgery were not available, 21% (26/123) of the total girls' knee injuries and 18% (16/89) of the knees required surgery. Both girls and boys were most likely to sustain moderate knee injuries.

Both girls and boys sustained the majority of their ankle injuries during the fourth quarter of games. No ankle injuries required surgery. There were slight differences between the genders; the girls sustained 62% minor, 30% moderate, and 8% major ankle injuries, while the boys sustained 71% minor, 22% moderate, and 8% major ankle injuries during both practice and games. Resprain rate was similar in both girls and boys.

Girls' basketball has been looked at at the high school level in Texas.[28] From the 1993–1994 season, 100 randomly selected 4A and 5A Texas high schools were evaluated for girls' high school basketball injuries. The ankle was most commonly injured (135; 31%), followed by the knee (86; 19%), the hip/thigh (49; 9%), and the hand/fingers (35; 8%). The rate of serious injury was 0.038 per athlete per year (34 serious injuries among 890 players), which surpasses the injury rate of 0.031 for varsity football. The rate for team exposure hours was 0.0035 serious injuries per team per hour. The knee injury severity was higher than expected in the population of female student athletes. Sixteen of 25 (64%) required surgery. Of these 16 knee injuries requiring surgery, 11% were ACL reconstructions. Therefore, ACL injuries accounted for 44% of the injuries requiring surgery and 32% of all severe injuries.[28]

Another study performed by the San Antonio, Texas, group involved 456 Class 4A and 5A high schools in Texas from the 1996–1997 season.[11] Data from this group were compared to those for the 1993–1994 season in female basketball. Types of injuries were similar in both groups. Sprains and contusions were the most common injury, and the ankle was the most common site of injury in both girls and boys. The girls had a significantly higher rate of lower extremity injuries (p = 0.003) and higher rate of knee injuries (p = 0.0001). The boys had a significantly higher rate of injuries to the face (p = 0.023). Knee injuries accounted for 10% of all injuries in boys and 20% of all injuries in girls. Based on exposure time, the risk of knee injury was 2.3 times greater in the female athlete than the male athletes (p = < 0.001). Upper extremity injuries tended to be more common in boys, but this was not statistically significant. Players are more likely to be injured during games. For boys, injury risk was 9.4 times higher in games than in practice and for girls it was eight times greater in games than in practice. Incidence of knee injuries was 0.71 knee injuries per 1,000 player-hours for girls and 0.31 knee injuries per 1,000 player-hours for boys. The risk of ACL injury among girls based on exposure time was 3.79 times greater than the risks in boys (0.091 per 1,000 player-hours vs. 0.024 per 1,000 player-hours).[11]

High School and College

Over two basketball seasons, 1994 to 1996, 4,940 female athletes and 6,840 male athletes from 95 high schools and colleges from the state of New Jersey were studied (Harner MF, Berson L, Hosea TM, et al, unpublished data, 1996). The female athletes sustained more total injuries including season-ending injuries ($p < 0.01$) and injuries requiring orthopaedic surgery ($p < 0.001$). The relative risk of female players sustaining a season-ending injury was 2.5 times that of male players and the risk of female players sustaining an injury requiring orthopaedic surgery was 3.4 times that of male players. ACL injuries were increased in female athletes with a relative risk of 2.6. Patellofemoral injuries in female players were two times greater and relative risk of meniscal injuries was 1.97 times greater. In contrast, ankle sprains and fractures were the same in both genders.

Over a 2-year period, 1988 to 1990, ACL injury statistics were kept for three college athletic conferences, the Atlantic Coast Conference (ACC), Pacific Ten Conference, and Big Ten Conference.[29] Using a denominator of the number of athletes playing the sport of basketball in the ACC, 16.5% of the female athletes (19/113) and 4.2% of the male athletes (3/119) sustained ACL injuries. The Pacific Ten statistics showed 12.3% of the female athletes (16/130) and 0.7% of the male athletes (1/138) sustained ACL injuries. In the Big Ten, 27 of 140 or 19.3% of female athletes sustained ACL injuries and 3/145 or 2.1% of male athletes. The odds ratio was 6.19% with women being six times more likely to sustain ACL injuries during their competitive season.

Knee injury rates in games are higher in every category (Fig. 2). In games, the ACL injury rate is five times greater in female athletes, the collateral ligament rate is 2.5 times greater, and the meniscus injury rate is 1.9 times greater. In practices, the rates are significantly lower; however, they continue to be greater in the female athlete. Vailas and associates[30] described injury patterns among NCAA male and female basketball players over one season with 23 teams consisting of 194 male and 182 female players. The injury rate per 1,000 hours in the female players was 2.02 compared to 1.95 in male players. The knee sprains consisted of 5% of the total injuries. Ankle sprains were more common in female players than in male players. Statistically significant differences were noted in the following categories. Male players had three times as many overuse injuries as did female players (21% to 8%). Strains were more common in the male players (28.9%) than in the female

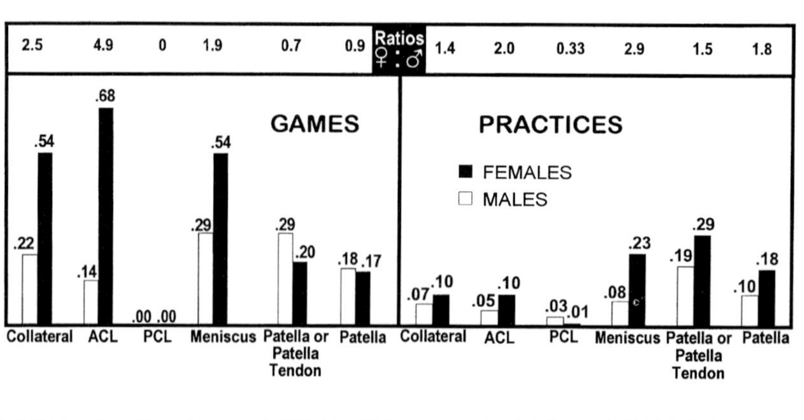

Fig. 2 Knee structure injury rates in basketball: 1997–1998. NCAA Injury Surveillance System, 1997–1998.[1]

players (14.7%). There were four times as many season-ending injuries in the female players (16%) compared to the male players (4%).

Assessment of Mechanism of Injury in Basketball

As the mechanisms of injury are captured on video, a common failure position occurs. It appears the individual is out of control in the air, thinking about many different things; often, the individual is on offense in the paint, charging toward the baseline, or rebounding, but usually there is an out-of-control, awkward landing. A typical video shows a female basketball player landing after a rebound. She is on her toes with her body weight forward. Her trunk moves forward as her hip internally rotates and the knee flexion increases. By the time the knee is in valgus and extension, the ACL has failed.

Figure 3 shows a male basketball player tearing his left ACL. He is at the baseline in the paint. As he decelerates, his left foot stays planted as his body

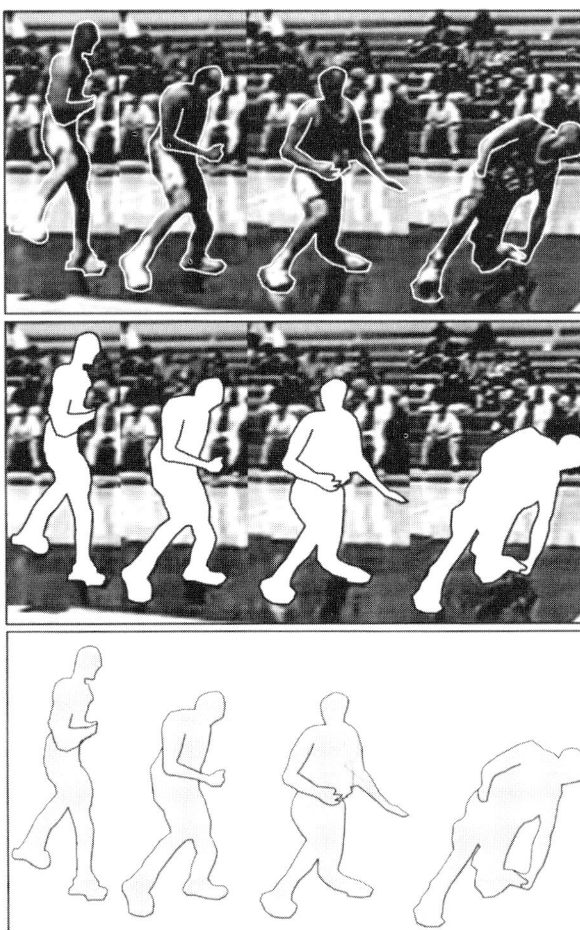

Fig. 3 *A male basketball player tearing his left ACL. (© Mary Lloyd Ireland, 2000)*

rotates, first to the opposite side, then to the same side. The athlete is upright as he lands. His hip goes into internal rotation and adduction as the tibia goes into external rotation and excessive knee valgus occurs. The ACL failure occurs between the second and third frames.

Analysis of mechanisms of injury in basketball shows a common position during an ACL injury. The ACL tears in less than 70 ms.[31] Commonalities are an awkward, out-of-control landing, forward body movement, back relatively straight, upright landing posture, hip internally rotated adducted, knee in slight flexion and valgus, tibia externally rotated, and foot pronated. In thinking about the position, it is possible to look at a safe landing position and an out-of-control position (Figs. 4 and 5). Protective joint positions are flexion of hip and knee, normal lumbar lordosis, and both feet neutral. Out-of-control position is one foot, less hip and knee flexion, forward and flexed back, and pronated externally rotated lower extremity. Agonist and antagonist muscle activity and joint position should be analyzed (Table 5). The more flexed

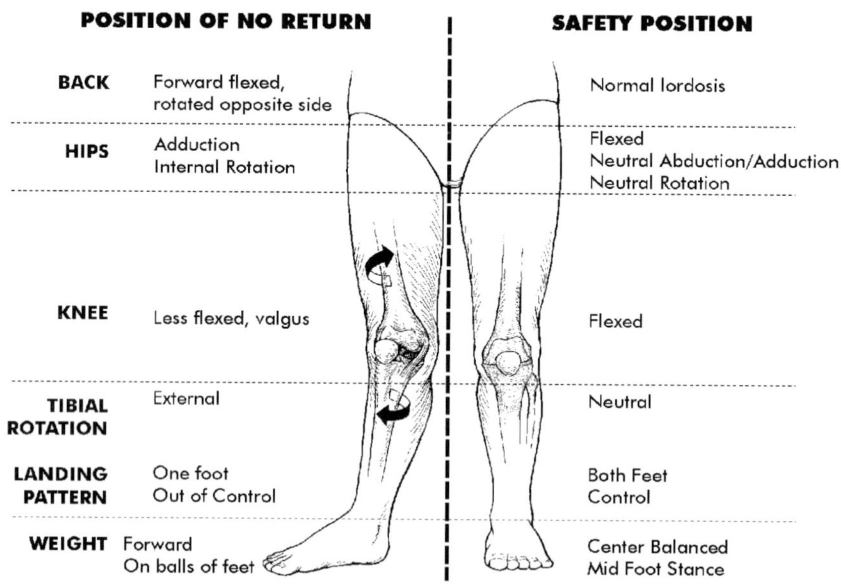

***Fig. 4** Position of no return versus safety position. On the left, this position of no return when the ACL tears is shown. Valgus and rotation forces and momentum forward are the significant factors causing the ACL to fail. The safety position is characterized by the pelvis in neutral, sacroiliac (SI) joint closed, hip flexed, neutral rotation, knee flexed, tibia neutral, center balanced, midfoot stance, and control on both feet. In the position of no return, the back is extended and rotated to the opposite side. The pelvis has an anterior tilt and forward rotation. The SI joint is open and unstable. The hips are adducted and internally rotated. The knees are less flexed in valgus. The tibia is externally rotated with a one-foot landing, with weight forward on the balls of the feet. The muscle firing patterns are altered and the individual is unable to get out of the position of no return because of the muscle not firing as quickly or being at a mechanical disadvantage due to the joint position. (© Mary Lloyd Ireland, 1998)*

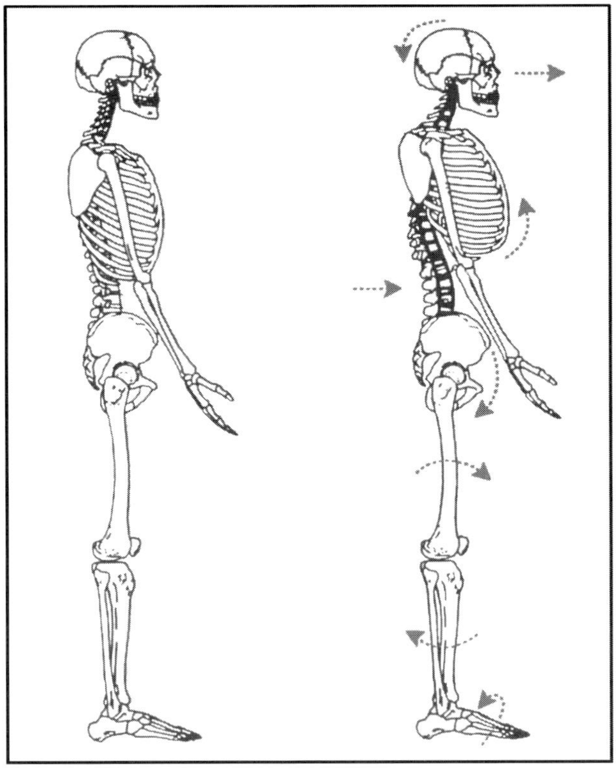

Fig. 5 *The optimal posture is shown on the left, with normal lumbar lordosis, neutral position pelvis with subsequent normal femoral rotation, neutral hemipelvis. On the right is the position of an anterior rotated pelvis. The anterior tilt or rotation of the pelvis increases lumbar lordosis of the lumbar and sacral spine, increases extension of the thoracic and lumbar spine, and increases hip flexion and femoral internal rotation. The subsequent lower extremity alignment is then genu valgum, genu recurvatum, subtalar eversion, and forefoot or rearfoot pronation. This creates a dissynchronism of agonist-antagonist muscles and subsequent tightness of the anterior hip capsule and hip flexors, which are then overused. The hamstrings and hip external rotators and extensors are then unable to function normally due to their new lengthened and less mechanically advantaged position. (Reproduced with permission from Hruska R: Pelvic stability influences lower-extremity kinematics.* Biomech *1998;5:24.)*

Table 5 Muscle activity

	No Return	Safety
Hip	Iliopsoas	Gluteus maximus
	Adductors	Abductors
Thigh	Quadriceps	Hamstrings
		Gastrocnemius soleus
Calf	Peroneals	Posterior tibialis
	Tibialis anterior	

hip and knee position of safety allows the gluteus maximus, abductors, hamstrings, gastrocnemius-soleus, and posterior tibialis to fire fast and function most efficiently. In basketball, the injury often occurs when the individual is driving for the basket, catching a ball, rebounding, and typically is in an out-of-control awkward landing position.[32-34]

Netball

In Commonwealth countries, netball is a very popular sport, particularly among women. Female basketball and netball player injury rates were compared.[34] Nine hundred seventy-two basketball athletes and 9,190 netball athletes were followed for injury. Rates were calculated by number of injuries per 1,000 participants. Netball players sustained severe injuries at a rate 3.3 times that of female basketball players. The rates of major and severe injuries occurred in 1:625 games in basketball and 1:250 games in netball.[34] Another study compared the kinanthropometric and performance variables to predict injury. The higher-risk netball athlete was thinner, fitter, and a more powerful jumping player.[35]

References

1. National Collegiate Athletic Association: *NCAA Injury Surveillance System*. Overland Park, Kansas, NCAA, 1998–1999.
2. Weir T: Hoops pioneers get home court. *USA Today* 1999;Thursday, June 3, p 3C.
3. High School Athletics Participation Survey. Kansas City, Missouri, The National Federation of State High School Associations 1998. www.nfhs.org.
4. *National Federation of State High School Associations Handbook: 1996 High School Athletics Participation Survey*. Kansas City, MO, National Federation of State High School Associations, 1997.
5. Powell JW, Barber-Foss KD: Injury patterns in selected high school sports: A review of the 1995-1997 seasons. *J Athletic Training* 1999;34:277–284.
6. Guyette RF, Facial injuries in basketball players. *Clin Sports Med* 1993;12:247–264.
7. Larrison WI, Hersh PS, Kunzweiler T, Shingleton BJ: Sports-related ocular trauma. *Ophthalmology* 1990;97:1265–1269.
8. Jeffers J: Sports-related eye injuries: Presentation, management, and prevention, in *Seventh Annual Professional Sports Care Sports Medicine Symposium*. Teaneck, New Jersey, 1994.
9. Zhaboedov GD, Bondareva GS: Traumatic rupture of the eyeball after radial keratotomy. Vestn *Oftalmol* 1990;106:64–65.
10. Vinger PF: Prescribing for contact sports. *Optom Clin* 1993;3:129–143.
11. Messina DF, Farney WC, DeLee JC: The incidence of injury in Texas high school basketball: A prospective study among male and female athletes. *Am J Sports Med* 1999;27:294–299.
12. Chandy TA, Grana WA: Secondary school athletic injury in boys and girls: A three-year comparison. *Phys Sportsmed* 1985;13:106–111.
13. DeHaven KE, Lintner DM. Athletic injuries: Comparisons by age, sport, and gender. *Am J Sports Med* 1986;14:218–224.

14. Garrick JG, Requa R: Medical care and injury surveillance in the high school setting. *Phys Sportsmed* 1981;9:115–120.

15. Garrick JG, Requa RK. Girls' sports injuries in high school athletics. *JAMA* 1978;239:2245–2248.

16. Ireland ML. Anterior cruciate ligament injury in female athletes: Epidemiology. *J Athletic Training* 1999:34:150–154.

17. Ferretti A, Papandrea P, Conteduca F, Mariani PP: Knee ligament injuries in volleyball players. *Am J Sports Med* 1992;20:203–207.

18. Keller CS, Noyes FR, Buncher CR: The medical aspects of soccer injury epidemiology. *Am J Sports Med* 1987;15:230–237.

19. Zelisko JA, Noble HB, Porter M: A comparison of men's and women's professional basketball injuries. *Am J Sports Med* 1982;10:297–299.

20. Wirtz PD: High school basketball knee ligament injuries. *J Iowa Med Soc* 1982;72:105–106.

21. Whiteside PA: Men's and women's injuries in comparable sports. *Phys Sportsmed* 1980;8:130–140.

22. Weesner CL, Albohm MJ, Ritter MA: A comparison of anterior and posterior cruciate ligament laxity between female and male basketball players. *Phys Sportsmed* 1986;14:149–154.

23. Shively RA, Grana WA, Ellis D. High school sports injuries. *Phys Sportsmed* 1981;9:46–50.

24. Lanese RR, Strauss RH, Leizman DJ, Rotondi AM: Injury and disability in matched men's and women's intercollegiate sports. *Am J Public Health* 1990;80:1459–1462.

25. Ireland ML, Wall C: Abstract: Epidemiology and comparison of knee injuries in elite male and female United States basketball athletes. *Med Sci Sports Exerc* 1990;22(suppl):S82.

26. Hutchinson MR, Ireland ML: Knee injuries in female athletes. *Sports Med* 1995;19:288–302.

27. Zillmer DA, Powell JW, Albright JP: Gender specific injury patterns in high school varsity basketball. *J Women's Health* 1992;1:69–76.

28. Gomez E, DeLee JC, Farney WC: Incidence of injury in Texas girls' high school basketball. *Am J Sports Med* 1996;24:684–687.

29. Malone TR, Hardaker WT, Garrett WE, Feagin JA, Bassett FH: Relationship of gender to anterior cruciate ligament injuries in intercollegiate basketball players. *J South Orthop Assoc* 1993;2:36–39.

30. Vailas JC, Moran MJ, Decoster LC, Bernier JN: Abstract: Injury patterns among NCAA male and female basketball players. *Med Sci Sports* 1998;30(suppl):S51.

31. Yasuda K, Erickson AR, Johnson RJ, Pope MH: Dynamic strain behavior in the medial collateral and anterior cruciate ligaments during lateral impact loading. *Trans Orthop Res Soc* 1992;17:127.

32. Hewett TE, Lindenfeld TN, Riccobene JV, Noyes FR: The effect of neuromuscular training on the incidence of knee injury in female athletes: A prospective study. *Am J Sports Med* 1999;27:699–706.

33. McKay GD, Payne WR, Goldie PA, Oakes BW, Stanley JJ: A comparison of the injuries sustained by female basketball and netball players. *Aust J Sci Med Sport* 1996;28:12–17.

34. Hopper DM, Hopper JL, Elliott BC: Do selected kinanthropometric and performance variables predict injuries in female netball players? *J Sports Sci* 1995;13:213–222.

Chapter 17

Tennis

W. Benjamin Kibler, MD

Introduction

Injuries are common in female tennis players at all levels of skill, age, and tournament play. Several studies of elite junior tennis players reveal that the injury incidence ranges from 42% to 78% of tennis players reporting an injury within the past 18 months.[1–4] Professional tennis players also have an injury incidence of about 24% over the past year.[5] Analysis of injury patterns and comparison to male tennis players reveals that the injuries are more sport specific than gender specific. The same sites of injury, the shoulder, the back, and the leg, seem to predominate, and there does not appear to be a difference in injury rate. Overload injuries are more common in girls and women, comprising 73% of the injuries in elite juniors[1,2] and 50% of the injuries in the professionals.[5] These rates are comparable to those in their male counterparts. This chapter will review risk factors that may predispose female tennis players to injury and will discuss selected injuries.

Risk Factors

The available literature on women's tennis injuries does not reveal specific cause and effect risk factors for these injuries. In general, the risk factors that appear to be common in the literature are imbalances in muscle strength or force couples or alterations in flexibility[1,6,7] that make the athlete predisposed to injury with further athletic exposure. These findings agree with Meeuwisse's theory[8] on microtrauma-induced causation of sports injuries (Fig. 1). The intrinsic risk factors, such as inflexibilities or strength imbalance, create a "predisposed" athlete who then interacts with the inherent demands of the sport, such as running, hitting, serving, or metabolic requirements. This interaction may create further risk and eventually produce an injury.

In general, girls and women are more flexible than boys and men.[9,10] Areas of increased flexibility include shoulder, elbow, low back, quadriceps, and hamstrings. However, female players appear to develop inflexibility patterns as a result of exposure to tennis in the same proportion and at the same rate as male players.[10,11] Predominant areas of muscle inflexibility include dominant shoulder internal rotation, low back inflexibility, and quadriceps and hamstring inflexibility. The dominant shoulder internal rotation inflexibility and lower extremity inflexibility have been associated with injury causation patterns in tennis and in other sports.[12–15] These

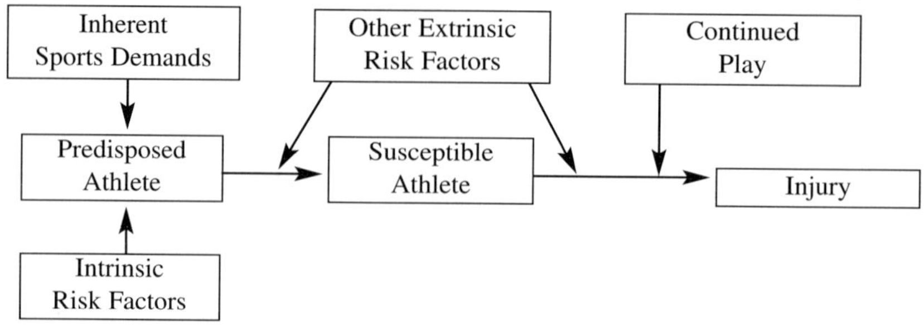

***Fig. 1** Multifactorial model for injury causation. Intrinsic risk factors create a predisposed athlete. (Adapted with permission from Meeuwisse WH: Assessing causation in sport injury: A multi-factorial model.* Clin J Sport Med *1994;4:166–170.)*

inflexibilities may be considered maladaptations to the demands of the sport in that they create extra stresses on the affected joints and decreased effective performance of motions that require the action of that joint.[15,16]

Strength imbalances also can be seen in female tennis players. Around the shoulder, the external rotators appear to have less strength and torque compared to the internal rotators, and the ratio of external rotation to internal rotation is less on the dominant side than the nondominant side.[17] The trunk extensor muscles seem to be relatively weaker than trunk flexors when compared to age-developed norms. Muscle activation patterns in the hip and leg also appear to be altered in female tennis players. The hamstrings and gluteal muscles have lower activation intensities than in males in the service motion. The result is that the trunk muscles work at higher levels of intensity in female than in male players, while the hip and leg muscles work at lower levels of intensity, especially on the nondominant side in the service motion. Muscle activation pattern alterations, or lower or upper extremity strength imbalances and inflexibilities, may predispose to injury by increasing loads on the musculotendinous structures[18] and may alter performance by decreasing maximum shoulder and arm rotational velocity.[19,20] Muscle activation alterations in the legs also may predispose to lower leg problems by not providing a stable base for muscle activity and by not creating stiffness of the entire leg to respond to flexion or rotation loads on the legs.[19] All of these potential sites of predisposition should be addressed in an injury evaluation or preparticipation examination for female tennis players and should be addressed in rehabilitation and conditioning programs.

Specific Tennis Injuries

There are no injuries that are specific to tennis or female tennis players. The following are the most common and illustrate the evaluation and treatment principles for tennis injuries.

Anterior Knee Pain

Anterior knee pain is quite common in tennis players, representing 22% of the injuries seen. Classic symptoms include pain, crepitus, swelling, weakness with flexion and rotation, inability to hit a shot that involves rotation, and occasional subluxation or dislocation of the patella. It is more common on the nondominant leg and usually is associated with twisting, especially on the service motion. Common associated physical alterations include hip and trunk weakness in the gluteal muscles, especially the gluteus medius, and in the hamstring muscles.[21] Hip muscular weakness creates a varus positioning of the femur on the pelvis and flexion of the hip. The varus positioning of the hip creates a slight valgus stress on the knee, increasing medial knee pain. There is also a common association of hip flexor and quadriceps inflexibility with anterior knee pain.

Evaluation of this injury should include evaluation of posture for leg length, asymmetry, or problems with femoral anteversion. The one-legged stability series consisting of a one-legged stance, one-legged squat, and one-legged step-up/step-down should be checked.[21] Trendelenburg positioning of the hip with one-legged stance or corkscrewing or excessive varus bending or rotation with one-legged squat or one-legged step-up/step-down are clues to muscle weakness of the hip abductors. Evaluation of knee varus and valgus in one-legged stance and step-up/step-down also should be checked, and knee strength should be evaluated by isokinetic measurement. Quadriceps and iliotibial band flexibility should be evaluated and patellofemoral tracking, alignment, and tilt should be evaluated in passive and active positioning of the knee. Imaging for anterior knee pain is best performed by anteroposterior, lateral, and Merchant views of the patella. Further evaluation can be accomplished by computed tomography scan or magnetic resonance imaging for evaluation of the patellofemoral congruence.

Treatment should start by correcting any of the alterations in flexibility and strength that are recognized in the physical examination. Quadriceps, iliotibial band, and hip flexor inflexibility can be corrected with appropriate stretching exercises. Hip strengthening can be done with closed-chain hip strengthening exercises. The most appropriate method of quadriceps strengthening involves closed-chain facilitated quadriceps activation (Fig. 2). This isolates the quadriceps in a closed chain or functional pattern as opposed to isolating the quadriceps in an open-chain or nonphysiologic pattern. Facilitated closed-chain quadriceps strengthening appears to be more efficacious in regaining quadriceps strength than the open-chain activation. Patellar taping has also been shown to be beneficial in the adjunctive care for this treatment. This appears to work by facilitating patellar positioning and by giving feedback to the quadriceps to allow it to be facilitated.

Glenoid Labral Injuries and Shoulder Instability

This combination of injuries is quite common in female tennis players, representing 46% of the injuries seen. They most commonly could be the result of microtrauma injury with repetitive overhead motions that create

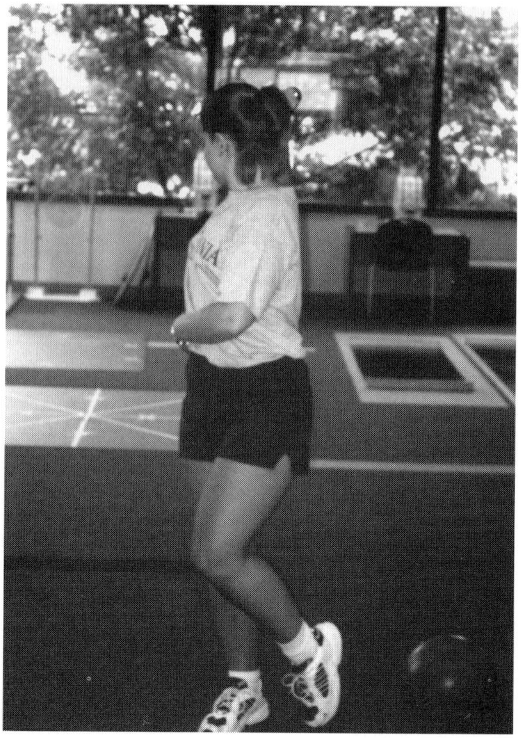

Fig. 2 *Closed-chain facilitated quadriceps activation. This requires the quadriceps to be active while the hip is extended and the foot is on the ground.*

shearing forces across the labrum and/or capsulolabral attachments. The clinical presentation is most commonly a gradual onset of soreness, tenderness, popping, and catching with rotation. The soreness is usually more common on overhead service motions or high volleys and is most commonly experienced either in acceleration out of cocking or at ball impact. Frank instability and dislocation are very rare in this set of injuries.

Associated physical alterations are quite common because of the gradual nature of the onset and the adaptations that the body attempts to overcome the functional limitations. Scapular dyskinesis or abnormal pattern of motion or position of the scapula with cocking or abduction is virtually universal in this condition.[22,23] This most commonly is due to lower trapezius and serratus anterior weakness, which is thought to be caused by an inhibition of their muscle activation as a result of the pain and instability demonstrated at the glenohumeral joint.[24] The result is a decrease in elevation of the acromion and retraction of the scapula so that the shoulder is unable to fully cock in cocking and unable to fully elevate in acceleration.[22] Also, the shoulder cannot normally track along with the movement of the humerus, thereby creating an increase in the glenohumeral angle in acceleration. The lack of scapular stability decreases the effectiveness of the scapula as an anchor for rotator cuff function. Rotator cuff strength often is apparently weak, decreasing the co-contraction/compression function of the rotator cuff.

Decreased glenohumeral internal rotation also is virtually universal in these individuals.[12,25] This decrease may be a result of the imposed demands of the sport with consequent adaptation, or it may be caused by guarding of the motion in the joint. Internal rotation changes the mechanics of the glenohumeral socket, decreasing normal rotary motion and increasing translation, both in anterosuperior and posterosuperior directions, creating extra shear on the glenohumeral surface and putting more stress on the labrum and on the biceps insertion.[15]

Rotator cuff weakness is also very common, appearing in 60% to 75% of the individuals. This strength weakness, measured by decreased strength in abduction or external rotation, can either be real, caused by actual injury of the rotator cuff tissue, especially in an undersurface fashion, or it can be apparent, as a result of neurologic inhibition secondary to pain and dysfunction or a disfacilitation due to lack of scapular stability.[24]

Evaluation of this problem should include kinetic chain as well as shoulder evaluation. Trunk posture should be checked for thoracic kyphosis or scoliosis, hip weakness, or abnormalities in hip posture or lumbar hyperextension or lordosis. The one-legged stability screening test can be used in this situation as well.

Scapular position to motion should be checked with arm forward flexion or abduction, both in the ascending and the descending phases. Lateral scapular slide measurements should be done to check for quantitative dynamic evaluation of muscle strength in the scapular stabilizers.[22] If impingement symptoms are present, the scapular assistance test[22] may be used to evaluate the contribution of lower trapezius weakness to impingement. If impingement symptoms are decreased or abolished by scapular assistance, lower trapezius weakness is present and its treatment should be included in the treatment plan. Glenohumeral inflexibility should be evaluated in a goniometric fashion rather than a spinal level fashion. True glenohumeral internal rotation is correlated with goniometric measurements rather than spinal level measurements and should be used as the basis for evaluation and treatment. External rotation should also be checked. Both internal and external rotation should be checked at 90° abduction for more functional evaluation. Rotator cuff strength should be tested in an isolated fashion; however, the strength testing should be done both in the normal scapular position and in the retracted stabilized scapular position. Apparent muscle weakness may be shown if the muscle strength becomes normal with scapular retraction.

Superior labral testing should include the anterior slide maneuver, O'Brien's maneuver, the biceps tension test for anterosuperior labral pathology, and the modified Jobe relocation test for posterosuperior labral instability. The modified Jobe relocation test maneuver is fairly specific for posterosuperior labral pathology. A positive test is pain localized to the posterosuperior joint area with external rotation and abduction that is not relieved by posterior pressure.

Instability testing should be done in the traditional fashion. Care should be taken in doing the examination because some of these instabilities are rather subtle. They will not show as frank dislocations. Anteroinferior testing with extra translation is most common. Posteroinferior instability with pain on horizontal adduction and slight extra translation is also common. If the patient presents with posterosuperior labral pathology, a pseudolaxity in the anteroinferior aspect may be present as a result of the lack of the tensioning effect of the biceps on the anterior capsule. Correction of the posterosuperior lesion often corrects the anterior pseudolaxity.

Treatment of these problems should start with rehabilitation of all of the observed deficits. The alterations in the leg, hip, and trunk can be addressed while decreasing the symptoms in the shoulder. Facilitated hip extension and trunk extension can increase control of the scapular muscles, especially the lower trapezius. Co-contraction closed-chain activation of the periscapular muscles is also beneficial in maintaining and increasing scapular control.[26] Rotator cuff exercises should be done in a facilitated fashion, with scapular retraction and stabilization, 90° of abduction of the arm, and closed-chain activation in a co-contraction/compression-type activation.[26] The traditional isolated rotator cuff exercises create extra shear across the joint and are more likely to cause injury and symptoms and should be done at a later stage of rehabilitation. If surgical stabilization is necessary, preoperative rehabilitation of the trunk and scapula should be performed, similar to the preoperative exercises performed before anterior cruciate ligament reconstruction. After surgical stabilization, trunk and leg exercises can be maintained. Facilitated scapular retraction can also be done early in the rehabilitation phase followed by integration of the glenohumeral rotation, motion, and stabilization as healing progresses.

Elbow Injuries

Elbow injuries, either epicondylitis or instability, comprise 24% of the injuries seen. Similar to male players, female tennis players get both medial and lateral symptoms. However, instability patterns on the medial side of the elbow are less common in female players than they are in male players. This difference is probably the result of the higher forces generated by male players in the forehand and service motions. Lateral elbow injuries are relatively uncommon in elite female players, predominantly because of the use of the two-handed backhand. Lateral epicondylar injuries are very common, however, in recreational one-hand backhand players as a result of poorer mechanics and more load on the lateral elbow due to proximal shoulder muscle weakness. The classic lateral symptoms of pain and stiffness over the lateral epicondylar area with point tenderness over the extensor carpi radialis brevis, with muscle strength weakness and increased pain with full extension, are common.[27] The shots that are most affected are the backhand ground stroke, the backhand volley, and occasionally the overhead service motion. Medial elbow symptoms are divided between epicondylitis symptoms, which include point tenderness over the medial epicondyle and over the pronator teres insertion, and valgus overload symptoms, with pain along the medial collateral ligament and in the posterior medial aspect of the elbow.

Physical alterations associated with elbow injuries include inflexibility or strength deficits in the shoulder muscles that decrease the rapid movement of the elbow through the hitting zone. In patients with lateral epicondylitis, the posterior deltoid and infraspinatus are often found to be weak. In patients with medial epicondylitis, scapular dyskinesis is common with internal rotation weakness and tightness and, on occasion, actual instability of the glenohumeral joint. Flexibility of the biceps with lack of full extension with the arm in supination is also seen. Decreased strength in the wrist extensors is common with lateral epicondylar symptoms, and decreased flexibility in the wrist flexors is common with medial epicondylitis symptoms.[27,28]

Treatment is almost always conservative with modification of activity, bracing, correction of the inflexibilities and strength deficits, and strengthening of the proximal musculature. Soft-tissue augmented massage has been noted to have benefit in patients with lateral epicondylitis. This technique of directed physical therapy with deep massage appears to be effective in improving healing response and decreasing stiffness. Elbow bracing may be of benefit in the acute situation to allow earlier return to play.

Surgical treatment is designed to obliterate the damaged tissue, to promote a healing response, and to restore integrity of the muscle-tendon unit so that force development can be maintained.[27] This classically has been achieved by open procedures that address the pathologic damage and do a repair with direct reattachment of tendon to tendon or tendon to bone. These treatment techniques have been very successful both in the first-time surgical treatment and in salvage operations.[27] More recently, arthroscopic resection techniques have been developed. This particular procedure has not been done much in high-demand tennis players, and because it does not reattach tissue, it may not have the same ultimate ability to allow force production and generation in the competitive tennis athlete.

Wrist Injuries

Triangular fibrocartilage complex injuries and tendinitis are very common in female tennis players and are becoming more prominent as new styles of tennis playing are evolving. These occur on the dominant hand in association with the forehand stroke and on the nondominant hand in association with the two-handed backhand stroke. The symptoms are usually related to pain along the ulnar aspect of the wrist, either over the extensor carpi ulnaris tendon or the triangular fibrocartilage complex. There is point tenderness, occasional crepitus, pain with ulnar deviation and supination of the wrist, and occasionally, a popping and catching with motion.[29] This occurs in the cocking phase of the tennis stroke and is relieved by decreased ulnar deviation with a brace.

Associated factors seen with pain with the forehand stroke include decreased shoulder internal rotation, increased forearm pronation with the racquet moving through the hitting zone, an extreme western grip of the racquet, and a consequent laying back of the wrist in supination and ulnar deviation to hit the ball. The problem is caused biomechanically by an increase in the use of forearm pronation to drive the racquet through the hitting zone because of weakness or tightness in shoulder internal rotation. As a result, to get extra movement and speed through the hitting zone, the wrist is cocked back in a hypersupinated and ulnar deviated position, creating extra compression on this side of the wrist as the racquet is brought from cocking into acceleration. The extreme western grip lays the hand into supination and exacerbates the impingement.

Associated factors seen with the two-handed backhand include pain and soreness over the nondominant ulnar area. The wrist is cocked in hyperextension and ulnar deviation to allow the nondominant hand to be the driver of the racquet through the hitting zone. The newest two-handed backhand strokes emphasize that the nondominant hand becomes the driver of the racquet rather than the dominant hand and dominant shoulder being the driver of the racquet through the hitting zone. The nondominant hand is usually weaker than the dominant arm; and, therefore, to get more power and to create more velocity through the hitting zone, the racquet is often held in a hypersupinated and dorsiflexed position that increases pressure on the ulnar side of the wrist.

Evaluation of tennis players with wrist injuries should include trunk rotational strength and flexibility, shoulder internal rotation strength and flexibility, forearm pronation tightness, and nondominant arm strength. All of these kinetic chain alterations can put extra stress on the wrist, creating a kinetic chain breakage and causing the wrist to have to do more work than normal to compensate.[28] At the wrist, the evaluation should include evaluation of impingement with the wrist in supination and dorsiflexion.[29] Pain over the ulnar aspect of the triangular fibrocartilage is a diagnostic sign. Tenderness along the extensor carpi ulnaris tendon and/or subluxation of the tendon should be evaluated as well. The distal radioulnar joint should be checked for dorsiflexion or palmar flexion instability, and a neurovascular examination should be done to rule out problems with the ulnar nerve at Guyon's canal or ulnar artery injury at the hook of the hamate.

Treatment is predicated on correcting the biomechanics of the stroke. Leg and trunk rotational strength should be maximized to allow for good hitting through the hitting zone. Shoulder weakness should be corrected so that the external rotators or internal rotators are strong to guide the racquet through the hitting zone. The motion of the arm through the hitting zone in the forehand should be one of internal rotation of the shoulder rather than pronation of the forearm. In the shoulder internal rotation dominant forehand, the elbow should be pointing toward the flight of the ball as the arm comes through. In the forearm pronation dominant type of forehand, the elbow goes out to the side because of the motion of the arm. Excessive wrist position should be checked. If this is a problem, then taping should be done to decrease the impingement with this excessive position, and the biomechanics should be corrected so that the arm rather than the wrist extends in cocking. Co-contraction wrist exercises should be performed to allow for stabilization of the wrist in the neutral position. Wrist taping can be beneficial in controlling the forces, and surgical repair of the triangular fibrocartilage complex or the subluxing extensor carpi ulnaris tendon can be performed if symptoms warrant.

Summary

Tennis injuries are common in female tennis players. There is no gender-specific injury pattern or causation to these injuries. If injuries occur, basic principles of kinetic chain evaluation and treatment should be performed to allow for normal return to athletic activities.

Because most tennis injuries are microtraumatic and are the result of a process of causation, preventative measures can be considered if predisposing physiologic and biomechanical factors are known. There is very little data on gender-specific kinetics or kinematics of tennis strokes, on other physiologic variables such as metabolic demands or the effect of rehabilitation exercises on recovery from injury, or on the effect of specific conditioning for female tennis players, either for injury prevention or increased performance. There is some evidence that there may be gender-associated differences in muscle activation in tennis strokes. These data must be confirmed and incorporated into evaluation and conditioning if found to be significant.

There is a huge increase in interest in women's tennis, both at the professional and the recreational level. Much more baseline information needs to be gathered to ensure that increased participation is associated with safe and enjoyable activity.

References

1. Kibler WB, McQueen C, Uhl T: Fitness evaluations and fitness findings in competitive junior tennis players. *Clin Sports Med* 1988;7:403–416.
2. Hutchinson MR, Laprade RF, Burnett QM II, Moss R, Terpstra J: Injury surveillance at USTA Boys' Tennis Championships: A 6-year study. *Med Sci Sports Exerc* 1995;27:826–830.
3. Verspeelt P: A review of tennis-related injuries in Flemish tennis players, in Pieper HG, Krahl H, Kibler WB, Renstrom P (eds): *Tennis: Sports Medicine and Science.* Düsseldorf, Germany, Rau, 1995, pp 47–51.
4. Kibler WB: Injuries to tennis athletes, in Renstrom P (ed): *IOC Encyclopedia of Sports Racquet Sports*, in press.
5. Winge S, Jorgensen U, Lassen Nielsen A: Epidemiology of injuries in Danish championship tennis. *Int J Sports Med* 1989;10:368–371.
6. Roetert EP, Brody H, Dillman CJ, Groppel JL, Schultheis JM: The biomechanics of tennis elbow: An integrated approach. *Clin Sports Med* 1995;14:47–57.
7. Zecher SB, Leach RE: Lower leg and foot injuries in tennis and other racquet sports. *Clin Sports Med* 1995;14:223–239.
8. Meeuwisse WH: Assessing causation in sport injury: A multi-factorial model. *Clin J Sport Med* 1994;4:166–170.
9. Griffin LY: The female athlete, in Renström PAFH (ed): *Sports Injuries: Basic Principles of Prevention and Care*. Oxford, England, Blackwell Scientific Publications, 1993, pp 194–202.
10. Kibler WB, Chandler TJ, Uhl T, Maddux RE: A musculoskeletal approach to the preparticipation physical examination: Preventing injury and improving performance. *Am J Sports Med* 1989;17:525–531.
11. Chandler TJ, Kibler WB, Uhl TL, Wooten B, Kiser A, Stone E: Flexibility comparisons of junior elite tennis players to other athletes. *Am J Sports Med* 1990;18:134–136.

12. Silliman JF, Hawkins RJ: Current concepts and recent advances in the athlete's shoulder. *Clin Sports Med* 1991;10:693–705.

13. Knapik JJ, Bauman CL, Jones BH, Harris JM, Vaughan L: Preseason strength and flexibility imbalances associated with athletic injuries in female collegiate athletes. *Am J Sports Med* 1991;19:76–81.

14. Ekstrand J, Gillquist J: The avoidability of soccer injuries. *Int J Sports Med* 1983;4:124–128.

15. Harryman DT II, Sidles JA, Clark JM, McQuade KJ, Gibb TD, Matsen FA III: Translation of the humeral head on the glenoid with passive glenohumeral motion. *J Bone Joint Surg* 1990;72A:1334–1343.

16. Chandler TJ, Kibler WB: Muscle training in injury prevention, in Renström PAFH (ed): *Sports Injuries: Basic Principles of Prevention and Care*. Oxford, England, Blackwell Scientific Publications, 1993, pp 252–261.

17. Chandler TJ, Kibler WB, Stracener EC, Ziegler AK, Pace B: Shoulder strength, power, and endurance in college tennis players. *Am J Sports Med* 1992;20:455–458.

18. Lieber RL, Friden J: Muscle damage is not a function of muscle force but active muscle strain. *J Appl Physiol* 1993;74:520–526.

19. Kraemer WJ, Triplett NT, Fry AC: An in-depth sports medicine profile of women college tennis players. *J Sport Rehab* 1995;4:79–98.

20. Elliott BC, Marshall RN, Noffal GJ: Contributions of upper limb segment rotations during the power serve in tennis. *J Appl Biomech* 1995;11:433–442.

21. Host JV, Craig R, Lehman RC: Patellofemoral dysfunction in tennis players: A dynamic problem. *Clin Sports Med* 1995;14:177–203.

22. Kibler WB: The role of the scapula in athletic shoulder function. *Am J Sports Med* 1998;26:325–337.

23. Warner JJ, Micheli LJ, Arslanian LE, Kennedy J, Kennedy R: Scapulothoracic motion in normal shoulders and shoulders with glenohumeral instability and impingement syndrome: A study using Moire topographic analysis. *Clin Orthop* 1992;285:191–199.

24. McQuade KJ, Dawson J, Smidt GL: Scapulothoracic muscle fatigue associated with alterations in scapulohumeral rhythm kinematics during maximum resistive shoulder elevation. *J Orthop Sports Phys Ther* 1998;28:74–80.

25. Kibler WB, Chandler TJ, Livingston BP, Roetert EP: Shoulder range of motion in elite tennis players: Effect of age and years of tournament play. *Am J Sports Med* 1996;24:279–285.

26. Kibler WB: Shoulder rehabilitation: Principles and practice. *Med Sci Sports Exerc* 1998;30(suppl 4):S40–S50.

27. Nirschl RP: Elbow tendinosis/tennis elbow. *Clin Sports Med* 1992;11:851–870.

28. Kibler WB: Pathophysiology of overload injuries around the elbow. *Clin Sports Med* 1995;14:447–457.

29. Rettig AC: Wrist problems in the tennis player. *Med Sci Sports Exerc* 1994;26:1207–1212.

Chapter 18
Rowing

Carol C. Teitz, MD

Rowing as an intercollegiate sport began in England in 1829 with the Oxford-Cambridge race. The first official intercollegiate competition in the United States was between Harvard and Yale in 1852. Although private rowing clubs existed even before these competitions, the fitness boom of the last two decades has markedly increased the popularity of rowing. Current estimates including recreational, club, high school, collegiate, and elite rowers exceeds 100,000 participants in the United States alone.

In spite of the large number of participants in this sport, published research on the injuries sustained in rowing is limited. Hickey and associates[1] studied elite rowers at the Australian Institute of Sport from 1985 to 1994 and analyzed their injury patterns retrospectively. The female athletes ranged in age from 14 to 36 years and the male athletes from 16 to 31 years. Hickey and associates[1] found an injury rate in female rowers of 1.58 injuries per year, and in male rowers of 0.85 injuries per year. The vast majority of injuries in both sexes were overuse injuries. The most prevalent sites of injury in the female rowers were the chest (22.6%) and the lumbar spine (15.2%). In the male rowers, the most prevalent sites were the lumbar spine (25%) and the wrist (15.5%).[1] Although complaints in the buttock region are less prevalent, they also present a particular problem for female rowers.

Background

Rowing is practiced at many levels, from the recreational rower to the elite international rower. It is divided into sweep rowing, in which each rower handles only one oar, and sculling, in which each rower handles two smaller oars. Sweep rowers compete in pairs and in shells (boats) of 4 or 8 rowers. Scullers compete alone, in pairs, or in four-person shells. Rowers also compete in different weight categories. The rowing stroke has been divided into four phases: the catch, in which the oar engages the water; the drive, in which the oar is pulled through the water; the finish, in which the oar is lifted from the water; and the recovery, in which the oar moves through the air in preparation for reentry into the water[2] (Fig. 1). In sweep rowing, the trunk is ever so slightly off center at the catch (Fig. 1, *A*) then brought back to the midline during the drive (Fig. 1, *B*). Consequently, at the catch, sweep rowers may stretch the ligamentous structures on the side opposite the oar and compress facet joints on the side adjacent to the oar. Moreover, sweep rowers tend to develop asymmetrical trunk musculature with the stronger side being opposite the side of the oar.[3] Rowing requires extremes of trunk motion at the same time as large muscle forces are generated. Ideally, when moving from the forward flexed position at the catch to the extended spine position at the finish, the pivoting should occur predominantly through the hip joint. This requires co-contraction of the quadriceps and hamstring muscles. The quadriceps must extend the knees and the hamstrings must extend the hips. When quadriceps muscles dominate, extension occurs in the spine instead of in the hips.

Back Pain

Background

Back pain, particularly in the lumbar region, is a major and costly problem for the population as a whole.[4] The percentage of athletes reporting low back

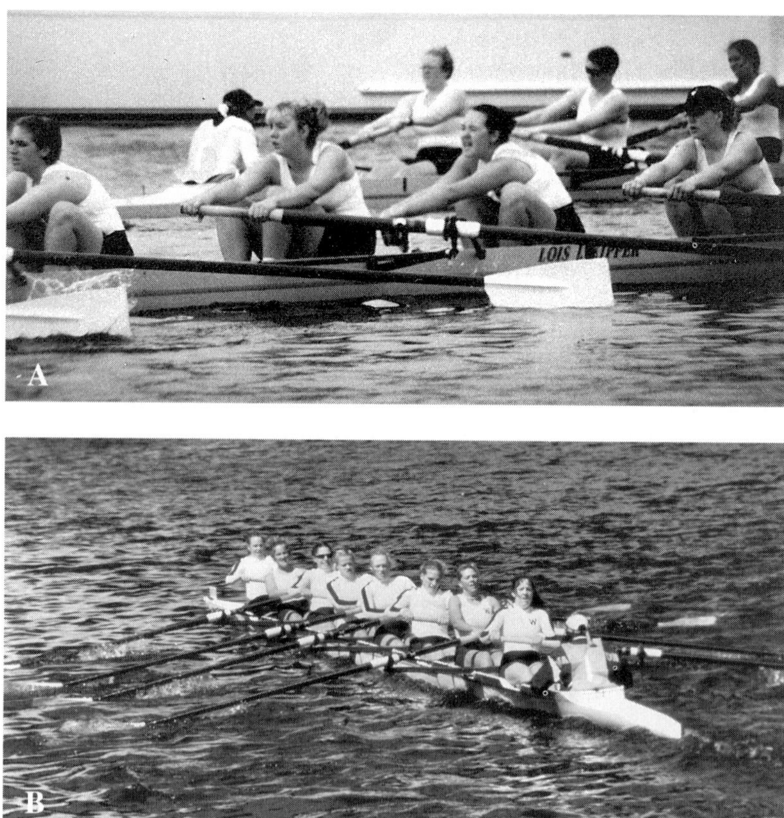

***Fig. 1 A**, In sweep rowing, the trunk is ever so slightly off center at the catch with the rower leaning toward the oar. **B**, The rower's trunk is in the midline during the drive.*

pain varies depending on the sport. In addition to rowing, the sports in which back pain is a prevalent problem are tennis, weightlifting, gymnastics, wrestling, football, and golf[5–10] (Table 1). In Hickey and associates'[1] study, lumbar spine problems were the most common acute problem (21.1%) and third most common chronic problem in the female rowers. In the male rowers, the lumbar spine was the most common site of chronic problems (29.6%). The conditions associated with the pain rarely require surgical treatment; however, low back pain can significantly interfere with training and competition. Much of the pain is attributed to muscular strains and ligamentous sprains, but diskogenic pain and spondylolysis also are frequently diagnosed. The forward flexed position of the rower at the catch likely produces high disk pressures. Nachemson[11] measured disk pressures in vivo with healthy subjects in various positions of lying, sitting, and standing. The second highest disk pressures recorded were found when the subjects were seated and bent forward 20° with a 10-kg weight in each hand, a position that closely simulates the position of the rower at the catch.[11]

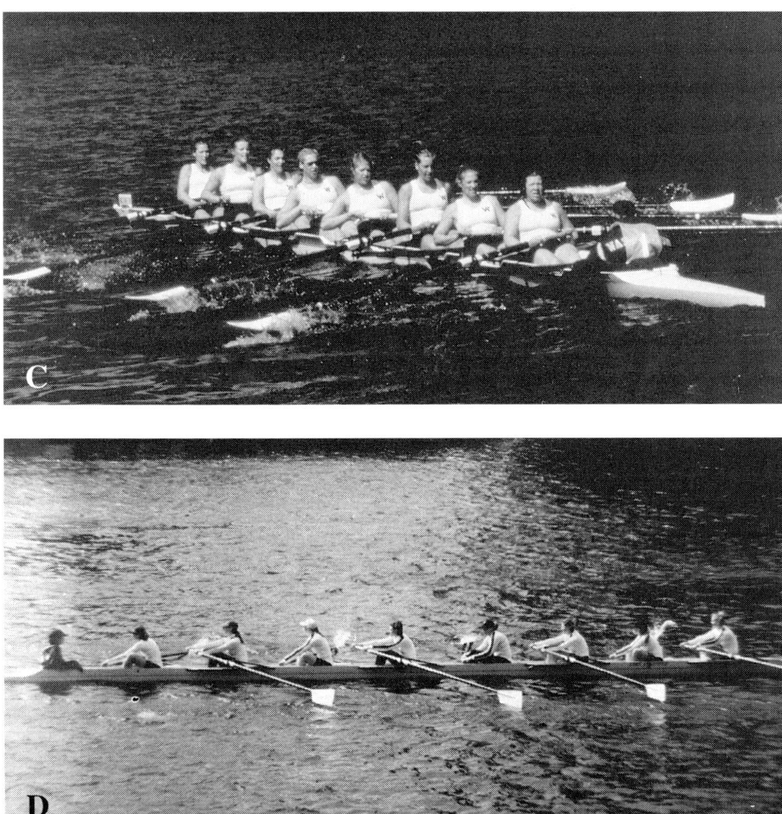

***Fig. 1 continued** C, The oar is lifted from the water during the finish. **D**, During the recovery, the oar moves through the air in preparation for re-entry into the water.*

Table 1 Sports in which back pain is a prevalent problem

Sport	Reporting Low Back Pain	Study
Tennis	50%	Sward, et al[5]
Weight lifting	40%	Aggrawal, et al[6]
Gymnastics	33%	Garrick and Requa[7]
Wrestling	32%	Wroble and Albright[8]
Football	27%	Semon and Spengler[9]
Golf	10% to 33%	Hosae and Gatt[10]
Rowing	15% to 25%	Hickey, et al[1]

Anatomy and Physiology of the Immature Spine

Because competitive rowing can begin in the high school years, the anatomy and physiology of the immature spine must be considered.[12] The immature intervertebral disk is more hydrated than that of the adult, and the fibers of the annular ligament are stronger than the vertebral end plate, which may remain cartilaginous until the age of 20 years. Therefore, compressive loading in the adolescent spine is more likely to damage the vertebral end plate and to produce a Schmorl's node than to produce an annular tear and a posterolaterally herniated disk, conditions that are common in adults.[13] Sward and associates[13] and Hellstrom and associates[14] found apophyseal injuries in wrestlers, gymnasts, football players, and tennis players, but in none of the nonathletes in their study populations. When disk herniations occur in adolescents, the disks often herniate vertically into the vertebral body (Schmorl's node) rather than through the anulus toward the neural foramen. Moreover, when adolescents have herniated disks, they often have a paucity of neurologic findings, making the diagnosis more difficult.[15] Although both Hellstrom and associates[14] and Sward and associates[13] found an equal frequency of Schmorl's nodes in athletes and nonathletes, Aggrawal and associates[6] found a much higher incidence in weight-training athletes. Micheli and Wood[16] found that low back pain in adolescents is more likely to be caused by posterior element problems such as spondylolysis than to disks or muscle strain. Therefore, when an adolescent rower presents with back pain, the physician must consider the diagnoses of growth plate injuries, spondylolysis, and disk herniations, as well as that of muscle strain. In the adult, physicians are usually more concerned about disk herniations, facet joint injury or arthritis, stress fractures, and muscle strain.

Diagnosis

Disk injuries are usually more symptomatic during forward bending (before the drive phase of rowing), and pain is increased during Valsalva maneuvers. Facet injuries, on the other hand, are more likely to be symptomatic during extension of the spine (the drive phase), and the associated pain is not exacerbated by Valsalva maneuvers. Facet injuries that are not fractures are usually not visible radiographically although facet arthritis will cause increased radioisotope uptake on bone scan. Stress fracture (usually of the pars interarticularis, ie, spondylolysis) is diagnosed either by bone scan or magnetic resonance imaging (MRI). Disk herniations can be diagnosed on MRI, although care must be taken not to overinterpret the MRI. Because disk degeneration is prevalent and not always symptomatic, the physician must be certain to correlate clinical symptoms and signs with the site of disk degeneration/herniation on MRI before considering a cause and effect relationship between the two sets of findings. The diagnosis of muscle strain tends to be one of exclusion after the diagnoses previously mentioned have been ruled out either clinically, with imaging, or both.

Rib Pain

Background

Rib stress fractures have been described in many sports, especially in golf and rowing.[17–21] In Hickey and associates' study,[1] chest wall injuries accounted for 22.6% of all injuries in the female athlete, with rib stress fractures making up 32.6% of these injuries. The remainder of chest injuries were ascribed to intercostal muscle strain, costochondral injury, contusions, or nonspecific chest wall pain. Rib stress fractures were diagnosed on 15 occasions in female rowers and on 2 occasions in male rowers and accounted for 7.4% of all female rowers' injuries. These fractures were first described in rowers by Holden and Jackson.[22] In a retrospective study at the 1996 US Olympic trials, 14 cases of rib stress fracture were found in 10 elite rowers, 7 of whom were women. The fractures were located in ribs 5 through 9 on the anterolateral to posterolateral aspects of the ribs. Nine of 14 occurred during training season when the emphasis was on high load per stroke. Seven of 9 fractures in the sweep rowers occurred on the side closer to the oar. Holden and Jackson[22] attributed these stress fractures to chronic pull by the serratus anterior muscle both during rowing and weight training. Christiansen and Kanstrup[20] thought the primary cause of rib stress fractures was an increase in training. Bojani'c and Desnica[18] reported a case thought to be due to change in technique rather than in training. Karlson[19] hypothesized that the increased frequency of stress fractures on the side of the oar in sweep rowers might be due to excessive use of the external oblique muscles on that side in order to lean toward the oar at the catch. She further hypothesized that a perceived increase in rib stress fractures in recent years may be related to a change in the shape of the oar blade.[19]

Rodriguez and associates[23] used electromyography to study muscle activity during the rowing stroke on an ergometer and found that the combined activity of 2 or more groups of muscles was more critical in producing a coordinated rowing stroke than the strength of any 1 muscle. Satou and Konisi,[24] using a fresh cadaver, electromyography, and finite element analysis, found that muscle forces generated by the scapulothoracic muscles were sufficient to cause rib stress fractures. Moreover, ribs 5 through 9 share insertional fibers of both the serratus anterior and the external oblique muscles. Both muscles insert in the lateral area of the rib where it bends around the thorax and where most of the fractures in rowers occur. The serratus posterior inferior also inserts in this area but has never been studied in rowers. Although the serratus anterior is considered a scapular stabilizer, it can also be thought of as a muscle that can pull the ribs up and back. The external oblique, on the other hand. pulls the ribs down and in. Boland and Hosea[25] thought that the serratus anterior contracted maximally at the catch when force is transferred from the legs and trunk to the arms. It may well be, however, that it is the eccentric contraction at the finish that creates greater forces than the concentric contraction at the catch. At the finish, because the trunk is behind the hips and the scapulae are maximally retracted, both the external oblique and the serratus anterior are acting eccentrically.

Diagnosis

Rib stress fractures present as either chest or thoracic back pain. Most occur in ribs 5 through 9 in the region between the anterior and posterior axillary lines. The site of fracture will be tender, and pain will increase with cough. Because strains can, on occasion, produce bony tenderness, imaging studies are recommended to confirm the diagnosis. Although many rib stress fractures are not initially visible on plain radiographs, they are easily seen on bone scan. Treatment includes cessation from rowing and chest muscle strengthening exercises until the rib is no longer tender. When the athlete complains of significant pain with deep breathing or coughing, a rib belt is prescribed.

Buttock Pain

Background

Female rowers have buttock pain that is different from the buttock pain associated with lower back problems. The latter is typically in the upper outer quadrant of the buttock and is thought to be referred from lumbar nerve root irritation or to be sclerotomal in origin. The rower's pain is more perineal, in the region of the ischial tuberosity or inferior pubic ramus. This area can be painful in runners as a result of hamstring origin avulsions, especially in adolescents who develop ischial apophysitis.[26] Pain in this area also is described in the medical literature in relation to bicycling.[27] Improperly fitting bicycle seats are known to produce ischial bursitis and stress on the pubic symphysis. Perineal pain presents problems to these athletes not only when they are training and competing, but also when they are sitting in classrooms or at work at other times during the day.

The shape of bicycle seats has been redesigned for the female perineum. In addition, seats made of various shock absorbing materials and bicycling shorts with built in perineal padding are available. In cycling, perineal problems affect both men and women. In crew, the problem predominates in female rowers (although epidemiologic studies are lacking). In an unpublished study at the University of Washington in the 1980s (NJ Smith, personal communication), stamp-pad prints were made of the buttocks of the women's crew team and compared to the shape of the seats in the rowing shells. These seats have openings in them that are meant to relieve the area of the ischial tuberosity and distribute the load-bearing area to the more fleshy areas of the buttocks (Fig. 2). Smith determined that, in fact, the seats did not fit female buttocks well. At the University of Washington, many female rowing athletes present with ischial tuberosity bursitis, and others present with tenderness along the inferior pubic ramus. These athletes noted no problems on the ergometers and also no problems in some shells but significant problems in other shells; ie, the problem seemed to be seat specific. Some athletes who had this problem unilaterally were found to have a leg-length discrepancy and therefore were slightly more forward in their seats on the side of the short limb. These athletes responded to correcting their leg-length discrepancies with orthoses. As a way of treating other symptomatic athletes, gel seats designed for kayaking were placed in the rowing shell. In addition to symptomatic relief, at the end of a workout it was possible to see ischial tuberosity impressions on the upper (buttock) side of the gel and seat impressions on the lower (seat) side of the gel. As suspected, the ischial tuberosities of these symptomatic rowers were rubbing against the edges of the openings in the seat. Although this improvisation proved helpful, gel seats designed for kayaks do not fit the seats in the shell exactly, and it was necessary to improvise methods of fixing the padding to the seats. There are pads designed for shells, but they are predominantly made of foam-like materials.

Diagnosis

The athlete with rowing-induced perineal pain will report that her pain occurs predominantly from rowing in the shell and often is not present on the ergometer or at other times during the day, unless it has been present for a long time. There are no associated bowel or bladder symptoms. Either the ischium or the inferior pubic ramus will be tender, but resisted use of hamstrings or adductors usually do not exacerbate the pain. Radiographs should be taken to rule out periosteal reaction or erosions.

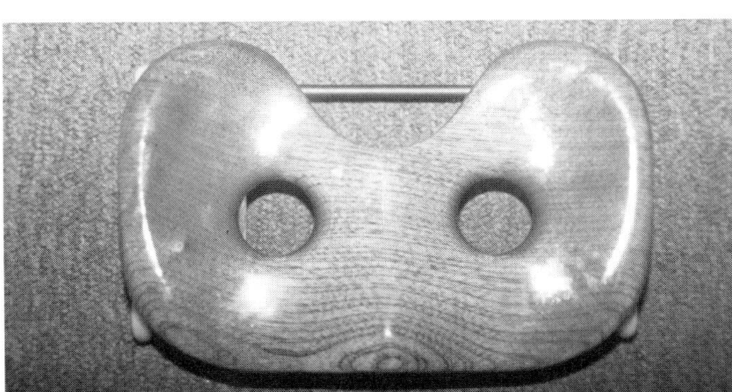

Fig. 2 *A typical seat from a rowing shell.*

Conclusion

Back pain, rib stress fractures, and perineal buttock pain are prevalent in the female rower. Although there is some knowledge transferable from other sports and from nonathletic patients with similar problems, there are clear avenues for futher research in defining etiologic factors and in developing prevention strategies.

References

1. Hickey GJ, Fricker PA, McDonald WA: Injuries to elite rowers over a 10-yr period. *Med Sci Sports Exerc* 1997;29:1567-1572.
2. Mickelson TC, Hagerman FC: Functional anatomy of the rowing stroke. *Oarsman* 1979;11:12.
3. Edgerton VR: Neuromuscular adaptation to power and endurance work. *Can J Appl Sport Sci* 1979;1:49-58.
4. Deyo RA, Phillips WR: Low back pain: A primary care challenge. *Spine* 1996;21:2826-2832.
5. Sward L, Hellstrom M, Jacobsson B, Peterson L: Back pain and radiological changes in the thoraco-lumbar spine of athletes. *Spine* 1990;15:124-129.
6. Aggrawal ND, Kaur R, Kumar S, Mathur DN: A study of changes in the spine in weight lifters and other athletes. *Br J Sports Med* 1979;13(2):58-61.
7. Garrick JG, Requa RK: Epidemiology of women's gymnastics injuries. *Am J Sports Med* 1980;8:261-264.
8. Wroble RR, Albright JP: Neck and low back injuries in wrestling. *Clin Sports Med* 1986;5:295-326.
9. Semon RL, Spengler D: Significance of lumbar spondylolysis in college football players. *Spine* 1981;6:172-174.
10. Hosea TM, Gatt CJ: Back pain in golf. *Clin Sports Med* 1996;15:37-53.
11. Nachemson AL: The load on lumbar disks in different positions of the body. *Clin Orthop* 1966;45:107-122.
12. Sward L: The thoracolumbar spine in young elite athletes: Current concepts on the effects of physical training. *Sports Med* 1992;13: 357-364.
13. Sward L, Hellstrom M, Jacobsson B, Nyman R, Peterson L: Disc degeneration and associated abnormalities of the spine in elite gymnasts: A magnetic resonance imaging study. *Spine* 1991;16:437-443.
14. Hellstrom M, Jacobsson B, Sward L, Peterson L: Radiological abnormalities in the spine of top athletes. *Acta Radiologica* 1990;31:127-132.
15. Epstein JA, Epstein NE, Marc J, Rosenthal AD, Lavine, LS: Lumbar intervertebral disc herniation in teenage children: Recognition and management of associated anomalies. *Spine* 1984;9:427-432.
16. Micheli LJ, Wood R: Back pain in young athletes: Significant differences from adults in causes and patterns. *Arch Pediatr Adolesc Med* 1995;149:15-18.
17. Lord MJ, Ha KI, Song KS: Stress fractures of the ribs in golfers. *Am J Sports Med* 1996;24:118-122.
18. Bojani'c I, Desnica A: Stress fracture of the sixth rib in an elite athlete. *Croat Med J* 1998;39:458-460.
19. Karlson KA: Rib stress fractures in elite rowers: A case series and proposed mechanism. *Am J Sports Med* 1998;26:516-519.

20. Christiansen E, Kanstrup IL: Increased risk of stress fractures of the ribs in elite rowers. *Scan J Med Sci Sports* 1997;7:49-52.
21. Brukner P, Khan K: Stress fracture of the neck of the seventh and eighth ribs: A case report. *Clin J Sport Med* 1996;6:204-206.
22. Holden DL, Jackson DW: Stress fracture of the ribs in female rowers. *Am J Sports Med* 1985;13:342-348.
23. Rodriguez RJ, Rodriguez RP, Cook SD, Sandborn PM: Electromyographic analysis of rowing stroke biomechanics. *J Sports Med Phys Fitness* 1990;30:103-108.
24. Satou S, Konisi N: The mechanism of fatigue fracture of the ribs. *Nippon Seikeigeka Gakkai Zasshi* 1991;65:708-719.
25. Boland AL, Hosea TM: Rowing and sculling and the older athlete. *Clin Sports Med* 1991;10:245-256.
26. Kujala UM, Orava S, Karpakka J, Leppavuori J, Mattila K: Ischial tuberosity apophysitis and avulsion among athletes. *Int J Sports Med* 1997;18:149-155.
27. Weiss BD: Non-traumatic injuries in amateur long distance bicyclists. *Am J Sports Med* 1985;13:187-192.

Chapter 19

Rehabilitation of Shoulder and Knee Instability in Female Athletes: Principles and Practice

W. Benjamin Kibler, MD

Introduction

Rehabilitation is best considered as a series of activities that prepare the athlete to return to athletic function at the highest level of achievement for the individual athlete. Rehabilitation is not a specific program of exercises that should be used in every instance but should be individualized for the athlete depending on the type of injury, the musculoskeletal base, and the desired function of the athlete. This chapter will present several salient principles that underlie this rehabilitation framework. It will present the basic science underlying the principles and the rationale for using the principles, and then will illustrate specific practices for implementing the principles around the knee and the shoulder. The practices will be illustrated by certain exercises that are not inclusive but should be used as starting points for development of the exercise programs. This chapter will specifically address rehabilitation of the knee from a knee instability reconstruction and rehabilitation of the shoulder following shoulder instability treatment.

Rehabilitate for Function, Not Only for Resolution of Symptoms

Rehabilitation is most efficacious when it addresses the specific activities or specific sports that the athlete wishes to return to. In some female athletes, these may be very specific, such as downhill skiing, kicking a soccer ball, or throwing a softball. At other times, it may be more general in that the athlete may play several sports or wish to do several activities. However, these goals should be recognized and identified before starting rehabilitation because different activities have different biomechanical and physiologic requirements for function. Maximum performance has both biomechanical and physiologic parameters that need to be identified in the rehabilitation plan.

Biomechanically, athletic function is the result of an activation of a series of links or individual body segments that produces force to achieve that function.[1,2] The link activation sequence is specific for the activity. Jumping has a different activation sequence than running, and throwing has a different activation sequence than swimming or shooting a basketball. The purpose of the link activation sequence is to place the delivery mechanism for the developed force, the hand or the foot, in the most appropriate position and at the most appropriate velocity to achieve the desired athletic function, whether it be kicking, jumping, or throwing. These activation sequences are called kinetic chains, and this should be considered the total body contribution to the athletic activity. There are probably many different ways of activating the sequences; however, there are only one or two most efficient ways given the individual's athletic ability and anatomy, and these should be reproduced as closely as possible. Alterations in link sequence activation can occur either as a result of injury or as a prelude to injury, and these must be modified or the rehabilitation effort will be limited. Because of the link activation sequencing and the integration of each link with another, link activation abnormalities in distant areas may also have an impact on the area of weakest link or the area of injury.

The muscle activation patterns that create link sequence activation are also specific for the physical activity and are part of the skill function. There are two major types of activation patterns.[3] The length-dependent patterns operate locally around joints, are modulated by muscle spindle receptors, work in co-contraction patterns to stabilize the joint against pertubations, and react with real-time feedback as the joint moves. The force-dependent patterns integrate the activation of different segments, are responsible for force production in the kinetic chain, are controlled by Golgi tendon receptors, are very commonly operated through the two-joint muscle linkage, and operate more efficiently at faster speeds of rotation. They are also highly dependent on individual joint position and, therefore, are interdependent with the length-dependent patterns to produce a certain joint position so that the force-dependent patterns can produce force.

Muscle activation sequencing can be altered by several anatomic and physiologic factors. Change in joint position of 15° alters the pattern, and the eccentric functions of muscle activation are sensitive to fatigue and injury and will become less intense at an early stage of fatigue or following injury. Muscle activation alterations then produce different kinetic chain activation sequences and produce adaptations in motions or positions of joints that can be deleterious to both function and return of function and can be productive of injury.

Several studies have shown that there appear to be some gender differences in the way that key hip and leg muscles are activated in normal running or cutting activities,[4] in landing from a jump,[5] and in response to pertubations.[4] It appears there is less hip abductor activation, less hamstring activation, and consequently less leg stabilization and force absorption in females than in males. Optimum activation is not known, but based on the principles outlined, more gluteus and hamstring activation would be desirable to optimally restore function of the central core of stability and force generation.

Injury involves the production and recognition of pain impulses by the athlete, and these are some of the major sources of athletic dysfunction. However, function also involves disorders of biomechanical sequencing and physiological activation. These will still be present after the pain is reduced or eliminated and must be restored to normal before the normal functional patterns and functional performance can be demonstrated.

Practice: Knee

The ultimate goal of knee rehabilitation is to return to the kicking, jumping, running, or stabilization activities that are required for the knee in the different athletic functions.[6] The kinetic chains of kicking, jumping, running, or stabilization require that the foot be on the ground for most of the cycle, that there be control of the knee, the hip, and the trunk over the foot while the foot is on the ground, and that there be a sequencing of these stance or stability patterns so that the appropriate functional activities of moving the leg forward, kicking, or stabilization can be achieved. The knee functions in coordination with the other segments of the leg and trunk to allow these kinetic chains to happen. In running, the knee is most efficiently modeled as a spring with the entire leg working as a unit.[7] The knee is then seen as a part of the whole leg in terms of stance, stability, or motion. In jumping, the knee once again is seen as a part of the entire leg stability.[2,8] The stance leg of kicking requires that the entire leg be stable with little change in joint angle or in stiffness while the kicking leg develops a sequence of torques, starting at the hip, going through the knee to the foot, to allow the foot to have maximum power, velocity, and position.[2] In both biomechanical situations, the moments and forces seen at the knee are generated not only by the knee, but also by the hip and ankle.[8] In running, the stability and stiffness of the leg is based off of the hip activation and then is transferred through the two-joint muscles of the quadriceps and the hamstrings to the knee to stabilize the knee.[9] In jumping, the moment that the knee generates and that the knee sees is "slaved" to the moment of the hip.[8]

The rehabilitation of normal biomechanical function of the knee involves normalization of the forces and positions of both the hip and the ankle, as well as the knee. The isolation of the knee to improve its biomechanics does not seem to be the most efficient pattern of rehabilitation because of this interdependence and this necessity of proper positioning of the hip and the ankle to allow the knee to have normal position, normal stiffness, and normal biomechanical function.

Similarly, physiologic activation of the muscles around the knee depends on hip and leg activation. The patterns for knee stiffness develop out of the position and function of the hip musculature. The one-joint muscles of the hip, the gluteus medius and maximus, act as stabilizing braces for the function of the knee both from the biomechanical standpoint of putting the hip joint in the proper position and also to stabilize the pelvis so that the quadriceps and hamstrings, which attach to the pelvis, will have a firm base of activation. There is also a physiologic facilitation of force production by the hip muscles for the quadriceps and hamstrings so that they can generate more force in a contraction.[8,9] Active hip extension through the activation of the hip extensors increases quadriceps torque by 21%, and as the hip is stabilized, the torque transferred by the hamstrings to the knee is increased by 20%.[9] As the hip goes into more flexion, this facilitation is lost with a correspondingly decreased ability for efficient torque reduction by the quadriceps and hamstrings. Weak hip abductors create a varus positioning of the hip. This varus positioning of the hip increases the valgus load on the knee and increases the force along the medial retinacular area. Return to physiologic function requires activation of the musculature in the normal proximal-to-distal pattern and requires appropriate activation of the two-joint muscles and of the force-dependent muscle activation patterns. This can be done only by involving all of the segments of the leg in a coordinated fashion.

Practice: Shoulder

The shoulder works in the kinetic chain as a funnel for the forces that are developed in the legs and trunk, modulating and transferring the forces to the force delivery mechanism, the hand.[1] The shoulder rotates on the stabilized platform of the scapula and is efficient in allowing maximum rotational momentum to create maximum velocity of the hand. This rotational momentum must occur around a rather fixed axis at the glenohumeral joint. The kinetic chain of throwing involves ground reaction force through the legs and trunk to the stable base of the scapula through the funnel of the shoulder and out into the hand.[1] This requires coordinated activation of the links so that the hand becomes the cracking end of the whip and the smaller muscles of the distal segments do not have to create the motion but are more guidance factors for the forces developed in the larger and more central proximal musculature.[2,10] The scapula becomes a major component of the kinetic chain: it provides the stable base for the rotation of the humerus; it provides a congruent socket so that the ball and socket joint is anatomically and kinematically a ball and socket joint; and it provides a stable base for muscular attachment to allow the muscles of the shoulder to be most efficient and to facilitate their coactivation just as pelvis stability allows the hamstrings and quadriceps to be facilitated.[11]

Return to function in throwing requires that pain be eliminated because pain is a major inhibitor of muscle activation around the shoulder. Return to function also requires that the normal kinetics of the kinetic chain are reestablished so that the generated force goes from the hip to the trunk and to the arm and so that there is adequate transfer of rotational momentum to the arm and to the ball.

Determine the Extent of Anatomic, Biomechanical, and Physiologic Alterations as a Result of the Injury

Alterations can occur at several places in the kinetic chain in injuries to the knee and the shoulder. These alterations can come before the injury and actually be causative in the injury; they can occur as the result of an injury; or they can occur as a result of the treatment. These all must be addressed in the rehabilitation sequencing to allow for normal return of function.

Because of the importance of the kinetic chain and the muscle activation patterns in producing performance and the interdependence of all of the different segments, it is very common to see alterations in one area of the kinetic chain accompanying injuries to another part. In overload microtrauma injuries, the incidence is as high as 80%. These alterations may not be strictly causative problems, but they may be considered predisposing factors.[12] They may occur as a result of playing the sport, other incompletely rehabilitated injuries, or from adaptations required to play the sport. They can be considered as factors that "break" the kinetic chain, requiring that either the athlete accept the consequent loss of force that will occur in the distal end due to kinetic chain breakage, or that the athlete will have to "catch up" in the distal segments for the force decrement in the proximal segments.[1] The latter may have deleterious effects for the distal segments because they have neither the time nor the size to make up for the force deficits. In microtrauma injuries, this can be thought of as a problem of "victims and culprits."[13] The victim may be considered the site of clinical symptoms. The culprit may include not only a local anatomic alteration, but also a distant anatomic or biomechanical alteration that is predisposing the athlete or causing the athlete to have the injury or perpetuating the injury.

Examples of these distant deficits include hip abductor weakness with anterior knee pain,[14] hip extensor weakness in patients with anterior cruciate ligament (ACL) deficiencies, quadriceps and hamstring energetics weakness with hip abductor energetic overcompensation in ACL deficiency,[15] scapular dyskinesis with abnormal scapular position and motion with patients with shoulder injuries,[11,16] hip and trunk stiffness and weakness in patients with shoulder injury, and tightness of internal rotation in patients with shoulder injury.[17] The evaluation prior to initiation of the rehabilitation program should emphasize evaluation of the appropriate kinetic chains, the appropriate joint flexibilities, joint positions, muscle strength, and muscle activation patterns for the individual and for the function that is being rehabilitated.

Practice: Knee

Evaluation of the patient before starting and continuing during the knee reconstruction and rehabilitation program would include evaluation of hip abductor and hip extensor weakness, both in the glutei and in the hamstrings, and hip muscle activation alterations by means of the hip stability series, consisting of one-legged stance, one-legged squat, and one-legged step-up and step-down. Hip muscle inflexibility, especially in flexors and external rotators, and persistent hip flexion on standing or walking should be evaluated. This inflexibility may be due to hip extensor weakness or hip flexor muscle tightness. A Trendelenburg sign with a varus positioning of the hip with one-legged stance is a key finding that should be evaluated and checked at several occasions during the rehabilitation program.

Practice: Shoulder

The extent of inflexibility should be evaluated in both glenohumeral internal rotation and pectoralis major and minor inflexibility. Glenohumeral internal rotation should be measured goniometrically to obtain the most accurate value of true glenohumeral limitation, as compared with the spinal level method, which measures several components of shoulder rotation. The pectoralis major and minor should be tested to determine the extent of lack of extension of the shoulder and scapular retraction.

Scapular dyskinetic patterns should be evaluated statically with the arm at the side and dynamically with the arm in forward flexion and in abduction in the scapular plane in both the ascending and the descending phase.[11] Patterns of scapular dyskinesis include prominence of the entire medial border of the scapula with upper and lower trapezius weakness, prominence of the inferior medial border of the scapula, associated with lower trapezius and serratus anterior weakness and pectoralis major and minor tightness, and elevation of the entire scapula due to upper trapezius/lower trapezius muscle imbalance with hyperactivity in the upper trapezius and lack of activity in the lower trapezius. These patterns create abnormal conditions for scapular stability and decrease the stability of the biomechanical axis for shoulder rotation. In addition, this creates impingement symptoms if the acromion is not elevated properly. It also creates an unstable base of attachment of the muscles, causing the muscles to be weak and also inhibiting the activation of the muscles that originate on the scapula. Two specific tests of scapular stability can be done.[18] The scapular assistance test helps to determine if weakness of the lower trapezius and serratus anterior is causing lack of elevation of the acromion. In this test, patients with impingement or muscle weakness in abduction are made better if the scapula is assisted in elevation by pushing against the medial border of the scapula as the arm is elevated. In the scapular retraction test, the scapula is manually retracted against the thorax and held in position while the arm is abducted or while the rotator cuff muscles are tested. Improvement in function of the rotator cuff or decrease in impingement symptoms is a positive test.

Rotator cuff muscle strength should be evaluated. Weakness of the rotator cuff can be due to three separate mechanisms: (1) disuse as a result of injury; (2) actual muscle damage, as can be seen with impingement or instability problems; and (3) dysfacilitation in which the muscles do not have an adequate neurologic drive. This weakness often can be seen in scapular dyskinetic patterns or in pain-based inhibition. Therefore, rotator cuff testing should be done both in the normal shoulder position and in the scapular retracted position to judge whether there is a dysfacilitation of the muscles.[18]

Hip and trunk flexibility and hip strength should be evaluated through some of the same hip stabilization techniques that were outlined for the knee evaluation. The one-legged stability series of one-legged stance, one-legged squat, and one-legged step-up and step-down are good tests to evaluate hip strength. Trunk flexibility should be measured by rotational as well as sit-and-reach measurements. Trunk strength should be measured in both flexion and extension.

Once the kinetic chain evaluation has been accomplished, rehabilitation can then be instigated. A lot of the kinetic chain techniques can be used early in the rehabilitation process while the injured or surgically-repaired tissues are healing. The rehabilitation sequencing can then progress to the injured areas as healing goes on. In this way, the proximal base will be normalized, and the kinetic chain progressions can be started to be continued up to the injured area.

Rehabilitation from Central to Peripheral

This rehabilitation principle is consistent with the biomechanical principle of proximal stability for distal mobility. The central core of the body, the hip, pelvis, and trunk is the platform of stability for motion of the peripheral segments whether it be the legs or the arms. This is the area in which maximum power is generated, where maximum rotation momentum is generated, and in which the kinetic energy is reacquired after the physical activity so that the body recalibrates itself and is ready to do the activity again.[19] Biomechanically, the central core is the area of force generation, and physiologically the central area is the core for facilitation of peripheral muscle activation patterns.

Practice: Knee

Hip and trunk flexibility should be established early in the rehabilitation process. The iliopsoas is quite commonly tight in these individuals; therefore, hip extension and external rotation should be advocated early in the process. This should be both a passive and an active process. The trunk extensors and hip extensor activations should accompany the active trunk flexor stretching. These patterns should be ipsilateral so that they go up one side of the spine and also diagonal because most activations are in a diagonal direction. Hip and trunk stability activations should also be started early. This can be started by two-legged activation with minimal stress on the knee through balance by external objects (Fig. 1). These activations can then progress to one-legged activations, both supported and unsupported. The sequencing would be stance activities, squat activities, step-up and step-down movements, and sideways and rotational movements (Fig. 2). Quadriceps activation should be the last part of the central to peripheral activation both because of the need to allow good healing of the injured tissue and the need to create a strong proximal base to allow facilitation of the quadriceps. Classic open-chain quadriceps activation with open arcs or short arcs does not seem to activate the quadriceps muscle maximally in the rehabilitation sequence.[14] Similarly, classic closed-chain activation does not maximally activate the quadriceps.[15] Therefore, the quadriceps must be selectively facilitated so that it will maximize its activation. This may be accomplished by putting a closed-chain load on the knee, isolating the knee in slight degrees of flexion, and positioning the hip in extension (Fig. 3). A stretch-shortening plyometric-type load is then applied to the quadriceps muscle. This selective facilitation of the quadriceps will allow it to be reorganized into the normal closed-chain patterns.

Practice: Shoulder

The central core of activation needs to progress from the contralateral leg and hip to the trunk and to the ipsilateral shoulder. This diagonal pattern of activation, called the serape effect,[19] can be undertaken early in the rehabilitation while the shoulder is still being protected. Hip and trunk extension should be emphasized, and control of the trunk over the hip can be implemented. These patterns involve

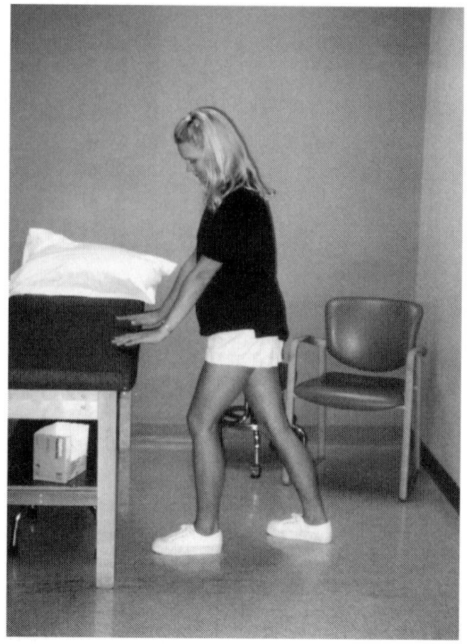

Fig. 1 *Two-leg balance closed-chain exercise with external support.*

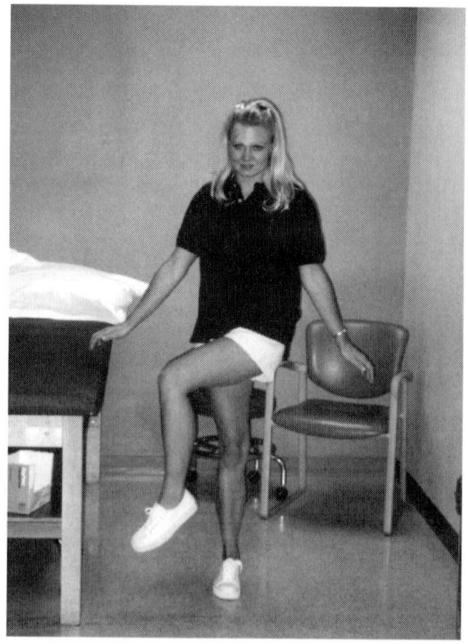

Fig. 2 *One-leg balance with rotational movement and hip control.*

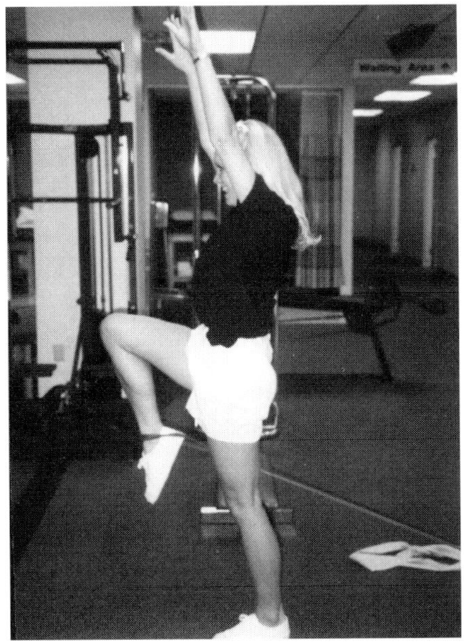

Fig. 3 Selective facilitation of quadriceps activation by closed-chain loading and hip extension.

hip extension, trunk extension, and scapular retraction or hip rotation, trunk extension, and scapular elevation[20] (Fig. 4). Legs, hip, or trunk flexibility should also be addressed at this time.

Scapular control is a key element of shoulder function. Scapular control can be started early with scapular retractions, isometric scapular pinches, and scapular roll-downs. Closed-chain activation of the scapula can be started in positions that are not harmful to the shoulder repair at less than 60° of abduction and less than 45° of flexion. These can then progress to patterns at 90° of abduction or 90° of flexion with the hand on the wall (Fig. 5). These activation patterns can then progress to scapular retraction and protraction and scapular elevation and depression. These are very safe patterns in that they do not promote shear across the joint, they decrease tension on the surgical repair, and they eliminate the deltoid as a deforming force.[20]

Rotator cuff activation can then progress when the scapula is stabilized. The rotator cuff muscles should be activated at 90° abduction. This is their normal plane of activation in throwing or serving, and they can work in their physiologic function as a "compressor cuff," helping to maintain the humeral head in the glenoid socket. Progression of activation in this manner allows the rotator cuff to be activated very smoothly and will eliminate the shrug that occurs when the arm is elevated by a strong deltoid against a weak rotator cuff. This progression also eliminates the shear across the joint that occurs with the shrug motion.

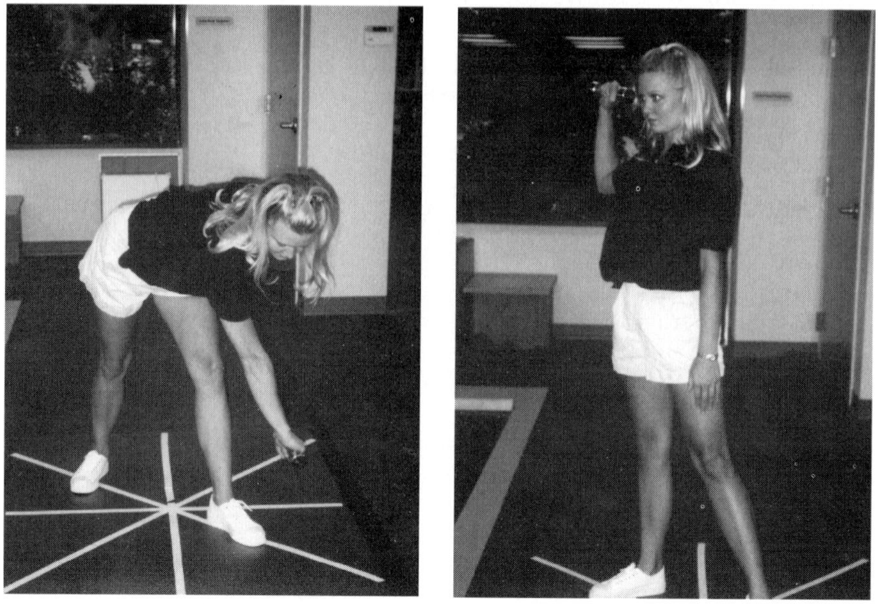

Fig. 4 Hip/trunk/scapula facilitation by trunk extension and simultaneous scapular retraction.

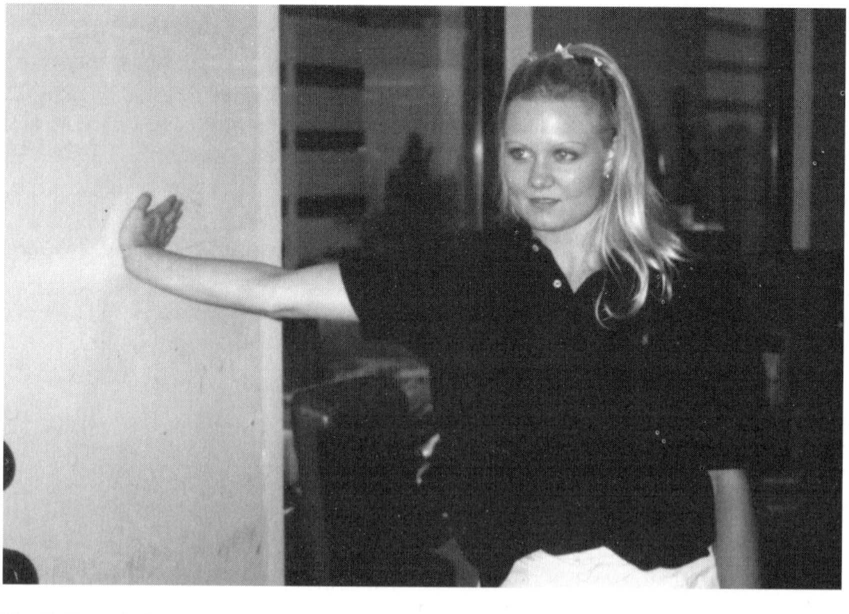

Fig. 5 Closed-chain scapula and rotator cuff activation by scapular "clock" exercises.

Closed-Chain Rehabilitation With Facilitation of Specific Muscles

Closed-chain rehabilitation, in which the distal end of a body segment is stationary or meets considerable resistance, most closely mimics the normal biomechanics and physiology of the leg and also very closely simulates the normal functional needs around the shoulder. This method creates a normal progression of activated links and muscle activation patterns due to the stabilization of the distal end and allows for a progression of muscle activation in a co-contraction joint-stabilizing method. Although the arm and hand are moving in an open-chain pattern in the throwing motion, the shoulder is functioning as a funnel, with co-contraction muscle activations and a need for stabilization at this proximal end.[1,2] From a rehabilitation standpoint, closed-chain protocols decrease the shear forces on the repairs or the reconstructions and are probably the major factor in allowing accelerated rehabilitation protocols. Use of closed-chain protocols is probably the major reason why the rehabilitation protocols are now allowing athletes to return to play much faster than in the past.

However, exclusive emphasis on these closed-chain activation patterns can allow some muscles to get lost in the rehabilitation sequence in both knee and shoulder rehabilitation.[15] Because these patterns emphasize activation of many muscles in very similar patterns, some muscles that are inhibited or weak will be compensated for by other stronger, more tonically-oriented muscles, and they will never develop the proper activation and proper force development characteristics. Prominent examples of this are the quadriceps around the knee and the lower trapezius, supraspinatus, and serratus anterior around the shoulder. These muscles continue to be weak, continue to create force-couple imbalances around the involved joints, and continue to decrease the joint's normal biomechanical function. They can also create alterations that have to be made up in other areas of the kinetic chain and can actually cause problems in other areas of the chain. Examples are patellar tendinitis in patients with weak quadriceps following ACL reconstructions and elbow injuries in patients with weak shoulder internal rotators and abductors following shoulder reconstruction. The whole chain may look good in terms of kinematics, but it does not function well in terms of kinetics or energetics.[15] The hip abductors and extensors are activated at higher levels of intensity, thereby allowing the entire leg to move well and actually to absorb loads in a fairly normal fashion; however, the knee energetics and kinetics are still extremely weak, thereby exposing the knee joint itself to higher loads in running and jumping activities. Similarly, the arm and hand may move in a functioning arc, but scapular dyskinesis and lack of acromial elevation create impingement problems with abduction. Elbow problems may occur because of lack of protective influence of shoulder internal rotation from the valgus loads that occur during pitching or throwing.[2]

I have adopted the practice of facilitating the muscles that need to be worked on with some extra degree of emphasis. Facilitation is defined as isolating muscles but helping them activate in their normal patterns. I do this by creating an activation stimulus on a specific muscle, decreasing the importance of the proximal stabilizing muscle, but still putting the entire kinetic chain in the normal position. This procedure unmasks the targeted muscle and requires that it work in its normal fashion and normal activation sequence.

Practice: Knee

The stability progressions for the knee start with the foot on the ground. I allow protected weightbearing with crutches or a knee brace as soon as the patient is comfortable but emphasize hip extension as soon as possible. I find that hip flexion leads to knee flexion, and I want to eliminate knee flexion as a predominant pattern of stance or of gait. The progressions then start with two-legged side-to-side and front-to-back movements, once again with the hip extended, going from supported to unsupported activations. I then go to one-legged activations with support and nonsupport, and then to hip rotation activities with two legs progressing to one leg and then support and nonsupport. To promote kinesthetic feedback, I put pertubations on the leg, first by side-to-side movements, and then when muscle strength is appropriate, my patients do trampoline, medicine ball, or wobble Biomechanical Ankle Platform System (BAPS) board stance. Facilitation exercises include step-up and step-down with the hip extended off of a step board (Fig. 6). Patients then do step-up, step-downs on inclines with the hip extended with the leg in a stretch-shortening activation, and then do hip rotations with the hip in extension with activations and medicine balls (Fig. 2).

Loading progressions include running, jumping, and then starting and stopping. This is done under controlled circumstances and then progressed to play conditions. These are done after teaching the athlete to move in a more biomechanically good position with hip extensor muscle activation and control of hip flexion and knee flexion.

Practice: Shoulder

Closed-chain shoulder rehabilitation starts with establishment of the central core with hip/trunk stabilization progressions (Figs. 1 and 2). Diagonal leg/hip/trunk/scapula exercises are instituted to maximize the serape effect (Fig. 4). As scapular control is achieved and the shoulder is healing, closed-chain rotator cuff progressions are instituted. These are all done with the hand on a table or the wall, with loads being passed from central to peripheral (Fig. 5). Gentle mobilizations and proprioceptive neuromuscular facilitation patterns are used to allow abduction and flexion. As the arm acquires 90° abduction, scapular clock exercises are introduced (Fig. 5).

Summary

Rehabilitation after athletic injury requires anatomic restoration, followed by normalization of physiology and biomechanics. Female athletes respond to the rehabilitation sequence in the same manner as male athletes. Extra effort

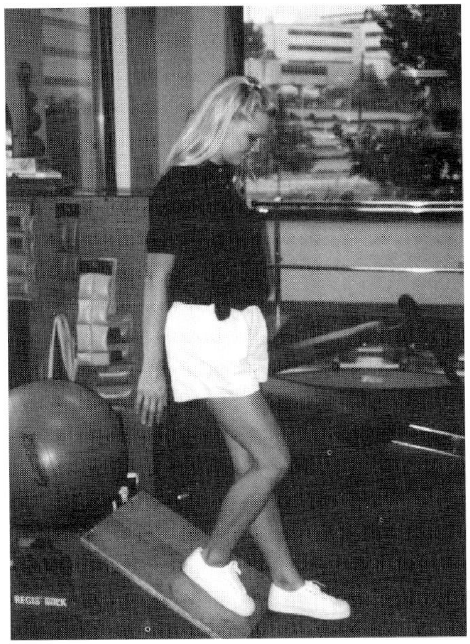

Fig. 6 Proprioceptive guided quadriceps facilitation off slant board.

should be made to evaluate and normalize certain problems that are more prevalent in female athletes. They include increased joint laxity, generalized muscle strength deficits, and hip and leg muscle activation alterations. Closed-chain, whole-body activation rehabilitation protocols are the most efficient methods to restore normal patterns and normal kinetic chains of function.

References

1. Kibler WB: Biomechanical analysis of the shoulder during tennis activities. *Clin Sports Med* 1995;14:79–85.
2. Putnam CA: Sequential motions of body segments in striking and throwing skills: Descriptions and explanations. *J Biomech* 1993;26(suppl 1):125–135.
3. Nichols TR: A biomechanical perspective on spinal mechanisms of coordinated muscular action: An architecture principle. *Acta Anat (Basel)* 1994;151:1–13.
4. Huston LJ, Wojtys EM: Neuromuscular performance characteristics in elite female athletes. *Am J Sports Med* 1996;24:427–436.
5. Hewett TE, Stroupe AL, Nance TA, Noyes FR: Plyometric training in female athletes: Decreased impact forces and increased hamstring torques. *Am J Sports Med* 1996;24:765–773.
6. Kibler WB, Chandler J: Baseball and tennis, in Griffin LY (ed): *Rehabilitation of the Injured Knee*, ed 2. St Louis, MO, Mosby-Year Book,1995, pp 219–226.
7. Heise GD, Martin PE: "Leg spring" characteristics and the aerobic demand of running. *Med Sci Sports Exerc* 1998;30:750–754.

8. Bobbert MF, van Zandwijk JP: Dynamics of force and muscle stimulation in human vertical jumping. *Med Sci Sports Exerc* 1999;31:303–310.
9. van Ingen Schenau GJ, Bobbert MF, Rozendal RH: The unique action of bi-articular muscles in complex movements. *J Anat* 1987;155:1–5.
10. Atwater AE: Biomechanics of overarm throwing movements and of throwing injuries. *Exerc Sport Sci Rev* 1979;7:43–85.
11. Kibler WB: The role of the scapula in athletic shoulder function. *Am J Sports Med* 1998;26:325–337.
12. Meeuwisse WH: Assessing causation in sport injury: A multi-factorial model. *Clin J Sport Med* 1994;4:166–170.
13. MacIntyre JG, Lloyd-Smith DR: Overuse running injuries, in Renstrom P (ed): *Sports Injuries: Basic Principles of Prevention and Care*. London, England, Blackwell, 1993, pp 139-160.
14. Host JV, Craig R, Lehman RC: Patellofemoral dysfunction in tennis players: A dynamic problem. *Clin Sports Med* 1995;14:177–203.
15. DeVita P, Hortobagyi T, Barrier J: Gait biomechanics are not normal after anterior cruciate ligament reconstruction and accelerated rehabilitation. *Med Sci Sports Exerc* 1998;30:1481–1488.
16. Warner JJ, Micheli LJ, Arslanian LE, Kennedy J, Kennedy R: Scapulothoracic motion in normal shoulders and shoulders with glenohumeral instability and impingement syndrome: A study using Moire topographic analysis. *Clin Orthop* 1992;285:191–199.
17. Silliman JF, Hawkins RJ: Current concepts and recent advances in the athlete's shoulder. *Clin Sports Med* 1991;10:693–705.
18. Burkhart SS, Morgan CD, Kibler WB: Shoulder injuries in overhead athletes: The "dead arm" revisited. *Clin Sports Med* 2000;19:125–158.
19. Young JL, Herring SA, Press JM, et al: The influence of the spine on the shoulder in the throwing athlete. *J Back Musculoskeletal Rehab* 1996;7:5–17.
20. Kibler WB: Shoulder rehabilitation: Principles and practice. *Med Sci Sports Exerc* 1998;30(suppl 4):S40–S50.

Directions for Future Research

Investigate whether sport-specific equipment and protective devices enhance safety and performance. Determine whether equipment designed for men is appropriate for the female athlete.

Sport-specific equipment either as part of the sport or for protective purposes is necessary for optimal participation. Before protective equipment is mandated, however, justification for its need and its effect on sports performance must be validated.

Many braces, protective pads, and other protective items such as soccer shin guards were designed for men. Smaller sizes of the devices have been used for women, but few studies have examined whether merely downsizing equipment made for men provides adequate protection and support for women.

Increase overall standards and qualifications of coaches. Provide coaches with gender-specified information on training and conditioning, injury rates, and injury prevention and rehabilitation protocols.

There presently exists no required or standardized education for most coaches. Most coaches are unaware of gender-specific sports issues.

Further define at-risk injury positions for women's sports and develop strategies to prevent these at-risk situations and to respond more appropriately when they occur.

Recent research has shown that there exist "at-risk positions" in certain sports. Early data appear to indicate that educating participants about these at-risk positions and ways to avoid them decreases injury rates. However, much more information is needed in this area.

Determine if there are gender-specific differences in movement patterns and if such differences exist, whether they affect injury risks and are alterable.

Most injuries appear to be more sport-specific than gender-specific, which implies that even though there may be differences in body mechanics between men and women these differences do not typically result in unique gender-specific injuries. However, there are not sufficient data at this time to verify this conclusion.

Identify differences in propriception and neuromuscular motor control and how these relate to injuries and injury prevention techniques.

There appear to be gender differences in muscle activation, movement patterns, and resultant load absorption. These may be modulated by neural factors such as proprioception or control of muscle stiffness. There is a need to see if these differences are gender- or fitness-related and to explore their interaction with injury patterns.

More specifically define what is meant by sport-specific rehabilitation.

Rehabilitation goals should include return to function as well as resolution of symptoms. Functional return to sports or physical activity is best achieved when the rehabilitation program allows and facilitates return of normal muscle activation patterns. At this time, there is sparse information about the most efficacious rehabilitation programs for all sports or activities.

Investigate whether sport floor surfaces or foot-surface interfaces influence injury rates, and whether gender-specific footwear or sport surfaces or a combination of both can improve safety.

During sports and exercise, large external loads are placed on the musculoskeletal system of the female athlete. Understanding these loads and ways to dissipate them is critical to injury prevention.

Continue to investigate anterior cruciate ligament (ACL) injuries in women to (1) improve public and participant awareness of the risk of ACL injury and the possibilities of prevention; (2) identify specific neuromuscular proprioceptive and motor control factors associated with ACL injury; and (3) implement training and prevention programs, assessing and improving them while more specifically defining predictive and protective factors.

Although epidemiologic research exists, only recently has the public become aware of the strong association of ACL injuries with certain activities. Programs emphasizing neuromuscular control of body positioning have shown promise in decreasing injury rates, particularly in female athletes. Further delineation of these interventions is vital.

Investigate in female soccer players the effects of heading the ball on the cervical spine and on immediate and long-term cognitive function.

There are few prospective, well-controlled studies of female soccer players that assess the short- and long-term effects of heading the ball on cognitive function. Furthermore, understanding the biomechanical demands of heading on the cervical spine is also critical and needs further investigation.

Determine the anatomic, physiologic, and psychological effects of sports participation during the adolescent years, including whether injuries are more likely at this time and if so, what the long-term effects of such injuries are.

The duration of puberty for women is brief, and there are many physical, physiologic, and psychological adaptations that must occur during this time, all of which may directly influence sports participation. Present treatments for injuries in adolescent athletes allow them to return to sports, but what is the long-term significance of these injuries on the adolescent athlete, her family, and society in general?

Encourage further epidemiologic studies to quantify and identify injury rates by sport, age, and gender.

Epidemiologic data provide the basic starting point for determining "areas of concern." Although a lot of epidemiologic data is available for some sports, few data exist for others such as tennis and rowing. Moreover, studies frequently lack gender and age stratification.

Gather additional data on the epidemiology of stress fractures exploring the effects of (1) gender, (2) hormonal status, (3) nutrition, (4) training techniques, and (5) sport specificity.

The epidemiologic data on the frequency of stress fractures and factors influencing this frequency are conflicting and need to be clarified.

Examine the value of single-sport versus multiple-sport participation by young women, assessing the effect of such on (1) injury rates, (2) continued participation in fitness activities as an adult, (3) levels of fitness, and (4) coping skills (psychological well-being).

With the advancement of and availability of sports participation for girls, there has been a recent trend for single sport specialization at an early age. Nowhere is this more apparent than in soccer and gymnastics, where year-round participation is common, almost to the point of being mandated. How such specialization at an early age impacts the female athlete is not well understood.

Section Four

Musculoskeletal Fitness

Section Editor:
Donald T. Kirkendall, PhD

Marybeth Brown, PT, PhD
James F. Clapp III, MD
William E. Garrett, Jr, MD, PhD
Laura J. Huston, MS
Terry R. Malone, EdD, PT, ATC
Margaret E. Stone, MS, CSCS
Michael H. Stone, PhD, CSCS
Travis Triplett-McBride, PhD, CSCS
Edward M. Wojtys, MD

Overview

Most of the sections in this volume deal with injuries, mechanisms of injury, and the similarities and dissimilarities between men and women. In contrast, this section focuses on the adaptations of the musculoskeletal system to regular exercise. Although some sections focus on specific injuries according to anatomic location or within particular sports, it is important to remember that all exercise is a request of the whole body. When a person exercises, the entire body participates, responds, and subsequently adapts. In fact, the athlete relies on these adaptations for ultimate success in competition. It is this constellation of adaptations that makes exercise such a useful primary or secondary intervention in numerous clinical settings. The benefits of training have been praised by numerous professional associations.

A common theme throughout the conference on which this volume is based dealt with the proper application of training principles. Properly applied, the basic tenets of training will lead to predictable adaptations in all systems—cardiovascular, neuromuscular, neurohormonal, musculoskeletal, etc.—that are beneficial in athletic competition. However, improper applications of training principles can lead to injuries that take an athlete out of training and competition.

Nonathletes, on the other hand, may have more modest goals for participation in sports and exercise: weight loss, stress reduction, and general improvement in overall health. However, regardless of the goal, the principles of training still apply. It is these principles that are addressed in this section. The systematic manipulation of frequency, intensity, duration, pattern, and progression leads to an increase in function and reserve. The difference in training between the athlete and the healthy adult nonathlete is a matter of degree, not the basic foundations of training.

Men and women differ in the ultimate level of performance. This section examines the absolute and relative performance of men and women. In addition, the basic principles of aerobic training are outlined and serve as the groundwork for the remaining chapters. Some basic training principles also are outlined. These training principles are the product of research and trial and error by coaches and are frequently ignored by inexperienced coaches and people eager to reach a higher plane of fitness.

The other end of the intensity extreme is resistance training. Probably no other aspect of training can elicit more emotion over training regimens than does resistance training. Sets, repetitions, intensity, initial starting points, and periodization are common points of discussion and contention among those who use weights as a primary training tool as well as among those who use resistance training as a supplement to other training modes. Chapter 21 outlines what is currently accepted by the scientific community on the practice, adaptation, and application of resistance training.

In the athletic community, the general feeling about flexibility is like many other aspects of training: more is better. Both athletes and the general public seem to have accepted that improved flexibility is good for injury prevention. The questions about flexibility training revolve around the details: how long to hold the stretch, which joints should be the focus of attention, how many repetitions of each stretch, and what are the other benefits of flexibility training. Chapter 22 points out the appropriate direction for maximum benefit for the joints most in need, and describes what to expect from proper application of a flexibility training program.

Appropriately, much of the attention in training has been directed toward the responses and adaptation of skeletal muscle. One of the major roles of muscle is locomotion, and it is important to determine just how this important part of the human "motor" operates. But it is equally important to remember that muscle only does as instructed by the central nervous system. To perform any physical activity efficiently requires training the central nervous system to recruit the appropriate motor units. This training process requires much repetition to select only those motor units that will best execute the desired pattern of movement. As this selection process proceeds, the central nervous system eventually directs the adaptations to regular exercise toward specific motor units. The concept of these motor programs has been an interest of professionals in motor learning for some time, but it has become a particular interest area in injury prevention because of the amount of injuries to the knee that do not involve contact. It is quite likely that a disruption of the normal motor pattern during some activity that the athlete has performed thousands of times can put the athlete at risk for damage to the anterior cruciate ligament. Chapter 23 points out the current concepts of basic motor control and the biomechanics of selected athletic skills that have been pinpointed as potential risks of knee injury.

The motor pattern has been implicated in knee injuries when a planned activity has been altered, perhaps by a change in the surface, a minor bump just prior to landing, or some other unexpected stimulus. When such a disruption occurs, the neuromuscular system executes a series of steps to try to correct the planned movement in response to the new condition. Some of these corrections are proprioceptive and some are spinal reflexes, but all lead to a change in muscular response to the new, unexpected situation. How the body responds to a change in the planned maneuver given the gender differences in muscle mass and recruitment patterns is the focus of Chapter 24, on neuromuscular performance.

Two special applications of training for women are the heart of the last two chapters in this section. Chapter 25 directs attention to the application of training principles to the pregnant woman and the adaptations that the woman undergoes during this time in her life. Pregnancy itself is a challenge for the woman, and to add or maintain training places additional stress on her. The very insightful research in this area covers the beneficial effects of physical activity on both the mother and the fetus.

Finally, the demographics of society point toward an increasingly aging population. With women living an average of 7 years longer than men, and the problems with the musculoskeletal system that occur with aging, it is imperative that possible interventions be explored to minimize the public health impact of aging and subsequent inactivity. Chapter 26 presents a body of work that justifies the application of training well into the life span in the attempt to delay frailty and the negative responses that are coincident with frailty and therefore to minimize the eventual social and economic impact on society.

Donald T. Kirkendall, PhD

Chapter 20

Aerobic and Anaerobic Performance in Men and Women

Donald T. Kirkendall, PhD

The most basic way to look at anaerobic and aerobic performance in women is first to compare the performance of men and women in identical activities. Next, it is important to look at the physiologic differences between men and women in an attempt to describe the observed differences in performance. Within this myriad of variables may be some clues to understanding the differences in performance between men and women.

Performance Differences

The simplest comparison is also the most instructive. In track and field, men and women compete at identical distances against the clock or the measuring tape. Thus, comparisons of men's and women's world records give some insight as to the uppermost levels of performance.

Table 1 lists world records in track and field for 1998. To get a relative measure of performance, the women's record is divided by the men's record.[1] The closer to a ratio of 1.0, the closer the two records are to each other (for the high jump and long jump, the men's record is divided by the women's record). As a comparison, the ratios from world records in 1991 are also offered. As the ratios move further from 1.0, the more divergent are the performances between men and women. Notice that beyond the sprints, there is little change in the ratio of women's to men's records. The differences are reduced as the running distances

Table 1 Current world records in track and field events and performance ratios for 1991 and 1998

Event	Men	Women	Ratio* 1998	Ratio* 1991
100 m	9.84	10.49	1.066	1.064
200 m	19.32	21.34	1.105	1.082
400 m	43.29	47.60	1.087	1.100
800 m	1:41.11	1:53.28	1.120	1.114
1,500 m	3:26.00	3:50.46	1.119	1.149
Marathon	2:06:05	2:20:47	1.117	1.107
High jump (m)	2.45	2.09	1.173	1.167
Long jump (m)	8.95	7.52	1.190	1.198

*Ratio is women's record divided by men's record; for jumping events, the men's record is divided by the women's record

increase to the marathon distance. Table 2 shows similar data for current records in freestyle, long-course swimming. Within these differences lie both subtle and obvious mechanisms for performance differences between men and women.

Table 2 Current world records in freestyle, long-course swimming and performance ratios for 1998

Distance	Men	Women	Ratio* 1998
50 m	21.81	24.51	1.124
100 m	48.21	54.01	1.120
200 m	1:46.69	1:56.78	1.094
400 m	3:43.80	4:03.85	1.090
800 m	7:46.00	8:16.22	1.064
1,500 m	14:41.66	15:52.10	1.080

*Ratio is women's record divided by men's record

Improvement in Human Performance

Accurate records for running performance by men have been kept for around 100 years and for women over the last 20 to 30 years (Fig. 1). Statisticians have viewed the improvement in performance to be linear or curvilinear with time.[2–5] From such investigations, it can be seen that the current 1,500-m pace for men is faster than the 800-m pace of the earlier years of this century (Fig. 1, *A*). For women, the rate of improvement has been faster because the most recent 1,500-m pace is about the same as the 800-m pace of about 40 years ago (Fig. 1, *B*). If these lines are superimposed and extrapolated (assuming a continuing linear improvement in performance), it appears that at the distances cited, women will eventually outperform the men (Fig. 1, *C*). In fact, women hold the fastest times for multilap swims of the English Channel.

Factors Affecting Performance Differences

Endurance performance tends to be viewed in terms of maximal oxygen consumption. The formula for maximum oxygen consumption is:

$$Vo_{2max} = A - Vo_2diff \times \text{cardiac output} \qquad \text{(Eq. 1)}$$

where Vo_{2max} is maximum oxygen consumption and $A - Vo_2diff$ is arteriovenous oxygen difference. When the heart rate and stroke volume are substituted for cardiac output, the equation becomes:

$$Vo_{2max} = A - Vo_2diff \times \text{heart rate} \times \text{stroke volume} \qquad \text{(Eq. 2)}$$

Within this equation are the major factors governing endurance performance: the ability of the muscles to use oxygen and the ability of the heart to deliver oxygen. Each major factor can influence the aerobic performance differences seen between men and women.

The differences in performance may fall within the interaction of structural, metabolic, and physiologic variables. The relationship among these three major classes of variables in women will influence the degree of improvement from training.

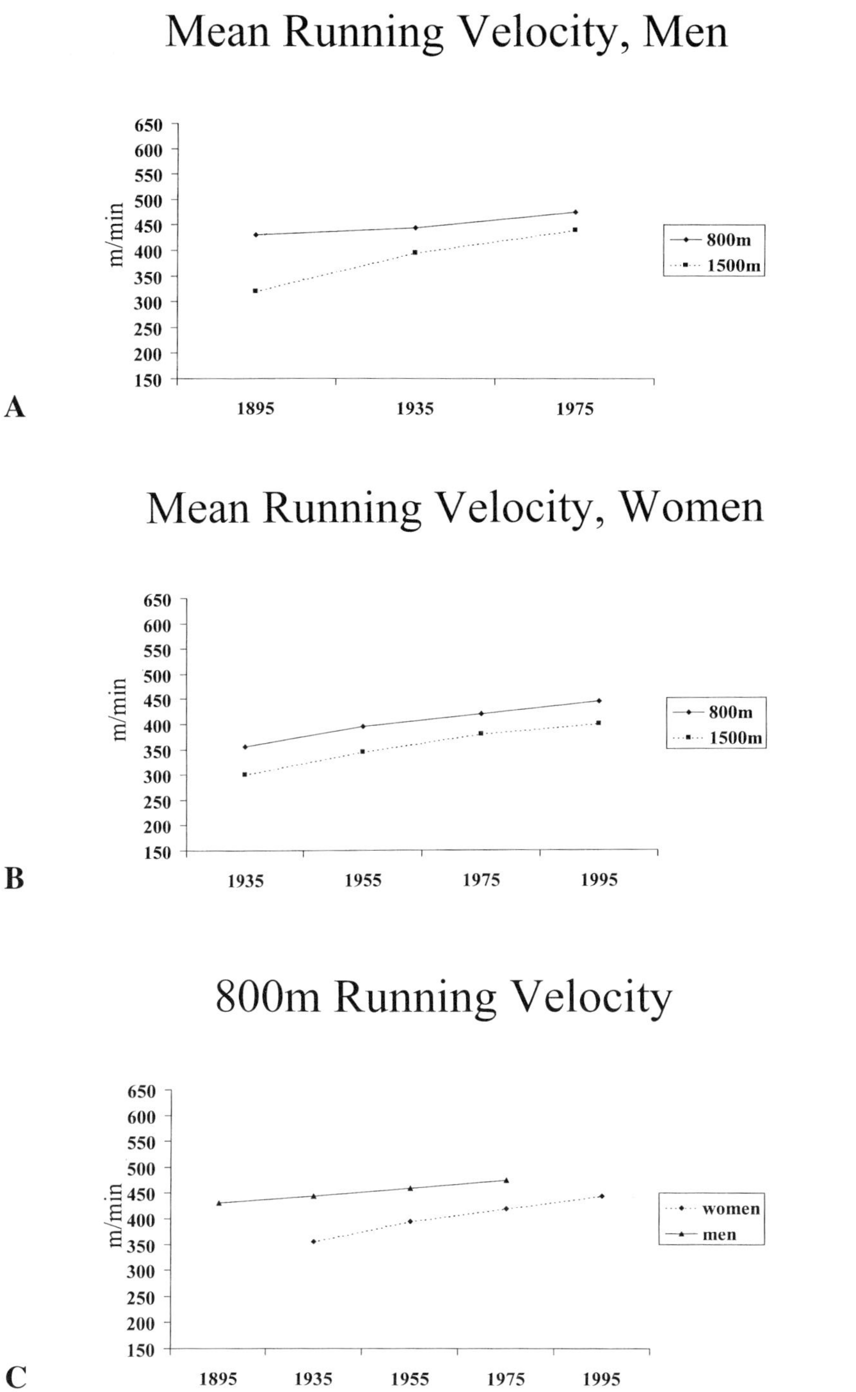

*Fig. 1 Progression in world running velocity for the 800 m and 1,500 m for men (**A**) and women (**B**). **C**, A and B are superimposed and regression lines extrapolated to point of intersection. (Adapted with permission from Whipp BJ, Ward SA: Will women soon outrun men?* Nature *1992;355:25.)*

Structural Factors

Height and Weight

Probably the first thing that the spectator notices is the difference in height and weight between men and women. Women, in general, are 3 to 4 in shorter and 25 to 30 lb lighter than men,[6] and they have increased body fat and reduced lean muscle tissue. Thus, the female athlete is trying to do the same activity with less muscle mass; naturally, women will not perform equally with men simply because they lack muscle mass.

It is obvious that women compete with men on a "level playing field" with no corrections for differences in body mass or height. Only in weightlifting is mass considered; when 2 lifters tie on total weight lifted, the lighter athlete is placed higher. However, if selected events are corrected for height and weight, some interesting relationships appear. For example, Figure 2 shows the relative jump height for the high jump corrected for height and mass. Notice that the woman record holder actually jumps higher relative to her height than the man. A similar relationship is also seen for the long jump.

Body Fat

The excess body fat that a woman carries is a blessing in swimming and a burden in running. For the swimmer, the extra body fat aids in buoyancy so the women has less "drag" while swimming. In fact, the female swimmer expends about 20% less energy for the same pace and distance as her male counterpart.[7] However, for the runner this extra tissue that is not involved in locomotion is a burden that has to be carried around. Body fat is probably a major factor in why the differences between women's and men's swimming records are less than the differences between their records in running events.

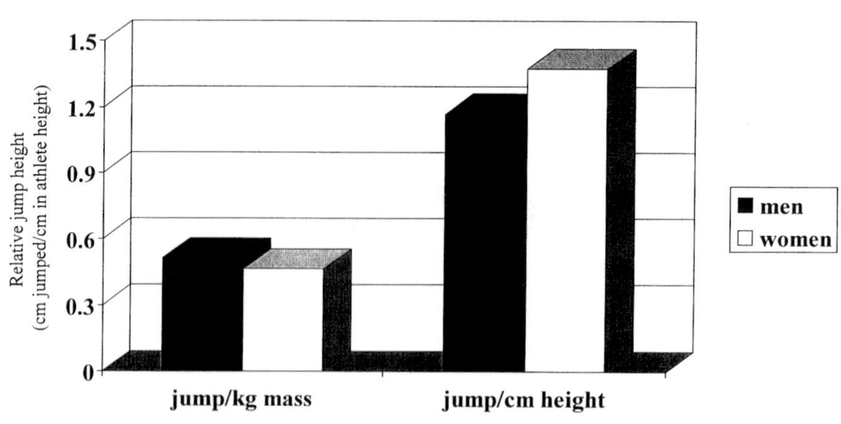

***Fig. 2** Jump height relative to athlete's height. (Adapted with permission from Fox EL, Bowers RW, Foss ML (eds):* The Physiological Basis for Exercise and Sport, *ed 5. Madison, WI, Brown & Benchmark, 1993.)*

Metabolic Factors

The ability to generate energy is critical in the performance of any athletic endeavor, and it is possible that there are inherent differences is metabolic production of adenosine triphosphate (ATP) by both anaerobic and aerobic mechanisms.

Anaerobic Metabolism

Adenosine Triphosphate-Phosphocreatine System The concentrations of ATP and phosphocreatine (PC) in skeletal muscle are similar in men and women. The skeletal muscle concentration of ATP and PC is 4 mmol/kg and 16 mmol/kg, respectively.[8] But the total content of the phosphagens is less in women because of their reduced muscle mass.

The difference in muscle mass and subsequent total content is reflected in performance testing. During exhaustive testing, the fast component of the recovery oxygen curve reflects replenishment of ATP and PC. Figure 3 depicts some sample values for this alactacid component of recovery. The lowest values are for untrained women; trained women and untrained men are about the same; and male oarsmen (rowing requires a very high anaerobic-aerobic requirement) have the highest values.[9–11] These values are reported per kilogram of body mass. These differences would be reduced if the data were reported per kilogram of lean muscle mass.

The Margaria-Kalamen Anaerobic Power Test[12] makes estimates of the ability to use stored ATP and PC. The athlete is required to run up a flight of stairs touching the third, sixth, and ninth steps. The time from the third to the ninth step is recorded by electronic timing (usually 0.3 to 0.6+ s). With stair height, mass, and time as variables, a power measure is determined (in kg-m/s). When power values (corrected for body mass) are plotted with age, there is a reasonably linear increase with age until the age of 25 years when power values begin to decrease.[13] For direct

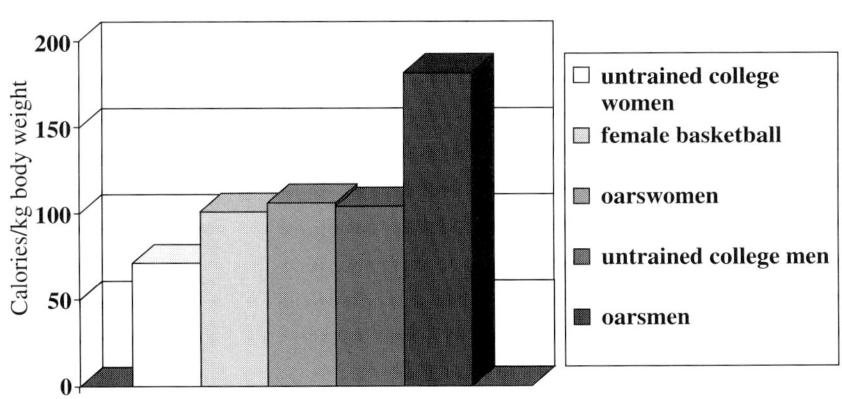

Fig. 3 *Maximal alactacid capacity. (Adapted with permission from Fox EL, Bowers RW, Foss ML (eds):* The Physiological Basis for Exercise and Sport, *ed 5. Madison, WI, Brown & Benchmark, 1993.)*

comparison using a familiar unit of analysis, the data from this stair-climbing task can be converted to horsepower, with men generating 2.1 hp and women generating 1.7 hp. This difference is largely due, again, to differences in muscle mass.

Return again to Tables 1 and 2 for performance ratios. Notice that in running, the best ratio is for the 100-m sprint, an event that is predominantly fueled by stored phosphagens. With stored concentrations being similar, the differences in performance should not be too great. Again, a primary factor in the differences in performance is likely due to the differences in muscle mass.

Glycolysis To test the glycolytic system, blood lactic acid levels after maximal, exhaustive exercise are measured. In nearly every case, postexercise lactic acid is lower in women than in men, suggesting a lower capacity in women (Fig. 4). Again, the differences are partly attributable to differences in muscle mass. Correction of these data per kilogram of lean muscle mass would further reduce the differences.[1]

Aerobic Metabolism

Aerobic capacity is determined by measuring oxygen consumption during progressive exercise to exhaustion. The data typically are reported as L/min in sports when the body mass is supported (eg, swimming, cycling, rowing) or as mL/kg/min when the body weight is not supported (eg, running, walking). It is not surprising to realize that the aerobic capacity of women is less than that of men by around 15% to 25%.[1] Figures 5, *A* through *C* show the relationship of maximal oxygen consumption and age by gender. When oxygen consumption is expressed in some relative term (eg, mL/kg/min in Fig. 5, *B* or mL/L leg volume/min in Fig. 5, *C*), the sex differences are fairly small. Also, there is an inverse relationship between

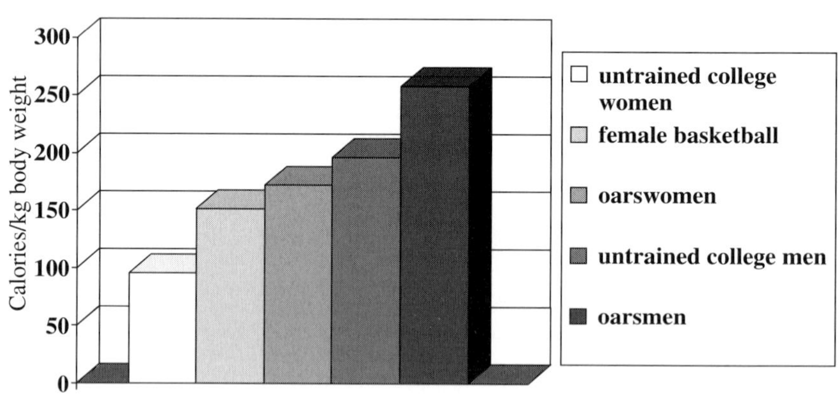

Fig. 4 *Maximal lactacid capacity. (Adapted with permission from Fox EL, Bowers RW, Foss ML (eds):* The Physiological Basis for Exercise and Sport, *ed 5. Madison, WI, Brown & Benchmark, 1993.)*

oxygen consumption and age. Although Figure 5, *A* and *B* show the differences in oxygen consumption on a whole body basis, if oxygen uptake is corrected even further for the active muscle mass involved (Fig. 5, *C*), the differences between men and women become even less with age. If oxygen consumption is plotted against the volume of the leg performing cycle ergometer exercise, there really is hardly any difference between men and women.

While some of the differences between genders and the relationship between age and oxygen uptake can be credited to the differences in muscle mass or the age-related decline in muscle mass, physiologic factors are implicated in aerobic differences.

Physiologic Factors

Hemoglobin and Blood Volume

Because hemoglobin has a critical role in the transport of oxygen, it should not be surprising to realize that the relationship between whole body oxygen consumption and hemoglobin is linear and positive. When plotted, the lines for men and women are identical. The only difference is the length of the lines due to the reduced overall content and concentration of hemoglobin.[14]

One of the adaptations to training is an increase in blood volume and related components (Table 3). With this increase in volume comes an increase in total hemoglobin content and hemoglobin concentration as both g/kg and g/100 mL blood. While increases in blood volume and hemoglobin improve the eventual maximum oxygen uptake, the values for women are still below those of men[15,16] (Table 3). A similar relationship can be seen for total blood volume.

In addition, the heart hypertrophies with training, but the adaptation is specific to the type of training performed. Resistance training leads to an increase in the mass of the left ventricle, whereas endurance training increases the volume of the left ventricle.[17,18] When these increases are corrected for lean muscle mass, it can be seen that resistance training increases the cardiac mass in proportion to the total muscle mass, whereas endurance training leads to a cardiac mass that is proportionately greater than the lean muscle mass: a true hypertrophy.[18] With a larger heart and greater stroke volume, Equation 2 is increased, and overall oxygen consumption is increased. Of course, the reverse is also true and can be seen during detraining and anorexia nervosa.[19]

Physiologic Characteristics When Men and Women Are Matched on Performance

Thus far, the discussion has looked at the performance differences between men and women and the factors that might be influential in these differences. An interesting project was led by Russell Pate at the University of South Carolina, where subjects were recruited because they were all matched on their 15-km time,[20] maximal oxygen consumption, maximal heart rate, and blood

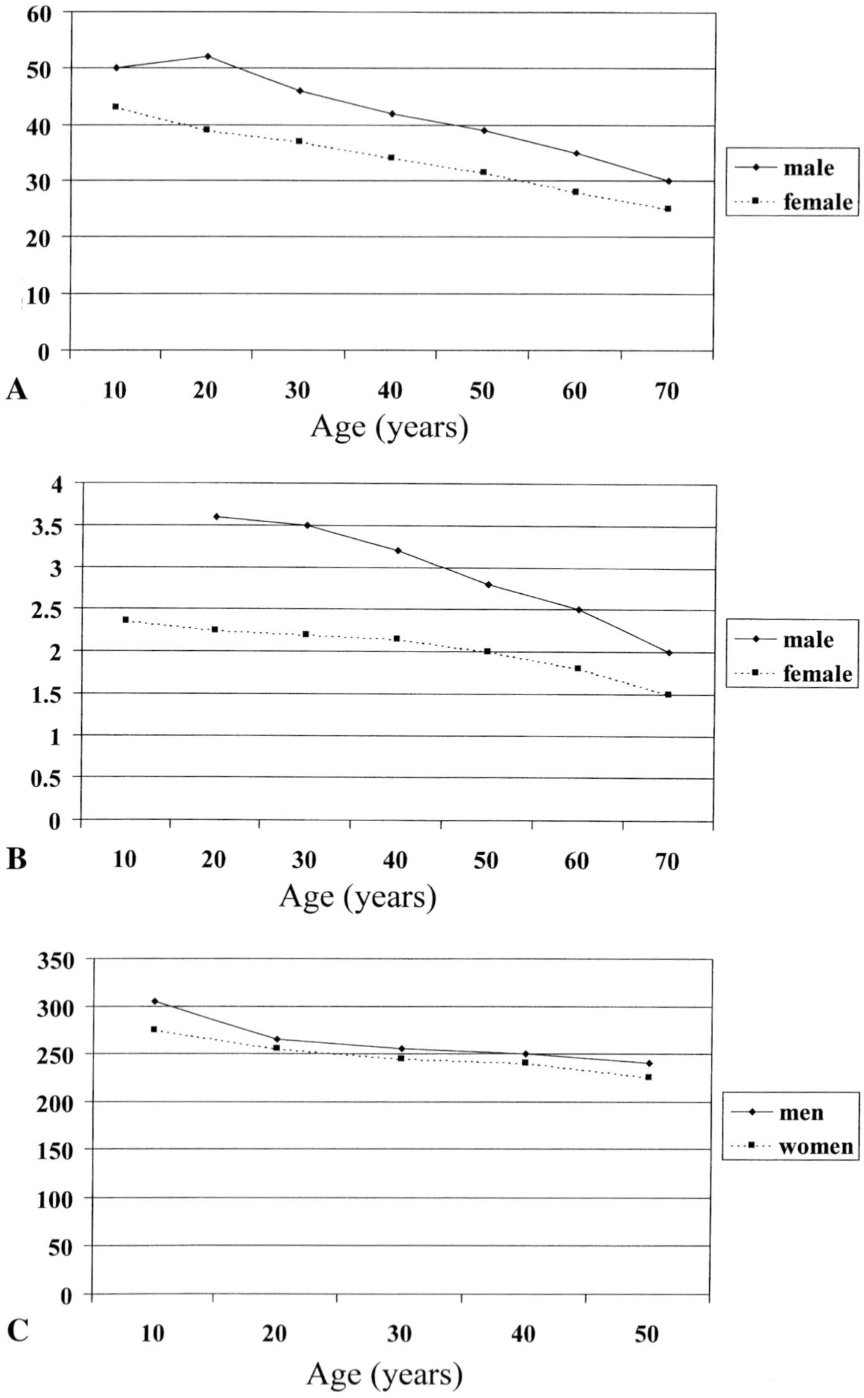

Fig. 5 *Maximal aerobic capacity by age and gender.* ***A****, maximal oxygen consumption expressed as L/min.* ***B****, expressed in mL/kg/min.* ***C****, Expressed in mL/L of leg volume. (Reproduced with permission from Fox EL, Bowers RW, Foss ML (eds):* The Physiological Basis for Exercise and Sport, *ed 5. Madison, WI, Brown & Benchmark, 1993.)*

Table 3 Physiologic variables by level of training and gender[15,16]

Variable	Untrained Women	Trained Women	Trained Men	Untrained Men
Hemoglobin (g)	555	800	805	995
Hemoglobin (g/kg)	8.5	12.5	11.6	13.7
Hemoglobin (g/100 mL blood)	13.6	14.1	15.3	15.1
Blood volume (L)	4.07	5.67	5.25	6.58
Blood volume (L/kg)	62.1	88.6	75.0	90.1
Heart volume (mL)	560	790	785	930
Heart volume (mL/kg)	8.5	12.3	11.2	12.7

parameters, such as hematocrit, hemoglobin, 2,3-diphosphoglycerate (2,3-DPG), and lactic acid. To the surprise of no one, the men were taller and heavier. There were no statistically significant differences between men and women on any of the variables studied. Only when 2,3-DPG was expressed per unit of hemoglobin were the women significantly greater than the men. Thus, with similar training patterns and performances, there was little in the way of any physiologic difference. It might even be argued that the women outperformed the men because they performed at an equal level with a reduced muscle mass. On the other hand, the men may have been more efficient because they were not taxing their full capacity in terms of muscle mass.

Concepts of Endurance Training

Training is a systematic manipulation of the primary training variables of frequency, duration, and intensity of training. There are many thorough reviews on the physiologic responses to physical training.[21–24] A complete summary of the responses to physical training can be found in every textbook on exercise physiology. A full treatment of this topic is beyond the scope of this chapter. In addition, broader topics in training theory such as specificity of training and periodization of training are also beyond the scope of this chapter. The general principles of endurance training and responses to endurance training will be discussed. It should come as no surprise that the principles of training apply to both men and women. Responses and adaptations to weight training will be discussed elsewhere in this section. In general, the more frequent, longer, and more intense the training sessions, the greater the improvement in fitness. However, there are restrictions to this concept to prevent injury or overtraining.

Frequency of Training

If a person works out 2 days/wk, will that person get over double the benefit from working out 5 days/wk? The number of days per week of training may be considered the least important variable in terms of improving fitness, yet most clinicians would cite training days as a critical variable in overuse injuries. Starting with 1 day/wk, training promotes improvement in Vo_{2max} up to 3 days/wk. From 3 to 5 days/wk, further improvements are seen, but these improvements are not as dramatic.[25] Training daily brings about smaller improvements in endurance, but at the cost of overuse injuries. Therefore, the common recommendation is to train 3 to 4 days/wk (I prefer 4 days so if 1 day/wk is missed, the preferred minimum of 3 days is still met).

Duration of Training

The threshold amount of daily training has not been well established. Earlier recommendations were for 20 to 40 min during each workout.[26,27] Now recommendations are for a total of 30 min/day of physical exercise and that these need not be consecutive minutes.[28] To avoid confusion, there are training recommendations for improvement in Vo_{2max} (the prior suggestion) and recommendations for improvement in general health (the latter suggestion). In many cases, the desired duration of training is dictated by the initial level of fitness (for very poorly fit people, multiple 3- to 5-min sessions) and the desired training intensity (the higher the training intensity, the shorter the duration; remember that training duration and training intensity are inversely related). It is interesting to note that excessive training volume does not always lead to improvement in fitness. For example, in a swimming study, there was no difference in endurance, power, or performance between a group who swam 1.5 hr/day and the other group that trained 2 × 1.5 hr/day.[29]

Intensity of Training

The bulk of the work on training methods has focused on the intensity of training. It is generally accepted that the relationship between training intensity and improvement in Vo_{2max} is a sigmoid curve.[30,31] Training at low intensities leads to small improvements in Vo_{2max}. At some threshold, small increases in training intensity lead to larger improvements in Vo_{2max}. Then at the highest intensities, there are small improvements in Vo_{2max}; not enough for the recreational athlete, but enough that the competitive athlete would desire to improve their performance.

The main questions about this curve are the threshold level of training and how to measure that threshold to ensure that a person is training in that "training zone." In many cases, the low and high intensity limits of this training zone depend on the method used to determine intensity. For example, heart rate and percent of Vo_{2max} can be used as indictors of training intensity (Table 4). With a training zone between 60% and 85%, if the Vo_{2max} were used as the method, the person would be training between 70% and over 90% of maximal heart rate response. Or, looking at it the other way, training at 60% to 85% of heart rate response would be training between 40% and around 75% of Vo_{2max}.[32]

There are a variety of methods for determining intensity of exercise. They are heart rate response, Vo_{2max} (this would include metabolic

Table 4 Comparison of Vo_{2max} and maximal heart rate responses as a means of determining training intensity

% of Vo_{2max}	% of Maximal Heart Rate
28	50
40	60
58	70
70	80
83	92
100	100

equivalents [METS] and caloric cost), rating of perceived exertion, and blood lactate.

Heart Rate

Most training studies use heart rate as the primary method of determining intensity because of the ease of measurement. To use heart rate, the trainer needs to know the maximal heart rate of the person training. It is best to use a known maximum heart rate from a progressive exercise test that usually is done before entering an exercise program. If an actual maximal heart rate is not known, then using the popular 220 – age relationship is appropriate.

Two methods for heart rate can be used: % of maximal heart rate response or % of maximal heart rate reserve. If 70% to 90% is the appropriate training zone, then the heart rate range for a person with a maximal heart rate (maxHR) of 180 would be 126 to 162 ($0.7 \times 180 = 126$; $0.9 \times 180 = 162$). The heart rate reserve method[33] takes into account the resting pulse rate (restHR) of the athlete.

$$\text{Training heart rate} = \text{restHR} + 0.7 \times (\text{maxHR} - \text{restHR}) \quad \text{(Eq. 3)}$$

The appropriate training percentages (0.7 and 0.9 in this example) are multiplied by the heart rate reserve (maxHR – restHR) then added to the resting heart rate. In the example of the person with a maximal heart rate response of 180 and a resting heart rate of 60, the training zone would be a much more narrow heart rate range:

$$144 = 60 + 0.7 \times (180 - 60) \quad \text{(Eq. 4)}$$

$$168 = 60 + 0.9 \times (180 - 60) \quad \text{(Eq. 5)}$$

The heart rate reserve method is the most widely used method to prescribe training intensity.

Vo_{2max}

In the laboratory, the gold standard for endurance is the maximal oxygen consumption test. If this figure is known, then percentages of Vo_{2max} can be prescribed and modes of activity suggested. For activities such as running, walking, cycling, and swimming among others, the energy cost (oxygen consumption) is known and many tables are published. Pace suggestions can then be made based on the known Vo_{2max} and the oxygen cost of a variety of training paces. Expensive equipment and technical expertise are needed to determine oxygen consumption and make training intensity prescriptions based on the known oxygen consumption. The values from oxygen consumption can be converted to more understandable units like METS (eg, 1 MET = energy expenditure at rest) or calories, either as total calories expended or calories relative to some time unit (usually per minute or per hour).

Rating of Perceived Exertion

When people exercise, they tend to train to a certain perception of intensity; how hard does this exercise feel? Numerous tables have been published to get the person's subjective opinion of the intensity of exercise. Two such examples are included in Table 5. The 6 to 20 scale was the first to gain wide acceptance and largely relates to heart rate by a factor of 10 (a perceived exertion of 13 would correspond to a heart rate of around 130). The second example was developed because people tended to rate exercise based not how hard their heart was beating, but rather how hard they were breathing. Minute ventilation during progressive exercise is exponential; there are small increases in ventilation up to some threshold beyond which breathing increases out of proportion to an increase in exercise intensity. Thus, the keywords are staggered at the higher numbers to take this fact into account. Appropriate training intensities using perceived exertion would be 12 to 15 or 3 to 5, depending on the scale used.[34]

Blood Lactate

There are many different titles and definitions for the point at which blood lactate accumulation begins to increase exponentially with increases in exercise intensity. Basically, there is a point where the production of pyruvic

Table 5 Two rating scales for perceived exertion

Rating of Perceived Exertion			
6		0	Nothing at all
7	Very, very light	0.5	Just noticeable
8		1	Very light
9	Very light	2	Light
10		3	Moderate
11	Fairly light	4	Somewhat hard
12		5	Hard
13	Somewhat hard	6	
14		7	Very hard
15	Hard	8	
16		9	
17	Very hard	10	Very, very hard
18		*	Maximal
19	Very, very hard		
20			

Use keywords and respond numerically to the question, "How hard is the exercise?"
*Person may rate exercise intensity as higher than 10 if they choose

acid by glycolysis exceeds the uptake of pyruvic acid by the Krebs cycle. The excess pyruvic acid is reduced to lactic acid, and this excess lactic acid diffuses into the blood and other tissues. A major goal of endurance training is to be able to run at higher and higher percentages of Vo_{2max} without lactic acid building up and being a culprit in fatigue. Thus, knowing the point where lactic acid begins to spill into the blood would be important. This determination is a complicated laboratory procedure in which the person exercises at progressively higher and higher intensities and blood samples are taken at each intensity and then plotted. The training pace at 2 and 4 mmol/L are determined. There are a variety of options for determining the appropriate training pace from blood lactic acid measurements.[35,36]

Observing how the world's elite athletes use such measures is sometimes instructive. For example, the Norwegian cross-country skiers typically perform their high volume-low intensity training at an intensity that elicits a blood lactate of 2 mmol/L or less. They do their low volume-high intensity training at paces that result in lactate levels well in excess of 4+ mmol/L and rarely train at intensities with lactates between 2 and 4 mmol/L (S. Seiler, PhD, personal communication, 1999). Obviously, an important point is how these intensities are applied in a year-long periodized training scheme.

One final word on intensity. There is frequent discussion of a method loosely termed the "talk test." A person's aerobic training would be at an intensity where he or she could carry on a conversation without getting winded. This is very effective because this level of exercise is within the perceived exertion limits suggested, right around the lactic acid threshold and within the prescribed heart rate reserve training range.

Rate of Improvement

A factor frequently overlooked is when to increase the training dosage. There are 3 primary variables; therefore, to improve, a person need increase only 1 of the variables: add a day, go a little longer, or train a little harder. The question is when to increase the training stimulus. It is surprising that there is no real consensus on this, but 2 primary opinions seem to be common. One opinion is that the training stimulus (usually training volume: a combination of frequency and duration) can be increased no more than 10% per week. The other opinion uses more conservative age-related criteria. Follow the training guidelines for 2 to 3 weeks for a person in his or her 20s. At the end of the 2 to 3 weeks, the person would add a day, distance, or intensity (only 1 factor, never 2 or all 3) and continue for the next 2 to 3 weeks and so on. The number of weeks between additions to training is increased 1 week for each decade: 3 to 4 weeks for people in their 30s, 4 to 5 weeks for people in their 40s, and so forth.[31]

Clinicians will often state that training errors are a frequent cause of overuse injuries. That usually means that the patient increased 2 or all 3 of the primary training variables at the same time. These same clinicians will also state that training errors can be extended to include shoes, training surface, and the environment. Consider the following scenario. A runner trains 3 days/wk, 20 to 30 min/day at a perceived exertion of 3 to 5 on a mulched trail in a neighborhood park. He or she jogs on Friday, then that evening travels to a professional meeting being held at altitude. Of course, new running shoes are purchased for the trip. The runner meets friends and they go for a run on Saturday morning on the back roads. The meeting is sponsoring a 10-km "fun run" Sunday morning, also on the roads. Our meeting-goer has now run 3 days in a row, on harder surfaces, in new shoes, at altitude, probably at a faster pace than normal, and definitely a longer distance. This scenario is a setup for an overuse injury. Change only 1 thing at a time to reduce the risk of training-induced injuries.

Some Training Theory

Thus far, the discussion has focused on the most basic aspects of training. When training for athletic performance, a few other generalizations are necessary to optimally prepare an athlete for competition and to avoid the possibility of overreaching or overtraining.

Ramping of Training

This first concept is somewhat related to the rate of progression above. Many coaches feel that the faster an athlete progresses in their training, the lower the eventual level of performance and the shorter the length of time that level of performance can be maintained before some reduction in performance (eg, injury or some level of staleness or overtraining). However, should the athlete's training be developed over a longer period of time, the greater will be the adaptation that will lead to a higher level of performance that can be maintained for a longer period of time. Current university and scholastic rules limit the amount of preseason training time before competition. If the athlete does not assume some personal responsibility in independent training before a training camp, then he or she will be exposed to a very fast ramp of training, which can lead to overreaching, overtraining, fatigue, injury, or poor performance.

Periodization of Training

Periodization is discussed in detail in chapter 21. Athletes who use resistance traning have made the most use of this concept, with other individual sport athletes also following periodized training programs. Team sports are somewhat sporadic in their use of these principles. The systematic manipulation of training volume, intensity, and emphasis on technique is planned out so that the athletes reach their peak level of performance with minimal risk of injury or overtraining. Refer to chapter 21 for a more detailed description. In addition, there are many sources on the internet that may be of interest; search using the keyword overtraining.

Within any discussion of overtraining is the relationship of intensity and duration of training. A common training error is trying to train long and hard. The relationship of training volume and intensity is inverse. The longer a training distance or volume, the lower the intensity. High-intensity training can be performed only for short volumes or distances.

This discussion has been directed to the general concepts of physical training. These factors are universal and apply to both men and women. Selected factors that are influenced by training will be discussed in multiple chapters throughout this volume.

Adaptations to Training

There are a number of chapters in this volume that address specific adaptations to training in women. In addition, there are a number of excellent reviews of physical training in the professional literature. I will summarize physical training from a general viewpoint and discuss adaptations that are seen at rest, during submaximal exercise, and during maximal exercise.

Cardiovascular Adaptations

One of the most notable adaptations to physical training is a reduction in resting heart rate that is due to a variety of factors. For example, following endurance training, there is cardiac hypertrophy that is secondary to increased cavity dimensions of the left ventricle.[17] This would mean that the stroke volume of the left ventricle should be increased, likely due to Starling mechanisms that increase myocardial contractility. Cardiac output and oxygen consumption are highly correlated, and resting oxygen consumption does not change with training. Therefore, if cardiac output stays constant and stroke volume increases, then heart rate has to go down. Neural factors that influence the left ventricle include a reduction in the intrinsic rate of the atria, an increase in the parasympathetic tone (vagus nerve), and a decrease in sympathetic influence.[1,32]

Other training-induced changes include an increase in the total blood volume and hemoglobin.[14] This will help with oxygen transport as well as heat dissipation.[1] Capillary density of the trained muscles is increased, effectively reducing the diffusion distance of oxygen from the capillaries to the working muscle fibers.[37–39] In fact, the degree of change in local capillaries is highly correlated with change in Vo_{2max}.[39] Muscle hypertrophy is localized to the recruited muscle fibers where endurance training increases metabolic (as opposed to contractile) proteins to improve the ability of the muscle to use oxygen to generate ATP from metabolism of carbohydrates, fats, and to a lesser degree, proteins.[1,32] These changes are summarized in Outline 1.

One of the best ways to document training adaptations is to observe the responses of the body to submaximal exercise, train, then repeat the same exercise and determine the changes due to training. Table 6 contains a summary of the primary adaptations to endurance training.

Submaximal Exercise

The caloric cost of running 7 mph should be the same before and after a training program. Therefore, there should be little difference in terms of oxygen consumption.[40] If submaximal oxygen consumption does decrease, this decrease is most likely due to improvements in performing the exercise technique. However, a significant reduction in blood lactic acid is a confirmation of improvement in training.[40,41] Numerous factors enter into this result. Any reduction in lactic acid production would indicate that oxidative metabolism is accounting for a greater fraction of the total energy production. The increases in blood volume and hemoglobin mean greater oxygen-carrying capacity of the blood. The increase in capillary density

Outline 1 Cardiovascular adaptations to endurance training

- Left ventricular hypertrophy
    - Increased internal dimension of the left ventricle
        - Increased overall mass of the left ventricle
        - Increased stroke volume
            - Increased myocardial contractility
    - Decreased heart rate
        - Reduced atrial rate
        - Increased parasympathetic tone
        - Decreased sympathetic tone
- Increased total blood volume and hemoglobin
    - Expansion of plasma volume
    - Increased red cell count
- Increased muscle hypertrophy and capillary density
    - Increased metabolic proteins
    - Decreased diffusion distance for oxygen

around the working muscle fibers reduces the diffusion distance of oxygen. Myoglobin, the storage location for oxygen in the muscle, increases in response to endurance training, thereby increasing the amount of oxygen stored locally in the muscle and making more oxygen available to the mitochondria. Endurance training increases the metabolic proteins of the trained muscle fibers; this would include the mitochondria and enzymes of the Krebs cycle and electron transport. If all these enzymes are functioning at a higher level of activity, then the Krebs cycle can more effectively compete for pyruvic acid, leading to a reduction in lactic acid production. In addition, endurance training teaches the muscle to use fats as an energy source that spares glycogen depletion.

Central cardiovascular changes seen during submaximal exercise mirror that seen at rest. Cardiac output shows little change or a slight decrease for the same reasons as stated above for oxygen consumption. Yet there is a significant reduction in exercise heart rate and a significant increase in stroke volume.[21] Stroke volume is increased due to the increased filling time and the subsequent improvement in contractility from the decreased heart rate. The training-induced bradycardia is a result of such variables as a reduction in exercise-induced catecholamines and a decrease in the sympathetic drive during exercise.

Local muscle blood flow (in mL/unit of muscle tissue) actually decreases following training.[42] The body makes more blood available for heat dissipation at the skin. Therefore, to compensate for the reduction in local blood flow, the muscle fibers extract more oxygen leading to an increased arteriovenous oxygen difference.[43]

Table 6 Summary of training responses to submaximal and maximal exercise[1,32]

	Submaximal Exercise	Maximal Exercise
Metabolic		
Oxygen consumption	No change or significant decrease	Significant increase
Lactic acid	Significant decrease	Significant increase
Glycogen use	Significant decrease	
Total blood flow		
Cardiac output	No change or significant decrease	Significant increase
Stroke volume	Significant increase	Significant increase
Heart rate	Significant decrease	No change or significant decrease
Local blood flow		
Muscle blood flow	Significant decrease	No change
A – Vo_2 difference	Significant increase	Significant increase

When all these variables are considered collectively, it is seen that the performance of the same submaximal exercise after training becomes physically and physiologically easier. These changes are summarized in Table 6.

Maximal Exercise

To determine just how effective a training program has been, a maximal exhaustive task usually is performed. The most obvious change is an increase in total work output; it takes longer to reach exhaustion.

Maximal oxygen consumption is the "gold standard" of aerobic fitness, so it should be expected that endurance training will yield a significantly improved Vo_{2max}. This is a result of both an increased oxygen delivery by the central cardiovascular system and peripheral use of the delivered oxygen. This increase in central delivery is a result of the improvement in cardiac output[44] that is driven by the increased stroke volume,[44,45] not heart rate. The improvement in stroke volume is driven by cardiac hypertrophy and contractility. A significant increase in lactic acid production is a common finding that may be caused either by an increase in the flux of the intermediates of glycolysis or by the fact that the person is better able to withstand the discomforts of exhaustive exercise.[1] This greater cardiac output is distributed over a larger working muscle mass, so the relative local muscle blood flow is relatively unchanged,[46] but all the increases in the local handling of oxygen yield a greater arteriovenous oxygen difference.[45]

This general discussion on the adaptations to physical training is applicable to both men and women. The relative degree of changes may vary slightly, but the overall patterns of adaptations are the same.[1] In subsequent chapters, the effects of training on selected topics specific to women will be discussed in detail.

References

1. Fox EL, Bowers RW, Foss ML (eds): *The Physiological Basis for Exercise and Sport*, ed 5. Madison, WI, Brown & Benchmark, 1993.
2. Whipp BJ, Ward SA: Will women soon outrun men? *Nature* 1992;355:25.
3. Joyner MJ: Physiological limiting factors and distance running: Influence of gender and age on record performances. *Exerc Sport Sci Rev* 1993;21:103–133.
4. Mognoni P, Lafortuna C, Russo G, Minetti A: An analysis of world records in three types of locomotion. *Eur J Appl Physiol* 1982;49:287–299.
5. Ryder HW, Carr HJ, Herget P: Future performance in footracing. *Sci Am* 1976;234:109–114, 118–119.
6. Medved R: Body height and predisposition for certain sports. *J Sports Med Phys Fitness* 1966;6:89–91.
7. Pendergast DR, Diprampero PE, Craig AB Jr, Wilson DR, Rennie DW: Quantitative analysis of the front crawl in men and women. *J Appl Physiol* 1977;43:475–479.
8. Hultman E, Bergstrom J, Anderson NM: Breakdown and resynthesis of phosphorylcreatine and adenosine triphosphate in connection with muscular work in man. *Scand J Clin Lab Invest* 1967;19:56–66.
9. Fox EL: Differences in metabolic alterations with sprint vs endurance interval training, in Howald H, Poortmans JR (eds): *Metabolic Adaptation to Prolonged Physical Exercise*. Basel, Switzerland, Kirkhäuser, 1975, pp 119–126.
10. Fox EL: Measurement of the maximal alactic (phosphagen) capacity in man. *Med Sci Sports* 1975;6:66–69.
11. Hagerman FC, Fox EL, Conners M, Pompei J: Metabolic responses of women rowers during ergometric rowing. *Med Sci Sports Exerc* 6:87–91.
12. Kalamen JL: Measurement of maximum muscular power in man. Columbus, OH, Ohio State University, 1968, Thesis.
13. Margaria R, Aghemo P, Rovelli E: Measurement of muscular power (anaerobic) in man. *J Appl Physiol* 1966;21:1662–1664.
14. Astrand PO (ed): *Experimental Studies of Physical Working Capacity in Relation to Sex and Age*. Copenhagen, Denmark, E Munksgaard, 1952.
15. Kjellberg SR, Rudhe U, Sjöstrand T: Increase of the amount of hemoglobin and blood volume in connection with physical training. *Acta Physiol Scand* 1949;19:146–151.
16. Kjellberg SR, Rudhe U, Sjöstrand T: The amount of hemoglobin and the blood volume in relation to the pulse rate and cardiac volume during rest. *Acta Physiol Scand* 1949;19:136–145.
17. Morganroth J, Maron BJ, Henry WL, Epstein SE: Comparative left ventricular dimensions in trained athletes. *Ann Intern Med* 1975;82:521–524.
18. Longhurst JC, Kelly AR, Gonyea WJ, Mitchell JH: Echocardiographic left ventricular masses in distance runners and weight lifters. *J Appl Physiol* 1980;48:154–62.
19. Kirkendall DT, Lemon PWR, Street G: Abstract: Aerobic power and body composition in anorexia nervosa patients. *Med Sci Sports Exerc* 1983;15:106.
20. Pate RR, Barnes C, Miller W: A physiological comparison of performance-matched female and male distance runners. *Res Q Exerc Sport* 1985;56:245–250.
21. Scheuer J, Tipton CM: Cardiovascular adaptations to physical training. *Annu Rev Physiol* 1977;39:221–251.
22. Viru A: Mechanism of general adaptation. *Med Hypotheses* 1992;38:296–300.
23. Matoba H, Gollnick PD: Response of skeletal muscle to training. *Sports Med* 1984;1:240–251.

24. Roy RR, Baldwin KM,,Edgerton VR: The plasticity of skeletal muscle: Effects of neuromuscular activity. *Exerc Sport Sci Rev* 1991;19:269–312.
25. Gettman LR, Pollock ML, Durstine JL, Ward A, Ayres J, Linnerud AC: Physiological responses of men to 1, 3, and 5 day per week training programs. *Res Q* 1976;47:638–646.
26. Milesis CA, Pollock ML, Bah MD, Ayres JJ, Ward A, Linnerud AC: Effects of different durations of physical training on cardiorespiratory function, body composition and serum lipids. *Res Q* 1976;47:716–725.
27. Pollock ML: The quantification of endurance training programs. *Exerc Sport Sci Rev* 1973;1:155–188.
28. American College of Sports Medicine Position Stand: The recommended quantity and quality of exercise for developing and maintaining cardiorespiratory and muscular fitness, and flexibility in healthy adults. *Med Sci Sports Exerc* 1998;30:975–991.
29. Costill DL, Thomas R, Robergs RA, et al: Adaptations to swimming training: Influence of training volume. *Med Sci Sports Exerc* 1991;23:371–377.
30. King CN; Senn MD: Exercise testing and prescription: Practical recommendations for the sedentary. *Sports Med* 1996;21:326–336.
31. Kirkendall DT: Exercise prescription for the healthy adult. *Prim Care* 1984;11:23–31.
32. McArdle WD, Katch FI, Katch VL (eds): Exercise Physiology*: Energy, Nutrition and Human Performance*, ed 3. Philadelphia, PA, Lea & Febiger, 1991.
33. Karvonen M, Kentala E, Mustala O: The effects of training on heart rate: A longitudinal study. *Ann Med Exper Biol Fenn* 1957;35:307–315.
34. Dishman RK: Prescribing exercise intensity for healthy adults using perceived exertion. *Med Sci Sports Exerc* 1994;26:1087–1094.
35. Kindermann W, Simon G, Keul J: The significance of the aerobic-anaerobic transition for the determination of work load intensities during endurance training. *Eur J Appl Physiol* 1979;42:25–34.
36. MacDougall JD: The anaerobic threshold: Its significance for the endurance athlete. *Can J Appl Sport Sci* 1977;2:137–140.
37. Hermansen L, Wachtlova M: Capillary density of skeletal muscle in well-trained and untrained men. *J Appl Physiol* 1971;30:860–863.
38. Saltin B, Henriksson J, Nygaard E, Andersen P, Jansson E: Fiber types and metabolic potentials of skeletal muscles in sedentary man and endurance runners. *Ann NY Acad Sci* 1977;301:3–29.
39. Andersen P: Capillary density in skeletal muscle of man. *Acta Physiol Scand* 1975;95:203–205.
40. Ekblom B, Astrand PO, Saltin B, Stenberg J, Wallstrom B: Effect of training on circulatory response to exercise. *J Appl Physiol* 1968;24:518–528.
41. Karlsson J, Nordesjo L-O, Jorfeldt L, Saltin B: Muscle lactate, ATP, and CP levels during exercise after physical training in man. *J Appl Physiol* 1972;33:199–203.
42. Klassen GA, Andrew GM, Becklake MR: Effect of training on total and regional blood flow and metabolism in paddlers. *J Appl Physiol* 1970;28:397–406.
43. Holloszy JO: Biochemical adaptations to exercise: Aerobic metabolism. *Exerc Sport Sci Rev* 1973;1:45–71.
44. Ekblom B, Hermansen L: Cardiac output in athletes. *J Appl Physiol* 1968;25:619–625.
45. Saltin B: Physiological effects of physical training. *Med Sci Sports* 1969;1:50–56.
46. Grimby G, Haggendal E, Saltin B: Local xenon 133 clearance from the quadriceps muscle during exercise in man. *J Appl Physiol* 1967;22:305–310.

Chapter 21

Strength Training for Women: Intensity, Volume, and Exercise Selection Factors

Michael H. Stone, PhD, CSCS
Travis Triplett-McBride, PhD, CSCS
Margaret E. Stone, MS, CSCS

Introduction

Resistance training has been an integral part of the training for most athletes for at least 25 years. More recently resistance training has become widely accepted as a training method that can enhance various health aspects for all ages.[1,2]

In the past, with a few exceptions, most exercise and sports scientists focused their research on the physiologic and performance effects of aerobic training. It only has been in the past 5 to 10 years that a relatively large amount of research time has been concentrated on resistance training. Consequently, factors concerned with the subtleties of training effects and gender differences are only just now beginning to emerge. Whereas adaptations in performance and health parameters as a result of long-term training appear to be similar between the genders, differences can occur in the magnitude of the training effect. These quantitative differences in adaptation between genders appear to have multifactorial causes including physical, psychological, and physiologic factors, but may also be influenced by the method and mode of training.

The purpose of this chapter is to discuss briefly health and performance adaptations to resistance training, make comparisons between genders, and suggest training modes and methods that can enhance specific adaptations. The primary focus of this chapter will deal with current knowledge of strength training for female athletes.

Basic Training Principles

Before a discussion of differences in trained state or gender differences can be adequately discussed, an understanding of basic training principles is necessary. Stone and associates[3] have outlined the basic training principles and their application to resistance training. The training method (repetitions and sets, velocity of movement, appropriate variation, and so forth) can make a considerable difference in the outcome of a resistance training program.[3–6] For example, high volume programs generally have a greater influence on body composition and endurance factors compared to low volume programs.[2,3,7,8] It also is probable that the choice of training mode (type of equipment) can influence the adaptations to a training program. There are three basic training principles: overload, variation, and specificity.[3]

Overload

Overload deals with providing a proper stimulus for attaining a desired level of physical, physiologic, or performance adaptation. Overload can be conceptualized as exercise and training that goes beyond normal levels of physical performance. Each exercise will have some level of intensity, frequency, and duration of application. Thus, all overload stimuli will have some level of intensity, relative intensity (percent of maximum), and volume.

For resistance exercise, intensity factors are associated with the rate of performing work and the rate at which energy is expended.[3] Intensity factors can be separated into two aspects: training intensity and movement or exercise intensity.[3] Training intensity is the rate at which a training exercise or a training session proceeds and can be estimated by the average mass (weight) lifted per exercise, per day, per week, and so forth. The relative intensity is a percentage of the one repetition maximum (1RM). The 1RM is stable only in advanced strength trainers, thus using relative intensity to plan training programs must be done with care. Exercise intensity is the actual power output of a movement. The hyperbolic force-velocity curve represents the inverse relationship between force and power. Power can be defined as a work rate or as the product of force and velocity. The product of force and velocity forms an inverted U with peak power occurring at approximately 35% of the peak isometric force. For well-trained strength/power athletes, evidence indicates that peak power may represent a somewhat higher percentage (45% to 60%) of peak isometric force.[5,9] Peak power has been shown to be associated with approximately 35% to 65% of the 1RM depending upon the type of exercise and the level of training.[4,5,9] Thus, the relative intensity can be used to estimate (and manipulate) the exercise intensity, with very heavy or very light weights producing lower power outputs than those in the middle range.

The volume of training is a measure or estimate of how much total work is performed and is related to total energy expenditure. Intensity (and relative intensity) can be provided by the amount of weight lifted. The volume of training is related to the number repetitions and sets per exercise, the number and types of exercises used (large versus small muscle mass), and the number of times per day, week, month, and so forth that these exercises are repeated. Volume load (repetitions times the mass lifted) is the best estimate of the amount of work accomplished during training and is commonly used in both research and practical settings. The application of training intensity and volume can be considered in terms of the overall workout (ie, all exercises performed during a specified period) or in terms of individual exercises. An understanding of overload factors can aid in the programming of training, including methods (sets and repetitions), velocity of exercise, and in exercise selection.

Variation

Variation is concerned with appropriate manipulation in training intensity, speed of movement, volume, and exercise selection. Appropriate variation is an important consideration for the continuation of adaptations over long-term training programs[10,11] Furthermore, appropriate sequencing of volume, intensity, and exercise selection, including speed-strength exercises in a periodized manner, can lead to superior enhancement of a variety of performance abilities.[4]

Specificity of Exercise and Training

Specificity of exercise and training is the most important consideration when selecting both methods and modes for resistance training, especially if athletic performance enhancement is a primary goal. Specificity includes both bioenergetics and mechanics of training.[5] This discussion will be concerned with mechanical aspects of specificity.

Mechanical specificity refers to the kinetic and kinematic associations between a training exercise and a physical performance. This includes movement patterns, peak force, rate of force development, acceleration, and velocity parameters. The more similar a training exercise is to the actual physical performance the greater the probability of transfer.[3,12–17] Mechanical specificity has been extensively studied as it affects strength training exercise. Of particular importance is explosive strength and power.

Specificity and Transfer of Training Effect

Using untrained subjects, heavy weight training can produce a rightward shift and beneficial effects in the entire force-velocity curve.[6,18] However, considerable evidence suggests that in strength trained subjects, high-velocity training is necessary to make additional alterations in the high-velocity end of the force-velocity curve.[4,6,18]

Although isometric training can result in an increased peak rate of force production and velocity of movement, especially in untrained subjects,[16] the isometric training effect on dynamic explosive force production is relatively minor.[18] Traditional heavy weight training primarily increases maximum strength, especially measured by a 1RM. In contrast, the primary effect of ballistic training is an increased rate of force production and velocity of movement.[4,5,14,18] Additionally, high power training can alter a wide range of athletic performance variables to a greater extent than does traditional heavy weight training, especially in subjects with a reasonable initial level of maximum strength.[19] Examination of longitudinal and cross-sectional studies[3,18,20] suggests that sequenced training, heavy weight training over a few weeks followed by speed strength training or combination training (heavy training plus high power or high speed), can produce superior results in strength and power gains compared to heavy weight training or speed-strength training alone. More importantly, evidence indicates that this type of sequenced training (a form of periodization) can beneficially alter a wide variety of athletic performance variables to a greater extent than either heavy weight training or speed-strength training.[4,21]

Movement Patterns: Modes of Training and Exercise Selection

Modes of Training

Free weight training applies resistance by use of a freely moving body. It includes the use of barbells, dumbbells, associated benches and racks, medicine balls, throwing implements, and body mass, and it allows for resistance/force production accommodation. Machine training applies resistance in a guided or restricted manner. It includes the use of plate-loaded and selectorized devices, electronically braked devices, springs, and rubber band devices.

Exercise Selection

Even though machine training is popular in many health clubs, there are few data to support its use over free weights, especially as it concerns athletes. Although it is a common belief, there is no evidence that machine training is safer than training with free weights.[22] Although programming (sets and repetitions) for a specific exercise is independent of exercise mode, the resulting overall total work (accomplished per session, week, month, and so forth) is not independent. For example, in general, changes in body composition, particularly decreases in body fat, are related to the total energy expenditure (during and after exercise) and, therefore, to the volume of training.[3] With a few exceptions, most machines use single-joint small muscle mass exercises, and most training programs using machines are centered on several small muscle mass exercises that can result in a smaller energy expenditure than if larger muscle mass exercises were used.[2,3,23] Thus, we make the argument that large muscle mass exercises and, therefore, larger energy expenditures are much more readily accomplished using free weights (ie, squats, jumps, pulling movements, and variations).

Although changes in volume and intensity are possible with machines, proper application, sequencing and variation of movement patterns, speed-strength, and speed oriented exercises are limited at best. This is a consequence of the limitations in the movement pattern and movement characteristics of the machines themselves.

Studies and reviews of the literature have consistently noted that the magnitude of measured maximum strength gains (and other variables such as power) depends on the similarity between the strength test and the actual training exercise.[14–16,24–27] Furthermore, mechanical and theoretical considerations suggest that training with free weights can have a greater transfer of training to athletic and ergonomic tasks than machines.[17,28–33] This transfer occurs primarily because free weight movements can be used to mechanically mimic athletic and ergonomic tasks more effectively than machines. Although there are relatively few studies that actually compare alterations in performance using various devices for training, the data generally support the concept of movement specificity and the use of free weights as the primary mode of training.[17]

The present understanding of training principles indicates that power and speed of movement specificity (as well as appropriate variation) are necessary considerations in the formulation of training programs leading to increased power and speed of movement. Even a cursory examination of most machines indicates that high speed and high power training may be compromised because of limitations on acceleration patterns (particularly in variable resistance and semi-isokinetic devices), friction, inappropriate movement patterns, and limited ranges of motion.[30,32–35] Most athletes typically center their training on free weights, using machines as assistance exercises.

Programming: Sets and Repetitions

Single Sets Versus Multiple Sets

Although there has been recent controversy,[36] most studies that have carefully examined training with one set versus training with multiple sets, with both men and women, indicate superior results can be obtained in a wide variety of performance and physiologic variables by using multiple sets.[3] The superior effects of multiple sets are particularly apparent among advanced weight trainers.[10,11] Furthermore, these effects can be enhanced by the use of periodization/variation techniques along with the multiple set protocols.

Periodization

Periodization can be defined as "a logical phasic method of manipulating training variables in order to increase the potential for achieving specific performance goals."[37,38] Thus, a basic tenet of periodization is training nonlinearity. The primary goals of periodization are: (1) reduction of overtraining potential and (2) peaking at the appropriate time or providing a maintenance program for sports with a specific season. The goals are met by appropriately manipulating volume and intensity factors and by appropriate exercise selection. Briefly, periodized training can be divided into three stages or levels: the macrocycle (long length cycle), the mesocycle (middle length cycle), and the microcycle (short length cycle). Each macro- and mesocycle generally begins with a high volume, low intensity of training and ends with a high intensity, low volume of training. The macro- and mesocycles can contain four phases: (1) preparation (general and special), (2) competition, (3) peaking, and (4) transition or active rest. Each of these phases can have different goals and require different degrees of variation in training variables.

General preparation is a high volume phase, usually lasting a few weeks, designed to enhance sports-specific fitness and associated physiologic parameters. Special preparation deals with relatively high volume training in which the exercises are more specific to the activity in terms of movement pattern and velocity. It is used as a transition phase linking high, less specific general preparation training to high intensity, very specific training associated with competition. During the competition phase, intensity factors are adjusted in keeping with the characteristics of the sport. For example, in a sport requiring high power outputs, more time is spent on using high exercise intensities; for a sport in which great strength is required, a greater emphasis can be placed on high training intensities. Volume during the competition phase is decreased. The competition phase can last several months. Peaking is a short phase (usually < 4 wks). During the early portion of peaking, volume is typically reduced as training intensity (or exercise intensity) is increased. During the last few days before competition, intensity factors are also reduced to encourage adequate recovery. The latter portion of peaking, when volume and intensity are markedly reduced, is referred to as a "taper." Active rest is a phase in which volume and intensity are decreased markedly to facilitate recovery from the training cycle. Recovery includes healing and rehabilitation of any injuries that may have occurred as well as recovery from the emotional rigors of competition. Complete rest allows sports-specific fitness to deteriorate to a degree from which it is difficult to recover without extensive training. Compared to complete rest, active rest allows for less deterioration of fitness and a faster return to peak fitness during the next cycle. Active rest usually lasts about 1 week. A modification of the typical scheme can be made for sports with a definite season in which winning all contests (games) is a goal, such as basketball. A typical modification for seasonal sports is to prolong the competition phase and remove the peaking phase. Most elite athletes typically use some form of periodization. For a more detailed discussion of periodization of training, see Stone and associates.[3,37,38]

Comparisons of Male and Female Strength Levels

Trained Versus Untrained

Comparisons of maximum strength levels among untrained men and women[39–42] are presented in Table 1. These values are a summary of different methods and modes of testing (ie, isometric versus freely moving; machines versus free weights; eccentric versus concentric). Thus, some differences may be observed when different testing devices are used. These values are also independent of body mass and muscle distribution differences. When body mass and lean body mass are accounted for, the differences between men and women are not as great.

Generally the differences between men and women appear to be similar among elite weight lifters and power lifters.[43] Table 2 shows the absolute values and relative values for 1RM lifts among track and field athletes (shot put). These data suggest that: (1) there is a relationship between strength/power performance

Table 1 Strength comparisons of untrained women to untrained men

	Absolute (%)	Relative to Body Mass (%)	Relative to Lean Body Mass (%)
Total body	64	72	87
Upper body	56	60	75
Lower body	74	85	100

as measured by the squat, clean, snatch, and bench press and throwing ability; (2) gender strength differences are greater in the upper body than lower (bench versus squat); and (3) lower level (collegiate) athletes show greater strength differences between genders than higher level athletes. Although the numbers are small, these data suggest that a major consideration for a women to reach the upper levels of throwing (and likely other strength/power sports) is a marked increase in strength/power. The strength differences in upper and lower body between men and women are likely related to differences in total muscle distribution. Men have a larger relative distribution of muscle in the upper body.[6,39]

Aging

Aging results in approximately a 9% loss in isometric and dynamic maximum strength per decade after age 40 years among untrained men and women.[44,45] These results are similar to the 5% to 15% decrease in strength

Table 2 Strength levels of throwers

	Squat	Clean	Snatch	Bench
Male Shot-Put (1997–1998)*				
National level (Automatic)	290.3 ± 38.8 (n = 3)	186.0 ± 12.0 (n = 3)	129.3 ± 28.9 (n = 2)	226.8 ± 0 (n = 3)
National level (Provisional)	283.5 ± 11.3 (n = 3)	155.3 ± 1.8 (n = 3)	106.8 ± 9.3 (n = 2)	189.0 ± 15.9 (n = 3)
Collegiate level	266.0 ± 38.4 (n = 7)	137.3 ± 17.3 (n = 7)	84.9 ± 39.3 (n = 6)	180.2 ± 23.9 (n = 7)
Female Shot Put (1997–1998)†				
National level (Automatic)	168.8 ± 11.7 (n = 7)	106.5 ± 6.7 (n = 7)	76.5 ± 7.1 (n = 7)	112.8 ± 9.6 (n = 7)
National level (Provisional)	147.0 ± 12.3 (n = 2)	100.0 ± 5.8 (n = 2)	71.1 ± 5.3 (n = 2)	101.5 ± 5.5 (n = 2)
Collegiate level	84.5 ± 10.0 (n = 5)	61.4 ± 4.3 (n = 5)	46.3 ± 5.9 (n = 5)	79.8 ± 0 (n = 1)
Percent Strength Comparison (Women/Men)				
National (Automatic)	65	57	59	50
National (Provisional)	52	64	67	54
Collegiate level	32	45	54	44
Elite weightlifters	—	63	65	—

*Data from UCLA, USC, Wyoming (mean ± SD; kg)
†Data from UCLA, USC, Wyoming, ASU (mean ± SD; kg)

per decade after age 40 years in both male and female competitive track and field athletes.[46] However, among competitive weightlifters aging appears to affect women more than men. In 1997, the women's world records for the both the snatch and clean and jerk averaged about 68% of the men's records over 5 weight categories.[47] At ages 40 to 54 years, this ratio decreases to about 50%; during ages 55 to 59 years, the ratio drops to about 30%. Because weight lifting movements have a large speed and power component, this observation could indicate a loss of speed and power at a faster rate among women. However, due to small numbers of women competing in the older age groups it is not possible to draw definitive conclusions.

Power

Power is highly related to performance in a number of sports and is a key characteristic that separates winning and losing.[6] Peak power output for women is about 65% that of men during the snatch and clean[48] and various jumping tasks.[39] Both untrained and trained women appear to generate lower power outputs per volume of muscle and generate lower peak rates of force development compared to men.[49,50]

Factors Affecting Strength Gains in Women: Implications for Training

Upper Body Versus Lower Body

Because of the relatively lower strength values for upper body movements, it has been suggested that more emphasis should be placed on upper body training for women (National Strength and Conditioning Association position stance). This may improve performance in tasks that depend in part or whole on upper body strength. Part of the reasoning for the greater emphasis on upper body strength training is the assumption that the weaker upper body musculature may limit strength gains in the lower body (ie, squats, cleans, etc). Recent evidence supports this assumption.[51]

Menstrual Cycle Effects

Alterations in hormones can affect physiologic parameters that, in turn, can affect force production parameters.[52,53] Indeed, strength gains in women have been correlated to serum concentrations of both total and free testosterone.[54] The menstrual cycle is characterized by large variations in several hormones on a regular (or nearly) basis. Because these hormones (ie, estradiol, progesterone, etc) affect metabolic and neuromuscular function, it is possible that training/performance can be affected during different phases of the cycle. Although most studies do not show profound effects of the menstrual cycle on various parameters of performance, some evidence suggests that strength gains may be negatively affected during the early follicular phase and positively affected during the late follicular and early luteal phases.[55] Increases in strength gains noted during the late follicular and early luteal phases were correlated with increases in serum estradiol and testosterone. Additionally, Reis and associates[55] suggest that altering the number of training sessions (reduced during the luteal phase) during various phases of the cycle may enhance the training effect. Obviously, more study is necessary.

Compromises with Aerobic Training

Endurance is also an important component for many sports. It is commonly believed that aerobic exercise is necessary to develop endurance even for highly anaerobic activities. However, evidence indicates that a combined training program (aerobic plus resistance training) can markedly compromise gains in strength and especially power and speed.[56–59] The mechanisms are unclear but may involve hormonal or neural adaptations.[59]

Health Parameters

A primary area of study in recent years has been the health effects of resistance training. Evidence suggests that, depending upon the type of resistance training used, a wide variety of health-related variables may be beneficially affected. In this discussion the magnitude of both physiologic responses to resistance exercises as well as training adaptations are influenced by a number of factors including training and exercise intensity, the muscle mass involved, and the volume load.[2,6]

Strength

Reduced physiologic stress as a result of increased strength is one of the most obvious benefits of resistance training. For example, when attempting to lift a heavy object (such as a couch), if the effort is stressful because the object represents a relatively large percentage of the person's maximum strength, elevations in heart rate (HR), blood pressure (BP), rate pressure product (RPP), hormonal responses, and so forth can be quite large. Higher strength levels can reduce these responses because the object to be lifted will be relatively lighter, producing less physiologic stress.[2,60] Indeed, increased strength generally enhances functional capabilities; this can be especially important in the elderly.[61]

Cardiovascular Effects

HR increases as a result of resistance exercise. Furthermore, because of the metabolic characteristics of resistance exercise, HR does not necessarily relate in a linear manner to oxygen consumption.[6] Additionally, the intermittent nature of resistance training results in the mean HR being influenced by the length of the rest periods. Thus, average HRs do not accurately reflect exercise intensity nor can they be used to accurately gauge cardiovascular stress. Cross-sectional data show that highly resistance-trained athletes have normal or lower than normal resting HRs.[2] Longitudinal studies generally show decreases in resting heart rates of about 3% to 12%.[2,39]

Training has also been shown to reduce exercise HR during submaximal box stepping, cycle, and treadmill exercise[62–66] and to enhance HR recovery to baseline.[53,65,67,68]

Both systolic and diastolic blood pressures rise during resistance exercise. The degree of increase is influenced by the intensity of contraction, amount of muscle engaged, and the contraction time.[2] Although exceptionally heavy loads and large muscle mass exercises can produce high blood pressures (330/250 mm Hg),[69] these values have not been reproduced in other studies that have shown typical elevations of 230/130 mm Hg.[2,68] Cross-sectional studies of strength-trained athletes generally show little difference in blood pressure compared to untrained subjects.[2] Meta-analyses of training studies generally show small decreases in both systolic (4.5 mm Hg) and diastolic (3.8 mm Hg) pressures due to resistance training.[70] These values compare favorably with meta-analyses of changes resulting from aerobic training of 4.7 mm Hg (systolic) and 3.1 mm Hg (diastolic).[71] Resistance training has also been shown to reduce blood pressure during resistance exercise[2,68,72] and during treadmill and cycle exercise.[2,68,73,74]

RPP, which equals HR × systolic BP (SBP), estimates myocardial oxygen consumption and work and may be of considerable importance in evaluating ischemic heart disease (IHD). IHD results from an imbalance of myocardial oxygen supply and demand. Thus, a decreased RPP would be a beneficial alteration that reduces risk of IHD. A cross-sectional study of body builders showed that they had lower resting and exercise RPPs[75] and several longitudinal studies have reported lower resting and exercise RPPs compared to controls.[64,68,69,76] These findings for HR, BP, and RPP indicate that there can be carryover from resistance training to other activities, thus providing a reduced potential for ischemic events during physical activity.

Although aerobic power ($\dot{V}o_{2max}$) has not been directly associated with disease, it is a good measure of cardiovascular function. Although resistance training has not generally been associated with increases in aerobic power, highly weight-trained athletes performing little or no aerobic training have higher $\dot{V}o_{2max}$ than untrained controls.[77–79] Short-term longitudinal studies, including circuit weight training, suggest changes in $\dot{V}o_{2max}$ are typically $< 5\%$.[2,80,81] However, when using large muscle mass, multijoint exercises, larger increases in $\dot{V}o_{2max}$ (8% to 10%) can be accomplished. Although the gains in aerobic power are lower than that expected from aerobic training, these data suggest that aerobic metabolic function can be enhanced as a result of high volume resistance training.[2]

Body Composition

Higher levels of lean body mass (LBM) and lower total and percent body fats are typically related to better performance. Excess body fat has been related to many different types of disease states including hypertension, hyperlipidemia, IHD, insulin resistance, diabetes mellitus, and osteoarthritis. Although resistance training is anaerobic in nature, both intramuscular[82] and serum triglycerides[83] have been shown to decrease following resistance exercise. Decreased postresistance exercise respiratory exchange ratios (RER) have been noted up to 3 hours[53,84,85] and during sleep. A decreased RER indicates an increase in fatty acid oxidation. These data indicate that resistance exercise may increase fatty acid oxidation to an extent during exercise and markedly postexercise.

An increased fatty acid oxidation over time (training) can result in body fat reductions. Highly weight-trained athletes, performing little or no aerobic exercise, show body fats ranging from 6% to 12% in men and 13% to 20% in women and when matched by age and weight with normal controls (14% to 17% in men; 20% to 25% in women), display lower total and percent fats.[2,39] Longitudinal studies also indicate that marked decreases in total and percent body fat and increases in LBM are possible in short periods of time (5 to 10 weeks).[2,39] The loss of percent fat, approximately 2.5% in 12 weeks, as a result of resistance training compares favorably with endurance training, which shows about a 2% decrease in 15 to 20 weeks.[86] Abdominal obesity may be particularly important in that it is believed to be a first step leading to insulin resistance, glucose intolerance, lipid-lipoprotein abnormalities, and hypertension.[61] Resistance training has been shown to provide substantial losses in abdominal fat in both men and women.[87–89] As with other variables, the training intensity and volume can markedly influence changes in body composition.[2]

Blood Lipids

High cholesterol, low high density lipoprotein-C (HDL-C), and high low density lipoprotein-C (LDL-C) are related to an increased incidence of a number of diseases including coronary heart disease, atherosclerosis, diabetes mellitus, and nephrotic syndrome. Although aerobic training is generally believed to have positive effects on blood lipids, the exact nature of the alterations is unclear.[2]

In cross-sectional studies that have not adequately controlled for androgen use, or type, volume, and intensity of training, little difference is noted in blood lipid profiles compared to sedentary subjects.[90–92] Positive lipid profiles have been noted in strength athletes when androgen use was controlled.[93–96] Furthermore, an epidemiologic study controlling for a variety of factors including smoking, alcohol use, body mass index, and age concluded that strength training can reduce total cholesterol and that the reductions increase with the volume of training.[97] Longitudinal studies have not always shown beneficial alterations in blood lipids as a result of either aerobic or resistance training.[2] However, evidence suggests that beneficial adaptations in blood lipids can occur over relatively short strength training periods (8 to 15 weeks) in both men and women.[2,39,98]

As with aerobic training, the exact effects of resistance training on lipid profile adaptations are not totally understood. Part of the problems with these studies, which have led to an incomplete understanding of blood lipid alterations with training, are concerned with design errors in some studies as well as differences in volume, intensity, and exercise selection.[2]

Gastric Motility

Impaired gastric motility is related to diseases such as diverticulosis and colorectal cancers. Improvement in gastric motility can reduce the potential for gastrointestinal tract diseases, and motility is improved through physical activity, including resistance training.[99]

Glucose Tolerance

Poor glucose tolerance and high blood glucose concentrations are associated with a number of diseases including noninsulin dependent diabetes mellitus, coronary artery disease, stroke, retinopathy, nephropathy, and risk of infection. Physical activity may enhance glucose tolerance. Muscle contraction increases glucose uptake by muscle cells by enhancing the translocation of glucose transporter proteins from the cytoplasmic pool to the cell membrane and in this manner mimics the effects of insulin.[100] Thus, muscle contraction facilitates glucose entry into the cell. Over time, as a result of training, this increased "sensitivity" to glucose may reduce the degenerative effects of high circulating glucose concentrations. Additionally, if the amount of muscle can be increased through training, this beneficial effect may be potentiated through improved insulin sensitivity and glucose uptake.[96]

Cross-sectional data indicate that bodybuilders have improved glucose tolerance and insulin sensitivity compared to control subjects.[96] Short-term longitudinal studies agree with the cross-sectional data,[2,61] and comparisons indicate that improved insulin sensitivity is greater following resistance training than aerobic training.[101] Furthermore, it has been shown that hemoglobin A1c, an indicator of long-term glucose control, is reduced in diabetic patients engaged in resistance training.[102,103] Thus, resistance training should be encouraged in diabetics.

Tissue Tensile Strength

Increased tissue strength can be an important factor in reducing the potential for injury.[104] Strength training offers advantages over other forms of training in that it can markedly increase the size and tensile strength of connective tissue including bone, thus reducing the potential for injury.[104] Of special importance for women is the potential effect of resistance training on bone. Osteoporosis is a disease state that is characterized by a progressive loss of bone material. Osteoporosis predominantly affects the elderly, particularly postmenopausal women, and it is related to changes in hormone status. Loss of bone material and subsequent decreases in bone mineral density (BMD) weaken the tissue and increase the potential for fractures.

Imposed mechanical stress on bone is critical for maintaining or increasing BMD.[104] A minimal effective strain (MES) is necessary to maintain or increase BMD; furthermore, it appears that a relative high strain rate may be the most important factor in stimulating new bone growth.[104] As a result of both relatively high forces and rates of force development, resistance training, provided appropriate exercise selection is used, is particularly suited for maintaining or promoting BMD.

Highly strength-trained athletes have higher values for BMD than sedentary controls or athletes in endurance sports.[105,106] Although not all longitudinal studies have shown increases in BMD, several recent studies have shown beneficial alterations in adult[107–109] and elderly women.[110–112] It is also important to note that increases in BMD in specific areas appear to be strongly related to the types of exercises performed and the movement patterns involved (ie, axial loading; closed versus open kinetic chain movements).

Flexibility

Flexibility is the range of motion about a joint. Flexibility decreases with inactivity and as a result of aging. Loss of flexibility (and strength) can be related to both athletic and daily task performance dysfunction and a decline in health status.[2,113] Hurley and Hagberg[61] have criticized strength training studies that show improved flexibility, pointing out design flaws in some of the studies. They suggest that there is no evidence that strength training can enhance flexibility. A key point overlooked by Hurley and Hagberg[61] is exercise selection. If the exercise used requires movement through a range of motion not typically encountered, then flexibility can be enhanced. For example, most people can already perform a leg extension through its full range of motion; however, many cannot perform a parallel squat through its full range of motion. Performing squats as part of a strength-training program will improve flexibility and the same arguments can be made for a variety of movements. Based on both cross-sectional and longitudinal studies, resistance training, with appropriate exercise selection, can maintain or enhance flexibility.[2,39,114,115] Appropriate exercise selection would include movements beyond normal ranges and training both sides (agonist and antagonist) of the joint.[2]

Risk of Injury

Properly planned and implemented weight training and weightlifting programs are safe and have very low injury rates compared to most sports and recreational activities.[116,117] It is commonly believed that machines are safer than free weights; however, there are no data to support this idea.[22] Performing maximum attempts (1RMs) has also been discouraged on the assumption that there is an increased risk of injury during their performance. However, this has not been confirmed experimentally and evidence suggests that injuries are rare.

Additionally, resistance training has been associated with a reduction in rate and severity of injury when participating in other activities and sports.[118–122] This effect is partially due to strengthening of musculoskeletal components, including muscle, ligaments, tendons, and cartilage, and to improved ability to perform specific movements.

Summary

Although much of the information currently available dealing with resistance training is based on studies using men, there is little reason to believe that similar general effects do not occur in women. Training data indicate that there is a high degree of specificity in strength training, including force production characteristics, velocity, and movement patterns. Thus, exercise selection should address performance needs. Periodization of training offers distinct advantages over nonperiodized programs, particularly for athletes.

Improved force generating capabilities are a primary consideration for most sports, particularly those requiring great strength and power such as weightlifting, throwing events, and sprinting. Appropriate resistance training is a requirement for most sports; proper integration of strength training requires detailed and circumspect planing.

Appropriate training with sufficient volume and intensity can beneficially alter a wide variety of health and performance parameters. From a health standpoint, resistance training should be started at an early age and be viewed as a preventive mechanism. When properly performed, resistance training is a safe and effective tool.

References

1. Holloway JB: A summary chart: Age related changes in women and men and their possible improvement with training. *J Strength Cond Res* 1998;12:126–128.
2. Stone MH, Fleck SJ, Triplett NT, Kraemer WJ: Health- and performance-related potential of resistance training. *Sports Med* 1991;11:210–231.
3. Stone MH, Plisk SS, Stone ME, Schilling BK, O'Bryant HS, Pierce KC: Athletic performance development: Volume load. 1 set vs multiple sets, training velocity, and training variation. *Strength Cond* 1998;20:22–31.
4. Harris G, Stone MH, O'Bryant HS, Proulx CM, Johnson R: Short-term performance effects of high speed, high force, and combined weight training. *J Strength Cond Res* 2000;14:14–20.
5. McBride JM, Triplett-McBride T, Davie A, Newton RU: A comparison of strength and power characteristics between power lifters, Olympic lifters and sprinters. *J Strength Cond Res* 1999;13:58–66.
6. Stone MH, O'Bryant HS (eds): *Weight Training: A Scientific Approach.* Minneapolis, MN, Burgess Publishers, 1987.
7. Frobose I, Verdonck A, Duesberg F, Mucha C: Effects of various load intensities in the framework of postoperative stationary endurance training on performance deficit of the quadriceps muscle of the thigh. *Z Orthop Ihre Grenzgeb* 1993;131:164–167.
8. Conley M, Rozenek R: Health aspects of resistance exercise and training. *Strength Cond*, in press.
9. Newton RU, Kraemer WJ, Hakkinen K, Humphries BJ, Murphy AJ: Kinematics, kinetics, and muscle activation during explosive upper body movements. *J Appl Biomech* 1996;12:31–43.
10. Kramer J, Stone MH, O'Bryant HS, et al: Effects of single versus multiple sets of weight training: Impact of volume, intensity and variation. *J Strength Cond Res* 1997;11:143–147.
11. Kraemer WJ: A series of studies: The physiological basis for strength training in American Football. Fact over philosophy. *J Strength Cond Res* 1997;11:131–142.
12. Cratty BJ: *Teaching Motor Skills.* Englewood, CA, Prentice Hall, 1979.
13. Knapp B (ed): *Skill in Sport: The Attainment of Proficiency.* London, England, Routledge and K. Paul, 1963.
14. Sale DG: Neural adaptation to resistance training. *Med Sci Sports Exerc* 1988;20(suppl 5):S135–S145.
15. Sale DG: Neural adaptation to strength training, in Komi PV (ed): *Strength and Power in Sport.* Oxford, England, Blackwell Scientific Publications, 1992, pp 249–265.

16. Behm DG: Neuromuscular implications and applications of resistance training. *J Strength Cond Res* 1995;9:264–274.
17. Stone MH, Borden RA: Modes and methods of resistance training. *Strength Cond* 1997;19:18–24.
18. Hakkinen K: Neuromuscular adaptation during strength training, aging, detraining and immobilization. *Crit Rev Phys Rehab Med* 1994;6:161–198.
19. Wilson GJ, Newton RU, Murphy AJ, Humphries BJ: The optimal training load for the development of dynamic athletic performance. *Med Sci Sports Exerc* 1993;25:1279–1286.
20. Stone MH: Explosive exercises and training: Literature review. *Natl Strength Cond Assoc J* 1993;15:7–15.
21. Medvedev AS, Rodionov VF, Rogozkin VN, Gulyants AE: Training content of weightlifters during the preparation period. *Teoriya I Praktika Fizicheskoi Kultury* 1981;12:5–7.
22. Requa RK, DeAvilla LN, Garrick JG: Injuries in recreational adult fitness activities. *Am J Sports Med* 1993;21:461–467.
23. Scala D, McMillan J, Blessing D, Rozenek R, Stone MH: Metabolic cost of a preparatory phase of training for weightlifting. *J Appl Sports Sci Res* 1987;1:48–52.
24. Abernethy PJ, Jurimae J: Cross-sectional and longitudinal uses of isoinertial, isometric, and isokinetic dynamometry. *Med Sci Sports Exerc* 1996;28:1180–1187.
25. Fry AC, Powell DR, Kraemer WJ: Validity of isometric testing modalities for assessing short-term resistance exercise strength gains. *J Sport Rehab* 1992;1:275–283.
26. Rasch PJ, Morehouse LE: Effect of static and dynamic exercises on muscular strength and hypertrophy. *J Appl Physiol* 1957;11:29–34.
27. Rutherford OM, Jones DA: The role of learning and coordination in strength training. *Eur J Appl Physiol* 1986;55:100–105.
28. Canavan PK, Garrett GE, Armstrong LE: Kinematic and kinetic relationships between an Olympic-style lift and the vertical jump. *J Strength Cond Res* 1996;10:127–130.
29. Garhammer J: Equipment for the development of athletic strength and power. *NSCA J* 1981;3:24–26.
30. Kovaleski JE, Heitman RH, Trundle TL, Gilley WF: Isotonic preload versus isokinetic knee extension resistance training. *Med Sci Sports Exerc* 1995;27:895–899.
31. Nosse LJ, Hunter GR: Free weights: A review supporting their use in rehabilitation. *Athletic Training* 1985;Fall:402–413.
32. Stone M: Considerations for gaining a strength-power training effect. *NSCA J* 1982;4:22–24.
33. Stone MH, Garhammer J: Some thoughts on strength and power: The nautilus controversy. *NSCA J* 1981;3:24–40.
34. Cabell L, Zebas CJ: Resistive torque validation of the Nautilus multi-biceps machine. *J Strength Cond Res* 1999;13:20–23.
35. Chow JW, Darling WG, Hay JG: Mechanical characteristics of knee extension exercises performed on an isokinetic dynamometer. *Med Sci Sports Exerc* 1997;29:794–803.
36. Carpinelli RN, Otto RM: Strength training: Single versus multiple sets. *Sports Med* 1998;26:73–84.
37. Stone MH, O'Bryant HS, Pierce KC, et al: Periodization: Effects of manipulating volume and intensity: Part 1. *Strength Cond* 1999;21:56–62.

38. Stone MH, O'Bryant HS, Pierce KC, et al: Periodization: Effects of manipulating volume and intensity: Part 2. *Strength Cond* 1999;21:54–60.
39. Fleck SJ, Kraemer WJ (eds): Designing Resistance Training Programs, ed 2. Champaign, IL, *Human Kinetics*, 1997.
40. Sanborn CF, Jankowski CM: Physiologic considerations for women in sport. *Clin Sports Med* 1994;13:315–327.
41. Miller AE, MacDougall JD, Tarnopolsky MA, Sale DG: Gender differences in strength and muscle fiber characteristics. *Eur J Appl Physiol* 1993;66:254–262.
42. Lewis DA, Kamon E, Hodgson JL: Physiological differences between genders: Implications for sports conditioning. *Sports Med* 1986;3:357–369.
43. Kraemer WJ, Koziris LP: Olympic weightlifting and powerlifting, in Lamb DR, Knuttgen HG, Murray R (eds): *Physiology and Nutrition for Competitive Sport*, Carmel, IN, Cooper Publishing, 1994, pp 1–54.
44. Lindle RS, Metter EJ, Lynch NA, et al: Age and gender comparisons of muscle strength in 654 women and men aged 20-93 yrs. *J Appl Physiol* 1997;83:1581–1587.
45. Harries UJ, Bassey EJ: Torque-velocity relationships for the knee extensors in women in their 3rd and 7th decades. *Eur J Appl Physiol* 1990;60:187–190.
46. Fung L, Ha A: Changes in track and field performance with chronological aging. *Int J Aging Hum Dev* 1994;38:171–180.
47. Rozenek R, Garhammer JJ: Male-female strength comparisons and rate of strength decline with age in weightlifting and powerlifting in *Conference Proceedings, International Symposium on Weightlifting and Strength Training*, Lahti, Finland, 1998, pp 287–288.
48. Garhammer JJ: A comparison of maximal power outputs between elite male and female weightlifters in competition. *Int J Sport Biomech* 1991;7:3–11.
49. Komi PV, Karlsson J: Skeletal muscle fiber types: Enzyme activities and physical performance in young males and females. *Acta Physiol Scand* 1978;103:210–218.
50. Ryushi T, Hakkinen K, Kauhanen H, Komi PV: Muscle fiber characteristics, muscle cross-sectional area and force production in strength athletes and physically active males and females. *Scand J Sport Sci* 1988;10:7–15.
51. Gotshalk L, Kraemer WJ, Nindl BC, et al: Contribution of upper body training on total body strength and power in young women. *Med Sci Sports Exerc* 1998;30(suppl):S162.
52. Kraemer WJ: Endocrine responses and adaptations to strength training, in Komi PV (ed): *Strength and Power in Sport*. Oxford, England, Blackwell Scientific Publications, 1992, pp 291–304.
53. McMillan JL, Stone MH, Sartin J, et al: 20-hour physiological responses to a single weight-training session. *J Strength Cond Res* 1993;7:9–21.
54. Hakkinen K, Pakarinen A, Kyrolainen H, Cheng S, Kim DH, Komi PV: Neuromuscular adaptations and serum hormones in females during prolonged power training. *Int J Sports Med* 1990;11:91–98.
55. Reis E, Frick U, Schmidtbleicher D: Frequency variations of strength training sessions triggered by the phases of the menstrual cycle. *Int J Sports Med* 1995;16:545–550.
56. Dolezal BA, Potteiger JA: Concurrent resistance and endurance training influence basal metabolic rate in nondieting individuals. *J Appl Physiol* 1998;85:695–700.
57. Dudley GA, Djamil R: Incompatibility of endurance- and strength-training modes of exercise. *J Appl Physiol* 1985;59:1446–1451.
58. Hennessy LC, Watson AWS: The interference effects of training for strength and endurance simultaneously. *J Strength Cond Res* 1994;8:12–19.

59. Kraemer WJ, Patton JF, Gordon SE, et al: Compatibility of high-intensity strength and endurance training on hormonal and skeletal muscle adaptations. *J Appl Physiol* 1995;78:976–989 .
60. Pierce K, Rozenek R, Stone MH: Effects of high volume weight training on lactate, heart rate, and perceived exertion. *J Strength Cond Res* 1993;7:211–215.
61. Hurley BF, Hagberg JM: Optimizing health in older persons: Aerobic or strength training? *Exerc Sport Sci Rev* 1998;26:61–89.
62. Blessing D, Stone MH, Byrd R, et al: Blood lipid and hormonal changes from jogging and weight training of middle-aged men. *J Appl Sports Sci Res* 1987;1:2–29.
63. Goldberg L, Elliot DL and Kuehl KS: Cardiovascular changes at rest and during mixed static and dynamic exercise after weight training. *J Appl Sports Sci Res* 1988;1:42–45.
64. Parker ND, Hunter GR, Treuth MS, et al: Effects of strength training on cardiovascular responses during a submaximal walk and a weight-loaded walking test in older females. *J Cardiopulm Rehabil* 1996;16:56–62.
65. Stone MH, Blessing DL, Byrd R, et al: Physiological effects of short-term resistive training on middle-aged sedentary men. *NSCA J* 1982;4:16–20.
66. Stone MH, Nelson JK, Nader C, Carter D: Short-term weight training effects on resting and recovery heart rates. *Athletic Training* 1983;18:69–71.
67. Kusinitz I, Keeney CE: Effects of progressive weight training on health and physical fitness of adolescent boys. *Res Q* 1958;29:294–301.
68. Stone MH, Pierce K, Godsen R, et al: Heart rate and lactate levels during weight-training exercise in trained and untrained men. *Phys Sportsmed* 1987;15:97–105.
69. MacDougall JD, Tuxen D, Sale DG, Moroz JR, Sutton JR: Arterial blood pressure response to heavy resistance exercise. *J Appl Physiol* 1985;58:785–790.
70. Kelley G: Dynamic resistance exercise and resting blood pressure in adults: A meta-analysis. *J Appl Physiol* 1997;82:1559–1565.
71. Halbert JA, Silagy CA, Finucane P, Withers RT, Hamdorf PA, Andrews GR: The effectiveness of exercise training in lowering blood pressure: A meta-analysis of randomised controlled trials of 4 weeks or longer. *J Hum Hypertens* 1997;11:641–649.
72. Fleck SJ, Dean LS: Resistance-training experience and the pressor response during resistance exercise. *J Appl Physiol* 1987;63:116–120.
73. Goldberg L, Elliot DL, Kuehl KS: A comparison of the cardiovascular effects of running and weight training. *J Strength Cond Res* 1994;8:219–224.
74. Copeland SR, Mills MC, Lerner JL, Crizer MF, Thompson CW, Sullivan JM: Hemodynamic effects of aerobic vs resistance exercise. *J Hum Hypertens* 1996;10:747–753.
75. Colliander EB, Tesch PA: Abstract: Long-term effect of heavy resistance training on rest and exercise blood pressure response. *Med Sci Sports Exerc* 1985;17:184.
76. Coale JA, Butler JJ, Santa Maria DL, Ostrove SM, Hurley BF: Abstract: Weight training and running reduce myocardial oxygen demand (MVO_2) but not by reducing sympathetic response. *Med Sci Sports Exerc* 1987;19(suppl):S42.
77. Fahey TD, Akka L, Rolph R: Body composition and Vo2max of exceptional weight-trained athletes. *J Appl Physiol* 1975;39:559–561.
78. Saltin B, Astrand PO: Maximal oxygen uptake in athletes. *J Appl Physiol* 1967;23:353–358.
79. Stone MH, Smith D, Ward T, Carter D: Olympic weightlifting: I. Physiological characteristics of the athlete, in Terauds J (ed): *Science in Weightlifting*. Del Mar, CA, Academic Publishers, 1979, pp 45–54.

80. Hickson RC, Rosenkoetter MA, Brown MM: Strength training effects on aerobic power and short-term endurance. *Med Sci Sports Exerc* 1980;12:336–339.

81. Fahey TD, Brown CH: The effects of an anabolic steroid on the strength, body composition, and endurance of college males when accompanied by a weight training program. *Med Sci Sports* 1973;5:272–276.

82. Essen-Gustavsson B, Tesch PA: Glycogen and triglyceride utilization in relation to muscle metabolic characteristics in men performing heavy-resistance exercise. *Eur J Appl Physiol* 1990;61:5–10.

83. Wallace MB, Moffatt RJ, Haymes EM, Green NR: Acute effects of resistance exercise on parameters of lipoprotein metabolism. *Med Sci Sports Exerc* 1991;23:199–204.

84. Melby C, Scholl C, Edwards G, Bullough R: Effect of acute resistance exercise on postexercise energy expenditure and resting metabolic rate. *J Appl Physiol* 1993;75:1847–1853.

85. Van Etten LM, Westerterp KR, Verstappen FT: Effect of weight-training on energy expenditure and substrate utilization during sleep. *Med Sci Sports Exerc* 1995;27:188–193.

86. Wilmore JH: Body composition in sport and exercise: Directions for future research. *Med Sci Sports Exerc* 1983;15:21–31.

87. Treuth MS, Ryan AS, Pratley RE, et al: Effects of strength training on total and regional body composition in older men. *J Appl Physiol* 1994:77:614–620.

88. Treuth MS, Hunter GR, Kekes-Szabo T, Weinsier RL, Goran MI, Berland L: Reduction in intra-abdominal adipose tissue after strength training in older women. *J Appl Physiol* 1995;78:1425–1431.

89. Ross R, Rissanen J, Pedwell H, Clifford J, Shragge P: Influence of diet and exercise on skeletal muscle and visceral adipose tissue in men. *J Appl Physiol* 1996;81:2445–2455.

90. Berg AJ, Ringwald G, Keul J: Lipoprotein cholesterol in well-trained athletes: Preliminary communication: Reduced HDL-cholesterol in power athletes. *Int J Sports Med* 1980;1:137–138.

91. Clarkson PM, Hintermister R, Fillyaw M, Stylos L: High density lipoprotein cholesterol in young adult weight lifters, runners and untrained subjects. *Hum Biol* 1981;53:251–257.

92. Farrell PA, Maksud MG, Pollock ML, et al: A comparison of plasma cholesterol, triglycerides, and high density lipoprotein-cholesterol in speed skaters, weightlifters and non-athletes. *Eur J Appl Physiol* 1982;48:77–82.

93. Cuppers HJ, Erdman D, Schubert H, et al: Glucose tolerance, serum insulin and serum lipids in athletes, in Berger M (ed): *Diabetes and Exercise*. Bern, Switzerland, Hans Huber, 1982, pp 115–165.

94. Hurley BF, Seals DR, Hagberg JM, et al: High-density-lipoprotein cholesterol in bodybuilders vs powerlifters: Negative effects of androgen use. *JAMA* 1984;252:507–513.

95. Yeater R, Reed C, Ullrich I, Morise A, Borsch M: Resistance-trained athletes using or not using anabolic steroids compared to runners: Effects on cardiorespiratory variables, body composition, and plasma lipids. *Br J Sports Med* 1996;30:11–14.

96. Yki-Jarvinen H, Koivisto VA, Taskinen MR, Nikkila E: Glucose tolerance, plasma lipoproteins and tissue lipoprotein lipase activities in bodybuilders. *Eur J Appl Physiol* 1984;53:253–259.

97. Tucker LA, Silvester LJ: Strength training and hypercholesterolemia: An epidemiologic study of 8499 employed men. *Am J Health Promot* 1996;11:35–41.

98. Boyden TW, Pamenter RW, Going SB, et al: Resistance exercise training is associated with decreases in serum low-density lipoprotein cholesterol levels in premenopausal women. *Arch Intern Med* 1993;153:97–100.

99. Koffler KH, Menkes A, Redmond RA, Whitehead WE, Pratley RE, Hurley BF: Strength training accelerates gastrointestinal transit in middle-aged and older men. *Med Sci Sports Exerc* 1992;24:415–419.

100. Hayashi T, Wojtaszewski JF, Goodyear LJ: Exercise regulation of glucose transport in skeletal muscle. *Am J Physiol* 1997;273:E1039–E1051.

101. Eriksson J, Tuominen J, Valle T, et al: Aerobic endurance exercise or circuit-type resistance training for individuals with impaired glucose tolerance? *Horm Metab Res* 1998;30:37–41.

102. Eriksson J, Taimela S, Eriksson K, Parviainen S, Peltonen J, Kujala U: Resistance training in the treatment of non–insulin-dependent diabetes mellitus. *Int J Sports Med* 1997;18:242–246.

103. Honkola A, Forsen T, Eriksson J: Resistance training improves the metabolic profile in individuals with type 2 diabetes. *Acta Diabetol* 1997;34:245–248.

104. Stone MH: Connective tissue and bone response to strength training, in Komi PV (ed): *Strength and Power in Sport*. Oxford, England, Blackwell Scientific Publications, 1992, pp 279–290.

105. Nilsson BE, Westlin NE: Bone density in athletes. *Clin Orthop* 1971;77:179–182.

106. Conroy BP, Kraemer WJ, Maresh CM, et al: Bone mineral density in elite junior Olympic weight lifters. *Med Sci Sports Exerc* 1993;25:1103–1109.

107. Dornemann TM, McMurray RG, Renner JB, Anderson JJ: Effects of high-intensity resistance exercise on bone mineral density and muscle strength of 40-50-year-old women. *J Sports Med Phys Fitness* 1997;37:246–251.

108. Lohman T, Going S, Pamenter R, et al: Effects of resistance training on regional and total bone mineral density in premenopausal women: A randomized prospective study. *J Bone Miner Res* 1995;10:1015–1024.

109. Snow-Harter C, Bouxsein ML, Lewis BT, Carter DR, Marcus R: Effects of resistance and endurance exercise on bone mineral status of young women: A randomized exercise intervention trial. *J Bone Miner Res* 1992;7:761–769.

110. Kerr D, Morton A, Dick I, Prince R: Exercise effects on bone mass in postmenopausal women are site-specific and load-dependent. *J Bone Miner Res* 1996;11:218–225.

111. Menkes A, Mazel S, Redmond RA, et al: Strength training increases regional bone mineral density and bone remodeling in middle-aged and older men. *J Appl Physiol* 1993;74:2478–2484.

112. Yarasheski KE, Campbell JA, Kohrt WM: Effect of resistance exercise and growth hormone on bone density in older men. *Clin Endocrinol (Oxf)* 1997;47:223–229.

113. Gehlsen GM, Whaley MH: Falls in the elderly. Part II: Balance, strength, and flexibility. *Arch Phys Med Rehabil* 1990;71:739–741.

114. Leighton JR: An instrument and technique for the measurement of range of joint motion. *Arch Phys Med Rehabil* 1955;36:571–577.

115. Beedle B, Jesse C, Stone MH: Flexibility characteristics among athletes who weight train. *J Appl Sports Sci Res* 1991;5:150–154.

116. Hamill B: Relative safety of weightlifting and weight training. *J Strength Cond Res* 1994;8:53–57.

117. Powell KE, Heath GW, Kresnow MJ, Sacks JJ, Branche CM: Injury rates from walking, gardening, weightlifting, outdoor bicycling, and aerobics. *Med Sci Sports Exerc* 1998;30:1246–1249.

118. Dominguez RH: Shoulder pain in age group swimmers, in Eriksson BO, Furberg B (eds): *Swimming Medicine IV*, Baltimore, MD, University Park Press, 1978, pp 105–109.

119. Gruchow HW, Pelletier P: An epidemiologic study of tennis elbow: Incidence, recurrence, and effectiveness of prevention strategies. *Am J Sports Med* 1979;7:234–238.

120. Hawkins RJ, Kennedy JC: Impingement syndrome in athletes. *Am J Sports Med* 1980;8:151–158.

121. Kulund DN, McCue FC III, Rockwell DA, Gieck JH: Tennis injuries: Prevention and treatment: *A review. Am J Sports Med* 1979;7:249–253.

122. Lehnhard RA, Lehnhard HR, Young R, Butterfield SA: Monitoring injuries on a college soccer team: The effect of strength training. *J Strength Cond Res* 1996;10:115–119.

Chapter 22

Flexibility and Conditioning in Women

Terry R. Malone, EdD, PT, ATC

Flexibility

Flexibility is easily perceived but may be a somewhat abstract measure. Kendall[1] defines this term as: "The ability to readily adapt to changes in position or alignment; may be expressed as normal, limited, or excessive." This definition presents the challenge of what is to be perceived and actually measured as normal, limited, or excessive. Clinical assessment often requires the comparison of side-to-side measures and thus permits the individual to serve as his or her control. This assessment must use the opposite limb but also consider the expected in the population. Specific activities require significantly more adaptability than others, and thus some populations (gymnastics, ballet, swimming, etc) will display very different levels than others. DeVries[2] defines flexibility in a more measurable sense: "Flexibility may be most simply defined as the range of motion available in a joint, such as the hip, or a series of joints, such as the spine." This definition leads to measurement via goniometer but begs the question as to what is causing restriction when seen in side-to-side comparison or when compared with specific population norms. Zachazewski[3] provides an eloquent synopsis of this problem, defining a person's flexibility as being dependent on actual joint range of motion (dictated by the deformation properties of the periarticular connective tissues and the arthrokinematics of the specific joint) and the muscle flexibility (ability of a muscle to lengthen enabling the joint or series of joints to go through their available range). Total flexibility is the sum of these two components with either being able to be restricted or enhanced.[3]

The periarticular tissues are the passive structures (eg, ligaments, capsules, fascias) that control and maintain the congruity of the joint enabling the active element (muscle-tendon unit) to provide movement or to absorb or dissipate forces. Influencing these actions are the neurophysiologic structures that gain information related to movement, speed of movement, and tension but also enable efferent drive to the muscle-tendon unit to protect joint structures from damaging and deforming forces. These structures and their interactions are described by Rowinski[4] (Figs. 1 and 2 and Table 1).

The passive structures are primarily collagen based with some ligaments having significant stiffness and thus being somewhat inelastic[5] while the active element is metabolically active and sensitive to normal, resting length.[6] Clinicians often attempt to use stretching patterns or techniques to effect lasting deformation of these tissues. Basic science evaluation demonstrates the viscoelastic properties of such collagen, with Taylor and associates[7] providing a description of these properties. Several significant concepts are displayed as tension and length responses show the phenomena of force-relaxation and creep-hysteresis of viscoelastic muscle-tendon units. It is interesting to note that significant differences were seen in repeated stretches 1-4 but no differences thereafter in 5-10. This pattern is also seen in the other force-tension sequences reinforcing the often cited concept of requesting a patient to perform 3 repetitions of 10 counts. Bandy and Irion[8] demonstrated this as well, with the hamstring muscle-tendon unit of humans responding in a similar pattern.

Patterns of flexibility training have typically been divided into static (joint position maintained placing collagen-based tissues on stretch), ballistic (quick, active movement into a stretched position), and neuromuscular patterns frequently described as proprioceptive neuromuscular facilitation. These techniques use reciprocal innervation and inhibition. Each of these may be effective and result in gains in flexibility.[3,8]

Flexibility should probably be represented in its dynamic as well as passive state. Although it is measured in a passive state, people function dynamically and at high velocities in sports activities. This process is often underemphasized in rehabilitation and preparticipation routines. The active elements require neurologic drive and are sensitive to temperature as is the collagen tissue as well.[9,10] This points to the introduction of a dynamic portion of stretching (use of the active element to move the joint through its range of

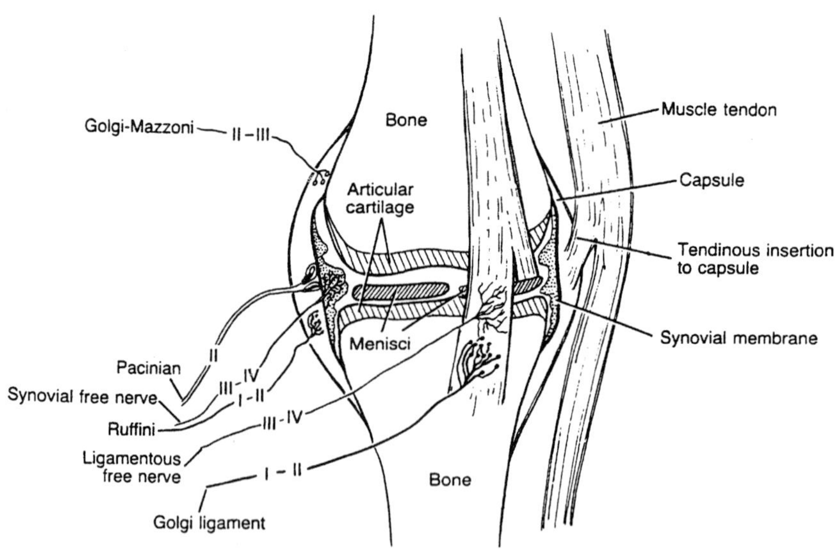

Fig. 1 Composite diagram of total joint innervation pattern, showing interrelations of afferent receptors. (Reproduced with permission from Malone TR, McPoil TG, Nitz AJ (eds): Orthopedic and Sports Physical Therapy, *ed 3. St. Louis, MO, Mosby-Year Book, 1997, p 51.)*

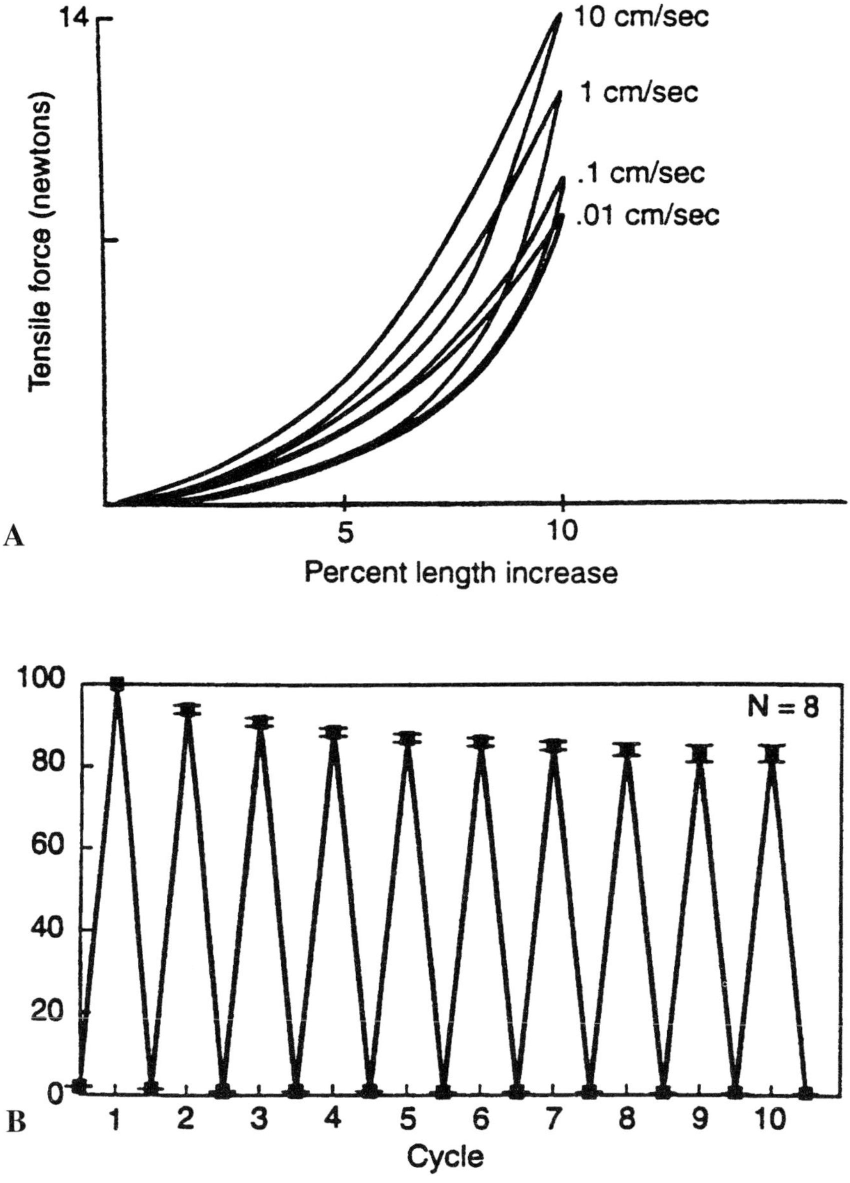

***Fig. 2 A**, Tension curves of extensor digitorum longus muscle-tendon units repeatedly stretched to 10% beyond resting length. Each of the peak tensions for the first four stretches showed a statistically significant* (p < *0.05) difference from the other peak tensions. The overall tension decrease was 16.6%. **B**, Hysteresis loops observed in thyroarytenoid muscle during loading and unloading at constant rates of 0.01, 0.1, 1, and 10 cm/s. (Reproduced with permission from Taylor DC, Dalton JD, Seaber AV, et al: Viscoelastic properties of muscle-tendon units: The biomechanical effects of stretching.* Am J Sports Med *1990;18:300–309.)*

Table 1 Joint receptors

Receptor	Location	Sensitivity	Distribution (of receptor types)	Functional classification
Pacinian corpuscles	Fibrous layer of capsule, on capsule-synovium border, close to small blood vessels	Sensitive to high frequency vibration (> 60 Hz), acceleration, and high velocity changes in joint position; possible sensitivity to hemohydraulic, transient events of adjacent muscles	Found in all joints examined; sole corpuscular receptor in laryngeal and middle ear joints; greater density in distal than in proximal joints	Very rapidly adapting; very low mechanical threshold
Golgi-Mazzoni corpuscles	Inner surface of joint capsule between fibrous layer and subcapsular fibroadipose tissue	Sensitive to compression of joint capsule in plane perpendicular to its inner surface; insensitive to stretching capsule	Knee joint and many others likely; may have specific distribution within joint capsule	Slowly adapting; response is linear function of compressive stress on capsule; low mechanical threshold
Ruffini endings	Fibrous layer of capsule; few present in extrinsic ligaments	Sensitive to capsule stretching along either of its long axes within capsular plane, direction and speed, of capsular stretch, intracapsular fluid pressure change, amplitude and velocityof joint-position change	Few present in distal joints; greater density in proximal joints; concentrated in capsular regions of most stress	Slowly adapting; low mechanical threshold; response is linear function of axial components of capsular plane stress
Golgi ligament endings (Golgi tendon organlike)	Extrinsic and intrinsic ligaments; adjacent to bony attachments of ligaments	Sensitive to tension or stretch on ligaments	Present in most joints except cervical vertebral, laryngeal, and ossicular	Slowly adapting; low-to-high mechanical threshold
Free nerve endings (nociceptive and nonnociceptive)	Fibrous capsule, ligaments, subsynovial capsule, synovium, fat pads	One type sensitive to nonnoxious mechanical stress; other type sensitive to noxious mechanical or biochemical stimuli	Present in all joints examined but density varies with joint component; most joints have relatively higher density in ligaments	Slowly adapting; low-to-high mechanical threshold

(Reproduced with permission from Malone TR, McPoil TG, Nitz AJ (eds): *Orthopedic and Sports Physical Therapy*, ed 3. St. Louis, MO, Mosby-Year Book, 1997, p 51.)

motion) to build on the appropriate passive or static flexibility as assessed in clinical environments. This is described as a progression by Zachazewski[3] with static stretch being performed first then progressively followed with slow controlled end range movements, slow full range of motion patterns, and rapid end range movements, culminating in rapid full range actions. This process prepares the participants for their specific activities enabling an emphasis to the primary functional patterns.

An important question is does gender affect this process, placing specific or different requirements into consideration. Women typically present with greater flexibility and have a higher percentage of athletes rated as hypermobile.[11] Although Decoster and associates[11] found female lacrosse players often presenting with hypermobility, no significant difference in injury rate was seen in these athletes. National Collegiate Athletic Association Division 1 basketball players exhibit significantly greater hamstring flexibility as measured statically when compared to their male counterparts.[12] Female basketball players typically perform in a more upright position (less hip/trunk flexion and often less knee flexion) than male athletes (TR Malone, unpublished data, 1992; KE Wilk, PT, ATC, unpublished data, 1993). When considering gender specificity, frequently sport or activity demand will be the overriding factor. Thus, there are some differences in how women may accomplish a movement pattern in contrast to their male counterparts. These changes may predispose these athletes to specific injuries.

Wojtys and associates[12–14] and Huston and Wojtys[15] have pursued additional areas of performance differences. These investigators have demonstrated that women have decreased hamstring strength, increased ligamentous laxity, altered muscular recruitment patterns, and specific alterations related to the menstrual cycle. Each of these parameters impacts on the ability of female athletes to perform sports activities within their controlled state of "flexibility."

Conditioning

A common misconception has been that women will not benefit from conditioning and resistance training in an equivalent pattern to men. In many ways this is true as women may actually have a greater response. This is often an area of misinterpretation because gains must be viewed as relative to body mass or pretraining status rather than evaluated on absolute numbers. A classic study of this was done by Cureton and associates[16] who demonstrated the effects of a 16-week program of resistance training on men and women. They found men and women gain strength equally when performing identical programs. Other body composition measures provide data to support similar gains in women related to increased lean body mass, increased oxygen maximum, and increased muscular cross-sectional areas.[16–18] Although early results are similar, there is evidence that long-term gains in women slow when compared with gains in men in similar programs.[19–22] Several explanations based on this observation are possible, including: women have significantly lower testosterone levels leading to a less pronounced hypertrophy; women often have not used as varied a training regimen; women may have hormonal adjustments to training that alter the long-term response; or a combination of these factors as individual responses vary. Fleck and Kraemer[21] offer a comprehensive review of these factors in their book on designing weight training programs.

Upper body muscle mass is significantly greater in men than in women. This is true on both relative and absolute measures.[21] However, when examining lower extremity values, leg strength in women is 90+% that of men's relative to body mass; it is greater than 100% when normalized to lean body mass.[21]

When power measures are used, women frequently are 60% to 80% of men's values. These discrepancies are greatest when upper body contributions are required and least when the lower body is the focus.[21]

Conditioning factors related to endurance demonstrate both a difference in maximal values and cardiac limitations that decrease women's maximal values. Londeree[23] describes these gender differences as being related to decreased heart size (limiting stroke volume), oxygen carrying capacity, body fat percentage, and muscle mass.

Neuromuscular factors of training indicate a general gender "equality of response" with fatigue and recruitment being the focus of several investigations.[12–15,24,25] Huston and Wojtys[15] demonstrated the increased quadriceps reliance and decreased hamstring contributions in female athletes. Hewett and associates[25] instituted a plyometric lower extremity program with female jumping athletes that resulted in increased jumping ability with decreased impact loads. Colby and associates[26] showed that female athletes perform movements that place the anterior cruciate ligament at risk (ie, cutting) in a more erect posture than do male athletes.

Training should be sport specific rather than gender specific. Women can make significant gains in resistance programs with lower extremity values being relatively equal to or greater than those of men. Upper extremity values increase but are not capable of approaching those of the male athlete. Conditioning should also use periodization concepts, which should encourage continual improvement.[21] Although neural factors dominate some female adaptations, some relative muscle hypertrophy and fat loss occur.

Case Presentation

This case is presented to illustrate the concepts of flexibility and conditioning in female athletes and the specific approach that should be applied.[27]

Sample: Intercollegiate Division 1 Female Basketball Program

The goals of the program were as follows: (1) Increase the quickness of the backcourt players; (2) Increase the jumping ability of the frontcourt players; and (3) Decrease the likelihood of anterior cruciate ligament injuries (2 had occurred the previous year; prevalence of 4).

The problem is multifactorial. These athletes need a base program using periodization (strength-building phase, high-volume, off-season; strength and power phase, moderate volume-increasing intensity, off-season; peaking, in-season phase; active rest, early off-season).

The base program is supplemented by the specific needs of each athlete, thereby customizing the program. If flexibility deficits are identified, a specific stretching program is implemented. All preparticipation stretching is static to dynamic but with control.

Numerous hip and positioning drills are used to get these athletes into a more flexed posture. Plyometric routines are used in the off-season program, much as described by Hewett and associates.[25] Backward running drills and forced flexion hop-and-stop maneuvers are included. If swimming pools are available, a high-knee running routine in the pool, both forward and backward, is recommended. It is not enough to work only in isolated activities. Often these athletes have completed their season and are told to play as much as possible to work on their game rather than being given a comprehensive sequence of activities designed to enhance their performance the next season.

This program was implemented with strong acceptance by coaches and athletes. Although data are short term (3 years), significant improvements in individual and team outcomes have been made. Importantly, there has not been an anterior cruciate ligament injury during this time.

Summary

Flexibility and overall conditioning should be viewed as sport specific, not gender specific. Women respond equivalently in most circumstances. Integration of training techniques with sport skill enhancement and injury reduction should be the goal for the female athlete.

References

1. Kendall FP: Definitions/glossary, in Kendall FP, McCreary EK, Provance PG (eds): *Muscles: Testing and Function: With Posture and Pain*, ed 4. Baltimore, MD, Williams & Wilkins, 1993, pp 411–420.
2. DeVries HA: Flexibility, in DeVries HA (ed): *Physiology of Exercise for Physical Education and Athletics*, ed 3. Dubuque, IA, William C Brown, 1980, pp 462–472.
3. Zachazewski JE: Flexibility for sports, in Sanders B (ed): *Sports Physical Therapy*. Norwalk, CT, Appleton & Lange, 1990, pp 201–238.
4. Rowinski MJ: Neurobiology for orthopedic and sports physical therapy, in Malone TR, McPoil TG, Nitz AJ (eds): *Orthopedic and Sports Physical Therapy*, ed 3. St Louis, MO, Mosby-Year Book, 1997, pp 47–63.
5. Amiel D, Billings E Jr, Akeson WH: Ligament structure, chemistry, and physiology, in Daniel DM, Akeson WH, O'Connor JJ (eds): *Knee Ligaments: Structure, Function, Injury, and Repair*. New York, NY, Raven Press, 1990, pp 77–91.
6. McComas AJ (ed): *Skeletal Muscle: Form and Function*. Champaign, IL, Human Kinetics, 1996.
7. Taylor DC, Dalton JD Jr, Seaber AV, Garrett WE Jr: Viscoelastic properties of muscle-tendon units: The biomechanical effects of stretching. *Am J Sports Med* 1990;18:300–309.
8. Bandy WD, Irion JM: The effect of time on static stretch on the flexibility of the hamstring muscles. *Phys Ther* 1994;74:845–852.
9. Lehmann JF, De Lateur BJ: Therapeutic heat, in Lehmann JF (ed): *Therapeutic Heat and Cold*, ed 3. Baltimore, MD, Williams & Wilkins, 1982, pp 404–562.
10. Strickler T, Malone T, Garrett WE: The effects of passive warming on muscle injury. *Am J Sports Med* 1990;18:141–145.

11. Decoster LC, Bernier JN, Lindsay RH, Vailas JC: Generalized joint hypermobility and its relationship to injury patterns among NCAA lacrosse players. *J Athletic Training* 1999;34:99–105.

12. Wojtys EM, Wylie BB, Huston LJ: The effects of muscle fatigue on neuromuscular function and anterior tibial translation in healthy knees. *Am J Sports Med* 1996;24:615–621.

13. Wojtys EM, Huston LJ, Taylor PD, Bastian SD: Neuromuscular adaptations in isokinetic, isotonic, and agility training programs. *Am J Sports Med* 1996;24:187–192.

14. Wojtys EM, Huston LJ, Lindenfeld TN, Hewett TE, Greenfield ML: Association between the menstrual cycle and anterior cruciate ligament injuries in female athletes. *Am J Sports Med* 1998;26:614–619.

15. Huston LJ, Wojtys EM: Neuromuscular performance characteristics in elite female athletes. *Am J Sports Med* 1996;24:427–436.

16. Cureton KJ, Collins MA, Hill DW, McElhannon FM Jr: Muscle hypertrophy in men and women. *Med Sci Sports Exerc* 1988;20:338–344.

17. Wilmore JH: Alterations in strength, body composition, and anthropometric measurements consequent to a 10-week weight training program. *Med Sci Sports* 1974;6:133–138.

18. Staron RS, Karapondo DL, Kraemer WJ, et al: Skeletal muscle adaptations during early phase of heavy-resistance training in men and women. *J Appl Physiol* 1994;76:1247–1255.

19. Hakkinen K, Pakarinen A, Komi PV, Ryushi T, Kauhanen H: Neuromuscular adaptations and hormone balance in strength athletes, physically active males and females during intensive strength training, in Gregor RJ, Zernicke RF, Whiting WC (eds): *Proceedings of the XII International Congress of Biomechanics*, No. 8. Champaign, IL, Human Kinetics, 1989.

20. Kraemer WJ, Fleck SJ, Dziados JE, et al: Changes in hormonal concentrations after different heavy-resistance exercise protocols in women. *J Appl Physiol* 1993;75:594–604.

21. Fleck SJ, Kraemer WJ (eds): *Designing Resistance Training Programs*, ed 2. Champaign, IL, Human Kinetics, 1997.

22. Kraemer WJ, Gordon SE, Fleck SJ, et al: Endogenous anabolic hormonal and growth factor responses to heavy resistance exercise in males and females. *Int J Sports Med* 1991;12:228–235.

23. Londeree BR: Gender differences in circulorespiratory and metabolic variables related to endurance performance, in Pearl AJ (ed): *The Athletic Female*. Champaign, IL, Human Kinetics, 1993, pp 149–164.

24. Rozzi SL, Lephart SM, Fu F: Effects of muscular fatigue on knee joint laxity and neuromuscular characteristics of male and female athletes. *J Athletic Training* 1999;34:106–114.

25. Hewett TE, Stroupe AL, Nance TA, Noyes FR: Plyometric training in female athletes: Decreased impact forces and increased hamstring torques. *Am J Sports Med* 1996;24:765–773.

26. Colby S, Francisco A, Yu B, Kirkendall DT, Finch M, Garrett WE Jr: Electromyographic and kinematic analysis of cutting maneuvers. Implications for anterior cruciate ligament injury. *Am J Sports Med* 2000,28:234-240.

27. Malone TR, Hardaker WT, Garrett WE, Feagin JA, Bassett FH: Relationship of gender to anterior cruciate ligament injuries in intercollegiate basketball players. *J South Orthop Assoc* 1993;2:36–39.

Chapter 23

Motor Learning and Sports Injury: A Role in Anterior Cruciate Ligament Injury

Donald T. Kirkendall, PhD
William E. Garrett Jr, MD, PhD

The study and scientific basis for human movement and its disorders is a field still in its relative youth. Several factors have developed that have made this field more productive and of more general interest. The study of movement has been increasingly associated with theories regarding motor control by the nervous system and the complex interaction of mechanics, sensory feedback, and the existing framework of the central nervous system. In addition, the field is easier to study with technical improvement in the ability to perform motion analysis, to detect and record muscle activation, and to measure relevant biomechanical factors. Certainly, the study of movement has received cross-fertilization from increasing efforts to improve and apply robotics where the control and efficiency of movement are so important.

High-speed biomechanical studies and motion analysis of skilled athletic maneuvers has received significant attention from scientists and athletes in recent years. Analysis of the baseball pitch,[1] golf swing,[2,3] cycling,[4] gymnastics,[5,6] and track and field[7] are among many studies that have helped to assess skill and experience in sports performance. Some studies have reported differences in motion and muscle activation as a function of skill or injury.[1–3] These analyses make it clear that there is a very rapid and highly coordinated set of physical and muscle forces that interact in ballistic athletic maneuvers. It is also striking that the speed with which these motions occur does not allow for continuous sensory feedback in the gross control of movement. For example, a baseball batter swings a bat in approximately 100 ms. The minimum reaction time for the initiation of a response to visual stimuli is on the order of 150 to 200 ms. There is too little time for a "closed loop" concept of motor control to be effective wherein the body has continuous ability to adapt to sensory feedback and to adjust motion.

The field of motor control has evolved towards the concept that both predictions of response and a set of "open loop" motions must be made to achieve the desired motion or athletic reaction. Further, these motions occur with a speed possible only if their performance stems from a learned or preprogrammed set of motion control commands in the central nervous system. This set of "hard wired" commands or responses has been termed a motor program. The concept is frequently discussed with respect to motor skills from athletic to artistic to occupational experiences.[8]

In considering the study of movement, there has not been much attention to the movement control factors that might be involved with the control and, ultimately, the prevention of injury. Many athletic injuries occur without violent external forces and at times of breakdown or dysfunction of normal muscle control. For example, falling or pivoting awkwardly or landing are major causes of athletic injury. An examination of motor control and response to environment may be a fruitful way to consider injury cause and prevention.

An important element of the analysis of motor control and injury would be to evaluate differences in motor control in populations who might be at more or less risk of injury. Recent studies have pointed out the relatively increased risk of female athletes with respect to some injuries, most notably injury to the anterior cruciate ligament (ACL) of the knee. Surprisingly, few studies have evaluated gender differences in motion analysis and motor control. It would seem promising to look at differences in motor control and motion as they relate to differences in risks of acute injury.

Many studies that attempt to determine the mechanism of injury to the ACL point out that up to 75% of injuries are not from a direct blow to the knee.[9] In the absence of direct contact, it is puzzling why this ligament is so vulnerable to injury. At least two main schools of thought interact in this multifactorial injury. One theory points toward intrinsic factors that put the ligament at risk. These factors might include ligament thickness and strength, the angles between the femur and tibia, the amount of room within the femoral notch that contains the cruciate ligaments, and various hormonal influences on ligaments. Another theory implicates the basic control of motion and the ability to react to extrinsic forces that put the ligament at risk. These extrinsic factors must be accommodated by the central nervous system during unfamiliar activities. A result might be an uncoordinated sequence of events that, in just the right circumstances, could place the ligament at risk. The theories behind motion control during situations at risk of injury are critical to understanding the role of these extrinsic factors in ACL injury. To gain a better understanding of these injuries, it might be instructive to ask patients to give details on just how they remember their injury. In addition, viewing videotapes of actual injuries might also provide more clues to understanding the injury.

One sport that has been looked at in some detail is downhill skiing.[10,11] Three common causes have been discussed. One method of ACL failure called the "phantom-foot" mechanism[10] occurs when a skier falls backwards on an internally rotated, flexed knee. This is seen more frequently in women and could be related to the skiing equipment, particularly the bindings. The combination of a strong contraction of the quadriceps (to maintain balance) and a rigid boot that does not release may lead to an ACL disruption.[12] As a result, an ACL disruption occurs during a hard landing when the skier is off balance. The second mechanism happens when the skier lands on the ski's tail, and the stiff posterior shell of the boot combines with a strong quadriceps contraction to maintain balance while displacing the tibia anteriorly, leading to strain of the ACL. The third mechanism, a valgus-rotation, seems more common in men during downhill or cross-country skiing when the inside (medial) edge of the front of the ski gets caught in the snow. The leg is abducted and externally rotated while the skier is driven forward by momentum. High-speed skiing and poorly kept ski slopes are also implicated in this type of injury.

Little attention has been directed to the mechanism of ACL injuries in other sports. Sudden deceleration, an abrupt change of direction, and a fixed foot have been described as key elements of an ACL injury.[12] Mechanisms of injury were reported in 23 athletes[13] in whom 70% of the injuries were noncontact injuries and only 30% involved direct contact to the knee. Patients who could fully describe the injury said their knee flexion angle was full extension to 20° combined with tibial internal rotation. Thus, the prominent mechanism involved a slightly flexed knee and internal rotation of the tibia at footstrike.

ACL injury factors have been divided into intrinsic and extrinsic factors.[14] Intrinsic factors include such factors as a narrow intercondylar notch, weak ACL, generalized overall joint laxity, and lower extremity malalignment. Extrinsic factors include abnormal quadriceps-hamstring interactions, altered neuromuscular control, shoe-surface interface, the playing surface, and the athlete's playing style. The interaction of this multitude of factors has led to the observation of a greater incidence of ACL injuries in women for such sports as basketball and soccer.[15]

Interviews and Videotapes

Currently, groups at the University of North Carolina and the University of Kentucky, among others, have been studying lower limb kinetics and kinematics during athletic maneuvers that seem to be implicated in ACL injuries. While the specific activities leading to an ACL tear in skiing have been described, we are only just beginning to get a better understanding of the specific activities and movement patterns that seem to be injurious to the ACL.

Boden and Garrett[9] interviewed over 100 patients with ACL tears using a standardized questionnaire about what common characteristics might be found. Eighty-nine patients (105 knees) were able to recall details of their injury (no skiing injuries included). A physician administered the questionnaire, and the interview focused on lower extremity position at the time of injury. The questions requested information regarding contact versus noncontact, foot and tibia position, knee flexion, direction of knee collapse, direction that the body was twisting, and so forth. Hamstring flexibility and knee recurvatum were measured. In addition to the questionnaires, 28 videotapes of separate ACL injuries were obtained from Division I National Collegiate Athletic Association (NCAA) collegiate programs. These videotapes were reviewed and compared to the information acquired from the patients.

In Boden and Garrett's data, contact was involved only 29% of the time, typical with other reports. The most common activities were basketball (25%), football (21%), and soccer (21%). Half the injuries (50%) happened on natural grass and one fourth were on an indoor court. The level of sports participation was fairly equally distributed across levels (recreational, 41%; varsity, 34%; and intramural, 23%).

Nearly three fourths of the patients heard a popping sound, and all but three had to be removed from play at the time of their injury. The injured subjects recalled the knee being near full extension, usually with an average angle of 21° of flexion. However, there was a wide range of knee flexion angles (range, −10° to 110°). If the few hyperextension injuries are excluded, the average knee flexion angle at the time of injury did not change greatly (to 24°). The body was recalled to be decelerating in 34 injuries, landing in 30 injuries (another form of deceleration), accelerating in 13 injuries, falling backwards in four injuries, and 19 could not recall.

Twenty-one athletes felt that their injury was due to the interface between the shoe and the surface. Of these 21 athletes, 15 thought their cleats became fixed to the ground. The other six thought their shoes didn't allow them to pivot. Only three players were unable to touch the ground with their fingers, knuckles, or palms, suggesting good hamstring flexibility. If good hamstring flexibility is combined with minimal activation, the tibia could well have sufficient room to slide anteriorly.

The interviews showed a number of different mechanisms with two broad classifications garnering the majority of injuries. For example, in 39 injuries, tibial rotation was implicated. The body was twisting in a direction opposite from the tibial rotation. Thirty-one of the injuries involved landing (varus, valgus, or hyperextension).

There were videotapes of 22 injuries that could be studied in comparison to the interviews. From videotapes, it was found that two out of three injuries were noncontact. In these injuries, the athletes were in close proximity to an opposing player. Thus while there was not direct contact with the knee, frequently there was some contact that may have thrown the athlete off balance. The leg's position before collapse was near footstrike with the knee flexed between 10° and 30°. A single-leg landing in valgus led to four injuries. The other noncontact injuries were during deceleration or pivoting.

Motor Learning and Ligament Injury

These interviews and videotapes indicate that there appear to be circumstances that make ACL injury likely during noncontact activity. This may be explained by some alteration in the normal pattern of activation of the lower extremity muscle groups. Alternatively, it is possible that relatively normal patterns of activation occur in circumstances that are not anticipated in time for an appropriate motor response in a "closed-loop" system. To understand this it is important to remember the differences between an open-loop and a closed-loop system. The open-loop system has two components, the command and the effector components, whereas the closed-loop system incorporates sensory feedback and the continuous ability to alter the signals from command to effector (eg, central nervous system to muscle). Open-loop systems are less flexible because changing situations can inappropriately modify the sequence of events. Closed-loop systems accept feedback and modify actions based on the feedback.

The delay in response to an unexpected stimulus is called reaction time and can range from 0.15 (to kinesthetic stimuli) to 0.30 (to visual and auditory stimuli) seconds. The human is often termed a "single channel" organism. Consider a reaction time to a stimulus of 0.20 s. If there is a pause before a second stimulus, the reaction time will still be 0.20 s. If the second stimulus arrives during the reaction time for the first stimulus, the reaction time to the second stimulus is delayed more than the expected 0.20 s.[8] This delay indicates that humans cannot process two overlapping stimuli at the same rate; the second stimulus is processed after the completion of the reaction time to the first stimulus. This reaction time delay to a second stimulus beyond the normal reaction time may be important in the consideration of injuries that happen in reaction to an environmental stimulus.

When discussing athletes, a further consideration is the time needed to alter movement. Many coordinated maneuvers are a reaction to the opponent or to the conditions of the performance. If the will to change a motor activity comes during the reaction, it can be changed only after completing some portion of the response to the initial stimulus. A common occurrence during ACL injury is a sudden attempt to change movement during the performance of previously commanded motor sequence.

Three elements make up reaction time.[8] At the outset, 1 unit of reaction time is required for the athlete to process information presented while a movement is already in progress. Second, if the stimulus requires the athlete to change movement, another unit of reaction time is necessary to begin to change the movement. Finally, the initial 0.20 to 0.30 s of any movement is preprogrammed and any change from the originally intended movement cannot begin until the movement has been underway for about 0.30 to 0.50 s. Given the less than ideal setting of a sport such as skiing, ligament damage has been estimated to occur 79 ms after loading. The muscle does not begin to contract until 213 ms after loading.[16] This difference indicates that the ligament is already damaged before the muscles can respond and compensate.

To counter this lag, athletes use anticipation to reduce some of the delays. For example, from many practice sessions, a batter knows how long it takes to swing the bat so the time to begin a swing is not dependent solely on the response to seeing the ball (also called effector anticipation). The batter also needs to preview (ie, predict) where and when the ball will cross the plate to initiate the swing at the correct time. This would all be delayed by at least one unit of reaction time (when a pitched ball is visible for only 0.60 s, every unit of reaction time is precious) if the swing was purely in response to seeing the ball. Superior athletes are the ones who anticipate their opponent or the physical demands of the competition. Skilled athletes can also disguise their own movement and deprive their opponent of valuable clues, effectively lengthening the opponent's reaction time.

The Motor Program

The length of the reaction times just discussed indicates that motor activities in sports cannot be solely in response to environmental stimuli (ie, the opponent or the ball). Thus, it is possible to see the concept of a motor program: a stored set of muscle commands that research has not conclusively been able to prove. Nevertheless, how could an athlete begin and end a movement on a specific target in 0.10 s if a preprogrammed set of instructions had not been activated? If visual or kinesthetic information were needed to stop the movement, then the issuance of the command to *stop* the movement would have to have begun *before* the movement actually began. A motor program would have within it the commands to start, carry out, and stop the motion. In some movement patterns, this would argue against the closed-loop command discussed earlier.

Consider an activity that takes 0.60 s. The activity might be underway for 0.30 s before the athlete must modify the movement. The new reaction time of about 0.20 s plus the first part of the movement means that at best the alteration would not occur for 0.50 s. With the duration of sporting activities such as hitting and kicking being less than 0.50 s, the role of motor programs becomes more important in skill performance.

Moving from a sensory based closed-loop system toward the open-loop system is the reason for practice. Given a new task (eg, juggling), the subject will use sensory (eg, visual) feedback to control the balls. With successful practice, a motor program will be developed for a more efficient motor pattern. In one sense, the motor program uses only those motor units appropriate for the movement by ruling out unnecessary pathways.

Looking at an athletic maneuver, like cutting, provides further evidence that motor programs must be evident. While running, from some environmental influence (often an opponent), the athlete rapidly changes direction. Prior to planting the cut foot, a series of events has already taken place that will influence the success of the cut. Immediately before ground impact of the planted foot, the leg is flexed (an attempt to protect internal ligaments?) and the quadriceps is activated because there is some deceleration upon impact. At impact, quadriceps activation increases in response to the eccentric load on the muscle. This activation from impact through the following milliseconds is quite high, often larger than seen during a maximal voluntary contraction (I have seen activation levels as high as 250% of maximal voluntary contraction when the quadriceps contracts during the cutting motion). Activation levels this high show there are incredibly high forces acting on the knee from the activation of the quadriceps when the foot is planted and the tibia is relatively fixed.

Maximum activation of the quadriceps from heelstrike to contraction takes only 12 s.[17] What would happen if, slightly before or during the cut, the player was bumped slightly just before heelstrike? Based on the discussions above, the motor program for that step would be put into place, but any chance for a correction of the movement would likely begin well after heelstrike. So, the player set a pattern of muscle action into effect and would be unable to change this pattern until after a ligament would tear.

Two more examples might be illustrative. Consider the player who expects to step on level ground, but ends up stepping into a small divot in the grass. A pattern of events begins, but the deviation in the surface means the program is no longer appropriate. When the player steps into the hole, his or her proprioceptive response likely will be unsuitable, and the response could well be a reactive contraction by the quadriceps. With these patterns happening with the knee near full extension, excess tibial shear forces are likely and can tear the ACL. Or consider the volleyball player who goes up to hit a quick set at the net. He or she jumps and begins a series of preprogrammed events to perform the skill and then land. However, if the set is a little high and behind, a midair correction must be made, which means the player will not be landing as planned. Upon heelstrike for take-off, the preplanned program can begin and the quadriceps could be performing normally. But with the changes in the air, the landing may take place off balance with the knee in an unfavorable position, leading to tibial shear tearing the ACL.

From this discussion, it is possible to see that there are factors contributing to ACL injuries that are beyond gender-specific intrinsic and direct trauma factors. Although these patterns seem to make some sense, there probably is a need to test whether these concepts truly are implicated in injury mechanisms. Then, it might be necessary to see if the motor program for risky maneuvers is different between men and women and, if so, how the motor program of the at-risk athlete might be changed to reduce the risk of injury.

Is the Extensor Mechanism Implicated?

The interviews and videotapes give insight into the circumstances surrounding noncontact ACL injuries. In these interviews and videotapes, the quadriceps is implicated. Perhaps it would be appropriate to see if the quadriceps has the necessary capabilities to exert an anterior drawer sufficient to tear the ACL.

There have been earlier reports that the quadriceps was capable of loading the ACL throughout the full motion of the knee.[18] But, there is a more important need to know if the forces on the ACL from the quadriceps are capable of producing sufficient force to tear the ACL. In most cases, these studies were done on cadavers in an "open chain" setting.[19,20] To estimate these forces, the patellar tendon-tibial shaft angle must be determined. These studies typically show that the patellar tendon-tibial shaft angle depends on the knee flexion angle. The quadriceps force can strain the ACL only in the arc of motion from 45° flexion to full extension.

Although these prior reports are very well defined, they may not be applicable to a closed-chain setting where the athlete is cutting or landing. First, there are the obvious difficulties in generalizing from the cadaver to the performing athlete and second, from interviews and the literature, it is known that ACL injuries do not occur in an open-chain setting. Therefore, an estimate of the in vivo forces on the ACL during closed-chain activities is needed.

To try to fill this void, Noonan and associates (unpublished observations) took sagittal plane radiographs of 9 men at 5°, 30°, 45°, and 60° of knee flexion (as defined by Van Eijden and associates[21]) while the subjects were bearing about 50% of their body weight and patellar tendon and tibia vectors at each angle were determined from the radiographs. The angle between these two vectors was defined as the patellar tendon-tibial shaft angle. An inverse linear relationship between resultant force vector and knee flexion angle was seen; the force vector increased as the knee flexion angle decreased. Using these measurements, the shear force exerted on the tibia by the patellar tendon could be estimated using data from prior work.[19,22–24] It was estimated that the resultant force on the patellar tendon at footstrike, when the quadriceps is contracting eccentrically, could exceed 5,000 N. During running and cutting, these loads can exceed 2,000 N, which is near the published ACL failure load.[25] These data are limited to men and knee angles between 15° and 60° of knee flexion. It is unknown at this time whether this relationship would be the same for women over a wider range of knee flexion angles. In addition, there was wide variability between the subjects, suggesting that it may be possible to determine who is at risk based on the patellar tendon-tibial shaft angle.

Motor Control of Athletic Maneuvers

Based on the interviews and review of videotapes, an idea of the type of maneuvers that put the ACL at risk is becoming apparent. As just pointed out, there is sufficient force within the quadriceps to cause an anterior drawer that could exceed the rupture force of the ACL. How the quadriceps and hamstrings interacted while performing risky activities may indicate how these maneuvers become so risky.

Malinzak and associates[26] studied the kinematics of running and cutting in male and female athletes. Motion capture was used to measure knee, hip, and ankle flexion angles and knee varus-valgus. Electromyography was used to record muscle activity of the quadriceps and the medial and lateral hamstrings. The data on muscle activation was reported as relative activation (the ratio of the quadriceps/hamstring). The subject would run along a runway and continue, or perform a side cut or a crosscut.

In comparison with men, data from the women showed they performed the cutting maneuvers in an erect posture with less knee and hip flexion and more knee valgus. Thus, the knee was in a position that favored a quadriceps-induced anterior drawer. Women also had greater relative quadriceps activation. Thus, the women performed cutting maneuvers in a manner that potentially places the ACL at risk for an injury.

If women do perform these actions with a more erect posture, could coaching women to play in a more crouched position reduce the incidence of ACL injuries? The results of an insightful project by Griffis and associates were presented to the American Orthopaedic Society for Sports Medicine meeting in Traverse City, MI, in 1989. The authors trained NCAA Division I female basketball players to perform their cuts in a three-step pattern that kept the knee flexed and the feet more under the hips, and ACL injuries were reduced by 89% over a 2-year period.

From the interviews and videotapes, it was mentioned that in many cases there was another player nearby at the time of injury. While it is not reproducible in the laboratory, it is possible that if a player is slightly thrown off balance just before a cut or jump stop, the movement the player intended to do is changed to one that can favor the quadriceps activation, placing the ACL at risk. The forces on the ACL during this slightly unplanned maneuver may be sufficient to tear the ACL.

At this point, it is not possible to say that any one mechanism is responsible for ACL injuries. The variety of intrinsic and extrinsic factors makes focusing on one variable difficult, if not impossible. However, given that most injuries to this ligament are noncontact and that there are predictable movement patterns that, if slightly disrupted, can place the ACL at risk, it is possible that preventive strategies might be developed.

These data indicate that motor programs may well be a real factor in dealing with both athletic performance and as a contributor to injury. The understanding of the interaction of closed and open loop programs helps the understanding of performance and injury. In the future, such theories may better indicate many mechanisms of injury that will suggest what measures must be taken to improve the safety of all sports.

References

1. Gowan ID, Jobe FW, Tibone JE, Perry J, Moynes DR: A comparative electromyographic analysis of the shoulder during pitching: Professional versus amateur pitchers. *Am J Sports Med* 1987;15:586–590.
2. Watkins RG, Uppal GS, Perry J, Pink M, Dinsay JM: Dynamic electromyographic analysis of trunk musculature in professional golfers. *Am J Sports Med* 1996;24:535–538.
3. Kao JT, Pink M, Jobe FW, Perry J: Electromyographic analysis of the scapular muscles during a golf swing. *Am J Sports Med* 1995;23:19–23.
4. Gregor RJ, Broker JP, Ryan MM: The biomechanics of cycling. *Exerc Sport Sci Rev* 1991;19:127–169.
5. Takei Y, Dunn JH: A 'kickout' double salto backward tucked dismount from the horizontal bar performed by elite gymnasts. *J Sports Sci* 1997;15:411–425.
6. Takei Y, Dunn JH: A comparison of techniques used by elite gymnasts in performing the basket-to-handstand mount. *J Sports Sci* 1996;14:269–279.
7. Mero A, Komi PV, Gregor RJ: Biomechanics of sprint running: A review. *Sports Med* 1992;13:376–392.
8. Shumway-Cook A, Woollacott MH (eds): *Motor Control: Theory and Practical Applications*. Baltimore, MD, Williams & Wilkins, 1995.
9. Boden BP, Garrett WE Jr: Abstract: Mechanisms of injury to the anterior cruciate ligament. *Med Sci Sports Exerc* 1996;28(suppl):S26.
10. Elmqvist L-G, Johnson RJ: Chapter 20: Prevention of cruciate ligament injuries, in Feagin JA Jr (ed): *The Crucial Ligaments: Diagnosis and Treatment of Ligamentous Injuries About the Knee*, ed 2. New York, NY, Churchill Livingstone, 1994, pp 495–505.
11. Feagin JA Jr, Lambert KL, Cunningham RR, et al: Consideration of the anterior cruciate ligament injury in skiing. *Clin Orthop* 1987;216:13-18.
12. Ettlinger CF, Johnson RJ, Shealy JE: A method to help reduce the risk of serious knee sprains incurred in alpine skiing. *Am J Sports Med* 1995;23;531–537.

13. Feagin JA Jr, Lambert KL: Mechanism of injury and pathology of anterior cruciate ligament injuries. *Orthop Clin N Am* 1995;16:41–45.

14. McNair PJ, Marshall RN, Matheson JA: Important features associated with acute anterior cruciate ligament injury. *NZ Med J* 1990;103:537–539.

15. Arendt E, Dick R: Knee injury patterns among men and women in collegiate basketball and soccer: NCAA data and review of literature. *Am J Sports Med* 1995;23:694–701.

16. Foerster O: The motor cortex in man in the light of Hughlings Jackson's doctrines, in Payton OD, Hirt S, Newton RS (eds): *Scientific Bases for Neurophysiologic Approaches to Therapeutic Exercise: An Anthology.* Philadelphia, PA, FA Davis, 1977, pp 13–18.

17. Pope MH, Johnson RJ, Brown DW, Tighe C: The role of the musculature in injuries to the medial collateral ligament. *J Bone Joint Surg* 1979;61A:398–402.

18. Colby SM, Malinzak RA, Garrett WE: Abstract: Electromyographic and kinematic analysis of the jump stop maneuver. *Med Sci Sports Exerc* 1998;30(suppl):S183.

19. Grood ES, Suntay WJ, Noyes FR, Butler DL: Biomechanics of the knee-extension exercise: Effect of cutting the anterior cruciate ligament. *J Bone Joint Surg* 1984;66A:725–734.

20. Buff HU, Jones JC, Hungerford DS: Experimental determination of forces transmitted through the patello-femoral joint. *J Biomech* 1988;21:17–23.

21. van Eijden TM, de Boer W, Weijs WA: The orientation of the distal part of the quadriceps femoris muscle as a function of the knee flexion-extension angle. *J Biomech* 1985;18:803–809.

22. Winter DA (ed): *Biomechanics and Motor Control of Human Movement*, ed 2. New York, NY, John Wiley & Sons, 1990.

23. Huberti HH, Hayes WC, Stone JL, Shybut GT: Force ratios in the quadriceps tendon and ligamentum patellae. *J Orthop Res* 1984;2:49–54.

24. Smidt GL: Biomechanical analysis of knee flexion and extension. *J Biomech* 1973;6:79–92.

25. Perry J, Antonelli D, Ford W: Analysis of knee-joint forces during flexed-knee stance. *J Bone Joint Surg* 1975;57A:961–967.

26. Malinzak RA, Colby SM, Kirkendall DT, Garrett WE Jr: Abstract: Electromyographic and 3-dimensional kinematic analysis of cutting maneuvers in men and women: Implications for anterior cruciate ligament injury. Proceedings of the American Academy of Orthopaedic Surgeons 66th Annual Meeting, Anaheim, CA. Rosemont, IL, American Academy of Orthopaedic Surgeons, 1999, p 12.

Chapter 24

Neuromuscular Differences Between Male and Female Athletes Contributing to Anterior Cruciate Ligament Injuries

Laura J. Huston, MS
Edward M. Wojtys, MD

Introduction

Anatomy, biomechanics, and hormones are three leading research areas that hold potential for explaining the epidemic of anterior cruciate ligament (ACL) injuries in female athletes. Of these, biomechanics appears to offer the most hope for improvement in this medical problem. Recently, Hewett and associates[1] demonstrated that changing some of these biomechanical factors can have a positive effect on this startling injury rate.

Essential to this discussion on ACL injuries in women is an understanding of how the active and passive restraint systems of the knee function. Passive restraints (eg, ligaments) can resist the relatively low forces seen during activities of daily living,[2] but the active restraints (eg, muscle) must be mobilized for successful protection of the knee joint during high loading activities such as sports or physical work.[3,4]

Several studies have established the crucial role that muscle activation plays at the knee in dynamic knee joint stability.[3–9] Unfortunately, when dynamic stability is inadequate or slow to develop, high forces are placed on the passive restraints of the knee and failure can occur. To make this neuromuscular system work, several components are necessary: (1) The afferent side of the neuromuscular system must detect hazardous joint movement or subluxation. (2) Once a deforming force is detected, there must be an adequate timely muscle response. (3) Joint stiffness must be generated dynamically through muscle contraction and joint positioning.

One of the problems that has hampered development in this area is that for years it was assumed that the neuromuscular systems of men and women were similar. In fact, they appear to be quite different. Gender differences in these neuromuscular characteristics may play a role in the high rate of ACL injuries seen among women. Recent studies of landing and pivoting movements show that these activities are performed differently by men and women.

Gender Differences in Muscle Strength

Gender differences in absolute muscle strength are well documented in the literature.[10–17] Factors that affect maximum strength include cross-sectional area (CSA) of the muscle, fiber type distribution, and the ability of the subject to fully activate the motor units (neuromuscular efficiency). Men generally have larger (based on CSA) and stronger muscles than women, although considerable gender overlap exists.[17–19] Table 1 summarizes a review of the literature in the area of relative muscle strength of the lower extremity between men and women.[15,20,21]

Interestingly, when muscle strength is normalized for body weight or lean body mass, these discrepancies diminish[10,13,16,17,22,23] (Table 2).

Table 1 Literature review of female strength as a percent of male strength in knee extension and flexion

Author	Knee Extension	Knee Flexion
Asmussen et al[20]	78%	77%
Nordgren[21]	78%	64%
Laubach[15]	57%	—

Table 2 Comparison of female strength as a percent of male strength in the lower extremity

Author	Absolute Value	Relative to Body Weight	Relative to Lean Body Mass
McBride*	74%	85%	100%
Castro et al[24]			
Untrained	79%	102%	112%
Trained	73%	97%	105%

*Unpublished data, 1999

Factors that Influence Muscle Strength

Muscle CSA

Several studies have reported that gender differences in muscle strength are explained primarily by differences in size or CSA, and not quality of the tissue.[10,17,24–26] Muscle CSA is determined by both the size and number of muscle fibers. Although it is generally accepted that untrained women have smaller fiber areas than untrained men,[13,17,27–29] studies in which fiber numbers have been estimated are somewhat contradictory. Several authors have reported significantly fewer muscle fibers in female biceps brachii and tibialis anterior compared to those muscles in males,[27,29] but such findings have not been supported by investigations of the triceps brachii or vasus lateralis.[30] If a significant gender difference in muscle fiber numbers exists, it probably represents a true biologic difference, because fiber number is determined genetically.[31]

Muscle Fiber Type Distribution

Part of the reason for the strength differences between men and women may lie in the composition of muscle and in the differing contractile properties of various fiber types. There is a considerable amount of evidence that muscle in women has, on average, a higher proportion of type I fibers compared to muscle in men.[17,32,33] In a longitudinal study of untrained men and women, Glenmark and associates[34] found that the percentage of type I muscle fibers did not differ between genders at age 16, but at age 27, women had a significantly higher percentage of type I fibers than did men. No difference appears to exist in the capacity to generate isometric force between type I and type II muscle fibers in untrained subjects,[18] but differences in dynamic (isokinetic) contractions have been demonstrated, with type II fibers able to generate a higher force, particularly at high angular velocities.[35,36]

It is generally accepted that fiber types are genetically determined.[37–40] Muscle fibers are highly adaptable and subtle alterations take place throughout life.[41] The nerve innervating the muscle fiber determines its type, so activity history and sports can influence the relative percentage of fiber type distribution.[41–45] For example, sprinters and shot putters have a high percentage of type II fibers (fast twitch), whereas distance runners have a higher percentage of type I fibers (slow twitch).

Neuromuscular Efficiency

Komi and Karlsson[14] studied muscle strength, fiber composition, and neuromuscular efficiency in young male and female twins and found that boys demonstrated more efficient neuromotoric output during contraction and more pronounced contractile profiles compared with their twin sisters.[14] However, this study did not consider the individual's previous level of physical activity. Research has shown that physical training has a profound impact on the level of neuromuscular efficiency.[46,47] In 1983, Hakkinen and Komi[46] found that 16 weeks of lower extremity strength training significantly improved activation of the knee extensor muscles. They believed that an increase in physical activity improves the sensitivity of the muscle spindle.[46] Castro and associates'[24] work suggested that trained subjects increased their neural activation.

Factors that Influence Muscle Composition

Physical activity has the most direct influence on the muscle composition of an individual.[46,47] However, hormonal influences, such as testosterone, also increase muscle mass, fiber recruitment, and the proportion of type II fibers, all favoring muscle strength.[48] Ramos and associates[48] investigated the relationship between muscle strength and hormone levels in activity-matched male and female teenagers. They concluded that the strength of men is influenced by both testosterone and physical activity. In women, physical activity was thought to have more influence on muscle strength because of the low levels of circulating testosterone in the body.

Muscle Reaction Time

Muscle reaction time (MRT) is the interval between the onset of a stimulus and the start of an action potential at the intended muscle. MRT is a valuable tool in determining how well a joint detects a disturbance and how quickly muscles respond to a stimulus or perturbation. MRT can be a good test of the afferent and efferent nervous system. Unfortunately, it is difficult to separate the afferent and efferent limbs of the neuromuscular system, posing problems for research work.

Several studies have reported no difference in lower extremity MRT between young, healthy men and women.[49–51] Winter and Brookes[50] used an acoustic signal delivered through headphones to compare the MRT of the soleus in a group of young active men and women and found no significant gender differences. Wojtys and Huston[51] investigated lower extremity MRT in a group of young, healthy men and women using an anteriorly directed mechanical stimulus at the proximal tibia. They found no gender differences in either spinal or cortical MRT in the quadriceps, hamstrings, or gastrocnemius muscle groups. Similarly, Huston and Wojtys[49] reported no differences in MRT between elite level male and female athletes.

Muscle Recruitment Order/Muscle Activation Patterns

Some female athletes appear to use different muscle activation patterns compared with their male counterparts.[49] In 1996, Huston and Wojtys[49] reported differences in muscle recruitment patterns between elite male and female athletes in response to anterior tibial translation. Female athletes preferred to contract their quadriceps first in response to anterior tibial translation (quadriceps dominant), whereas the male athletes as well as male and female nonathlete controls, responded to anterior tibial translation by first contracting their hamstrings (hamstrings dominant). Hamstring function is critical to dynamic knee stability. That is, if the quadriceps fire without the hamstrings, the tibia may sublux anteriorly and significantly increase the load on the ACL.[8,52,53] If these quadriceps muscle contractions are very powerful and are not balanced by a hamstrings co-contraction, the ACL may be injured by the quadriceps alone. Conversely, if the hamstrings fire without a quadriceps contraction, anterior tibial translation is decreased, and loads on the ACL are significantly decreased.[8,52–54] Thus, a "quadriceps dominant" pattern in a female athlete may place significantly more strain on the ACL compared with an individual who simultaneously co-contracts the quadriceps and hamstring muscles, or contracts the hamstring muscles before the quadriceps muscles in response to anterior tibial translation.

Gender differences in muscle coactivation patterns in young subjects have also been investigated.[3] Baratta and associates[3] quantified the coactivation patterns of the knee flexor and extensor muscles of nonathletic, recreational, and highly competitive male and female athletes. Electromyographic (EMG) data were collected during an isokinetic strength evaluation producing maximal muscle contractions. High-performance athletes with hypertrophied quadriceps demonstrated strong inhibitory effects on the coactivation of the hamstrings compared with a group of nonathletic, healthy subjects. Athletes who routinely exercised their hamstrings, however, had a coactivation response similar to that of the nonathletic subjects. Baratta and associates[3] concluded that the coactivation of the hamstrings with quadriceps was necessary to aid the dynamic component of joint stability, to equalize articular surface pressure distribution, and to regulate the joint's mechanical impedance. They suggested that high-performance athletes with a muscular imbalance could reduce their risk of knee injuries by performing complementary resistive exercises of the hamstring muscles.

Muscle Stiffness

Muscle stiffness across the knee joint may represent an important component of knee joint stability and injury prevention. Mechanoreceptors in the knee ligaments and the joint capsule regulate muscle stiffness by influencing muscle spindle afferents from agonist and antagonist muscles with excitatory and inhibitory activity.[55–58] In order for the neuromuscular system to be effective in preventing ligament strain, muscle tension must be developed in a timely fashion. As muscles that span the knee joint contract, they act to increase joint contact force and decrease tibial-femoral displacements, dissipate ground reaction forces, and may decrease strain in the ACL and other passive structures.

Muscle stiffness across the knee has both "intrinsic" and "extrinsic" components. The intrinsic component depends largely on the number of active actin-myosin cross bridges in the muscles at a specified time. Measures of intrinsic stiffening before reflexive muscular activation provide essential information regarding the adequacy of protective neuromuscular response mechanisms.[59,60] The extrinsic component depends on the excitation provided by the alpha and gamma motoneurons. It is important to note that a muscle's intrinsic muscle stiffness is probably the knee's first line of protection. However, the potential of the extrinsic component's protection is greater, and it can be modified with training. Markolf and associates[7] reported that varus-valgus knee stiffness in nonathletes could increase two to fourfold with isometric co-contraction of the hamstrings and quadriceps and that well-conditioned athletes were capable of increasing knee joint stiffness by a factor of ten.

Unfortunately, gender differences exist in the ability to produce adequate muscle stiffness.[61,62] In 1988, Bryant and Cooke[61] looked at the varus and valgus stiffness of 17 female and 24 male subjects. Female knees were found to rotate 66% more than male knees and were 35% less stiff. In 1998, Wojtys and associates (unpublished data, Vancouver, BC, 1998) investigated both passive and active components of knee joint stiffness (in the anteroposterior plane) in a group of healthy men and women. Although results were normalized for both body weight and height, a significant gender difference was found in the ability to voluntarily stiffen the knee joint in the anteroposterior plane. Men were able to increase their knee stiffness by an average of fourfold, while women were only able to double their joint stiffness with a voluntary muscle contraction (473% vsersus 217%; $p = 0.003$). Wojtys and associates concluded that the ability to increase knee stiffness may not be determined by a person's muscle strength or body height/weight ratio, but primarily by unknown factors relating to gender. This contradicts the work of Such and associates,[62] who tested 70 male and female knee joints and showed that even though women's knee joints exhibited lower values of stiffness than those of men, lower extremity muscle mass had the greatest influence on the stiffness properties of the knee.

Electromechanical Delay Time

Apparent gender differences in the generation of muscle stiffness may also be associated with differences in electromechanical delay time (EMD) and musculotendinous elasticity properties. EMD is the time lapse between the neural activation of the muscle and the actual force generation.[50,63] This delay can be quite variable as a result of factors such as fiber-type composition and firing rate dynamics of the muscle, velocity of movement, viscoelastic properties and length of the muscle and tendon tissues, activity state, and coactivity of other muscles.

Winter and Brookes[50] compared the delay in muscle force generation in young, healthy men and women and attributed these gender differences to muscle elasticity. In that study, a group of 22 men and women performed an ankle plantar flexion movement in the dominant leg as quickly as possible on hearing an acoustic signal delivered via headphones. Their results indicated no differences in myoelectric response times, but they did find significant differences in both the time from force generation to heel movement (electromechanical delay) and in the span from EMG activity to heel movement (elastic charge time). Similarly, Bell and Jacobs[63] compared myoelectric response times and electromechanical delay times in men and women during a maximal contraction of the elbow flexors after a visual stimulus. Results indicated no difference in myoelectric response time; however, the EMD in the men was significantly shorter than in the women. In 1978, Komi and Karlsson[14] reported that women have a 100% longer rise time in force development of muscles of the lower extremity. These studies suggest that intrinsic, mechanical properties within the muscle may differ between men and women, with men having the ability to generate muscle forces significantly quicker.[50]

Conclusion

Both the force and speed at which muscular activation can be generated may be an important determinant in providing dynamic stability and potential injury prevention at the knee. Neuromuscular differences in the lower extremity muscles appear to exist between men and women. Women have less muscle mass, less efficient contractile properties, and different muscle fiber compositions compared with men. These discrepancies may explain why women produce lower absolute strength values in the lower extremity compared with men. During training, female athletes are more likely to become quadriceps dominant, which may lead to increased strain on the ACL. The rate of muscle force development is significantly longer in women compared to men. Lastly, gender differences exist in the ability to produce muscle stiffness across the knee joint. Collectively, these neuromuscular differences may help explain the gender discrepancy seen in noncontact ACL injuries.

References

1. Hewett TE, Lindenfeld TN, Riccobene JV, Noyes FR: The effect of neuromuscular training on the incidence of knee injury in female athletes: A prospective study. *Am J Sports Med* 1999;27:699–706.
2. Butler DL, Noyes FR, Grood ES: Ligamentous restraints to anterior-posterior drawer in the human knee: A biomechanical study. *J Bone Joint Surg* 1980;62A:259–270.
3. Baratta R, Solomonow M, Zhou BH, Letson D, Chuinard R, D'Ambrosia R: Muscular coactivation: The role of the antagonist musculature in maintaining knee stability. *Am J Sports Med* 1988;16:113–122.
4. Solomonow M, Baratta R, et al: The synergistic action of the anterior cruciate ligament and thigh muscles in maintaining joint stability. *Am J Sports Med* 1987;15:207–213.
5. Hagood S, Solomonow M, Baratta R, Zhou BH, D'Ambrosia R: The effect of joint velocity on the contribution of the antagonist musculature to knee stiffness and laxity. *Am J Sports Med* 1990;18:182–187.
6. Louie JK, Mote CD Jr: Contribution of the musculature to rotatory laxity and torsional stiffness at the knee. *J Biomech* 1987;20:281–300.
7. Markolf KL, Graff-Radford A, Amstutz HC: In vivo knee stability: A quantitative assessment using an instrumented clinical testing apparatus. *J Bone Joint Surg* 1978;60A:664–674.
8. Renström P, Arms SW, Stanwyck TS, Johnson RJ, Pope MH: Strain within the anterior cruciate ligament during hamstring and quadriceps activity. *Am J Sports Med* 1986;14:83–87.
9. Walla DJ, Albright JP, McAuley E, Martin RK, Eldridge V, El-Khoury G: Hamstring control and the unstable anterior cruciate ligament-deficient knee. *Am J Sports Med* 1985;13:34–39.
10. Behm DG, Sale DG: Voluntary and evoked muscle contractile characteristics in active men and women. *Can J Appl Physiol* 1994;19:253–265.
11. Cureton KJ, Collins MA, Hill DW, McElhannon FM Jr: Muscle hypertrophy in men and women. *Med Sci Sports Exerc* 1988;20:338–344.
12. Frontera WR, Hughes VA, Lutz KJ, Evans WJ: A cross-sectional study of muscle strength and mass in 45- to 78-year-old men and women. *J Appl Physiol* 1991;71:644–650.
13. Kanehisa H, Okuyama H, Ikegawa S, Fukunaga T: Sex difference in force generation capacity during repeated maximal knee extensions. *Eur J Appl Physiol* 1996;73:557–562.
14. Komi PV, Karlsson J: Skeletal muscle fibre types, enzyme activities and physical performance in young males and females. *Acta Physiol Scand* 1978;103:210–218.
15. Laubach LL: Comparative muscular strength of men and women: A review of the literature. *Aviat Space Environ Med* 1976;47:534–542.

16. Maughan RJ, Watson JS, Weir J: Strength and cross-sectional area of human skeletal muscle. *J Physiol* (*Lond*) 1983;338:37–49.

17. Miller AE, MacDougall JD, Tarnopolsky MA, Sale DG: Gender differences in strength and muscle fiber characteristics. *Eur J Appl Physiol* 1993;66:254–262.

18. Maughan RJ: Relationship between muscle strength and muscle cross-sectional area: Implications for training. *Sports Med* 1984;1:263–269.

19. Maughan RJ, Nimmo MA: The influence of variations in muscle fibre composition on muscle strength and cross-sectional area in untrained males. *J Physiol (Lond)* 1984;351:299–311.

20. Asmussen E, Heeboll-Nielsen K: Isometric muscle strength of adult men and women. *Communications from the Testing and Observation Institute of the Danish National Association for Infantile Paralysis* 1961;11:1–44.

21. Nordgren B: Anthropometric measures and muscle strength in young women. *Scand J Rehabil Med* 1972;4:165–169.

22. Griffin JW, Tooms RE, vander Zwaag R, Bertorini TE, O'Toole ML: Eccentric muscle performance of elbow and knee muscle groups in untrained men and women. *Med Sci Sports Exerc* 1993;25:936–944.

23. Hakkinen K, Kraemer WJ, Newton RU: Muscle activation and force production during bilateral and unilateral concentric and isometric contractions of the knee extensors in men and women at different ages. *Electromyogr Clin Neurophysiol* 1997;37:131–142.

24. Castro MJ, McCann DJ, Shaffrath JD, Adams WC: Peak torque per unit cross-sectional area differs between strength-trained and untrained young adults. *Med Sci Sports Exerc* 1995;27:397–403.

25. MacDougall JD, Sale DG, Alway SE, Sutton JR: Muscle fiber number in biceps brachii in bodybuilders and control subjects. *J Appl Physiol* 1984;57:1399–1403.

26. Ryushi T, Hakkinen K, Hauhanen H, Komi PV: Muscle fiber characteristics, muscle cross-sectional area and force production in strength athletes, physically active males and females. *Scand J Sports Sci* 1988;10:7–15.

27. Henriksson-Larsen K: Distribution, number and size of different types of fibres in whole cross-sections of female m tibialis anterior: An enzyme histochemical study. *Acta Physiol Scand* 1985;123:229–235.

28. Ricoy JR, Encinas AR, Cabello A, Madero S, Arenas J: Histochemical study of the vastus lateralis muscle fibre types of athletes. *J Physiol Biochem* 1998;54:41–47.

29. Sale DG, MacDougall JD, Alway SE, Sutton JR: Voluntary strength and muscle characteristics in untrained men and women and male bodybuilders. *J Appl Physiol* 1987;62:1786–1793.

30. Schantz P, Randall-Fox E, Hutchison W, Tyden A, Astrand PO: Muscle fibre type distribution, muscle cross-sectional area and maximal voluntary strength in humans. *Acta Physiol Scand* 1983;117:219–226.

31. Van De Graaff KM (ed): *Human Anatomy*. Dubuque, Iowa, WC Brown, 1984.

32. Nygaard E: Skeletal muscle fibre characteristics in young women. *Acta Physiol Scand* 1981;112:299–304.

33. Simoneau JA, Bouchard C: Human variation in skeletal muscle fiber-type proportion and enzyme activities. *Am J Physiol* 1989;257:E567–572.

34. Glenmark B, Hedberg G, Kaijser L, Jansson E: Muscle strength from adolescence to adulthood: Relationship to muscle fibre types. *Eur J Appl Physiol* 1994;68:9–19.

35. Thorstensson A, Grimby G, Karlsson J: Force-velocity relations and fiber composition in human knee extensor muscles. *J Appl Physiol* 1976;40:12–16.

36. Coyle EF, Costill DL, Lesmes GR: Leg extension power and muscle fiber composition. *Med Sci Sports* 1979;11:12–15.

37. Costill DL, Daniels J, Evans W, Fink W, Krahenbuhl G, Saltin B: Skeletal muscle enzymes and fiber composition in male and female track athletes. *J Appl Physiol* 1976;40:149–154.

38. Gollnick PD, Armstrong RB, Saltin B, Saubert CW IV, Sembrowich WL, Shepherd RE: Effect of training on enzyme activity and fiber composition of human skeletal muscle. *J Appl Physiol* 1973;34:107–111.

39. Gollnick PD: Relationship of strength and endurance with skeletal muscle structure and metabolic potential. *Int J Sports Med* 1982;3(suppl 1):26–32.

40. Jansson E, Sjodin B, Tesch P: Changes in muscle fibre type distribution in man after physical training: A sign of fibre type transformation? *Acta Physiol Scand* 1978;104:235–237.

41. Staron RS: Human skeletal muscle fiber types: Delineation, development, and distribution. *Can J Appl Physiol* 1997;22:307–327.

42. Buller AJ, Eccles JC, Eccles RM: Differentiation of fast and slow muscles in the cat hind limb. *J Physiol (Lond)* 1960;150:399–416.

43. Burke RE, Levine DN, Zajac FE III: Mammalian motor units: Physiological-histochemical correlation in three types in cat gastrocnemius. *Science* 1971;174:709–712.

44. Dubowitz V: Cross-innervated mammalian skeletal muscle: Histochemical, physiological and biochemical observations. *J Physiol (Lond)* 1967;193:481–496.

45. Edstrom L, Kugelberg E: Histochemical mapping of motor units in experimentally re-innervated skeletal muscle. *Experientia* 1969;25:1044–1045.

46. Hakkinen K, Komi PV: Changes in neuromuscular performance in voluntary and reflex contraction during strength training in man. *Int J Sports Med* 1983;4:282–288.

47. Zappala A: Influence of training and sex on the isolation and control of single motor units. *Am J Phys Med* 1970;49:348–361.

48. Ramos E, Frontera WR, Llopart A, Feliciano D: Muscle strength and hormonal levels in adolescents: Gender related differences. *Int J Sports Med* 1998;19:526–531.

49. Huston LJ, Wojtys EM: Neuromuscular performance characteristics in elite female athletes. *Am J Sports Med* 1996;24:427–436.

50. Winter EM, Brookes FB: Electromechanical response times and muscle elasticity in men and women. *Eur J Appl Physiol* 1991;63:124–128.

51. Wojtys EM, Huston LJ: Neuromuscular performance in normal and anterior cruciate ligament-deficient lower extremities. *Am J Sports Med* 1994;22:89–104.

52. Draganich LF, Vahey JW: An in vitro study of anterior cruciate ligament strain induced by quadriceps and hamstrings forces. *J Orthop Res* 1990;8:57–63.

53. Dürselen L, Claes L, Kiefer H: The influence of muscle forces and external loads on cruciate ligament strain. *Am J Sports Med* 1995;23:129–136.

54. More RC, Karras BT, Neiman R, Fritschy D, Woo SL, Daniel DM: Hamstrings: An anterior cruciate ligament protagonist: An in vitro study. *Am J Sports Med* 1993;21:231–237.

55. Johansson H, Sjölander P, Sojka P: Activity in receptor afferents from the anterior cruciate ligament evokes reflex effects on fusimotor neurones. *Neurosci Res* 1990;8:54–59.

56. Sjölander P: A sensory role for the cruciate ligaments: Regulation of joint stability via reflexes onto the γ-muscle-spindle system. UmeÜö, Sweden, UmeÜö University, 1989. Dissertation.

57. Sojka P, Johansson H, Sjölander P, Lorentzon R, Djupsjobacka M: Fusimotor neurones can be reflexly influenced by activity in receptor afferents from the posterior cruciate ligament. *Brain Res* 1989;483:177–183.

58. Sojka P, Sjölander P, Johansson H, Djupsjobacka M: Influence from stretch-sensitive receptors in the collateral ligaments of the knee joint on the gamma-muscle-spindle systems of flexor and extensor muscles. *Neurosci Res* 1991;11:55–62.

59. Hoffer JA, Andreassen S: Regulation of soleus muscle stiffness in premammillary cats: Intrinsic and reflex components. *J Neurophysiol* 1981;45:267–285.

60. Kearney RE, Stein RB, Parameswaran L: Identification of intrinsic and reflex contributions to human ankle stiffness dynamics. *IEEE Trans Biomed Eng* 1997;44:493–504.

61. Bryant JT, Cooke TD: Standardized biomechanical measurement for varus-valgus stiffness and rotation in normal knees. *J Orthop Res* 1988;6:863–870.

62. Such CH, Unsworth A, Wright V, Dowson D: Quantitative study of stiffness in the knee joint. *Ann Rheum Dis* 1975;34:286–291.

63. Bell DG, Jacobs I: Electro-mechanical response times and rate of force development in males and females. *Med Sci Sports Exerc* 1986;18:31–36.

Chapter 25

Exercise During Pregnancy and Lactation

James F. Clapp III, MD

Introduction

At the present time approximately 25% of women planning pregnancy are involved in exercise regimens that involve strenuous, prolonged types of weight bearing exercise (running, aerobics, stair climbing, etc), and most continue their exercise throughout pregnancy and lactation at levels that exceed the current guidelines published by the American College of Obstetricians and Gynecologists.[1,2] A recent survey indicates that 42% of all women pregnant in the United States perform some type of exercise during pregnancy, and at least half of these continue beyond the sixth month.[3]

However, it is really unclear how much exercise a woman can do without compromising the growth and development of her fetus. This concern is based on the fact that, in the nonpregnant state, performance of sustained, moderate-intensity exercise reduces splanchnic blood flow by 50% or more,[4] often raises core temperature more than 1.5°C,[5] depletes glycogen stores,[6,7] and produces significant shear stress effects.[1] The obvious medical concern is that during pregnancy these exercise-associated changes in visceral blood flow, blood glucose levels, core temperature, and shear stress could produce abortion, malformation, fetal tissue hypoxia, and growth retardation as well as premature labor and direct fetal, placental, or maternal injury.

The purpose of this chapter is to summarize experiments done in my laboratory and those of others over the last 10 years that indicate that this is not the case and then to describe some of the maternal, fetal, and offspring benefits associated with regular exercise during pregnancy and lactation. I will conclude with a discussion of why this appears to be the case and point out how these findings may be applied to various aspects of health care delivery during pregnancy and lactation.

Pregnancy Outcomes: Research Findings

The Pregnancy

Early Pregnancy

There is concern that the mechanical and hormonal changes associated with regular exercise could increase the incidence of abortion and ectopic pregnancy.

Although little research has been done in this area, results from my laboratory show that regularly exercising women can continue their regular exercise regimen without increasing their risk in these two areas.[1,8,9] Whether or not the same is true for women who begin an exercise program very early in pregnancy is unknown. Thus, it is generally recommended that pregnant women who wish to start an exercise program for the first time wait until the twelfth week to begin.

Late Pregnancy

In late pregnancy, obstetric concerns regarding exercise focus on the effects of shear stress on the placenta, membranes, and uterus. Problems of this type should manifest themselves as placental separation with hemorrhage, premature rupture of the membranes, and premature labor. Fortunately, in my experience neither has occurred with any greater frequency in women who either begin or continue a regular exercise regimen throughout late pregnancy.[1,8]

Gestational Length

There is concern that regular exercise might precipitate premature labor because almost every woman who engages in sustained exercise in late pregnancy notes symptoms of increased uterine activity during and immediately after exercise. However, data from many investigators indicate that either continuing or beginning a regular exercise regimen during pregnancy does not increase the incidence of premature labor.[8–12] Nonetheless, the timing of the onset of labor at term (after the beginning of the thirty-eighth week) does appear to vary with the overall volume of exercise. In my experience, 80% of women who continue regular (three or more times a week), sustained (20 minutes or more), weightbearing exercise throughout late pregnancy above a maintenance training level (> 55% of maximal capacity) deliver before their due date, whereas the percentage is 50% in both physically active controls and women who perform at a lower level. This is viewed as a beneficial effect of exercise by most women and by those who care for them.

Length of Labor and Mode of Delivery

Most investigators find that beginning or continuing a regular exercise regimen during pregnancy has no consistent effect on the labor and delivery process, but several have observed that labor is shorter in women who have continued a fairly vigorous program throughout late pregnancy.[8–11,13,14] However, many of these studies simply have used retrospective chart reviews to look at the question, whereas in my laboratory, a member of the investigative team is present during the labor in order to document things as they occur. Using this approach, we find that fit women who continue vigorous weightbearing exercise throughout late pregnancy have labors whose active phase is one third shorter (because of a very low incidence of protraction disorders) and have one third the rate of surgical delivery as well. Thus, when compared to the controls, the exercising women have a 30% increase in the rate of uncomplicated spontaneous vaginal delivery and only a 10% rate of cesarean section.

The Mother

Fertility

While it is clear that marked increases in exercise load or the very high levels found in elite athletes produce both ovulatory dysfunction and infertility,[15,16] I have prospectively followed 250 women who continued to exercise at their regular preconceptional recreational level throughout the periconceptional period and compared them with 250 matched controls. The incidence of infertility was 5% in both groups.[8,9,17] As this is the identical incidence seen in the population as a whole, it is likely that the average woman who exercises recreationally is not at increased risk of experiencing difficulty with conception because she exercises.

Physical Complaints and Musculoskeletal Injury

Because pregnancy is associated with ligamentous relaxation, lordosis, a change in the center of gravity, and an increased number of physical complaints related to the low back, pelvic girdle, and legs, it had been assumed that exercise during pregnancy would increase the incidence of both physical complaints and musculoskeletal injury. However, several reviews that focused on physical complaints and accidental injury during pregnancy comment that there is no evidence that exercise during pregnancy increases the incidence of accidental injury, that even individual case reports are rare, and that exercise actually reduces physical complaints in most women during pregnancy.[18–21] Likewise, in my experience, the rate of exercise-induced injury is actually decreased during pregnancy, and there is a three-fold reduction in the incidence of physical complaints as well.[1,8,17] The reason for this is not entirely clear, but simple observation suggests that fit pregnant women who exercise have better muscle tone and posture, pay greater attention to their exercise environment, and avoid factors that increase injury risk.[9]

Body Composition

In my experience, women who continue regular (three or more times a week), sustained (20 minutes or more), weightbearing exercise at a moderate to high intensity level throughout pregnancy gain less weight (about 3.5 kg less) and retain significantly less fat.[22] In women who begin an exercise regimen for the first time, the exercise volume required to limit weight gain and fat retention exceeds 40 minutes 5 times a week at 50% to 55% of maximal capacity.[9] I believe that this difference simply reflects the differences in energy expenditure during training in the two groups (much less energy expended by the beginner versus the trained woman per hour of exercise at the same intensity).

Bone density is essentially unchanged by pregnancy, and exercise throughout pregnancy has no discernable beneficial effect.[23,24] During lactation, however, there is acute estrogen deficiency, which is accompanied by a pronounced loss of bone mineral with a fall in bone density of approximately 5% in the first three months. Again, regular postpartum exercise does not diminish this effect.[24]

During lactation, the rate of weight loss is not different in women who exercise for the first 3 to 6 months. The reason is that they simply eat enough to balance out the exercise-associated increase in caloric expenditure.[25,26] However, once lactation ceases, the women who continue to exercise readily regain their prepregnancy weight and percent body fat whereas those who do not exercise continue to retain both weight (2 to 4 kg) and fat (2% to 5%) at 1 year.[9,17]

Fitness

Many investigators have demonstrated that beginning a regular program of exercise during pregnancy improves multiple indices of fitness.[8] In addition, women runners who continue to run during pregnancy and lactation actually improve their maximal aerobic capacity by 8% to 10% compared to a group of nonpregnant runners followed over the same time period.[27] This suggests that pregnancy per se has a training effect that probably is a result of the cardiovascular remodeling of pregnancy that increases ventricular volume.[28]

Attitudes and Recovery

All studies that have evaluated the effects of exercise on various indices of feelings of well-being and attitude find that regular exercise has a beneficial effect, and the same is true during pregnancy.[9,17,20,21,29] The findings indicate that exercise improves daily productivity and self-image as well as fostering a positive attitude toward interpersonal relationships, daily life, and the pregnancy. Because most of the women who exercise during pregnancy also continue to exercise postpartum, these attitudes persist postpartum. In addition to the improved fitness noted above, women who exercise regularly postpartum report a more rapid recovery in the areas of general physical ability and emotional stability. They also are better at mastering the new coping skills required for dealing with a new infant.

Breast Feeding

One recent report indicated that exercise might interfere with breast feeding by increasing milk lactate, which altered taste and reduced infant acceptance.[30] However, additional studies clearly refute this contention and document that infant growth is normal and that milk constituents and milk volumes are unaffected in women who exercise at usual training intensities while breast feeding.[26,31]

The Offspring

Fetal Growth and Development

A widespread concern is that the increase in body temperature and reduced uterine blood flow during strenuous exercise in early pregnancy would increase the incidence of fetal congenital malformations. This has not been the case in the 250-odd women I have studied to date.[1,9] However, this question has not been addressed by others, and the normal prevalence of congenital malformations is low (2% to 3%), so that many more women need to be studied to be absolutely sure that there is no negative effect.

Multiple investigators have examined the effect on birth weight of beginning various exercise regimens (cycle ergometry, swimming, stretching, multimodality exercise) during midpregnancy and have not observed any clear positive or negative effect.[10,13,32–40] Multiple retrospective and epidemiologic studies, in which the consistency, intensity, and duration of the exercise was not measured, indicate that the same is true when regular walking and running are continued during pregnancy. However, carefully collected prospective data demonstrate that birth weight is reduced by about 300 g when fit women maintain a regimen of vigorous, sustained exercise (three or more sessions a week, at an intensity > 50% Vo_{2max} [maximum oxygen consumption], lasting a minimum of 20 minutes) throughout pregnancy and that birth weight is increased by a similar amount in those who stop or cut back in mid and late pregnancy.[8,9,17] The data indicate that most of these changes in birth weight are due to changes in fat mass and that the reduction in birth weight is directly related to the mother's level of exercise in the third trimester. Several other studies also note that high volumes of exercise decrease birth weight and that beginning a low intensity regimen of regular weight-bearing exercise appears to actually increase birth weight.[9,36,41,42] In the latter instance, the increase in birth weight is not due to an increase in percent body fat but represents an increase in both axial and circumferential growth with a normal ratio between lean body mass and fat mass.

Fetal Hypoxia

Obviously a major fetal concern is that exercise-induced decreases in maternal glucose levels and placental blood flow reduce fetal glucose and oxygen delivery to critical levels, especially during intense, prolonged exercise. Indeed, the reduction in birth weight with high exercise volumes in late pregnancy reinforces this concern because the reduction in birth weight probably is the result of recurrent transient decreases in fetal glucose availability.[43] Therefore, my associates and I have done a series of studies aimed at determining if maternal exercise induces a significant decrease in fetal oxygen availability. The first, a study of the fetal heart rate response to maternal exercise, indicated that the fetal heart rate increased, indicating some degree of hypoxic stress, and that the magnitude of the increase in heart rate varied directly with exercise intensity and duration.[44] The second examined the effects of maternal exercise on erythropoietin levels in cord blood and amniotic fluid.[45] Levels were no different from those obtained from the fetuses of physically active controls, indicating that the magnitude of the hypoxic stress was small. The third involved studies of fetal behavior, which again showed no evidence of significant hypoxia.[46] The fourth examined the fetal cerebral and renal circulation for evidence of flow redistribution and demonstrated that maternal exercise was associated with an increase in blood flow to both the brain and kidney.[47] Finally, we have completed three studies that assessed neurodevelopmental outcome at 5 days, 1 year, and 5 years of age and found that the neurodevelopment of the offspring of the exercising mothers was consistently equal to or better than that seen in the offspring of the physically active controls.[48–50] Thus, the data consistently indicate that maternal exercise does not induce significant fetal hypoxia in clinically normal pregnancies.

Cord Entanglement

The sudden postural changes and foot strikes associated with a variety of exercises produce fairly intense, sudden acceleration and deceleration forces. These could easily produce sudden postural changes in the fetus who is tethered by its umbilical cord, which raises concern that the fetus might get tangled up in the cord or actually form a true knot in the cord, leading to reductions in umbilical blood flow and fetal compromise. Most studies have not examined this possibility but delivery data from our 250 exercisers and 250 controls indicate that cord complications are significantly less frequent in the fetuses of women who exercise regularly throughout pregnancy.[1,8,17] Currently we are examining the issue with ultrasound to determine if the same is true during mid and late pregnancy.

Direct Fetal Trauma

It is also possible that either abdominal trauma or shear stress could produce direct fetal tissue injury. However, there are no case reports documenting this type of event in association with accidental injury during exercise, and our monitoring has not documented any findings that suggest that it actually occurs.

The Placenta

Studies show that regular weightbearing exercise during pregnancy has a positive effect on placental growth and development.[43,51,52] It increases the growth rate of placental volume in midpregnancy by about a third and, at term, anatomic indices of placental function are significantly higher in the placentae of regularly exercising women. Randomized studies indicate that this response requires only 20 minutes of exercise 3 to 5 days a week.

The Maternal and Fetal Benefits of Exercise During Pregnancy

The Mother

The data discussed above indicate that either beginning or continuing a regular exercise regimen during pregnancy improves multiple facets of maternal outcome and is not detrimental. All types of exercise studied improve a woman's sense of well being, fitness, and recovery after the birth. However, it takes a relatively large volume of exercise to provide the additional benefits of a reduction in weight gain and fat accretion, an earlier onset of labor, and a shorter, less complicated labor. If a woman is starting an exercise regimen and restricts the exercise intensity to 55% of maximum capacity, this means 40 to 60 minutes of exercise 5 days a week. If a woman is continuing a higher intensity regimen, then the volume of exercise necessary to attain these additional benefits must exceed 80% of the prepregnancy regimen.[9] If a woman exercises vigorously in early pregnancy and then cuts back or stops, then the latter benefits are lost.

The Offspring

Currently it appears that regular weightbearing maternal exercise has no identifiable fetal risks and multiple benefits. The first fetal benefit of regular maternal exercise is an increase in the rate of placental growth, which results in an improved functional capacity late in pregnancy. The second benefit is an improved tolerance to a variety of physiologic stresses, which probably relates to an increased blood volume and differences in autonomic response. The third appears to be a restriction in the growth of the fat organ, and the final benefit is evidence of behavioral imprinting, which alters behavior and perhaps long-term neurodevelopment after birth. Further studies are underway to examine that issue as well as the issues of maternal exercise initiating metabolic and cardiovascular imprinting that should alter disease risk later in life.

Why Maternal Exercise Is Beneficial

Regular maternal exercise during pregnancy produces these benefits because the physiologic adaptations to regular exercise and those of pregnancy either magnify one another or cancel one another. The physiologic end result is a very robust alteration in maternal function that protects both mother and fetus from many of the usual problems associated with pregnancy. Several specific examples follow.

Musculoskeletal Adaptations

With the exception of ligamentous laxity of the pelvic girdle,[53] the musculoskeletal adaptations to pregnancy have not been studied well. Objective evidence of an increase in ligamentous laxity around other joints indicates that peripheral changes are minimal.[54,55] Body mass increases by 15% to 25% and, in sedentary individuals, the protuberant abdomen coupled with lumbar lordosis changes the center of gravity, increases the loading of most joints, and is believed to be responsible for a high incidence of low back, hip, symphyseal, and leg pain.[8,56] Limited information on changes in bone mineral indicates that both calcium absorption and bone turnover are increased and that bone density is maintained.[23,24] Changes in muscle mass and contractile force of specific muscle groups have not been examined.

It is well known that regular exercise improves bone density, muscle mass, muscle tone, muscle strength, the velocity of contraction, and ligamentous tensile strength.[57–59] In women, the effects of estrogen and progesterone also interact with exercise and enhance bone mineral turnover and retention.[57]

When pregnancy and exercise are combined it appears that the endocrine changes of pregnancy enhance the effects of exercise on bone and that the effects of exercise act to balance the pregnancy-induced changes in mass, posture, and ligamentous laxity. Thus bone mineral is maintained, and the incidence of musculoskeletal complaints and injury are reduced.

Cardiovascular Adaptations

During pregnancy there are large (40%) increases in blood volume and cardiac output, with two- to twentyfold increases in regional blood flow within the cutaneous, renal, and uterine circulations.[28] These are initiated by the changing hormonal milieu within 2 weeks of conception by a generalized and persistent decrease in vascular tone and reactivity that reduces both preload and after-load, increases heart rate, and triggers salt and water retention. End-diastolic volume and stroke volume increase by 15% to 20%, vascular compliance increases, and total peripheral resistance falls by about 40%. Both catecholamine release with stress and adrenergic vascular sensitivity are down-regulated during pregnancy.[8,60,61]

Classic studies have demonstrated that regular endurance exercise has similar effects on blood volume and ventricular volumes.[58] It also increases the cross-sectional area of the muscle capillary bed and lowers resting heart rate, cardiac output, arterial blood pressure, and the magnitude of the decrease in visceral blood flow during exercise.[58,62,63] Total peripheral resistance and regional perfusion patterns at rest appear unchanged, and all changes rapidly revert to baseline values if the exercise regimen is interrupted. However, during exercise blood flow is redistributed away from the splanchnic viscera to supply the needs of the exercising muscle. Fortunately that is not a problem during pregnancy because, when the physiologic adaptations to regular exercise are combined with those to pregnancy, many of the cardiovascular adaptations are complementary, producing a physiologic environment that ensures tissue perfusion and reduces the risk of fetal hypoxia. For example, the training effects on blood volume, end diastolic volume, and stroke volume are further enhanced by pregnancy. These changes act to maintain fetal oxygenation by minimizing the need for flow redistribution away from the splanchnic and uterine vascular beds during times of hemodynamic stress.[47,64] This assures that both the fetus and the muscle receive adequate amounts of oxygen during sustained vigorous exercise in pregnancy.

Thermoregulatory Adaptations

Pregnancy is associated with a progressive decrease in rectal temperature at rest and a dramatic increase in minute ventilation, blood volume, body mass, and skin blood flow.[5,65] Training also increases blood volume and decreases the core temperature threshold for both cutaneous vasodilatation and sweating.[58,66] Estrogen also enhances both heat storage capacity and heat dissipation by reducing resting core temperature and the thresholds for vasodilation and sweating.[67] All these adaptations improve the capacity for heat storage and dissipation in response to thermal stress. Thus, when exercise is continued during pregnancy, the thermoregulatory adaptations are additive, which dramatically reduces the magnitude of any thermal stress for both mother and fetus.[5]

Significance

These findings clearly indicate that exercise during pregnancy is safe and beneficial for healthy pregnant women. More importantly, however, they suggest that exercise during pregnancy may have long-term health benefits for both the mothers and the offspring. Furthermore, introducing exercise into routine obstetric care may prevent specific maternal symptomatology and be a logical preventive therapy for premature labor and disorders of both fetal under- and overgrowth. These should be considered as important directions for further research. It just may be that the key to reducing perinatal morbidity and mortality in our society lies in increasing the physical activity levels of most women at risk for poor outcomes. Most are currently managed by restricting physical activity. Only further research can determine which is the best approach.

Summary

As a whole, the data do not support a restrictive approach to strenuous recreational physical activity during pregnancy and indicate that the discrepancy between theoretical concerns and observed outcomes is a result of the fact that the physiologic adaptations to regular exercise enhance those to the pregnancy. In fact, the data strongly suggest that regular, sustained physical activity, sufficient to either maintain or improve fitness, has additional physiologic benefit to both the woman and the pregnancy. Therefore, it appears that the inclusion of recreational exercise with specific training objectives as a part of antenatal care for the motivated, healthy woman is not unreasonable. Finally, to be sure that this is the case at a societal level, there is a need for prospective, randomized studies with monitored, quantified exercise regimens that incorporate objective measures of physiologic effects and both short- and long-term outcome.

Acknowledgments

Many of the experiments reviewed in this chapter were supported by NIH grants RO1-21268, P50-211089, and MO1-RR00080, several grants from the National Foundation March of Dimes, and the generous support of MetroHealth Medical Center. In addition, the work would not have been possible without the work of a dedicated staff and the large number of women who gave freely of their time, energy, and sweat.

References

1. Clapp JF III: A clinical approach to exercise during pregnancy. *Clin Sports Med* 1994;13:443–458.
2. American College of Obstetricians and Gynecologists: *ACOG Technical Bulletin #189: Exercise During Pregnancy and the Postpartum Period.* Washington, DC, ACOG Press, 1994.
3. Zhang J, Savitz DA: Exercise during pregnancy among US women. *Ann Epidemiol* 1996;6:53–59.
4. Rowell LB, Blackmon JR, Martin RH, Mazzarella JA, Bruce RA: Hepatic clearance of indocyanine green in man under thermal and exercise stresses. *J Appl Physiol* 1965;20:384–394.

5. Clapp JF III: The changing thermal response to endurance exercise during pregnancy. *Am J Obstet Gynecol* 1991;165:1684–1689.
6. Clapp JF III, Capeless EL: The changing glycemic response to exercise during pregnancy. *Am J Obstet Gynecol* 1991;165:1678–1683.
7. Bonen A, Campagna P, Gilchrist L, Young DC, Beresford P: Substrate and endocrine responses during exercise at selected stages of pregnancy. *J Appl Physiol* 1992;73:134–142.
8. Clapp JF: Exercise during pregnancy, in Bar-Or O, Lamb DR, Clarkson PM (eds): *Exercise and the Female: A Life Span Approach*. Carmel, IN, Cooper Publishing, 1996, pp 413–451.
9. Clapp JF (ed): *Exercising Through Your Pregnancy*. Champaign, IL, Human Kinetics, 1998, pp 245.
10. Lokey EA, Tran ZV, Wells CV, Myers BC, Tran AC: Effects of physical exercise on pregnancy outcomes: A meta-analytic review. *Med Sci Sports Exerc* 1991;23:1234–1239.
11. Hatch MC, Shu XO, McLean DE, et al: Maternal exercise during pregnancy, physical fitness, and fetal growth. *Am J Epidemiol* 1993;137:1105–1114.
12. Kardel KR, Kase T: Training in pregnant women: Effects on fetal development and birth. *Am J Obstet Gynecol* 1998;178:280–286.
13. Beckmann CR, Beckmann CA: Effect of a structured antepartum exercise program on pregnancy and labor outcome in primiparas. *J Reprod Med* 1990;35:704–709.
14. Wong SC, McKenzie DC: Cardiorespiratory fitness during pregnancy and its effect on outcome. *Int J Sports Med* 1987;8:79–83.
15. Bullen BA, Skrinar GS, Beitins IZ, von Mering G, Turnbull BA, McArthur JW: Induction of menstrual disorders by strenuous exercise in untrained women. *N Engl J Med* 1985;312:1349–1353.
16. Loucks AB, Mortola JF, Girton L, Yen SS: Alterations in the hypothalamic-pituitary-ovarian and the hypothalamic-pituitary-adrenal axes in athletic women. *J Clin Endocrinol Metab* 1989;68:402–411.
17. Clapp JF III: Exercise during pregnancy: A clinical update. *Clin Sports Med* 2000;19:273–286.
18. Karzel RP Jr, Friedman MJ: Orthopedic injuries in pregnancy, in Mittelmark RA, Wiswell RA, Drinkwater BL (eds): *Exercise in Pregnancy*, ed 2. Baltimore, MD, Williams & Wilkins, 1991, pp 123–132.
19. Sherer DM, Schenker JG: Accidental injury during pregnancy. *Obstet Gynecol Surv* 1989;44:330–338.
20. Horns PN, Ratcliffe LP, Leggett JC, Swanson MS: Pregnancy outcomes among active and sedentary primiparous women. *J Obstet Gynecol Neonatal Nurs* 1996;25:49–54.
21. Koniak-Griffin D: Aerobic exercise, psychological well-being, and physical discomforts during adolescent pregnancy. *Res Nurs Health* 1994;17:253–263.
22. Clapp JF III, Little KD: Effect of recreational exercise on pregnancy weight gain and subcutaneous fat deposition. *Med Sci Sports Exerc* 1995;27:170–177.
23. Sowers M, Crutchfield M, Jannausch M, Updike S, Corton G: A prospective evaluation of bone mineral change in pregnancy. *Obstet Gynecol* 1991;77:841–845.
24. Little KD, Clapp JF III: Self-selected recreational exercise has no impact on early postpartum lactation-induced bone loss. *Med Sci Sports Exerc* 1998;30:831–836.
25. Little KD, Clapp JF, Ridzon SE: Abstract: Effect of exercise on post partum weight loss. *Med Sci Sports Exerc* 1994;26(suppl):S15.

26. Dewey KG, Lovelady CA, Nommsen-Rivers LA, McCrory MA, Lonnerdal B: A randomized study of the effects of aerobic exercise by lactating women on breast-milk volume and composition. *N Engl J Med* 1994;330:449–453.
27. Clapp JF III, Capeless E: The Vo2max of recreational athletes before and after pregnancy. *Med Sci Sports Exerc* 1991;23:1128–1133.
28. Clapp JF III, Capeless E: Cardiovascular function before, during, and after the first and subsequent pregnancies. *Am J Cardiol* 1997;80:1469–1473.
29. Wallace AM, Boyer DB, Dan A, Holm K: Aerobic exercise, maternal self-esteem, and physical discomforts during pregnancy. *J Nurse Midwifery* 1986;31:255–262.
30. Wallace JP, Inbar G, Ernsthausen K: Infant acceptance of postexercise breast milk. *Pediatrics* 1992;89:1245–1247.
31. Carey GB, Quinn TJ, Goodwin SE: Breast milk composition after exercise of different intensities. *J Hum Lact* 1997;13:115–120.
32. Collings CA, Curet LB, Mullin JP: Maternal and fetal responses to a maternal aerobic exercise program. *Am J Obstet Gynecol* 1983;145:702–707.
33. Hall DC, Kaufmann DA: Effects of aerobic and strength conditioning on pregnancy outcomes. *Am J Obstet Gynecol* 1987;157:1199–1203.
34. Kulpa PJ, White BM, Visscher R: Aerobic exercise in pregnancy. *Am J Obstet Gynecol* 1987;156:1395–1403.
35. Sibley L, Ruhling RO, Cameron-Foster J, Christensen C, Bolen T: Swimming and physical fitness during pregnancy. *J Nurse Midwifery* 1981;26:3–12.
36. Sternfeld B, Quesenberry CP Jr, Eskenazi B, Newman LA: Exercise during pregnancy and pregnancy outcome. *Med Sci Sports Exerc* 1995;27:634–640.
37. Pivarnik JM: Potential effects of maternal physical activity on birth weight: Brief review. *Med Sci Sports Exerc* 1998;30:400–406.
38. Kardel KR, Kase T: Training in pregnant women: Effects on fetal development and birth. *Am J Obstet Gynecol* 1998;178:280–286.
39. Wolfe LA, Mottola MF, Bonen A, et al: Abstract: Controlled randomized study of aerobic conditioning effects on neonatal morphometrics. *Med Sci Sports Exerc* 1999;31(suppl):S138.
40. Magann EF, Evans SF, Newnham JP: Employment, exertion, and pregnancy outcome: assessment by kilocalories expended each day. *Am J Obstet Gynecol* 1996;175:182–187.
41. Bell RJ, Palma SM, Lumley JM: The effect of vigorous exercise during pregnancy on birth-weight. *Aust NZ J Obstet Gynaecol* 1995;35:46–51.
42. Clapp JF, Tomaselli J, Rizdon S, Kortan M, Lopez B, Little KD: Abstract: Pregnancy training volume: Effect on placental growth and size at birth. *Med Sci Sports Exerc* 1997;29(suppl):S4.
43. Clapp JF: Diet, exercise, and feto-placental growth. *Arch Gynecol Obstet* 1997;261:101–107.
44. Clapp JF III, Little KD, Capeless EL: Fetal heart rate response sustained recreational exercise. *Am J Obstet Gynecol* 1993;168:198–206.
45. Clapp JF III, Little KD, Appleby-Wineberg SK, Widness JA: The effect of regular maternal exercise on erythropoetin in core blood and amniotic fluid. *Am J Obstet Gynecol* 1995;172:1445–1451.
46. Hatoum N, Clapp JF III, Newman MR, Dajani N, Amini SB: Effects of maternal exercise on fetal activity in late gestation. *J Matern Fetal Med* 1997;6:134–139.
47. Clapp JF, Stepanchak W, Tomaselli J, Kortan M, Fanselow S: Abstract: The effect of exercise training during pregnancy on flow redistribution in mother and fetus. *Med Sci Sports Exerc* 1999;31(suppl):S139.

48. Clapp JF III, Lopez B, Harcar-Sevcik R: Neonatal behavioral profile of the offspring of women who continued to exercise regularly throughout pregnancy. *Am J Obstet Gynecol* 1999;180:91–94.

49. Clapp JF III, Simonian S, Lopez B, Appleby-Wineberg S, Harcar-Sevcik R: The one-year morphometric and neurodevelopmental outcome of the offspring of women who continued to exercise regularly throughout pregnancy. *Am J Obstet Gynecol* 1998;178:594–599.

50. Clapp JF: The morphometric and neurodevelopmental outcome at age five years of the offspring of women who continued to exercise regularly throughout pregnancy. *J Pediatr* 1996;129:856–863.

51. Clapp JF III, Rizk KH: Effect of recreational exercise on mid-trimester placental growth. *Am J Obstet Gynecol* 1992;167:1518–1521.

52. Jackson MR, Gott P, Lye SJ, Ritchie JW, Clapp JF III: The effects of maternal aerobic exercise on human placental development: Placental volumetric composition and surface areas. *Placenta* 1995;16:179–191.

53. Abramson D, Roberts SM, Wilson PD: Relaxation of the pelvic joints in pregnancy. *Surg Gynecol Obstet* 1934;58:595–613.

54. Calguneri M, Bird HA, Wright V: Changes in joint laxity occurring during pregnancy. *Ann Rheum Dis* 1982;41:126–128.

55. Dumas GA, Reid JG: Laxity of knee cruciate ligaments during pregnancy. *J Orthop Sports Phys Ther* 1997;26:2–6.

56. Ellis MI, Seedhom BB, Wright V: A comparison of knee joint and muscle forces in women 36 weeks pregnant and four weeks after delivery. *Eng Med* 1985;14:95–99.

57. Drinkwater BL, Nilson K, Chesnut CH III, Bremner WJ, Shainholtz S, Southworth MB: Bone mineral content of amenorrheic and eumenorrheic athletes. *N Engl J Med* 1984;311:277–281.

58. Saltin B, Rowell LB: Functional adaptations to physical activity and inactivity. *Fed Proc* 1980;39:1506–1513.

59. Tipton CM, Vailas AC, Matthes RD: Experimental studies on the influences of physical activity on ligaments, tendons, and joints: A brief review. *Acta Med Scand* 1986;711(suppl):157–168.

60. Nisell H, Hjemdahl P, Linde B: Cardiovascular responses to circulating catecholamines in normal pregnancy and in pregnancy-induced hypertension. *Clin Physiol* 1985;5:479–493.

61. Barron WM, Mujais SK, Zinaman M, Bravo EL, Lindheimer MD: Plasma catecholamine responses to physiologic stimuli in normal human pregnancy. *Am J Obstet Gynecol* 1986;154:80–84.

62. Tipton CM: Exercise, training and hypertension: An update. *Exerc Sport Sci Rev* 1991;19:447–505.

63. Andersen P, Henriksson J: Capillary supply of the quadriceps femoris muscle of man: Adaptive response to exercise. *J Physiol (Lond)* 1977;270:677–690.

64. Clapp JF, Little KD, Rizk KH, Appleby-Wineberg S: Pregnancy alters the cardiovascular response to mock hemorrhage. *Proc Soc Gynecol Invest* 1994;41:280.

65. Katz M, Sokal MM: Skin perfusion in pregnancy. *Am J Obstet Gynecol* 1980;137:30–33.

66. Roberts MF, Wenger CB, Stolwijk JA, Nadel ER: Skin blood flow and sweating changes following exercise training and heat acclimation. *J Appl Physiol* 1977;43:133–137.

67. Stephenson LA, Kolka MA: Menstrual cycle phase and time of day alter reference signal controlling arm blood flow and sweating. *Am J Physiol* 1985;249:R186–R191.

Chapter 26

Fitness and Aging

Marybeth Brown, PT, PhD

It has been noted frequently that the fastest growing segment of the population is the 85+ year old group.[1] Approximately half of all the people in this age group have difficulty with activities of daily living and, thus, are limited in their ability to function within the community at large.[2] Most in the 85+ year old group are women, which suggests that women are living longer but not better. Current data indicate that during their final 4 years of life women require the assistance of others, with more than 50% requiring nursing home placement.[3] Longevity for most older women is not synonymous with quality of life. This finding is not unique to our western society. There are indicators that women around the globe are living longer but with more infirmity.

Many factors are associated with the loss of independence in older women, but chief among them is lifestyle, particularly inactivity.[4] Within this past decade several important studies with large sample sizes have clearly indicated that women who remain physically active are not nearly as likely as their sedentary counterparts to become physically incapable of completing their routine activities of dressing, grooming, and housekeeping.[4,5] It would appear that the incorporation of exercise into the daily routine would markedly improve final life outcomes for many women.[6]

In the past 20 years there has been a compression of mortality in the United States.[7] The improved diagnosis and treatment of hypertension, coronary artery disease, and cancer, among other medical conditions, has led to a reduction in premature death and an increase in longevity. The average life span has been shifted closer to the maximal possible life span. What is needed at this juncture is to more closely match longevity with physical independence, ie, the compression of infirmity (Fig. 1). The desired outcome is the postponement of physical frailty and infirmity to the final days of life. Frailty and infirmity can best be delayed by the incorporation of physical activity into the daily routine.[4–6]

Healthy Lifestyle

There is increasing awareness of the need for physical activity, at all ages, but particularly for the older adult.[8] For the past decade, the American Heart Association and the American College of Sports Medicine, for example, have exhorted older adults to exercise.[9] Although awareness of the need for activity has probably increased, there seems to be very little change occurring in

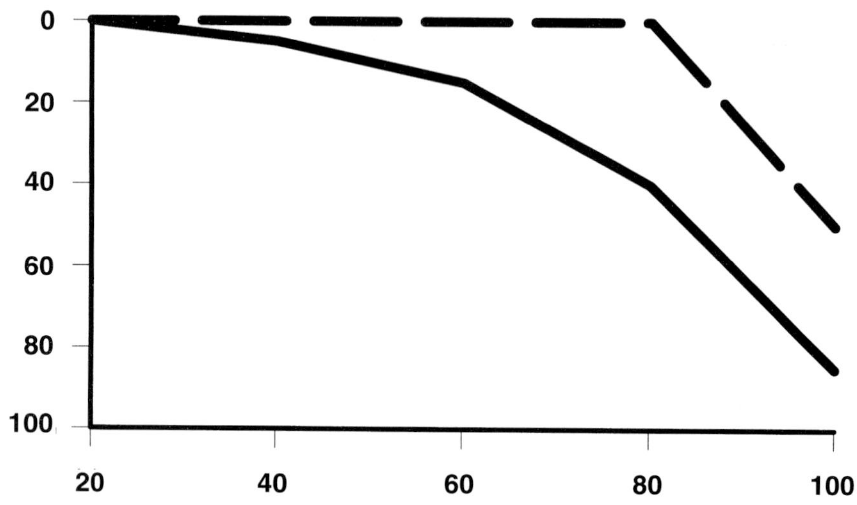

Fig. 1 Compression of infirmity with advancing age. Theoretical reduction of infirmity with aging if physical activity were incorporated into the daily routine (dashed line). The Y axis represents the percentage of those with physical infirmity. The X axis indicates age in years. (Adapted with permission from Fries I, Crapo L: Vitality and Aging. *San Francisco, CA, WH Freeman, 1981.)*

lifestyle. The number of women engaging in exercise, particularly after the age of 60 years, is still very low. Although the following is rather speculative, there appear to be 3 primary reasons for the lack of involvement in activity: (1) there are few programs appropriate for older women, (2) there are no standards or norms for performance of any physical activity at any age, and (3) it is difficult to access health care practitioners who understand the exercise needs of older adults.

Appropriate Programs

On the positive side, there has been an increase in activity programs for older adults in the past decade. In most major metropolitan areas there is an "active aging" column in the newspaper that includes opportunities for activity classes at such venues as the YMCA and older adult community center. These classes clearly serve a need because typically they are filled to capacity each session. Even with the availability of classes, there are many older women with transportation needs, many with frank disinterest in community-based programs, and many with fear of the unknown. What is needed is an opportunity for older women to become involved and knowledgeable about physical activity in all forms, not just exercise per se.

Exercise or sport do not need to be synonymous with physical activity. Increases in physical activity of any sort can achieve major improvements in physical well-being.[9] Making older women more aware of ways to make routine daily chores such as stair climbing, dusting, walking, washing, and shopping more of a physical challenge is an alternative way of influencing behavior. Enhancing awareness of the need to move periodically while sitting to watch television or play cards may be another approach. If women come to understand that lifestyle change can occur without engaging in sports, without exacerbating a medical condition, and without leaving home, there might be more willingness to embrace activity.

Age-Appropriate Norms

Curiously, there are no norms for physical capacity after high school. While in primary school, children may be acculturated to the President's Fitness Program, but unless one joins the Armed Services, there is no obligatory physical challenge for the remainder of life. Thus, there is no opportunity for women to become aware of their physical decline until the end of life, when it might be too late. Women have become aware in our society of the need to brush one's teeth, have PAP smears, have mammograms, and to have cholesterol and blood pressure taken periodically. Perhaps having physical capacity checked routinely should be incorporated as well. Becoming aware of deficiencies in getting down to and up from the floor, picking up an object from the ground, or lifting a weight overhead might serve as an impetus to eliminate inadequacies. It would not be a difficult task to establish norms for women of all ages, using routine activities as the challenge. These physical challenges, picking up an object, rising from a chair, walking quickly enough to cross the street in time (12.5 m in 10 s), and lifting an object overhead, can be evaluated in a minute or less. Thus, these three or four activities (as an example) could become part of a routine check-up in a medical office, at local health fairs, and at senior centers. Virtually anyone can be trained to administer the test reliably. Regardless of what is used to identify physical infirmity or impending frailty, there exists a need for the establishment of performance norms for women of all ages, but particularly those older than 60 years.

Access to Exercise Providers

Physical activity programs for older adults do exist, but finding an appropriate activity outlet for each individual is very difficult. For some a Jane Fonda or "Sit and Be Fit" videotape will suffice, but for other elders a more structured opportunity is imperative. Helping seniors find a successful venue needs to become the responsibility of all health care practitioners. More and more seniors are seeking help with exercise outside the traditional health care model (eg, hiring personal trainers, joining a gym) because those within the system are failing to provide the needed guidance. Older adults should be encouraged to exercise and assisted to exercise by everyone within the health care system. Along with encouragement should come sensible advice regarding safety and expected outcomes and some help with who can best provide the desired service.

Exercise Adaptations in Later Years

Although a lifetime of exercise is the most desirable to optimize well-being, there will always be women who will not engage in physical activity unless coerced by a family member or unless they become frightened by their lack of capability. What potential is there for older deconditioned women to modify their physical status after many decades of inactivity? There is an emerging body of evidence to support the efficacy of exercise even for the oldest. Although exercise can be a potent modifier of physical frailty, exercise cannot eliminate the condition. Preventing physical infirmity through a lifetime of activity should always be the emphasis.

Frailty is a complex phenomenon, characterized by deficits in strength, range of motion, balance, coordination, and speed of reaction. In addition, there may be visual and hearing deficits, peripheral sensory loss, and cognitive impairment. The remainder of this chapter will focus on the elements of frailty that are modifiable, such as strength and balance.

Balance

Balance impairments may be captured using a variety of tests, including the 14-item Berg test, the Romberg test (feet together, semitandem, full tandem positions), the forward reach test, standing on one leg, walking rapidly forward and backwards, characterizing sway, using a movable platform, and negotiating an obstacle course. Some of these balance tests capture static balance whereas others emphasize dynamic balance and weight shifting. Regardless of the method(s) used to capture balance trouble, there are encouraging indicators that balance can be enhanced through exercise. Wolfe and associates,[10] for example, found that older adults who underwent 10 weeks of T'ai Chi exercise had fewer falls 6 months later than control subjects who did not exercise. Shumway-Cook and associates[11] prescribed individualized home exercise programs for men and women older than 65 years of age with a history of two or more falls in the previous 6 months. A reduction in falls risk and an improvement in performance on five clinical tests of balance occurred.[11] Data from our laboratory[12] also indicate that in response to 12 weeks of low intensity exercise that includes a balance component, women are capable of showing improvements in performance on an obstacle course, one-limb stance time, the Romberg test for balance, and the Berg test. What is unknown at this juncture is whether aerobic activity or strength training can result in balance enhancement. Although there are studies that show no change in balance in older adults,[13,14] most intervention trials indicate that older women are capable of making improvements in balance.[10–12,15] In summary, there are encouraging results from balance studies except, perhaps, for the nursing home population.

Strength

Considerable attention has been placed on the enhancement of strength in the older adult, because of the association of strength loss and poor balance,[16] reduction in functional capacity[17] and aerobic capacity,[18] and loss of independence.[19] Frontera and associates[20] demonstrated a highly significant improvement in strength in younger men (age range 60 to 72 years) challenged to lift weights for 12 weeks. Gains in strength averaged more than 100%.[20] Comparable studies have not been conducted for women. More recently, Fiatarone and associates[21] demonstrated that even the oldest men and women, those in the ninth and tenth decades of life, are capable of making substantial increases in strength (~125%) with a concomitant (~10%) increase in lean mass. Reportedly, the improvements in strength were associated with a reduction in frailty as evidenced by faster stair climbing speeds and less reliance on assistive gait devices. Most recently, Chandler and associates[22] reported significant improvements in strength that were associated with improvement in physical performance (chair rise performance, gait speed) and mobility (transfers, stooping, stair climbing). Presumably the improvements noted were comparable for both men and women. Findings from our laboratory indicate that men and women show the same relative increase in strength with comparable training, but the absolute improvements for men are, on average, 50% greater than those for women (Fig. 2).

In summary, studies of strength training universally demonstrate that older adults are capable of marked improvements in force-generating capacity. Typically, gains in strength far exceed the gains in lean mass, which suggests that most of the strength increase is due to neural activation. Although significant increases in strength are possible for older adults with training, strength is never restored to values typical for young adults. What is not known to date is how much strength must change for improvements in strength to translate into changes in function. Also unclear is whether increases in strength lead directly to changes in balance, flexibility, or speed of reaction.

Flexibility

A loss in range of motion occurs with age[23] that may be due to an increase in collagen cross-linking, loss of muscle strength, inactivity, or joint deterioration.[24] Some of the loss in range of motion can be restored through a program of activity such as dance,[25] or more traditional flexibility exercise.[26] More research is needed, however, to determine the critical ranges required to accomplish routine activities and whether these ranges are recoverable with exercise. Also unclear is if improvements in flexibility translate to enhanced balance and functional ability, have an effect on poverty of movement and strength, or affect speed of movement.

Speed of Reaction

A slowing of movement with age has been demonstrated in a variety of ways. Gait speed is diminished[27] and simple and choice reaction times are prolonged. Slowness has been associated with increased risk of falling and car accidents.[28] Although reaction times have not been well studied, there is

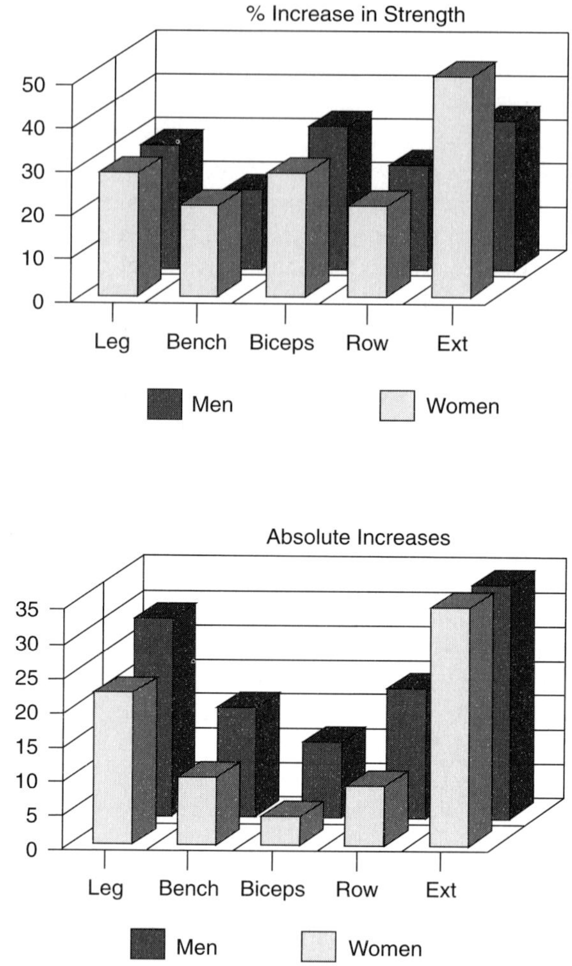

***Fig. 2** Relative increases in strength (%) in comparison to absolute increases for men and women with an average age of 83±4 years. Traditional strengthening exercises (three times a week for 12 weeks) were performed and included the leg press, bench press, biceps curl, seated row, and leg extension.*

little evidence thus far to indicate that older adults are capable of improving speed of reaction. Lord and Castell[29] showed an improvement in reaction time in young subjects (age = 62 years) following a 10-week physical activity program designed to improve speed of reaction, but Rooks and associates[30] did not find any improvement in reaction time in subjects who were older and more physically compromised. A previous study of young-old adults (60 to 70 years) indicates that isokinetic peak torque was reached more quickly following a year of aerobic exercise, but whether isokinetic performance translates to real life circumstances is unknown.[31] Currently, the group of older adults (age = 83 years) in our study that are exercise training exhibit mild to moderate frailty, and there is no indication thus far that reaction time is improved.

Aerobic Capacity

There is evidence that older men and women are capable of increases in aerobic capacity or VO_{2max} that, on a relative basis, are comparable to the gains made by young men and women. Kohrt and associates,[32] for example, found that women ranging in age from 60 to 72 years increased VO_{2max} by 22% with 9 months of aerobic training. Hagberg and associates[33] demonstrated that women from the ages of 70 to 79 years also are capable of increasing aerobic capacity significantly. Whether women older than 80 years are still "trainable" is not clear.

In summary, older adults are capable of responding to an exercise stimulus with improvements in strength, balance, flexibility, and aerobic capacity. Improvements in these domains are often associated with improvements in functional capability, which, for the oldest, are vital to the maintenance of community independence. However, even though exercise is effective at the end stages of life to reduce physical frailty, exercise will probably not, at this stage, eliminate frailty entirely. To prevent physical frailty, activity must be incorporated into the lifestyle at a young age. Women who are physically active throughout their lives are far less likely to require the assistance of others, require hospitalization or nursing home placement, or become infirm.[6] All health care practitioners need to encourage women to embrace activity as an important and integral part of their lives.

Acknowledgments

This project was supported by the Washington University Claude D. Pepper Older Americans Independence Center (AG13629) and by grant AG00585 from the National Institute on Aging.

References

1. Wolinsky FD, Callahan CM, Fitzgerald JF, Johnson R: The risk of nursing home placement and subsequent death among older adults. *J Gerontol* 1992;47:S173–S182.
2. Harris T, Kovar MG, Suzman R, Kleinman JC, Feldman JJ: Longitudinal study of physical ability in the oldest-old. *Am J Public Health* 1989;79:698–702.
3. Guralnik JM, LaCroix AZ, Abbott RD, et al: Maintaining mobility in later life: I. Demographic characteristics and chronic conditions. *Am J Epidemiol* 1993;137:845–857.
4. Blair S, Kohl III H, Paffenbarger Jr R, Clark D, Cooper K, Gibbons L: Physical fitness and all-cause mortality: A prospective study of healthy men and women. *J Am Med Assoc* 1989;262:2395–2401.

5. Seeman TE, Charpentier PA, Berkman LF, et al: Predicting changes in physical performance in a high-functioning elderly cohort: MacArthur studies of successful aging. *J Gerontol* 1994;49:M97–M108.
6. Chandler JM, Hadley E.: Exercise to improve physiologic and functional performance in old age. *Clin Geriatr Med* 1996;12:761–784.
7. Fries I, Crapo L: *Vitality and Aging*. San Francisco, CA, WH Freeman,1981.
8. Buchner D, Wagner EH: Preventing frail health. *Clin Geriatr Med* 1992;8:1–17.
9. American College of Sports Medicine Position Stand: Exercise and physical activity for older adults. *Med Sci Sports Exer* 1998;30:992–1008.
10. Wolfe S, Barnhart HX, Kutner NG, McNeely E, Coogler C, Xu T: Reducing frailty and falls in older persons: An investigation of Tai Chi and computerized balance training. Atlanta FICSIT Group. Frailty and Injuries: Cooperative studies of intervention techniques. *J Am Geriatr Soc* 1996;44:489–497.
11. Shumway-Cook A, Gruber W, Baldwin M, Liao S: The effect of multidimensional exercises on balance, mobility, and fall risk in community-dwelling older adults. *Phy Ther* 1997;77:46–57.
12. Brown M, Holloszy JO: Effects of a low-intensity exercise program on selected physical performance characteristics of 60- to 71-year olds. *Aging Clin Exper Res* 1991;3:129–139.
13. Mills EM: The effect of low-intensity aerobic exercise on muscle strength, flexibility, and balance among sedentary elderly persons. *Nurs Res* 1994;43:207–211.
14. Reinsch S, MacRae P, Lachenbruch PA, Tobis JS: Attempts to prevent falls and injury: A prospective community study. *Gerontologist* 1992;32:450–456.
15. Lord SR, Castel: Physical activity program for older persons: Effect on balance, strength, neuromuscular control, and reaction time. *Arch Phys Med Rehabil* 1994;75:648–652.
16. Whipple RH, Wolfson LI, Amerman PM: Relationship of knee and ankle weakness to falls in nursing home residents: An isokinetic study. *J Am Geriatr Soc* 1987;35:13–21.
17. Hyatt RH, Whitelaw MN, Bhat A, Scott S, Maxwell JD: Association of muscle strength with functional status of elderly people. *Age Ageing* 1990;19:330–336.
18. Fleg JL, Lakatta EG: Role of muscle loss in the age-associated reduction in Vo2max. *J Appl Physiol* 1988;65:1147–1151.
19. Jette AM, Branch LG: The Framingham disability study: II. Physical disability among the aging. *Am J Public Health* 1981;71:1211–1216.
20. Frontera WR, Meredith CN, O'Reilly KP, et al: Strength conditioning in older men: Skeletal muscle hypertrophy and improved function. *J Appl Physiol* 1988;64:1038–1042.
21. Fiatarone MA, O'Neill EF, Doyle N, et al: The Boston FICSIT study: The effects of resistance training and nutritional supplements on physical frailty in the oldest old. *J Am Geriatr Soc* 1993;41:333–337.
22. Chandler JM, Duncan PW, Kochersberger G, Studenski S: Is lower extremity strength gain associated with improvement in physical performance and disability in frail, community-dwelling elders? *Arch Phys Med Rehab* 1998;79:24–30.
23. Walker JM, Sue D, Miles-Elkousy N, Ford G, Trevelyan H: Active mobility of the extremities in older subjects. *Phys Ther* 1984;64:919–923.
24. Vandervoort AA, Chesworth BM, Cunningham DA, Patterson DH, Rechnitzer PA, Koval JJ: Age and sex effects on mobility of the human ankle. *J Gerontol A Biol Sci Med Sci* 1992;47:M17–M21.

25. Munns K: Effects of exercise on the range of joint motion in elderly subjects, in Smith EL, Serfass RC (eds): *Exercise and Aging*. Hillside, NJ, Enslow Publishers, 1981, pp 167–178.

26. Raab DM, Agre JC, McAdam M, Smith EL: Light resistance and stretching exercise in elderly women: Effect on flexibility. *Arch Phys Med Rehabil* 1988;69:268–278.

27. Murray MP, Kory RC, Sepic SB: Walking patterns of normal women. *Arch Phys Med Rehabil* 1970;51:637–650.

28. Wilkinson RT, Allison S: Age and simple reaction time: Decade differences for 5,325 subjects. *J Gerontol* 1989;44:29–36.

29. Lord AR, Castell S: Physical activity program for older adults: Effect on balance, strength, neuromuscular control, and reaction time. *Arch Phys Med Rehabil* 1994;75:648–652.

30. Rooks DS, Kiel DP, Parsons C, Hayes WC: Self-paced resistance training and walking exercise in community-dwelling older adults: Effects on neuromotor performance. *J Gerontol A Biol Sci Med Sci* 1997;52:M161–M168.

31. Brown M, Holloszy JO: Effects of walking, jogging and cycling on strength, flexibility, speed and balance in 60- to 72-year-olds. *Aging (Milano)* 1993;5:427–434.

32. Kohrt WM, Maley MT, Coggan AR, et al: Effects of gender, age, and fitness level on response of Vo2max to training in 60-71 yr olds. *J Appl Physiol* 1991;71:2004–2011.

33. Hagberg JM, Graves JE, Limacher M, et al: Cardiovascular responses of 70- to 79-year-old men and women to exercise training. *J Appl Physiol* 1989;66:2589–2594.

Directions for Future Research

Continuing research should be directed toward the appropriate types and levels of physical activity so that each individual can realize the benefits to each of the systems of the body. While much is known about training, it does not include all the information needed to gain the maximum benefits while avoiding the negative aspects of injury that forces people out of activity and down the road toward the recognized problems of inactivity. Specifically, within this construct, it is possible to explore this dose-response relationship in men and women across the life span—preadolescent, adolescent, young adult, and the aging adult—as it affects performance and injury prevention.

Revisit the athletic profile research.

Many of the current concepts on the differences and similarities between men and women are based on data collected when athletic profiling was popular, which was over 20 years ago. There is no doubt that the male or the female athlete of today is a superior performer. Perhaps it is time to reconsider expectations of the athletic profile within both individual and team sports for men and women.

Continue to refine the principles of physical training to maximize the adaptations to training and minimize the risk of injury.

The systematic manipulation of the variables of training, if complied with, will lead to predictable adaptations. However, the potential magnitude of the adaptations is still unknown, especially with respect to age, gender, and activity mode. Within sports, coaches still strive to further improve the level of performance through training modifications and improvements in technique and equipment. The overall goal should be to improve fitness, but not to be so aggressive at this improvement that athletes are led into overreaching, overtraining, or injury. A focus on training program research might also be directed toward the use of the principles of periodization across the spectrum of sport.

Focus on the need for and development of resistance training programs for the upper body in women.

The literature has shown repeatedly that the greatest difference between men and women in absolute and relative strength is in the upper body. Therefore, it may be necessary to emphasize upper body resistance training for women. There is increasing support for this concept as upper body strength (or lack thereof) may attenuate strength gains in the lower body in lifts that require some participation of the upper body.

Resistance training is beneficial for numerous systems. Determine the optimal programs for the most favorable adaptations and benefits for women.

Resistance training is known to have beneficial effects on strength, connective tissue, bone, neuromuscular facilitation, the cardiovascular system, and body composition as well as numerous psychological benefits. Most of these programs are based on what is known from studies on men. Perhaps there are refinements in the methods of resistance training that would offer more appropriate benefits in areas that are of particular interest to women, eg, bone density or osteoarthritis.

Longitudinal studies need to be conducted with regard to health benefits of long-term participation in resistance training programs.

It is possible that promoting resistance training as a lifetime activity will reduce the incidence and severity of osteoporosis and other debilitating diseases (eg, osteoarthritis) in the aging female. This theory needs support in the literature through longitudinal investigations and cross-sectional investigations of individuals who have used resistance training for many years (ie, competitive Master's weightlifters and power lifters).

Determine whether flexibility training has a real impact on decreasing injury rates.

It is reasonably well accepted that an improvement in flexibility is protective against selected injuries. However, there is some evidence to suggest that the people sustaining a noncontact injury to the anterior cruciate ligament (ACL) have greater hamstring flexibility than others. These clinical observations may be indicating some threshold. Flexibility training may prevent strain injury but increase the risk of ACL injury. Most surveys show that girls and women pursue flexibility training more aggressively than do boys and men; thus, they may be increasing their risk for ACL injury. Systematic examination of the efficacy of flexibility training in preventing injury has not been explored in detail.

Determine whether improvements in flexibility can have an impact on eventual motor patterns that are considered injurious.

Increasing the range of motion about a joint may lead to subtle changes in the motor pattern necessary to perform routine athletic maneuvers. It may be possible that these subtle changes, while obtained with good intentions, put athletes in a position of being at higher risk of injury. Although training/conditioning programs in males have generally predictable progressions in strength and performance, questions remain as to whether females have a similar ability to achieve continuous gain through the use of similar protocols.

Study the patterns of movement for walking, running, and athletic maneuvers for important variables associated with age, gender, and level of experience.

Investigators tend to react to injuries by looking at as many details as possible about the injury. For example, investigators wonder why women have so many more ACL injuries than men before looking to see why men (or any athletes) tear their ACL in the first place. Investigators report that women are more "quadriceps dependent" in the performance of complex athletic maneuvers. But they may need to look at motor patterns of even more basic movements such as walking and various speeds of running before making reasonable statements about the age, gender, and training influences on the more complicated athletic maneuvers.

Define the structural, neuromuscular, and motor control factors that lead to injury with respect to biomechanics.

Physicians attempt to understand injuries using the clinical methods available. However, these impressions really need to be explored in detail using whatever technological means can best help answer questions objectively. The field of sports biomechanics has long been focused on sport technique in order to optimize performance. These same methods can be used to explore the neural activation patterns and the kinetics and kinematics of simple and complex sporting movements.

Determine the optimal patterns of neural activation within each sport.

The continued improvement of skill performance in most activities suggests that the motor and neural activation patterns in the performance of these skills continue to be refined. Such refinements need to be studied in order to identify the patterns that might be injurious.

Determine whether motor patterns in women are inherent or are driven by experience.

A fundamental question is whether motor patterns are inherent or whether these are learned through the particular environment. If these patterns are inherent, then it must be determined why such patterns work better for women than for men. If the patterns are learned, then there is potential for changing such patterns. If it is determined that these patterns should be changed, it then becomes important to explore teaching and coaching strategies that are specific for women with respect to injury prevention.

Determine whether motor activation patterns change with different stages of development, eg, prepubescent, adolescent, early adult, elderly.

Once the patterns of routine and complex activities are determined, it is important to learn when these patterns might be set and how these patterns change across the spectrum of development. Learning more about when these patterns develop and how they change could influence not only participation in activity but also potential motor pattern modification, both of which might lead to the prevention of injury in daily activities throughout life.

Continue to investigate the multitude of physiologic, biochemical, and psychosocial responses to training during pregnancy.

The beneficial effect of physical training during pregnancy is not widely recognized or practiced in the clinic or the laboratory. Is there a threshold for the volume and intensity of exercise at the various stages of pregnancy, and at what point might risks become evident? Are the responses and adaptations mode specific? For example, how do various activities such as walking, running, swimming, and cycling affect the woman and the fetus? Which physiologic effects are positive or negative (eg, insulin sensitivity)? There is a need to investigate whether exercise might be used to offset some of the problems of pregnancy (eg, hypertension, gestational diabetes, etc). The long-term outcome of exercise on both the mother and the child and whether "fetal imprinting" extends to prenatal physical activity need to be explored.

Explore the guidelines for physical activity for the elderly to ensure that the range of benefits can be achieved.

In many interventions, there are people who undertake the regimen and do not achieve the expected result. This is a frustration for all concerned. More information is needed to guide the application of activity so that the benefits can be realized.

Continue the search for simple, low-cost, reliable methods that will alert individuals that they are on the path to frailty.

There currently is no easily administered tool that could be used as a "wake-up call" that a person is progressing toward frailty. The public health cost of injuries in the elderly is staggering, and while frailty may not be preventable, it can be delayed. Physicians, health clubs, health fairs, and so forth could have a wide impact on the aging population with simple tools that could be used to alert the person that they need to begin trying to delay their progression toward the risks associated with frailty.

Section Five

General Health Issues

Section Editor:
Steven N. Blair, PEd

Roger A. Fielding, PhD
Kenton R. Kaufman, PhD, PE
Wendy M. Kohrt, PhD

Overview

Thorough reviews of physical activity and health issues have been presented in recent reports from the American College of Sports Medicine, American Heart Association, Centers for Disease Control and Prevention, National Institutes of Health, and the Office of the Surgeon General. The general consensus presented in these reports is that physical inactivity is a major public health problem in the United States. This conclusion derives from the high prevalence of sedentary living patterns and the strong association of low levels of activity and fitness to numerous chronic diseases and conditions. Population attributable risks for physical inactivity are high and rival those of cigarette smoking and unhealthful dietary patterns as a cause of poor health, functional limitations, and decreased longevity.

Evidence for the effects of physical activity on health is from pathophysiologic investigations, clinical research, and epidemiologic studies. A thorough review of this evidence is beyond the scope of this section, and those seeking more information are referred to the "Surgeon General's Report on Physical Activity and Health" that was published in 1996 (available from the Centers for Disease Control and Prevention or the U.S. Government Printing Office). Drawing from the evidence reviewed in the Surgeon General's report and the other recent consensus statements and guidelines mentioned above, we can conclude that regular physical activity provides numerous health benefits. Active and fit individuals have greater longevity and are less likely to die from coronary heart disease, other cardiovascular diseases, and colon cancer, when compared with those who are sedentary and unfit. Inactivity also is implicated as a cause of overweight and obesity, type II diabetes mellitus, hypertension, and loss of function and independence that are often found in elderly individuals. There also is evidence suggesting that activity may protect against loss of bone mineral, development of depressive symptoms, and gall bladder disease. Regular physical activity appears to enhance general psychological well-being and promote better sleep patterns.

Many of the early studies on the health effects of regular exercise were conducted in populations of men, but much recent evidence comes from investigations of women. The benefits of exercise listed in the preceding paragraph appear to be similar for women and for men. In most studies where women and men are included, physiologic adaptations to exercise and health effects are comparable. This should not be surprising for the chronic health problems affected by exercise, in that the other risk factors for these diseases such as cigarette smoking, abnormal lipid profile, and blood pressure also seem to have comparable effects in women and men.

In this section, three detailed reviews of specific issues related to exercise and women's health are presented. Chapter 27 reviews the role of exercise in bone mineral density and overall skeletal health. Evidence is presented from studies of reduced loading of bone, cross-sectional comparisons of sedentary and active individuals, and prospective investigations. Although there are equivocal findings, it seems clear that regular exercise plays an important role in bone health, along with nutritional factors and hormonal conditions.

Chapter 28 examines the role of exercise in relation to osteoarthritis and notes that there is a paucity of well-designed published studies. Although women have a higher prevalence of osteoarthritis than men at all ages, the association between exercise and osteoarthritis appears to be similar in women and men. Participation in exercise and physical activity for health and recreation does not appear to cause osteoarthritis in individuals with normal joints. Strenuous competitive sports activities may increase risk of osteoarthritis, especially following overuse and acute injuries that are often part of competitive athletics in both women and men. Patients with osteoarthritis who exercise often improve functional status, decrease medication use, report less pain, and have psychological benefits; however, these findings are primarily from short-term studies. Patients with osteoarthritis who plan to start an exercise program should proceed carefully and discuss any unusual signs or symptoms with their health care professional.

Chapter 29 presents evidence that age-related changes in body composition, particularly the loss of skeletal muscle mass, are related to the prevalence of increased disability in the elderly. Older women are at increased risk for sarcopenia and the accompanying physical dysfunction. Nutritional status throughout the life span is associated with the development of sarcopenia. Intervention studies have examined the interaction between nutrient supplementation and resistance exercise training in frail older men and women and have demonstrated an enhancement of strength gains and type II muscle fiber hypertrophy. Nutritional status in women is an important covariate in assessing the relationship between age-related changes in body composition and disability.

In summary, physical activity provides many health and functional benefits for adult women. The prevalence of sedentary habits is high, increases with age, and is higher for women in minority groups. There are 20 to 25 million adult women in the United States who are sedentary and, thus, at substantially elevated risk for several chronic diseases and conditions. Therefore, low levels of activity and fitness constitute a major public health burden for women. A significant challenge is to develop and implement effective strategies to help these sedentary women adopt and maintain a more physically active way of life so that they can enjoy greater longevity and improved quality of life.

STEVEN N. BLAIR, PED

Chapter 27
Exercise and Bone Mass

Wendy M. Kohrt, PhD

Introduction

The notion that exercise prevents osteoporosis is prevalent among health care professionals and the lay community. However, although exercise is unquestionably an important determinant of bone mass, there is no direct evidence that it prevents osteoporotic fractures. The occurrence of an osteoporotic fracture depends both on the fragility of the bone and on an event, such as a fall, that causes the fracture. It is, therefore, conceivable that people who maintain high levels of physical activity are at increased, rather than decreased, risk for osteoporotic fractures because they are more likely to put themselves in situations where fractures can occur. Because of these issues, this chapter will focus on the effects of exercise on bone mineral density (BMD), which is the single most important determinant of bone strength.

A number of different approaches have been used by investigators to study the effects on BMD of the mechanical loading forces generated during exercise. These approaches include (1) the characterization of changes that occur under conditions of reduced loading (eg, bed rest, space flight, immobilization); (2) cross-sectional comparisons of sedentary and physically active individuals, of athletes and nonathletes, or of groups of athletes who participate in sports that vary in skeletal loading characteristics; and (3) prospective studies of changes that occur in response to various types of exercise training programs. Examples of each of these will be discussed, along with the types of exercises most likely to be beneficial to the skeleton and factors that may influence whether the benefits of exercise are realized. In general, this chapter will be limited to studies that involved humans, although findings from studies of animal models will be discussed where relevant.

Effects of Reduced Mechanical Loading

The deleterious change in bone mass that occurs when normal loading forces that act on the skeleton are eliminated or diminished provides the most compelling evidence that mechanical loading is a critical determinant of BMD. An excellent example of this is the study by Leblanc and associates[1] in which they measured changes in BMD in healthy young men in response to 17 weeks of bed rest. BMD decreased significantly at all sites measured except the forearm. Reductions at the femoral neck, greater trochanter, and lumbar spine averaged –3.6%, –4.6%, and –3.9%, respectively. These reductions are particularly important from a clinical perspective because osteoporotic fractures at these sites are associated with a high degree of morbidity and mortality in the elderly. Because young men would normally lose little, if any, bone mineral over a 4-month period, the 3% to 5% decreases that were observed reflected a more than 50-fold increase in the rate of loss.

More recently, Zerwekh and associates[2] examined the effects of 12 weeks of bed rest on BMD, bone histology, and biochemical markers of bone turnover in 9 men and 2 women, aged 20 to 53 years. They observed decreases in BMD of the femoral neck (–1.1%), greater trochanter (–3.8%), and lumbar spine (–2.9%), increases of more than 100% in the eroded surface of both cancellous and cortical bone, and increases in biochemical markers of bone resorption that remained elevated after 12 days of reambulation. Markers of bone formation were not significantly changed in response to bed rest, suggesting that mechanical loading forces are necessary to maintain appropriate coupling between bone resorption and formation.

Even more disturbing than the rapid and profound loss of bone mineral that occurs in response to bed rest is the observation that the mineral does not appear to be readily recovered upon reambulation. Ito and associates[3] reported that brief periods of bed rest subsequent to hip surgery led to significant bone loss in the tibia and that it took more than 1 year to recover to the baseline BMD. Although it might be postulated that the slow recovery of mineral was related to reduced physical activity levels of the patients after surgery, that would not be the case for the young, healthy men subjected to bed rest by Leblanc and associates.[1] In that study, there was no recovery of mineral at the hip or spine 6 months after the men returned to their usual activities. It seems plausible, based on Lanyon's error strain distribution theory of bone modeling and remodeling,[4] that the "usual activities" of the young men, which were presumably adequate for maintaining bone mass prior to bed rest, were also adequate only for maintaining, not increasing, bone mass after bed rest. The error strain distribution theory suggests that the strains of normal locomotion are ineffective in promoting new bone formation. Rather, it is "error strains," those to which bone cells are unaccustomed, that are theorized to stimulate the adaptive response. If this theory is correct, it has important implications for designing exercise programs targeted toward the prevention of osteoporosis. It also has important implications for older individuals, already at risk for osteoporosis, who undergo recurrent periods of bed rest or markedly reduced physical activity due to illness or injury, because it suggests that aggressive therapy may be necessary to restore the loss of bone mineral that is likely to occur.

Cross-Sectional Comparisons

In general, comparisons of BMD in physically active and sedentary individuals and in athletes and nonathletes support the contention that exercise has beneficial effects on bone mass.[5–9] Obviously, these cross-sectional comparisons must be interpreted cautiously, because it is impossible to determine whether observed differences in BMD are truly the result of differences in intensity, volume, or mode of exercise. For example, investigators have attempted to determine whether nonweightbearing sports (eg, swimming) are as effective as weightbearing sports (eg, running) in increasing or maintaining bone mass by comparing BMD values in groups of athletes who participate in these different activities. Results of these studies have been contradictory[10–13] and it is likely that the discordant findings are due, at least in part, to the fact that the activities of athletes are not necessarily limited to the sport in which they participate. Indeed, competitive swimmers may not be an appropriate model for studying the osteogenic effects of nonweightbearing exercise, because they typically participate in vigorous weight lifting and other weightbearing activities.

In spite of such limitations, there are certainly issues worth noting regarding information gleaned from cross-sectional studies of the effects of exercise on bone. Studies of highly trained athletes suggest that the osteogenic effects of a given exercise are specific to the skeletal regions stressed by the activity. Thus, runners have been shown to have increased leg, but not arm, BMD when compared with nonathletes,[14] and contralateral differences in arm BMD have been observed in volleyball, basketball, and tennis players, but not swimmers.[11,15] Perhaps the most uniform finding among studies of athletes is that BMD values are higher in strength- and power-trained athletes than in endurance-trained athletes,[6] with differences reaching approximately 15%. One factor that must be taken into consideration in this regard is that athletes who participate in endurance sports (eg, running) typically maintain relatively low body weights and that in women, low body weight frequently is associated with amenorrhea and low BMD. It is uncertain, therefore, whether the lower BMD values in endurance-trained versus resistance-trained athletes reflect differences in body weight and/or hormonal status, or whether resistance training is truly more effective in stimulating bone mineral accretion.

The most definitive information regarding the specific characteristics of mechanical loading forces (ie, intensity, frequency) that are important determinants of an osteogenic response has come from the work of Rubin and Lanyon,[16,17] who used an avian model. By manipulating the intensity and frequency of mechanical loading forces applied to bone, these investigators demonstrated that the extent of bone mineral accretion was positively related to the magnitude of the force applied (ie, the resulting strain) and that the peak osteogenic response was attained with relatively few loading cycles (~36/day). They further demonstrated that it was essential that the force be applied in a dynamic rather than static fashion, and that the adaptive response depended on whether the strain distribution was novel.[18] If these findings are relevant to humans, it would suggest that an activity such as walking would not be expected to induce an increase in bone mass in most individuals because it is a highly repetitious activity that does not stress the skeleton in a unique manner, either in terms of the magnitude of the loading forces or the distribution of the resulting strains. Resistance training (ie, weight lifting), on the other hand, might be expected to stimulate bone formation if the training regimen involves few repetitions (eg, 6 to 8) performed at a high relative intensity (eg, 80% of the maximal weight that can be lifted one time) and is carried out in a progressive manner, meaning that the training stimulus continues to increase as muscle hypertrophy occurs and strength increases. This may explain why, in cross-sectional studies, resistance-trained athletes consistently have higher BMD values than endurance-trained athletes.

Comparisons of sedentary and physically active individuals provide further support for the beneficial effects of physical activity on bone. An obvious limitation of these studies is that it is very difficult to quantify physical activity level and even more difficult to quantify the exposure to activities that are specifically likely to have an impact on bone mass. Although most physical activity questionnaires attempt to categorize activities according to intensity (eg, easy, moderate, vigorous), this categorization is usually a reflection of cardiovascular stress rather than bone stress. Current physical activity status typically is assessed by having individuals maintain written logs that describe their activities. Historical physical activity habits are usually assessed through the use of questionnaires than inquire about activities performed over the previous week, month, year, or even a lifetime. Obviously, these methods lack precision and are appropriate for use only in studies involving relatively large cohorts.

Greendale and associates[19] evaluated the relationships among lifetime physical activity habits, BMD, and osteoporotic fracture in 1,014 women and 689 men, 50 years or older at the time of the assessment. They found no association of either current or former exercise habits with BMD of the distal forearm and only a trend for lifetime exercise to be positively associated with lumbar spine BMD. However, they found that both current and former exercise habits were associated positively with BMD of the total hip and specific regions of the hip (ie, greater trochanter, neck). Despite the apparent positive effects of exercise on hip BMD, the risk of osteoporotic fracture was not associated with exercise habits in this study.

Potential benefits of exercise on the skeleton may not be realized in the absence of an appropriate nutritional environment. This fact was demonstrated by Uusi-Rasi and associates,[20] who studied 422 women ranging in age from 25 to 65 years, classified by level of physical activity (ie, low or high) and calcium intake (ie, low or high). Neither physical activity nor calcium intake was related to BMD of the forearm. However, both physical activity and calcium intake were significant determinants of total body bone mineral content and both were also associated with estimates of bone strength for the shaft of the femur. BMD of the femoral neck was greater in the high activity group, but was not significantly affected by calcium intake. In a similar study by Suleiman and associates[21] of 124 women, aged 52 to 62 years, women with the highest levels of calcium intake and physical activity had significantly higher BMD values at the hip and spine when compared with those with the lowest levels of calcium intake and physical activity. Physical activity level was also a significant independent determinant of femoral neck BMD in the 827 women older than 60 years studied by Nguyen and associates.[22] In that study, comparisons of women aged 60 to 69 years, 70 to 79 years, and 80 years or older suggested that the age-adjusted rate of decline in femoral neck

BMD was –1.4 ± 0.2%/yr in physically inactive women, but only –0.5 ± 0.3%/yr in those who were physically active.

The numerous published studies of physically active individuals and of athletes provide strong support for the positive effects of exercise on bone mass. However, more definitive information regarding expected increases in BMD in response to exercise and the types of exercise most likely to induce bone mineral accretion can be gained only from studies that involve exercise interventions.

Prospective Studies of Exercise Training

Studies of the effects of exercise training, which have been reviewed recently by others,[5,7] have yielded equivocal results, with reports of significant increases in BMD, a preservation of bone mass in exercisers relative to nonexercising controls, or an even an acceleration of bone loss. Even in those studies that have demonstrated significant increases in BMD in response to exercise training, the magnitudes of improvement have been relatively small, averaging 1% to 4%. However, for the postmenopausal woman, whose BMD may be decreasing by 1% to 2% per year,[22] this may represent a physiologically significant improvement, because exercise is likely to influence bone in a more mechanically and structurally appropriate manner than systemic agents that act throughout the skeleton.[4]

The reasons for the variable findings of the effects of exercise training on bone are not certain. However, a shortcoming of many of the studies in the literature is the absence of a detailed description of the exercise program and, even more importantly, the degree of compliance to the program. Thus, in many of the studies that yielded negative results, it is not possible to discern whether the exercise was performed but was ineffective in increasing bone mass, or whether bone mass failed to increase because the exercise was not performed as prescribed. Another factor that may contribute to the discordant findings in the literature is that the loading forces induced by an exercise program represent only a small fraction of the total forces to which the skeleton is subjected over the course of a day. Because it is the intensity, rather than the frequency, of the loading forces that is the most critical determinant of the bone modeling response,[16,17] whether an exercise program leads to an increase in bone mass may depend on whether the peak forces engendered by the exercise are sufficiently higher than those to which the skeleton is subjected outside of the exercise program. Such factors are difficult, if not impossible, to control and/or quantify.

Studies that have documented compliance to vigorous exercise training programs indicate that significant increases in BMD can be induced by exercise.[23–28] The type of exercise most likely to stimulate bone formation and prevent bone loss remains uncertain. However, the importance of high strain rates in inducing an osteogenic response in humans is particularly apparent in studies that have examined the effects of gymnastics training (ie, high-impact loading) on BMD. In female collegiate athletes, 6 to 12 months of gymnastics training resulted in increases in BMD of the spine (1.2% to 2.8%) and femoral neck (1.6% to 5.0%) that were larger than those that occurred over the same time period in swimmers,[29] runners,[29] or nonathletic controls.[29,30] The changes in gymnasts occurred despite high initial BMD values and were independent of reproductive hormone status.[29]

Gymnastics may be effective in inducing bone mineral accretion, but it is not an activity in which many people are likely to participate. It is therefore important to identify those lifetime activities that are most likely to be beneficial to the skeleton. Although higher BMD values are consistently reported for power- or resistance-trained, as compared with endurance-trained, athletes, prospective studies suggest that resistance exercise training is no more effective in increasing bone mass than weightbearing endurance exercise training.[24,31] In fact, in older postmenopausal women, exercise programs involving either walking, jogging, and stair climbing/descending or weight lifting and rowing, resulted in significant and similar increases in whole body and lumbar spine BMD.[24] However, only the more traditional endurance exercise program (walking, jogging, stepping) was effective in increasing BMD of the femoral neck.

There is some evidence that past participation in sports that increase BMD (ie, gymnastics) may confer residual positive effects on bone in adulthood.[32,33] Exercise during the developmental years may therefore be very important in maximizing peak bone mass. However, even though exercise training may initially increase and then help to sustain bone mass, it does not appear to prevent age-related declines in BMD. In a 9-year follow-up study of runners and nonrunning controls, the age-related rate of decline in lumbar spine BMD was similar in both groups, although BMD levels were higher in runners.[34] It now also is apparent that exercise cannot compensate for the menopause-related bone loss that occurs in women.[35] However, exercise and estrogen replacement have been shown to have independent and additive effects on total body and spine BMD, but not hip BMD, in postmenopausal women.[25,26,36]

The importance of estrogen in maintaining bone mass is apparent not only in postmenopausal women, but also in older men and in some young female athletes who have a history of oligomenorrhea or amenorrhea. In men aged 60 to 89 years, bioavailable estradiol levels have been shown to be more strongly associated with BMD than free testosterone and other endogenous sex hormone levels.[37] With respect to female athletes, there has been heightened awareness in recent years of a condition that has come to be known as the female athlete triad (see chapter 32), consisting of disordered eating, amenorrhea, and osteoporosis. The athletes at highest risk for this condition include those who participate in sports that emphasize low body weight, sports in which appearance may affect subjective scoring, and sports that use weight categories for participation.[38] In young women who have this disorder, it is likely that it is low energy intake and not exercise, per se, that causes the disruption in sex hormone metabolism that leads to the development of osteoporosis.[39] Importantly, even amenorrheic athletes can respond to exercise training with increases in bone mass.[29]

Summary

Exercise plays an important role in sustaining skeletal integrity. People with more physically active life styles maintain higher BMD levels in critical weightbearing regions of the skeleton than sedentary individuals. Drastic reductions in the mechanical loading forces that normally act on the skeleton result in a rapid and profound loss of bone mineral that is difficult to recover. Exercise training, involving either vigorous weightbearing endurance exercises or high-intensity resistance exercises, can induce significant increases in BMD, but the magnitude of the increase is likely to be relatively small, averaging 1% to 4% in the spine and hip regions. Furthermore, although exercise may attenuate the age-related decline in bone mass, habitual exercise, even when vigorous in nature, does not fully prevent either the age-related decline in BMD or the menopause-related loss of bone mineral in women. Thus, optimizing bone health depends not only on maintaining a physically active lifestyle, but also on maintaining appropriate nutritional and hormonal conditions.

Acknowledgments

The author was supported by NIH awards AG00663 and AG13629.

References

1. Leblanc AD, Schneider VS, Evans HJ, Engelbretson DA, Krebs JM: Bone mineral loss and recovery after 17 weeks of bed rest. *J Bone Miner Res* 1990;5:843–850.
2. Zerwekh JE, Ruml LA, Gottschalk F, Pak CY: The effects of twelve weeks of bed rest on bone histology, biochemical markers of bone turnover, and calcium homeostasis in eleven normal subjects. *J Bone Miner Res* 1998;13:1594–1601.
3. Ito M, Matsumoto T, Enomoto H, Tsurusaki K, Hayashi K: Effect of non-weightbearing on tibial bone density measured by QCT in patients with hip surgery. *J Bone Miner Metab* 1999;17:45–50.
4. Lanyon LE: Using functional loading to influence bone mass and architecture: Objectives, mechanisms, and relationship with estrogen of the mechanically adaptive process in bone. *Bone* 1996;18(suppl 1):37S-43S.
5. Snow-Harter CM: Bone health and prevention of osteoporosis in active and athletic women. *Clin Sports Med* 1994;13:389–404.
6. Suominen H: Bone mineral density and long term exercise: An overview of cross-sectional athlete studies. *Sports Med* 1993;16:316–330.
7. Chilibeck PD, Sale DG, Webber CE: Exercise and bone mineral density. *Sports Med* 1995;19:103–122.
8. American College of Sports Medicine position stand: Osteoporosis and exercise. *Med Sci Sports Exerc* 1995;27:i–vii.
9. Berard A, Bravo G, Gauthier P: Meta-analysis of the effectiveness of physical activity for the prevention of bone loss in postmenopausal women. *Osteoporosis Int* 1997;7:331–337.

10. Heinrich CH, Going SB, Pamenter RW, Perry CD, Boyden TW, Lohman TG: Bone mineral content of cyclically menstruating female resistance and endurance trained athletes. *Med Sci Sports Exerc* 1990;22:558–63.

11. Lee EJ, Long KA, Risser WL, Poindexter HB, Gibbons WE, Goldzieher J: Variations in bone status of contralateral and regional sites in young athletic women. *Med Sci Sports Exerc* 1995;27:1354–1361.

12. Fehling PC, Alekel L, Clasey J, Rector A, Stillman RJ: A comparison of bone mineral densities among female athletes in impact loading and active loading sports. *Bone* 1995;17:205–210.

13. Risser WL, Lee EJ, LeBlanc A, Poindexter HB, Risser JM, Schneider V: Bone density in eumenorrheic female college athletes. *Med Sci Sports Exerc* 1990;22:570–574.

14. Bennell KL, Malcolm SA, Khan KM, et al: Bone mass and bone turnover in power athletes, endurance athletes, and controls: A 12-month longitudinal study. *Bone* 1997;20:477–484.

15. Calbet JA, Moysi JS, Dorado C, Rodriguez LP: Bone mineral content and density in professional tennis players. *Calcif Tissue Int* 1998;62:491–496.

16. Rubin CT, Lanyon LE: Regulation of bone formation by applied dynamic loads. *J Bone Joint Surg* 1984;66A:397–402.

17. Rubin CT, Lanyon LE: Regulation of bone mass by mechanical strain magnitude. *Calcif Tissue Int* 1985;37:411–417.

18. Lanyon LE, Rubin CT: Static vs dynamic loads as an influence on bone remodelling. *J Biomech* 1984;17:897–905.

19. Greendale GA, Barrett-Connor E, Edelstein S, Ingles S, Haile R: Lifetime leisure exercise and osteoporosis: The Rancho Bernardo study. *Am J Epidemiol* 1995;141:951–959.

20. Uusi-Rasi K, Sievanen H, Vuori I, Pasanen M, Heinonen A, Oja P: Associations of physical activity and calcium intake with bone mass and size in healthy women at different ages. *J Bone Miner Res* 1998;13:133–142.

21. Suleiman S, Nelson M, Li F, Buxton-Thomas M , Moniz C: Effect of calcium intake and physical activity level on bone mass and turnover in healthy, white, postmenopausal women. *Am J Clin Nutr* 1997;66:937–943.

22. Nguyen TV, Sambrook PN, Eisman JA: Bone loss, physical activity, and weight change in elderly women: The Dubbo Osteoporosis Epidemiology Study. *J Bone Miner Res* 1998;13:1458–1467.

23. Kerr D, Morton A, Dick I, Prince R: Exercise effects on bone mass in postmenopausal women are site-specific and load-dependent. *J Bone Miner Res* 1996;11:218–225.

24. Kohrt WM, Ehsani AA, Birge SJ, Jr: Effects of exercise involving predominantly either joint-reaction or ground-reaction forces on bone mineral density in older women. *J Bone Miner Res* 1997;12:1253–1261.

25. Kohrt WM, Ehsani AA, Birge SJ Jr: HRT preserves increases in bone mineral density and reductions in body fat after a supervised exercise program. *J Appl Physiol* 1998;84:1506–1512.

26. Kohrt WM, Snead DB, Slatopolsky E, Birge SJ Jr: Additive effects of weight-bearing exercise and estrogen on bone mineral density in older women. *J Bone Miner Res* 1995;10:1303–1311.

27. Friedlander AL, Genant HK, Sadowsky S, Byl NN, Glüer CC: A two-year program of aerobics and weight training enhances bone mineral density of young women. *J Bone Miner Res* 1995;10:574–585.

28. Braith RW, Mills RM, Welsch MA, Keller JW, Pollock ML: Resistance exercise training restores bone mineral density in heart transplant recipients. *J Am Coll Cardiol* 1996;28:1471–1477.

29. Taaffe DR, Robinson TL, Snow CM, Marcus R: High-impact exercise promotes bone gain in well-trained female athletes. *J Bone Miner Res* 1997;12:255–260.

30. Nichols DL, Sanborn CF, Bonnick SL, Ben-Ezra V, Gench B, DiMarco NM: The effects of gymnastics training on bone mineral density. *Med Sci Sports Exerc* 1994;26:1220–1225.

31. Snow-Harter C, Bouxsein ML, Lewis BT, Carter DR, Marcus R: Effects of resistance and endurance exercise on bone mineral status of young women: A randomized exercise intervention trial. *J Bone Miner Res* 1992;7:761–769.

32. Bass S, Pearce G, Bradney M, et al: Exercise before puberty may confer residual benefits in bone density in adulthood: Studies in active prepubertal and retired female gymnasts. *J Bone Miner Res* 1998;13:500–507.

33. Kirchner EM, Lewis RD, O'Connor PJ: Effect of past gymnastics participation on adult bone mass. *J Appl Physiol* 1996;80:226–232.

34. Lane NE, Oehlert JW, Bloch DA, Fries JF: The relationship of running to osteoarthritis of the knee and hip and bone mineral density of the lumbar spine: A 9-year longitudinal study. *J Rheumatol* 1998;25:334–341.

35. Ryan AS, Elahi D: Loss of bone mineral density in women athletes during aging. *Calcif Tissue Int* 1998;63:287–292.

36. Notelovitz M, Martin D, Tesar R, et al: Estrogen therapy and variable-resistance weight training increase bone mineral in surgically menopausal women. *J Bone Miner Res* 1991;6:583–590.

37. Greendale GA, Edelstein S, Barrett-Connor E: Endogenous sex steroids and bone mineral density in older women and men: The Rancho Bernardo Study. *J Bone Miner Res* 1997;12:1833–1843.

38. Otis CL, Drinkwater B, Johnson M, Loucks A, Wilmore J: American College of Sports Medicine position stand: The Female Athlete Triad. *Med Sci Sports Exerc* 1997;29:i–ix.

39. Loucks AB, Verdun M, Heath EM: Low energy availability, not stress of exercise, alters LH pulsatility in exercising women. *J Appl Physiol* 1998;84:37–46.

Chapter 28

The Relationship Between Exercise and Osteoarthritis

Kenton R. Kaufman, PhD, PE

Introduction

Physical activity is an important component of a healthy lifestyle. Studies have shown that increased physical activity results in reduced risk of cardiovascular disease, improves blood pressure, assists in weight reduction, improves mood, and enhances emotional well being.[1–4] Although regular exercise provides health benefits through primary prevention, it also plays an important role in the treatment of many disease states and can be instrumental in reducing disability from chronic illness.[5,6]

In the United States, those older than 65 years represent the fastest growing segment of the population. Arthritis is the leading chronic condition of individuals in this age group.[7] The rate of functional disability increases with age, affecting over 50% of people 65 years and older.[8] A major factor of this disability seems related to the onset of osteoarthritis (OA). Degenerative changes in joints have been found in autopsy studies of patients in the second decade of life, with almost universal abnormalities noted in weightbearing joints by 40 years of age.[9] OA has been identified in 35% of populations younger than 30 years of age.[8] Radiographic changes of OA occur in most individuals by age 65 years and are present in more than 85% of people by age 75 years.[10] At present, 40.5 million adults are thought to have OA and 27 million of these adults have symptoms related to the disease.[8] Although the prevalence of OA increases with age, this pathologic process is thought to be different from the effects of aging itself.

The clinical management of OA involves two approaches, pharmacologic or nonpharmacologic. Therapeutic programs usually emphasize drug treatments. Treatment is often initiated with nonsteroidal anti-inflammatory drugs (NSAIDs). If symptoms are not satisfactorily managed with NSAIDs, analgesics usually are given. Occasionally, symptomatic joints that appear to have an inflammatory component are injected with intra-articular corticosteroids. Nonpharmacologic treatment involves recommendations for weight loss, activity modification, and exercise. Patients who cannot be managed successfully while on either of these programs and whose radiographic evaluations show sufficient damage are offered reconstructive surgery.

This chapter evaluates 3 areas in which exercise may have an impact on arthritis. The first area is the long-term effect of exercise on the joints. Second, the relationship between sports injury and the risk of OA is evaluated. Third, the therapeutic effects of exercise for patients with OA is discussed.

Long-Term Effects of Exercise on Osteoarthritis

Millions of people are exercising for one or more of several potential health benefits that include improved fitness, better emotional well-being, increased longevity, and decreased risk of cardiovascular disease. However, the long-term consequences of exercise on the musculoskeletal system are not fully understood. Recently, a number of studies have attempted to define this relationship. There is little definitive information about the impact of physical exercise and biomechanical factors on OA. Numerous retrospective studies have been performed to examine a possible relationship between occupation or sports participation and OA. However, until recent years there were no prospective, controlled studies examining effects of regular exercise on the human musculoskeletal system. Factors that contribute to exercise-related OA in joints without preexisting injury (primary OA) may differ from those factors that contribute to arthritis in joints with previous injury (secondary OA).

Numerous predisposing factors relating exercise to OA have been identified. However, few have been proven with well-controlled longitudinal studies. Most studies are retrospective or cross-sectional, or come from extrapolation of data that did not specifically incorporate exercise in the study design. Nonetheless, several predisposing factors have a major proven relationship, major influence, or potential for significant relationship with exercise-related OA.

Age

The age at which an individual begins participating in sports may influence the subsequent risk of developing OA. Several authors have noted premature closure of the distal radial epiphysis in gymnasts.[11–13] Pathologic changes in elbows of Little League pitchers have also been described.[14–17] Nevertheless, these studies have failed to demonstrate long-term sequelae in Little League pitchers with elbow pain and radiographic changes. Therefore, although there is clear evidence that repetitive forces to the skeletally immature elbow can result in damage to articular cartilage in subchondral bone, the long-term consequences of these pathologic changes have yet to be fully defined.

Conversely, the strong association between advancing age and OA seems to indicate that advancing age is a major factor affecting OA. Nonetheless, numerous differences exist between the changes associated with aging and those characteristic of OA (Table 1). Although dramatic differences exist, most individuals suffering from severe OA are members of the geriatric population. Therefore, until more well-designed studies can be performed, advancing age can be thought of as the major factor affecting OA.

Table 1 Osteoarthritis versus aging

	Aging	Osteoarthritis
Articular cartilage		
Water content	Decreased	Increased
Glycosaminoglycans		
Chondroitin sulfate	Normal or slightly decreased	Decreased
Chondroitin sulfate 4:6 ratio	Decreased	Increased
Keratan sulfate	Increased	Decreased
Hyaluronate	Increased	Decreased
Proteoglycans		
Aggregation	Normal	Diminished
Monomer size	Decreased	Decreased
Link Protein	Fragmented	Normal
Proteases	Normal	Increased
Inflammation	Absent	Present
Synthesis of collagen and proteoglycan	Normal	Increased
Enzymatic destruction of hard tissue	Normal	Present
Chondrocyte mitosis	Absent	Present
Pigment (cartilage)	Present	Absent
Eburnation	Absent	Present

(Reproduced with permission from McKeag DB: The relationship of osteoarthritis and exercise. *Clin Sports Med* 1992;11:471–487.)

Occupational Activities

Degenerative arthritis may follow repetitive trauma. Certain occupations result in increased mechanical stress on the joints. Studies have suggested an increased prevalence of OA in the elbows and knees of miners; the shoulders and elbows of pneumatic drill operators; the intervertebral disks of dock workers; and the hands of cotton workers, diamond cutters, seamstresses, and textile workers (Table 2). However, this association has not been confirmed. Burke and associates[18] failed to find an increased incidence of OA in pneumatic drill users. They criticized inadequate sample sizes, lack of statistical analyses, and omission of appropriate control populations in previous reports. They also commented that impact without injury or preceding abnormality of either joint contour or ligaments is unlikely to produce OA. Recent studies suggest a role for occupational physical stress in the development of OA in some subjects.[19–21]

Sports Participation

Numerous retrospective studies have suggested a possible relationship between sports activity and OA (Table 3). OA has been found in ballet dancers, baseball pitchers, boxers, cricketeers, cyclists, players of American football, gymnasts, lacrosse players, martial artists, parachutists, rugby players, downhill skiers, soccer players, weight lifters, and wrestlers. These studies should be considered uncontrolled observations that suggest, but do not prove, the hypothesis that regular exercise may be a factor leading to OA. The data are difficult to evaluate because of limitations of the studies. These limitations

Table 2 Occupational physical activity and possible associations with osteoarthritis (OA)

Occupation	Involved joints	Risk of OA
Miners	Elbow, knee, spine	Increased
Pneumatic drillers	Shoulder, elbow, wrist, MCPs	Increased/none
Dock workers	Intervertebral disks DIPs, elbow, knee	Increased
Cotton workers	Hand*	Increased
Diamond workers	Hand*	Increased
Seamstresses	Hand*	Increased
Textile workers	Hand*	Increased
Occupations requiring knee bending	Knee	Increased
Farmers	Hip, knee	Increased

MCPs = metacarpophalangeal joints, DIPs = distal interphalangeal joints
(Reproduced with permission from Panush RS, Lane NE: Exercise and the musculoskeletal system. *Baillieres Clin Rheumatol* 1994;8:79–102.)

Table 3 Arthritis and exercise: alleged association with osteoarthritis (OA)

Sport	Site (Joint)	Risk of OA
Ballet	Talus, ankle, cervical spine, hip, knee, metatarsophalangeal	Probably increased
Baseball	Elbow, shoulder	Possibly increased
Boxing	Hand (carpometacarpal)	Possibly increased
Cricket	Finger	Possibly increased
Cycling	Patella	Possibly increased
Football (American style)	Ankle, feet, knee, spine	Probably increased
Gymnastics	Elbow, shoulder, wrist, hip	Possibly increased
Lacrosse	Ankle, knee	Possibly increased
Martial arts	Spine	Possibly increased
Parachuting	Ankle, knee, spine	Probably increased
Rugby	Knee	Possibly increased
Running	Knee, hip	Little to none
Skiing (downhill)	Thumb	Possibly increased
Soccer	Ankle-foot, cervical spine, hip, knee, talus	Probably increased
Weight lifting	Spine	Possibly increased
Wrestling	Cervical spine, elbow, knee	Possibly increased

(Reproduced with permission from Panush RS: Does exercise cause arthritis? Long term consequences of exercise on the musculoskeletal system. *Rheum Dis Clin North Am* 1990;16:827–836.)

include the facts that controls were often not included, studies were retrospective, and standards of radiologic criteria for OA were not established. Until recent years, there have been no prospective, controlled clinical studies examining the effects of exercise on musculoskeletal disability.

A number of studies have examined the role of running as a possible cause of OA (Table 4). These studies retrospectively examined a group of former high-level runners and found no increased incidence of OA of the lower extremity as compared with control subjects.[22–25] In contrast, Marti and associates[26] and Knobloch and associates,[27] using a similar study design, did find that a history of long-distance running was predictive of radiographic

Table 4 Studies of running and risk of developing osteoarthritis (OA)

Reference	No. of Runners	Mean Age (Years)	Mean No. of Years Run	Miles/ Week	Comments
Puranen et al[23]	74	56	21	NA	Champion distance runners had no more hip OA than nonrunners in their sixth decade
De Carvalho and Langfeldt[25]	32	NA	NA	NA	Radiographs of runners' hips and knees were similar to those of control
Sohn and Micheli[22]	504	57	25	25	"No association between moderate long-distance running and the future development of OA" (of hips and knees)
Lane et al[29]	41	58	9	22	No differences between runners and controls in cartilage loss, crepitus, joint stability, or symptomatic OA
Panush et al[28]	17	56	12	28	Comparable low prevalence of OA in lower extremities of runners and nonrunners
Lane et al[30]	498	59	12	27	"No differences were found between groups in conditions thought to predispose to OA and musculoskeletal disability"
Marti et al[26]	27	42	NA	61	More radiologic changes of hip OA in former Swiss national long-distance runners than bobsledders and controls, few runners had clinical symptoms of OA, no differences noted in ankle joints
Konradsen et al[24]	27	58	40	12–24	No clinical or radiographic differences in hips, knees and ankles between runners and nonrunners
Lane et al[31]	28	66	17–20	17	Presence and progression of OA was similar for runners and nonrunners

NA = not available

degenerative hip disease as compared with controls. Several cross-sectional studies also found no association between running and OA.[28–30] Panush and associates[28] concluded, after looking at 17 middle-aged runners over a 12-year period, that there were no differences in arthritis between a group of runners and a group of sedentary, nonrunning control subjects. Likewise, Lane and associates[29] reported on 41 runners and an equal number of matched controls over a 5-year period, analyzing radiographs of the hands, lumbar spine, and the knees, as well as a computed topography scan of the first lumbar vertebra. Results of this study indicated that, although runners did have 40% more mineral content in the bone, there was no increased prevalence of clinical OA. A 9-year follow-up longitudinal study of 28 runners and 27 nonrunner control subjects matched for age, sex, years of education, and occupation was conducted by Lane and associates.[31] Both groups had significant progression of the individual radiographic features of OA. Although OA had developed in these subjects, running did not appear to have accelerated the development of OA in this population. Similarly, an 8-year follow-up conducted by Panush and associates[32] found that both runners and controls had some radiographic progression in joints, but cartilage thickness measurements over the 8-year period did not change within the two groups. It is now generally thought that runners without underlying biomechanical problems of the lower extremity do not appear to develop arthritis at a rate different from nonrunner, normal populations. However, some evidence suggests that high-intensity, high-impact sports in young adults may be a risk factor for later development of OA.[33] Further, those individuals who have underlying articular biomechanical abnormalities do appear to be at a greater risk of subsequent development of OA,[27,34] and these observations seem to be valid for other sport activities as well.[35] In addition, female runners were noted to have more sclerosis and spurs than matched control subjects.[29] Further, a higher rate of radiologic progression in knees of women with a history of long-distance running has been reported.[31–36]

Cumulative Exposure From Sports and Occupation

Very few studies have considered the cumulative effect of combined exposure to sporting activity and occupational workload. Two case-control studies by Vingård and associates[37,38] have investigated the relationship between sporting activities and OA of the hip in women and men. The study base comprised all 50- to 70-year-old men and women living in 5 counties in western Sweden. Sweden has a National Registry of total hip replacements. All orthopaedics departments report to the Registry. Cases were those individuals who received a total hip replacement due to primary OA. The control subjects were randomly selected from the study population. The subjects were matched for age and geographic region. Detailed information on different loads from occupational and home activities was collected by questionnaire. Physical loads from occupation were quantified as low, medium, and high for static and dynamic forces acting on the hip joint.[39] Exposure information on participation in different sporting activities was also collected. The study subjects were asked how many hours per week, how many weeks per year, during how many and which years, and at what level they participated in sports. Each exposure was aggregated to the age of 50 years. Three exposure classes were defined for total hours of sports activity. There were differences in the definition of sports exposure for men and women. Female subjects considered to have low exposure were those with less than 100 hours of sporting activities in total and women considered to have high exposure were those with 800 or more hours of

Table 5 Relative risk of developing hip osteoarthritis for women with different exposure to physical load from occupation and sports activities aggregated to the age of 50 years*

Exposure to Sports	Physical Load From Occupation		
	Low	Medium	High
Low	1.0	1.1 (0.5–2.0)†	1.7 (0.8–3.5)
Medium	1.1 (0.3–3.4)	1.8 (0.8–4.1)	2.7 (1.1–7.0)
High	2.0 (0.7–5.2)	2.7 (1.2–5.9)	4.3 (1.7–11.0)

*Relative risk adjusted for age and body mass index
†Numbers in parentheses represent the 95% confidence interval
(Reproduced with permission from Vingård E, Alfredsson L, Malchau H: Osteoarthrosis of the hip in women and its relationship to physical load from sports activities. *Am J Sports Med* 1998;26:78–82.)

Table 6 Relative risk of developing hip osteoarthritis for men with different exposure to physical load from occupation and sports activities aggregated to the age of 50 years*

Exposure to Sports	Physical Load From Occupation		
	Low	Medium	High
Low	1.0	2.1 (0.9–4.8)†	3.3 (1.4–7.7)
Medium	1.6 (0.6–3.7)	3.9 (1.5–10.1)	4.0 (1.7–9.6)
High	2.1 (0.9–4.9)	6.0 (2.7–13.0)	8.5 (4.0–17.9)

*Relative risk adjusted for age and body mass index
†Numbers in parentheses represent the 95% confidence interval
(Reproduced with permission from Vingård E, Alfredsson L, Goldie I, Hogstedt C: Sports and osteoarthrosis of the hip: An epidemiologic study. *Am J Sports Med* 1993;21:195–200.)

sporting activities. The definition for men was slightly different. Those men who did not participate in sports and the 5% with least participation were considered to have low exposure. The rest of the male subjects were divided into two equally large groups classified as having medium and high exposure. For women, adjustments were made in the analysis for age, body mass index at the age of 40 years, smoking, and hormone therapy. For men, data were adjusted for age, body mass index, and smoking habits. The results indicate a dose-response relationship for women (Table 5) and men (Table 6) between sporting activities, occupation, and OA of the hip. Both groups of individuals demonstrated increased relative risk of developing OA of the hip for increased exposure to sporting activity and occupational workloads. Across each activity level, relative risk increased with a higher level of the other activity. The highest relative risk was found for those individuals exposed to both high physical loads from work and sporting activities. The relative risk of developing OA in men was greater than the relative risk for women. The different levels of relative risk in men and women may depend on lower exposure rates among women compared with those in men. For instance, the number of hours in sports activities for women during life was low compared with those reported by men. Nonetheless, long-term exposure to strenuous sports activities combined with heavy workloads seems to be a risk factor for developing severe hip OA later in life.

Sports Injury and Osteoarthritis

Injuries may occur during athletic participation and competition. Joint injury may involve bony structures, menisci, articular cartilage, ligaments, and surrounding soft tissue. Ligamentous instability, abnormal joint motion, and prior injury are important in the premature development of OA associated with regular exercise. Study of individuals with cruciate, collateral ligament, and meniscal injuries is part of the concept that unstable or damaged knees are associated with the development of premature OA. Moretz and associates[40] demonstrated in a retrospective study that there is a strong correlation between high school football injuries and the development of knee OA. Injury to the meniscus or anterior cruciate ligament (ACL) of the knee has been shown to have a clear role in the development of premature OA in athletes. A 10% incidence of OA of the knee during long-term follow-up of 440 patients who underwent meniscectomies has been reported.[41] Radiographic changes of OA after meniscectomy were described by Fairbank.[42] Before 1980, meniscal injury was often treated by total meniscectomy, imposing a substantial risk of early OA.[43] Subsequently, arthroscopic partial meniscectomies have become the surgical standard for meniscal tears. The long-term effect of partial meniscectomies on the risk of subsequent OA remains to be fully understood.[44] Similarly, injuries to the ACL result in abnormal knee biomechanics and recurrent subluxations. Without intervention, individuals with these injuries are predisposed to early OA.[45,46] The effects of the ACL-deficient knee are well recognized today, and arthroscopic-assisted ACL reconstruction has become the standard of care for these patients. A 5-year follow-up study of 292 patients who had sustained an acute ACL injury demonstrated that patients who had undergone reconstruction had a higher level of arthrosis by radiograph and bone scan evaluation than those patients whose ACL had not been reconstructed.[47] This can be explained in part by a higher instance of meniscal surgery in the patients who have undergone knee reconstruction.

Exercise for Patients With Arthritis

Individuals with arthritis restrict joint motion and limit activity to decrease their symptoms. The reduced activity contributes to muscle atrophy, loss of proprioception, and decreased muscle strength and endurance, which further compromise joint integrity and accelerate the destructive process (Fig. 1). Consequently, the disuse and inactivity result in a deconditioned state that can be as incapacitating as the symptoms of the primary disease. It is assumed that function will be restored and/or a joint will be protected from further damage if joint mobility, muscle strength, and/or aerobic conditioning are

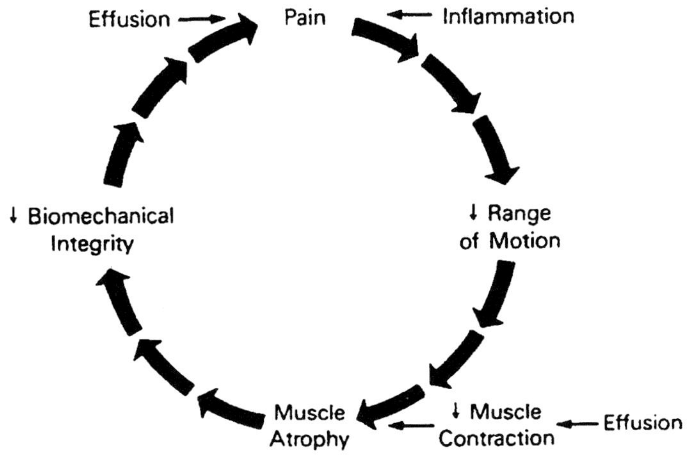

Fig. 1 The negative cycle that may develop in patients with arthritis. Patients will often respond to pain by restricting joint motion and increasing time at rest. This, in turn, leads to a decreased range of motion, muscle atrophy, and alterations in joint biomechanics. These deficits result in increased joint pain, perpetuating the cycle. (Reproduced with permission from Hicks JE: Exercise in patients with inflammatory arthritis and connective tissue disease. Rheum Dis Clin North Am *1990;16:846–870.)*

improved. However, there is little scientific evidence to support this logic. Clinical studies of exercise for OA are difficult to compare because study designs, exercise programs, and outcome measures have been different. Few exercise programs for patients with OA have been subjected to rigorous, well-controlled studies.

In general, exercise programs can be divided into either aerobic exercise or strengthening programs. Most studies examine a single, short-term therapeutic exercise intervention and have not directly compared the efficacy of these two broad exercise regimens. However, a study by Messier and associates[48] compared the long-term effects of aerobic walking, weight training, and health education (control) on the gait mechanics of 103 older adults afflicted with OA of the knee. Both intervention groups (aerobic exercise and weight training) exercised 3 days per week for 18 months. Exercise compliance was 53% for the aerobic exercise group and 65% for the weight training group. Each subject participated in a series of tests at baseline, 3 months, 9 months, and 18 months. Biomechanical measures of physical function included kinematic and kinetic analyses of gait. The results of this study suggest that long-term aerobic walking and weight training programs are safe and effective nonpharmacologic interventions for improving walking mechanics in older adults with OA of the knee. Both exercise groups had significantly less knee pain than the health education (control) group. Moreover, the results also demonstrated that the aerobic exercise group benefited more from exercise than did the

Table 7 Summary of studies on effect of aerobic exercise on osteoarthritis (OA)

Author	N	Exercise	Duration (months)	Conclusions
Minor et al[34]	120	Aerobic (walking, aquatics) or nonaerobic (range of motion)	3	Aerobic exercise groups showed significant improvement in aerobic capacity and 50-ft walk time; no significant difference in number of clinically active joints or duration of morning stiffness
Kovar et al[49]	102	Walking	2	Increase in walking distance, improvement in Arthritis Impact Measurement Scale, and decreased medication use
Afable et al[50]	10	Aerobic or strength training	3	Aerobic or strength training can improve strength, exercise capacity, and functional performance in elderly with knee OA
Peterson et al[51]	102	Walking	2	Increase in velocity, stride length, and distance walked
Coleman et al[52]	105	Cycling, strength training, or both	6	Exercise did not produce or exacerbate joint symptoms
Ettinger et al[53]	365	Walking or resistance exercise	18	Exercise groups reported less disability, less pain, and improved physical performance; aerobic exercise did slightly better than resistance exercise; No difference in radiograph scores among all groups
Michel et al[54]	51	Running and aerobic exercise	24	Inverse relationship between exercise and rate of spur formation on knee radiographs

weight training group. Therefore, aerobic exercise should be studied more extensively as a nonpharmacologic treatment for OA of the knee.

Several studies have demonstrated that patients can participate in low-impact aerobic conditioning exercises without exacerbating arthritic symptoms (Table 7). However, most observations are from very short-term studies. Minor and associates[34] studied 120 patients in a 12-week program of aerobic walking, aerobic aquatic exercise, or range of motion exercises. At the end of 12 weeks, aerobic capacity and exercise endurance were increased in the two aerobic exercise groups. Further, the pain and physical activity scores on the arthritis impact measurement scales (AIMS) were improved in the 2 aerobic groups. Most importantly, this study demonstrated no adverse joint consequences for the exercise programs. In a similar study, Kovar and associates[49] compared the effects of an 8-week fitness walking program with no exercise in a large group of patients with OA of the knee. The results showed reduction rather than an increase in knee pain, improvement in physical function, and improvement in the physical activity subscale of the AIMS. Afable and associates[50] compared the effects of aerobic training with strength training in 10 older people (mean age 68 years; 8 women, 2 men) who reported pain and disability from OA of the knee. The strength group used free weights and the aerobic group walked on a circular track. Both groups exercised for 30 minutes, 3 times a week for 12 weeks. The data showed that either aerobic training or strength training resulted in improvements in strength, exercise capacity, and functional performance. Peterson and associates[51] quantitatively analyzed the gaits of subjects with OA of the knee(s) before and after an 8-week walking program. Walking 4 times per week for 30 minutes per session resulted in significant increases in walking velocity and stride length, demonstrating improved gait patterns. The distance the subjects were able to walk was also increased without exacerbation of joint symptoms. Thus, gentle, short-term walking programs appear to confer measurable aerobic benefits and improve gait efficiency in individuals with OA of the knee.

Less currently is known about the long-term effects of exercise programs on the functional status of patients with OA. Coleman and associates[52] evaluated the effects of a cycling, strength training, or combined 6-month exercise program on OA of the knee. They concluded that exercise did not produce or exacerbate joint symptoms. However, no improvements in functional status were obtained. Ettinger and associates[53] studied 365 community-dwelling adults, aged 60 years or older, in an 18-month program. The program consisted of aerobic exercise, resistance exercise, or health education. The primary outcome was a self-reported disability score, with secondary measures of a knee pain score, performance measures of physical function, radiograph score, aerobic capacity, and knee muscle strength. The participants had modest improvements in measures of disability, physical performance, and pain from participating in either the aerobic or resistance exercise program. Michel and associates[54] analyzed the knee radiographs of 51 subjects with a mean age of 60 years who regularly practiced weight-bearing exercise over a 2-year period. The results showed a negative correlation ($r = -0.47$; $p < 0.001$) between rate of spur formation and change in weightbearing exercise. So, in general, it is thought that an exercise program can minimize or even reverse many of the processes that lead to loss of functional capacity in patients with OA. Nonetheless, these studies are either short term or have been based on an unsupervised home exercise program with low compliance. A rigorous assessment of the impact of delaying surgical intervention by exercise and other conservative modalities has not been performed. Studies attempting to determine the type of exercise and optimal range of exercise intensity for patients with OA are needed. Further, studies comparing the potential benefits of weightbearing to nonweightbearing exercise for these patients also need to be conducted.

Gender

Female gender is a significant risk factor for OA. A longitudinal study of OA of the knee showed that women have a 1.8 times greater risk of developing OA than do men.[55] Arthritis is more prevalent among women than among men at all ages.[56] These gender differences are most prominent when OA affects the knee (7.3% of women and 4.1% of men aged 55 through 64 years, 18% of women and 8.3% of men aged 65 through 74 years). For all grades of radiographic severity of OA, more women than men report knee pain. Among those older than 60 years, women are twice as likely to have symptomatic arthritis as men.[57]

Summary

Exercise carried out within the limits of normal joint motion and loading does not predispose individuals to OA. Normal joints in individuals of all ages appear to tolerate exercise without adverse consequences or accelerated development of OA. Risk of developing destructive joint disease from recreational activities is low. However, sports that subject joints to intermittent high or violent impact loads may increase the risk of OA, but well-designed studies are lacking, and this association is speculative. Joints with preexisting injury, anatomic or biomechanical variance are at increased risk of developing OA with repetitive loading. Individuals who have suffered injuries of ligaments, tendons, or menisci may have accelerated development of OA in weightbearing joints, even without increased stress to the joint from exercise. Finally, patients with arthritis can benefit from exercise programs. Short-term studies have documented improved functional status, decrease in medication use, and psychological benefits from exercise programs.

More research is needed. Well-designed, long-term studies are lacking. Studies that include appropriate patient and control populations and are of sufficient duration and sample size need to be performed. Studies need to standardize clinical and radiologic assessment of joint degeneration, quantify the patients' functional status, and assess the contributions of other risk factors. These studies are needed to identify subjects at risk for the development of OA, provide advice on the type, frequency, intensity, and duration of exercise; and develop successful rehabilitation programs for patients with OA.

References

1. Ekelund LG, Haskell WL, Johnson JL, Whaley FS, Criqui MH, Sheps DS: Physical fitness as a predictor of cardiovascular mortality in asymptomatic North American men: The Lipid Research Clinics Mortality Follow-up Study. *N Engl J Med* 1988;319:1379–1384.
2. Haskell W: Exercise and health, in Wyngaarden JB, Smith L Jr (eds): *Cecil Textbook of Medicine*, ed 18. Philadelphia, PA, WB Saunders, 1988, pp 45–48.
3. Harris SS, Caspersen CJ, DeFriese GH, Estes EH Jr: Physical activity counseling for healthy adults as a primary preventive intervention in the clinical setting: Report for the US Preventive Services Task Force. *JAMA* 1989;261:3588–3598.
4. Sandvik L, Erikssen J, Thaulow E, Erikssen G, Mundal R, Rodahl K: Physical fitness as a predictor of mortality among healthy, middle-aged Norwegian men. *N Engl J Med* 1993;328:533–537.
5. Buchner DM, Beresford SA, Larson EB, LaCroix AZ, Wagner EH: Effects of physical activity on health status in older adults: II. Intervention studies. *Annu Rev Public Health* 1992;13:469–488.
6. Morey MC, Cowper PA, Feussner JR, et al: Evaluation of a supervised exercise program in a geriatric population. *J Am Geriatr Soc* 1989;37:348–354.
7. Cassel CK, Brody JA: Demography, epidemiology, and aging, in Cassel CK, Riesenberg DE, Sorensen LB, Walsh JR (eds): *Geriatric Medicine*, ed 2. New York, NY, Springer-Verlag, 1990, p 20.

8. McKeag DB: The relationship of osteoarthritis and exercise. *Clin Sports Med* 1992;11:471–487.

9. Lowman EW: Osteoarthritis. *JAMA* 1955;157:487–488.

10. Moskowitz RW: Primary osteoarthritis: Epidemiology, clinical aspects, and general management. *Am J Med* 1987;83:5–10.

11. Dobyns JH, Gabel GT: Gymnast's wrist. *Hand Clin* 1990;6:493–505.

12. Mandelbaum BR, Bartolozzi AR, Davis CA, Teurlings L, Bragonier B: Wrist pain syndrome in the gymnast: Pathogenetic, diagnostic, and therapeutic considerations. *Am J Sports Med* 1989;17:305–317.

13. Tolat AR, Sanderson PL, DeSmet L, Stanley JK: The gymnast's wrist: Acquired positive ulnar variance following chronic epiphyseal injury. *J Hand Surg* 1992;17B:678–681.

14. Francis R, Bunch T, Chandler B: Little League elbow: A decade later. *Phys Sportsmed* 1978;6:88–94.

15. Grana WA, Rashkin A: Pitcher's elbow in adolescents. *Am J Sports Med* 1980;8:333–336.

16. Gugenheim JJ Jr, Stanley RF, Woods GW, Tullos HS: Little League survey: The Houston study. *Am J Sports Med* 1976;4:189–200.

17. Larson RL, Singer KM, Bergstrom R, Thomas S: Little League survey: The Eugene study. *Am J Sports Med* 1976;4:201–209.

18. Burke MJ, Fear EC, Wright V: Bone and joint changes in pneumatic drillers. *Ann Rheum Dis* 1977;36:276–279.

19. Lindberg H, Montgomery F: Heavy labor and the occurrence of gonarthrosis. *Clin Orthop* 1987;214:235–236.

20. Felson DT, Hannan MT, Naimark A, et al: Occupational physical demands, knee bending, and knee osteoarthritis: Results from the Framingham Study. *J Rheumatol* 1991;18:1587–1592.

21. Hannan MT, Felson DT, Anderson JJ, Naimark A: Abstract: Habitual physical activity and knee osteoarthritis (OA) in the Framingham study. *Arthritis Rheum* 1991;34(suppl):S171.

22. Sohn RS, Micheli LJ: The effect of running on the pathogenesis of osteoarthritis of the hips and knees. *Clin Orthop* 1985;198:106–109.

23. Puranen J, Ala-Ketola L, Peltokallio P, Saarela J: Running and primary osteoarthritis of the hip. *Br Med J* 1975;2:424–425.

24. Konradsen L, Hansen EM, Sondergaard L: Long distance running and osteoarthrosis. *Am J Sports Med* 1990;18:379–381.

25. De Carvalho A, Langfeldt B: Running practice and arthrosis deformans: A radiological assessment. *Ugeskr Laeger* 1977;139:2621–2622.

26. Marti B, Knobloch M, Tschopp A, Jucker A, Howald H: Is excessive running predictive of degenerative hip disease? Controlled study of former elite athletes. *Br Med J* 1989;299:91–93.

27. Knobloch M, Marti B, Biedert R, Howald H: Risk of arthrosis of the upper ankle joint in long distance runners: Controlled follow-up of former elite athletes. *Sportverletz Sportschaden* 1990;4:175–179.

28. Panush RS, Schmidt C, Caldwell JR, et al: Is running associated with degenerative joint disease? *JAMA* 1986;255:1152–1154.

29. Lane NE, Bloch DA, Jones HH, Marshall WH Jr, Wood PD, Fries JF: Long-distance running, bone density, and osteoarthritis. *JAMA* 1986;255:1147–1151.

30. Lane NE, Block DA, Wood PD, Fries JF: Aging, long-distance running, and the development of musculoskeletal disability: A controlled study. *Am J Med* 1987;82:772–780.

31. Lane NE, Oehlert JW, Block DA, Fries JF: The relationship of running to osteoarthritis of the knee and hip and bone mineral density of the lumbar spine: A 9 year longitudinal study. *J Rheumatol* 1998;25:334–341.

32. Panush RS, Hanson CS, Caldwell JR, Langley S, Stork J, Thoburn R: Is running associated with degenerative joint disease? An eight-year followup study. *J Clin Rheumatol* 1995;1:35–39.

33. Lane NE: Physical activity at leisure and risk of osteoarthritis. *Ann Rheum Dis* 1996;55:682–684.

34. Minor MA, Hewett JE, Webel RR, Anderson SK, Kay DR: Efficacy of physical conditioning exercise in patients with rheumatoid arthritis and osteoarthritis. *Arthritis Rheum* 1989;32:1396–1405.

35. Panush RS, Lane NE: Exercise and the musculoskeletal system. *Baillieres Clin Rheumatol* 1994;8:79–102.

36. Spector TD, Harris PA, Hart DJ, et al: Risk of osteoarthritis associated with long-term weight-bearing sports: A radiologic survey of the hips and knees in female ex-athletes and population controls. *Arthritis Rheum* 1996;39:988–995.

37. Vingård E, Alfredsson L, Malchau H: Osteoarthrosis of the hip in women and its relationship to physical load from sports activities. *Am J Sports Med* 1998;26:78–82.

38. Vingård E, Alfredsson L, Goldie I, Hogstedt C: Sports and osteoarthrosis of the hip: An epidemiologic study. *Am J Sports Med* 1993;21:195–200.

39. Vingård E, Hogstedt C, Alfredsson L, Fellenius E, Goldie I, Koster M: Coxarthrosis and physical work load. *Scand J Work Environ Health* 1991;17:104–109.

40. Moretz JA III, Harlan SD, Goodrich J, Walters R: Long-term followup of knee injuries in high school football players. *Am J Sports Med* 1984;12:298–300.

41. Appel H: Late results after meniscectomy in the knee joint: A clinical and roentgenologic follow-up investigation. *Acta Orthop Scand* 1970;133(suppl): 1–111.

42. Fairbank TJ: Knee joint changes after meniscectomy. *J Bone Joint Surg* 1948;30B:664–670.

43. Jackson JP: Degenerative changes in the knee after meniscectomy. *Br Med J* 1968;2:525–527.

44. Hamberg P, Gillquist J, Lysholm J: A comparison between arthroscopic meniscectomy and modified open meniscectomy: A prospective randomised study with emphasis on postoperative rehabilitation. *J Bone Joint Surg* 1984;66B:189–192.

45. Noyes FR, Mooar PA, Matthews DS, Butler DL: The symptomatic anterior cruciate-deficient knee: Part I: The long-term functional disability in athletically active individuals. *J Bone Joint Surg* 1983;65A:154–162.

46. Sommerlath K, Lysholm J, Gillquist J: The long-term course after treatment of acute anterior cruciate ligament ruptures: A 9 to 16 year followup. *Am J Sports Med* 1991:19:156–162.

47. Daniel DM, Stone ML, Dobson BE, Fithian DC, Rossman DJ, Kaufman KR: Fate of the ACL-injured patient: A prospective outcome study. *Am J Sports Med* 1994;22:632–644.

48. Messier SP, Thompson CD, Ettinger WH: Effects of long-term aerobic or weight training regimens on gait in an older, osteoarthritic population. *J Appl Biomech* 1997;13:205–225.
49. Kovar PA, Allegrante JP, MacKenzie CR, Peterson MG, Gutin B, Charlson ME: Supervised fitness walking in patients with osteoarthritis of the knee: A randomized, controlled trial. *Ann Intern Med* 1992;116:529–534.
50. Afable RF, Bailey E, Woodard M, et al: Abstract: Comparison of aerobic and strength training in persons with osteoarthritis (OA) of the knee. *J Am Geriatr Soc* 1992;40(suppl):SA17.
51. Peterson MG, Kovar-Toledano PA, Otis JC, et al: Effect of a walking program on gait characteristics in patients with osteoarthritis. *Arthritis Care Res* 1993;6:11–16.
52. Coleman EA, Buchner DM, Cress ME, Chan BK, de Lateur BJ: The relationship of joint symptoms with exercise performance in older adults. *J Am Geriatr Soc* 1996;44:14–21.
53. Ettinger WH Jr, Burns R, Messier SP, et al: A randomized trial comparing aerobic exercise and resistance exercise with a health education program in older adults with knee osteoarthritis: The Fitness Arthritis and Seniors Trial. *JAMA* 1997;277:25–31.
54. Michel BA, Fries JF, Bloch DA, Lane NE, Jones HH: Osteophytosis of the knee: Association with changes in weight-bearing exercise. *Clin Rheumatol* 1992;11:235–238.
55. Felson DT, Zhang Y, Hannan MT, et al: Risk factors for incident radiographic knee osteoarthritis in the elderly: The Framingham Study. *Arthritis Rheum* 1997;40:728–733.
56. Adams PF, Marano MA: *Current estimates from the National Health Interview Survey*, 1994. Vital & Health Statistics—Series 10: Data from the National Health Survey. Hyattsville, MD, US Department of Health and Human Services, 1995, vol 193, pp 83–84. DHHS publication (PHS) 95-1521.
57. Brandt KD: Nonsurgical management of osteoarthritis, with an emphasis on nonpharmacologic measures. *Arch Fam Med* 1995;4:1057–1064.

Chapter 29

Nutrient Metabolism During Exercise and Nutritional Considerations for Physically Active Women Throughout the Life Span

Roger A. Fielding, PhD

Introduction

Exercise and/or physical activity can cause up to a 20-fold increase in whole body energy expenditure. Adequate replenishment of these depleted energy stores has dramatic effects on the nutritional requirements of the individual. In addition to the increased energy requirements posed by exercise training, physically active women and female athletes need to be concerned about the adequacy of their usual diet. This chapter will focus on nutrient utilization during exercise and the unique aspects of the nutritional requirements of physically active women. Particular attention will be paid to the role of an adequate protein intake on maintaining the proper function of the musculoskeletal system throughout the life span.

Substrate Metabolism During Exercise: Gender Differences

Maximal Oxygen Uptake

The concept of the maximal oxygen uptake (Vo_{2max}) serving as an upper physiologic limit for aerobic exercise was first described by Hill and Lupton[1] and validated in classic studies by Taylor and associates.[2] These studies demonstrated a direct relationship between whole body oxygen consumption and exercise intensity. As the intensity of exercise increases, oxygen consumption also increases in a linear fashion. Clearly gender differences exist between this upper limit in exercise capacity.[3] On average, Vo_{2max} tends to be 20% to 40% lower in age- and weight-matched women compared to men. These differences in aerobic fitness between men and women can partially be explained by differences in body composition, particularly skeletal muscle mass.[4]

It is well established that whole body oxygen consumption is the product of maximal cardiac output and maximal peripheral oxygen extraction. These terms are usually considered the central and peripheral links in the oxygen transport chain, respectively. As discussed in other chapters, oxygen serves as the final electron acceptor during oxidative phosphorylation. Rates of adenosine triphosphate (ATP) turnover during energy production cannot be conveniently measured through direct means. Whole body oxygen consumption has traditionally been used as an indirect measure of energy expenditure during exercise and serves as the best correlate to the physical work of exercise.[3]

Physical exercise presents the most profound challenge to fuel homeostasis in normal humans. Whole body energy expenditure can increase 10- to 20-fold from rest to maximal exercise.[2] To maintain this increased rate of energy expenditure, the performance of physical activity is associated with a marked increase in the fuel and oxygen needs of working muscles. Because the available quantities of high-energy phosphate compounds, such as creatine phosphate (CP) and ATP, within muscle are relatively limited (26 $mmol \cdot kg^{-1}$ wet wt CP, and 8 $mmol \cdot kg^{-1}$ wet wt ATP), the availability of the necessary metabolic machinery and oxidizable substrate is a necessity for sustained muscular activity. Human skeletal muscle contains the necessary enzymes to oxidize carbohydrate in the forms of glucose and glycogen, nonesterified fatty acids transported from adipocytes and derived from intramuscular triglycerides, and to a small extent amino acids for energy.[5] To meet these requirements and at the same time maintain the fuel and energy supply to other vital organs, major metabolic, hormonal, and cardiovascular adjustments are essential. There are some gender-specific differences in substrate metabolism during exercise that have implications for the nutritional requirements of physically active women.

Carbohydrate Metabolism

Skeletal muscle glucose uptake is a carrier-mediated process initiated by the pancreatic hormone insulin.[6,7] At rest, permissive levels of insulin are necessary for glucose uptake to occur, but during exercise increases in glucose uptake occur despite declining circulating insulin concentrations.[8] It appears that the increased skeletal muscle glucose uptake during exercise occurs by noninsulin-dependent signaling mechanisms.[9] Blood glucose oxidation has been estimated to account for up to 40% of the total oxidizable substrate during prolonged submaximal exercise (ie, 40% to 50% Vo_{2max}). The decline in blood glucose concentrations observed at the end of prolonged exercise has been implicated as a possible cause of fatigue.[8,10,11]

Skeletal muscle glucose uptake increases linearly with increasing exercise intensity.[12] Despite this dramatic increase in glucose uptake by active muscle, plasma glucose concentration remains notably level in normal humans during exercise of low to moderate intensity. Feedback signals from plasma glucose sensors appear to elicit changes in neuroendocrine function so that hepatic glucose production increases.[13] Also, decreases in plasma glucose may directly stimulate hepatic glucose production. Feedback mechanisms are less involved during intense exercise because plasma glucose concentrations increase initially, then fall as hepatic glycogen stores are depleted.[13] Instead, the glycemic response during periods of intense exercise may be subject to a feed-forward regulation elicited by the central command that changes neuroendocrine function, and subsequently causes an initial overshoot in hepatic glucose production. For example, at the onset of exercise, impulses from the working muscles and motor centers increase neuroendocrine activity in an intensity dependent manner.[14]

Analogous to the blood glucose supply, intramuscular stores of glycogen are broken down to facilitate resynthesis of high-energy phosphate compounds. The direct availability of muscle glycogen to the contractile tissue eliminates the need for a circulatory response for its mobilization. Muscle glycogen utilization appears to be greatest at the onset of exercise, and then as other substrates become available the rate of muscle glycogen utilization decreases.[15] As with blood glucose uptake, the rate of muscle glycogen utilization will increase with increasing exercise intensity, reaching maximal rates well above the maximal oxygen uptake.[15] More recently, animal studies have indicated a close relationship between intramuscular availability of glycogen and its rate of utilization during contractile activity.[16] Several studies have noted a relationship between pre-exercise muscle glycogen concentrations and exercise time to exhaustion during submaximal endurance exercise.[15,17] In addition, fatigue during intermittent high-intensity exercise also has been shown to coincide with low intramuscular glycogen concentrations.[18,19] It is possible that with the depletion of muscle glycogen, selected muscle fibers may no longer be able to generate the necessary force to maintain a given power output.

Carbohydrate metabolism during exercise differs between men and women. At the same relative exercise intensity, studies have indicated that the respiratory exchange ratio is lower in women performing prolonged submaximal exercise, suggesting a decreased rate of carbohydrate oxidation.[20] In addition, subsequent work has shown that utilization of muscle glycogen is lower in women compared to men when the exercise is performed at the same relative exercise intensity.[21,22] However, in these studies the mechanism for this apparent carbohydrate sparing in women during exercise remains unclear. Carbohydrate metabolism in the post-exercise recovery period also appears to be altered in women. Tarnopolsky and associates[22] have reported that muscle glycogen stores are not increased in trained women in response to a standard carbohydrate loading regimen. This reduced capacity to resynthesize glycogen also appears to depend on menstrual cycle phase.[23]

Fat Metabolism

Skeletal muscle possesses the capacity to derive energy from blood-borne fatty acids and intramuscular stores of triglyceride in addition to the relatively smaller stores of carbohydrate available for oxidation. It has been estimated that in normal weight individuals, the total body stores of carbohydrate and fat account for 2,000 and 140,000 kcal of energy respectively.[5] Because of the large difference in the amounts of these substrates available for energy metabolism, the coordinated process of carbohydrate and fat metabolism is essential for the performance of prolonged muscular activity. During prolonged exercise and the resultant hypoinsulinemia and increased catecholamine release, free fatty acids (FFAs) mobilized from adipose tissue become a more important energy yielding substrate. The process of lipolysis occurring in adipose tissue results in the breakdown of triglycerides to FFAs and glycerol. In addition to its stimulatory effect on hepatic glucose output, epinephrine further stimulates lipolysis in an effort to preserve circulating glucose.[24] Transported in the plasma bound to albumin, FFAs are then taken up by contractile tissue independent of insulin, but not necessarily by passive diffusion.[13] Sorrentino and associates[25] and Stremmel[26] have isolated FFA binding proteins from plasma membranes of adipocytes, hepatocytes, and cardiac myocytes, and because antibodies raised against these proteins inhibit FFA uptake, it has been hypothesized that FFA transport across the plasma membrane is, in fact, carrier-mediated.

Rates of fatty acid oxidation increase progressively during prolonged exercise. Temporally, this increase appears to be related to the increases in circulating nonesterified fatty acid concentrations; however, there appears to be some dissociation between the rate of fatty acid lipolysis from adipose tissue and the increased rates of skeletal muscle fatty acid oxidation. In exercise-trained individuals, rates of fatty acid oxidation are higher than in untrained men during low intensity exercise despite similar increases in adipose tissue lipolysis and a fatty acid uptake.[27] Several possible mechanisms that explain the observed increase in fatty acid oxidation during exercise in trained individuals include increased oxidation of fatty acids derived from intramuscular triglycerides[28] and enhanced fatty acid extraction during exercise by trained skeletal muscle.[29]

As alluded to in the section on carbohydrate metabolism, fat oxidation appears to be increased in women compared to men at the same relative exercise intensity. Costill and associates[30] reported a lower capacity for the skeletal muscle of women to oxidize fatty acids in vitro compared to that of men. In addition, the increased fatty acid oxidation observed during exercise in women appears to be independent of differences in circulating fatty acid concentrations.[21]

Protein and Amino Acid Metabolism

Oxidation of specific amino acids such as the branched-chain amino acids leucine, isoleucine, and valine also can be increased during exercise, but is increased to a smaller extent than oxidation of fat and carbohydrate (10% to 15% of total oxidized substrate).[31] Women who exercise, however, have been shown to have lower rates of amino acid oxidation during prolonged exercise and reduced urea excretion following exercise compared to men.[20,21] Reports of several studies have indicated that the increased amino acid oxidation during prolonged exercise results in an increased dietary requirement for protein in physically active individuals.[32,33]

Women and "Sarcopenia"

Body Composition and Aging

The most visible and, perhaps, the most profound changes that occur with advancing age are the alterations in whole body composition. Throughout the life span there is a progressive decline in the fat-free mass and a corresponding increase in fat mass. Estimates from several studies have indicated that beyond the third decade of life fat mass increases and continues to increase well into the eighth decade.[34,35] Arm circumference and skinfold thickness measurements from 700 male participants in the Baltimore Longitudinal Aging Study who were aged 20 to 92 years revealed a slow progressive loss of lean tissue until age 65 years, followed by a more rapid decline.[36]

By far, the most important functional changes in body composition that occur with advancing age are the reductions in active skeletal muscle mass. Fat-free mass or body cell mass as measured by the ratio of total body potassium to nitrogen reveals that nonmuscle lean tissue is preserved at the expense of the loss of skeletal muscle mass.[35] Within each age group, fat-free mass and muscle protein content are lower in women compared to men (Table 1). Tzankoff and Norris[37] confirmed that skeletal muscle mass measured by 24-hour urinary creatinine excretion declines an average of 6% per decade, and that this decline in muscle mass is largely responsible for the age-related decrease in resting metabolic rate. Fleg and Lakatta[38] also have demonstrated that the decline in muscle mass observed with age as measured by 24-hour urinary creatinine excretion can explain approximately 50% of the age-related decline in maximal oxygen uptake in women. These findings indicate that the alterations in body composition and in particular, the declines in skeletal muscle mass have profound effects on basal metabolism and functional exercise capacity.

In light of the clinical and functional significance of this age-related decline in skeletal muscle mass, a new term, "sarcopenia" (from Greek: loss of flesh), has been adopted to characterize this age-associated syndrome.[39] The etiology of sarcopenia is unknown but it probably results from the interactions throughout the life span between nutritional status, functional capacity, and body composition (Fig. 1). More recently, Baumgartner and associates[40] have shown that the prevalence of sarcopenia is higher in women than men up to age 80 years, when it converges and is similar between men and women. In addition, in this same study sarcopenia was linked to an increased prevalence of physical disability in both men and women.

Table 1 Muscle protein (kg) in men and women throughout the life span

	Young	Middle-aged	Older
Men	4.5	3.8	2.5
Women	1.8	1.9	1.1

(Reproduced with permission from Cohn SH, Vartsky D, Yasumura S, et al: Compartmental body composition based on total-body nitrogen, potassium, and calcium. *Am J Physiol* 1980;239:E524–E530.)

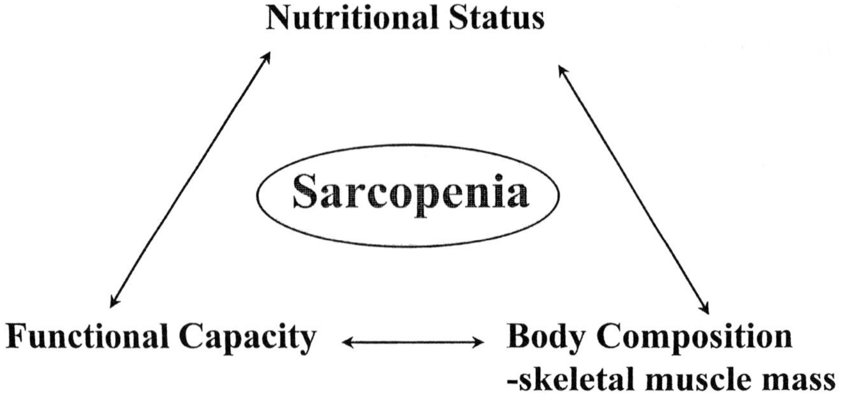

Fig. 1 Illustration of the relationship between nutrition, physical activity, body composition and sarcopenia.

Protein Utilization in Older Women

Suboptimal dietary protein intake along with a sedentary lifestyle may contribute to the increased prevalence of sarcopenia among older women. Data from a nutritional survey of older women living in the greater Boston area has revealed that greater than 25% of elderly women consume less than 0.81 $g \cdot kg^{-1} \cdot day^{-1}$ of dietary protein.[41] These results coupled with recent findings that the estimated protein requirement for older individuals should be approximately 0.91 + 0.04 $g \cdot kg^{-1} \cdot day^{-1}$ suggest a high prevalence of protein deficiency in older women.[42] More recently, Castaneda and associates[43] have examined the effects of chronic low protein intakes on body composition and function in older women. When elderly women were fed an isoenergetic diet with a protein intake of 0.45 to 0.81 $g \cdot kg^{-1} \cdot day^{-1}$ for 10 weeks, they observed a significant loss in fat-free mass, skeletal muscle function, and immune responses. Protein turnover and amino acid oxidation were also reduced in the low protein group as an apparent adaptation to attenuate the loss of lean tissue during the intervention period.[44] These results suggest that dietary protein intake plays a key role in the development of sarcopenia and that protein nutrition in many older women may be particularly inadequate.

Exercise and Sarcopenia

In both older men and women, exercise has been investigated as a possible intervention to reverse or attenuate age-related sarcopenia. Several studies in older men have shown that a program of high intensity progressive strength training can improve muscle strength and increase muscle size.[45] However, far fewer studies have examined the effects of progressive strength training on muscle size and function in older women.

Recently, Charette and associates[46] confirmed that dynamic resistance training (upper and lower body) of a similar intensity in healthy elderly women (mean age 69 years) results in significant increases in muscle strength (28% to 115%) and a 20% increase in type II muscle fiber area. In contrast to Frontera and associates,[47] they reported no change in type I fiber area following training. The apparent discrepancies regarding the magnitude of the change in type I fiber area may be related to the differences in the intensity and duration of the warm-up and cool-down period or to the initial pretraining activity patterns of the various subject populations. That the subjects in the study by Frontera and associates[47] were extremely sedentary prior to the start of the study is evidenced by the fact that the resistance training resulted in a significant increase in leg maximal oxygen uptake and a 38% increase in citrate synthase activity of the vastus lateralis muscle. This increased oxidative capacity is consistent with the type I muscle fiber hypertrophy observed. No measures of whole body or cellular oxidative metabolism were reported by Brown and associates[48] or by Charette and associates.[46] More recently, Pyka and associates[49] reported that a year-long strength training intervention in older men and women resulted in a 58% and 67% increase in type I and type II muscle fiber cross-sectional area, reflecting greater increases in muscle fiber size to strength training in the elderly over the course of a year than had previously been reported in several short-term studies lasting only a few months. Overall, these studies suggest that older women will respond favorably to a progressive strength training program with increases in strength and muscle mass.

Exercise and Nutritional Supplementation

Several studies have examined the effects of a dietary supplement in combination with resistance training exercise in older men and women. Studies in young individuals have failed to show an increase in skeletal muscle mass or enhanced strength gains when traditional strength training is coupled with a high protein supplement.[50,51] However, some studies in older individuals undergoing strength training have shown synergistic improvements in skeletal muscle mass with nutritional supplementation. Meredith and associates[52] observed a greater gain in body weight, muscle cross-sectional area, and subcutaneous fat accumulation in older men given a nutritional supplement (560 kcal/day; 17% protein, 43% carbohydrate, and 40% fat) and strength training compared with a group given strength training alone. In a recent study, Singh and associates[53] examined the combined effect of a 10-week strength training exercise program plus the provision of a multinutrient supplement (360 kcal, 60% carbohydrate, 23% fat, 17% soy-based protein) in frail nursing home residents (men and women). Gains in muscle strength were significantly higher in the strength training plus nutritional supplementation group compared to the strength training alone group (Fig. 2). In addition, the authors[53] observed a greater increase in type II muscle fiber cross-sectional area in response to the strength training plus nutritional supplementation compared to strength training alone (Fig. 3).

Despite these positive findings, not all studies have observed this effect. Campbell and associates[42] observed no difference in fat-free mass gains or increased muscle fiber cross-sectional area in older men and women consuming the RDA or twice the RDA for dietary protein during 12 weeks of strength training. However, this study is confounded by the adjustment of dietary energy intake to stabilize body weight throughout the exercise training program. It is possible that a relatively lower energy intake in this study may have blunted any potential benefits of the higher intake of dietary protein.

Taken together, the results of these studies suggest that our most frail older individuals may benefit from a combined nutritional and exercise intervention. This recommendation would be of particular importance to frail older women who appear to be at increased risk for sarcopenia-associated disability.

Summary and Conclusion

The evidence presented in this chapter suggests that there are unique nutritional requirements for physically active women that are superimposed on the already shifted nutritional requirements of physically active men and women. Throughout the life cycle, several major changes in body composition appear to affect women to a much greater degree than men, including the age-related decline in muscle mass, or sarcopenia. These changes may be

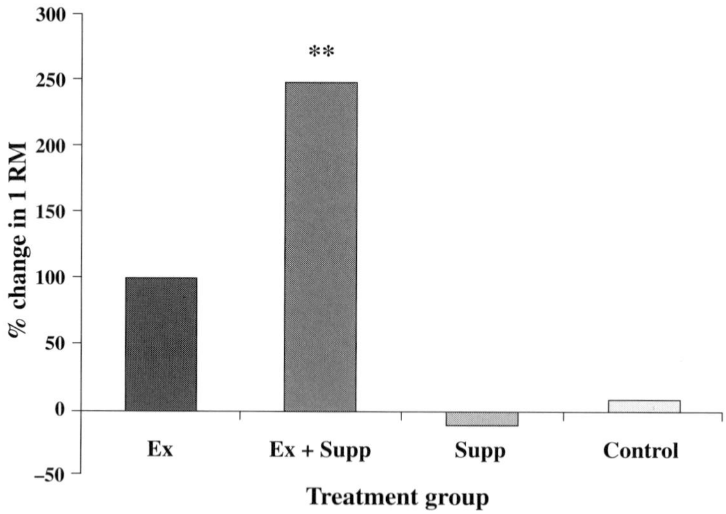

Fig. 2 Plot of the percentage change in the 1 repetition maximum (1 RM) muscle strength in frail older men and women following 10 weeks of strength training (Ex), strength training plus nutritional supplementation (Ex + Supp), nutritional supplementation alone (Supp), and control (Control). Asterisks indicate significant difference between Ex and Ex + Supp ($p < 0.01$). *(Reproduced with permission from Singh MA, Ding W, Manfredi TJ, et al: Insulin-like growth factor I in skeletal muscle after weight-lifting exercise in frail elders.* Am J Physiol *1999;277:E135–E143.)*

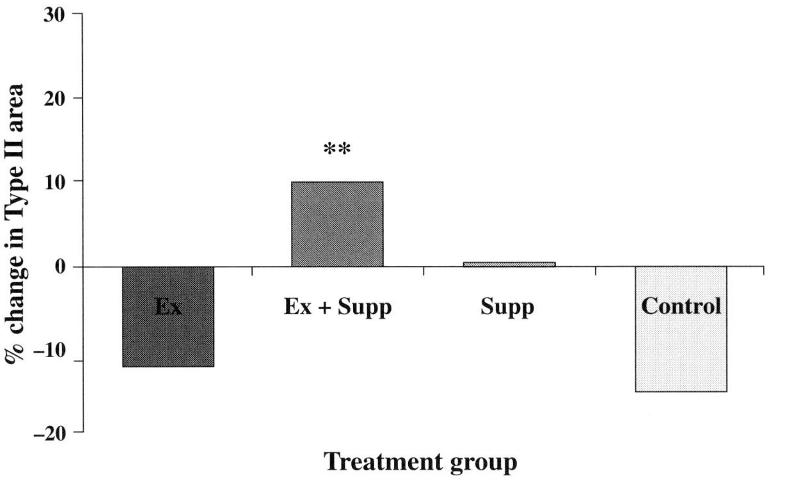

Fig. 3 *Plot of the percentage change in the type II muscle fiber areas in frail older men and women following 10 weeks of strength training (Ex), strength training plus nutritional supplementation (Ex + Supp), nutritional supplementation alone (Supp), and control (Control). Asterisks indicate significant difference between Ex and Ex + Supp* ($p < 0.033$)*. (Reproduced with permission from Singh MA, Ding W, Manfredi TJ, et al: Insulin-like growth factor I in skeletal muscle after weight-lifting exercise in frail elders.* Am J Physiol *1999;277:E135–E143.)*

influenced by the adequacy of protein. Physical activity and exercise may also impact on these specific age-related changes as has been discussed. Future research should focus on the optimal interaction between physical activity and proper nutrition on optimizing physical function and preventing disability throughout the life span. Specifically, intervention studies should examine the influence of protein and energy intake on accretion of skeletal muscle protein during resistance exercise training. The role of specific micronutrients such as calcium and vitamin D on muscle and bone metabolism and their interaction also warrant further study. Finally, effectiveness trials need to be conducted to assess the true impact of exercise and nutritional interventions on preventing or reversing age-associated sarcopenia.

References

1. Hill AV, Lupton H: Muscular exercise, lactic acid, and the supply and utilization of oxygen. *QJ Med* 1923;16:135–171.
2. Taylor HL, Buskirk E, Henschel A: Maximal oxygen uptake as an objective measure of cardio-respiratory performance. *J Appl Physiol* 1955;8:73–80.
3. Astrand I: Aerobic work capacity in men and women with special reference to age. *Acta Physiol Scand* 1960;169(suppl):1–92.

4. Kohrt WM, Malley MT, Dalsky GP, Holloszy JO: Body composition of healthy sedentary and trained, young and older men and women. *Med Sci Sports Exerc* 1992;24:832–837.
5. Newsholme EA, Start C (eds): *Regulation in Metabolism*. London, England, John Wiley & Sons, 1973, p 255.
6. Berger M, Hagg SA, Goodman MN, Ruderman NB: Glucose metabolism in perfused skeletal muscle: Effects of starvation, diabetes, fatty acids, acetoacetate, insulin, and exercise on glucose uptake and disposition. *Biochem J* 1976;158:191–202.
7. Ivy JL, Young JC, McLane JA, Fell RD, Holloszy JO: Exercise training and glucose uptake by skeletal muscle in rats. *J Appl Physiol* 1983;55:1393–1396.
8. Felig P, Cherif A, Minigawa A, Wahren J: Hypoglycemia during prolonged exercise in normal men. *N Engl J Med* 1982;306:895–900.
9. Goodyear LJ, Chang P-Y, Sherwood DJ, Dufresne SD, Moller DE: Effects of exercise and insulin on mitogen-activated protein kinase signaling pathways in rat skeletal muscle. *Am J Physiol* 1996;271:E403–E408.
10. Coyle EF, Hagberg JM, Hurley BF, Martin WH, Ehsani AA, Holloszy JO: Carbohydrate feeding during prolonged strenuous exercise can delay fatigue. *J Appl Physiol* 1983;55:230–235.
11. Coyle EF, Coggan AR, Hemmert MK, Ivy JL: Muscle glycogen utilization during prolonged strenuous exercise when fed carbohydrate. *J Appl Physiol* 1986;61:165–172.
12. Katz A, Broberg S, Sahlin K, Wahren J: Leg glucose uptake during maximal dynamic exercise in humans. *Am J Physiol* 1986;251:E65–E70.
13. Richter EA, Turcotte L, Hespel P, Kiens B: Metabolic responses to exercise: Effects of endurance training and implications for diabetes. *Diabetes Care* 1992;15:1767–1776.
14. Galbo H (ed): *Hormonal and Metabolic Adaptation to Exercise*. New York, NY, Thieme-Stratton, 1983.
15. Hermansen L, Hultman E, Saltin B: Muscle glycogen during prolonged severe exercise. *Acta Physiol Scand* 1967;71:129–139.
16. Richter EA, Galbo H: High glycogen levels enhance glycogen breakdown in isolated contracting skeletal muscle. *J Appl Physiol* 1986;61:827–831.
17. Bergstrom J, Hermansen L, Hultman E, Saltin B: Diet, muscle glycogen and physical performance. *Acta Physiol Scand* 1967;71:140–150.
18. Jacobs I: Lactate concentrations after short, maximal exercise at various glycogen levels. *Acta Physiol Scand* 1981;111:465–469.
19. Maughan RJ, Poole DC: The effects of a glycogen-loading regimen on the capacity to perform anaerobic exercise. *Eur J Appl Physiol* 1981;46:211–219.
20. Phillips SM, Atkinson SA, Tarnopolsky MA, MacDougall JD: Gender differences in leucine kinetics and nitrogen balance in endurance athletes. *J Appl Physiol* 1993;75:2134–2141.
21. Tarnopolsky LJ, MacDougall JD, Atkinson SA, Tarnopolsky MA, Sutton JR: Gender differences in substrate for endurance exercise. *J Appl Physiol* 1990;68:302–308.
22. Tarnopolsky MA, Atkinson SA, Phillips SM, MacDougall JD: Carbohydrate loading and metabolism during exercise in men and women. *J Appl Physiol* 1995;78:1360–1368.
23. Nicklas BJ, Hackney AC, Sharp RL: The menstrual cycle and exercise: Performance, muscle glycogen, and substrate responses. *Int J Sports Med* 1989;10:264–269.

24. Zinman B, Murray FT, Vranic M, et al: Glucoregulation during moderate exercise in insulin treated diabetics. *J Clin Endocrinol Metab* 1977;45:641–652.
25. Sorrentino D, Stump D, Potter BJ, et al: Oleate uptake by cardiac myocytes is carrier mediated and involves a 40-kD plasma membrane fatty acid binding protein similiar to that in liver, adipose tissue, and gut. *J Clin Invest* 1988;82:928–935.
26. Stremmel W: Fatty acid uptake by isolated rat heart myocytes represents a carrier-mediated transport process. *J Clin Invest* 1988;81:844–852.
27. Klein S, Coyle EF, Wolfe RR: Fat metabolism during low-intensity exercise in endurance-trained and untrained men. *Am J Physiol* 1994;267:E934–E940.
28. Hurley BF, Nemeth PM, Martin WH III, Hagberg JM, Dalsky GP, Holloszy JO: Muscle triglyceride utilization during exercise: Effect of training. *J Appl Physiol* 1986;60:562–567.
29. Turcotte LP, Richter EA, Kiens B: Increased plasma FFA uptake and oxidation during prolonged exercise in trained vs. untrained humans. *Am J Physiol* 1992;262:E791–E799.
30. Costill DL, Fink WJ, Getchell LH, Ivy JL, Witzmann FA: Lipid metabolism in skeletal muscle of endurance-trained males and females. *J Appl Physiol* 1979;47:787–791.
31. Rennie MJ, Edwards RH, Krywawych S, et al: Effect of exercise on protein turnover in man. *Clin Sci (Colch)* 1981;61:627–639.
32. Meredith CN, Zackin MJ, Frontera WR, Evans WJ: Dietary protein requirements and body protein metabolism in endurance-trained men. *J Appl Physiol* 1989;66:2850–2856.
33. Tarnopolsky MA, Atkinson SA, MacDougall JD, Chesley A, Phillips S, Schwarcz HP: Evaluation of protein requirements for trained strength athletes. *J Appl Physiol* 1992;73:1986–1995.
34. Parizkova J: Body composition and exercise during growth and development, in Rarick GL, Adams FH (eds): *Physical Activity: Human Growth and Development.* New York, NY, Academic Press, 1973.
35. Cohn SH, Vartsky D, Yasumura S, et al: Compartmental body composition based on total-body nitrogen, potassium, and calcium. *Am J Physiol* 1980;239:E524-E530.
36. Borkan GA, Norris AH: Fat redistribution and the changing body dimensions of the adult male. *Hum Biol* 1977;49:495–513.
37. Tzankoff SP, Norris AH: Longitudinal changes in basal metabolism in man. *J Appl Physiol* 1978;45:536–539.
38. Fleg JL, Lakatta EG: Role of muscle loss in the age-associated reduction in Vo2max. *J Appl Physiol* 1988;65:1147–1151.
39. Evans WJ, Campbell WW: Sarcopenia and age-related changes in body composition and functional capacity. *J Nutr* 1993;123(suppl 2):465–468.
40. Baumgartner RN, Koehler KM, Gallagher D, et al: Epidemiology of sarcopenia among the elderly in New Mexico. *Am J Epidemiol* 1998;147:755–763.
41. Hartz SC, Russell RM, Rosenberg IH (eds): *Nutrition in the Elderly: The Boston Nutritional Status Survey*. London, England, Smith-Gordon, 1992.
42. Campbell WW, Crim MC, Dallal GE, Young VR, Evans WJ: Increased protein requirements in elderly people: New data and retrospective reassessments. *Am J Clin Nutr* 1994;60:501–509.
43. Castaneda C, Charnley JM, Evans WJ, Crim MC: Elderly women accommodate to a low-protein diet with losses of body cell mass, muscle function, and immune response. *Am J Clin Nutr* 1995;62:30–39.

44. Castaneda C, Dolnikowski GG, Dallal GE, Evans WJ, Crim MC: Protein turnover and energy metabolism of elderly women fed a low-protein diet. *Am J Clin Nutr* 1995;62:40-48.

45. Fielding RA: Effects of exercise training in the elderly: Impact of progressive-resistance training on skeletal muscle and whole-body protein metabolism. *Proc Nutr Soc* 1995;54:665–675.

46. Charette SL, McEvoy L, Pyka G, et al: Muscle hypertrophy response to resistance training in older women. *J Appl Physiol* 1991;70:1912–1916.

47. Frontera WR, Meredith CN, O'Reilly KP, Evans WJ: Strength training and determinants of Vo2max in older men. *J Appl Physiol* 1990;68:329–333.

48. Brown AB, McCartney N, Sale DG: Positive adaptations to weight-lifting training in the elderly. *J Appl Physiol* 1990;69:1725–1733.

49. Pyka G, Lindenberger E, Charette S, Marcus R: Muscle strength and fiber adaptations to a year-long resistance training program in elderly men and women. *J Gerontol* 1994;49:M22–M27.

50. Weideman CA, Flynn MG, Pizza FX, et al: Abstract: Effects of increased protein intake on muscle hypertrophy and strength following 13 weeks of resistance training. *Med Sci Sports Exerc* 1990;22(suppl):S37.

51. Lemon PW, Tarnopolsky MA, MacDougall JD, Atkinson SA: Protein requirements and muscle mass/strength changes during intensive training in novice bodybuilders. *J Appl Physiol* 1992;73:767–775.

52. Meredith CN, Frontera WR, O'Reilly KP, Evans WJ: Body composition in elderly men: Effect of dietary modification during strength training. *J Am Geriatr Soc* 1992;40:155–162.

53. Singh MA, Ding W, Manfredi TJ, et al: Insulin-like growth factor I in skeletal muscle after weight-lifting exercise in frail elders. *Am J Physiol* 1999;277:E135–E143.

Directions for Future Research

Conduct randomized clinical trials and population-based investigations to more fully specify the types, modes, amounts, intensities and patterns of physical activity that are necessary to promote health and specific physiologic and metabolic adaptations and to facilitate recovery/rehabilitation from disease and injury.

Current evidence is sufficient to conclude that regular physical activity is beneficial to health in general. More detailed information is needed to describe details of the dose-response relationship between physical activity and specific outcomes. Because the dose-response relationship between exercise and health may well vary for different outcomes (such as coronary heart disease, osteoarthritis, osteoporosis, diabetes, and functional limitations), it will be important to conduct studies for specific outcomes. Emphasis should be directed toward determining whether the effectiveness of exercise interventions is dependent on the severity of the disease state.

Improve surveillance systems to (1) monitor population levels and trends of physical activity and fitness, especially for the current consensus public health recommendations for physical activity, and (2) document exercise-related health problems such as musculoskeletal injuries and sudden death associated with exercise.

Much more work is needed to establish the specific cost-benefit of regular exercise. It is important to enhance measurement of the effects of physical activity and fitness on nationally representative populations to monitor trends in this important determinant of health. Numerous benefits of regular participation in physical activity have been documented, but there are few data on exercise-related injuries and other problems. Information is needed on injury rates resulting from sedentary adults adopting and maintaining current public health recommendations for physical activity.

Establish prospective epidemiologic studies to define risk factors for exercise-related musculoskeletal problems.

Little is known about factors predisposing individuals to musculoskeletal injury if they follow current public recommendations for physical activity. This line of research must be developed before effective strategies for prevention and rehabilitation of musculoskeletal injuries can be developed.

Conduct long-term trials of physical activity interventions.

There is a substantial body of literature from exercise training studies, but controlled investigations on methods to help sedentary individuals adopt and maintain a healthful level of physical activity are lacking. Research studies are needed on the determinants of physical activity, how to influence these determinants and mediators of activity, and how to help individuals develop the behavioral skills that lead to increased exercise. These interventions should be based on established psychological theories and should include currently known determinants such as barriers to physical activity, health status, knowledge of health effects, environmental factors such as proximity of facilities for physical activity, lack of time, and socioeconomic characteristics. There is a special need to develop and evaluate intervention methods designed to help women who have increased their physical activity to maintain this new behavior over the long term. Few current studies include data on maintenance of physical activity longer than 1 year, and it is necessary to extend these observations over at least 5 years. It is important to conduct intervention studies in a variety of populations, including a broad age range, women from minority groups, and those who are healthy as well as those with a variety of diseases or conditions.

In the disease state of osteoarthritis, there is a need for standardized subjective and objective methods of assessing exposures, predisposing factors, and osteoarthritis outcomes.

There is a need to develop and validate better measurements of exercise, sport, and occupational exposures for use in clinical trials and epidemiologic studies on exercise and arthritis. These methods should include development of questionnaires to assess short-term and lifetime characteristics of muscle and joint loading. Additionally, objective monitoring of exercise exposures by accelerometers or other devices should be investigated. Various medical specialties and subspecialties currently use different rating scales, so there also is a need for better standardization of patient-reported outcome assessment. There is an additional need for research to identify valid biomarkers and radiographic and functional assessment techniques for objective evaluation of osteoarthritis development and progression throughout the life span.

Evaluate the role of nutritional and hormonal status on responses to exercise training in women throughout the life span.

Specific areas of emphasis should include the interaction of skeletal muscle mass and bone in relation to function, health, and disease. The efficacy of dietary supplements on optimizing responses to exercise training in individuals with chronic disease and disability should be investigated.

There is a need for more randomized clinical trials and methodologically rigorous observational studies in which the independent and combined effects of diet and activity are evaluated as they relate to progression and treatment of disease.

Healthful dietary patterns and regular physical activity are important components of health promotion and disease prevention. For example, diets high in saturated fat and low levels of physical activity are both predictors of colon cancer incidence. Additionally, sedentary individuals also eating a diet high in saturated fat had especially high risk in one report. Very little is known about how a low-fat diet and regular physical activity might act synergistically in relation to risk of coronary heart disease or type II diabetes.

Section Six

Psychosocial Health Issues

Section Editor:
Aurelia Nattiv, MD

Susan N. DiGrazia, BS
Cheryl Hug-English, MD, MPH
Anthony Margherita, MD
Jerry R. May, PhD
Heidi Prather, DO

Overview

The advent of Title IX legislation and the resultant involvement of strong, healthy women portrayed in the Olympics and in professional sports have inspired young girls and women to increase their participation in sports and exercise. This increased participation has, in turn, led to more knowledge about the physical and psychological health benefits of sport and physical activity, as well as the potential barriers. Regular physical activity for girls and young women can reduce risk of many chronic diseases of adulthood. Furthermore, female athletes do better academically, have lower drop-out rates, and are more likely to go on to college than their nonathletic counterparts. Regular physical activity has been demonstrated to enhance mental health, reduce symptoms of depression and stress, and improve self-esteem in young girls. According to the "Surgeon General's Report on Physical Activity and Health," however, almost half of our United States youth are not vigorously active on a regular basis and 14% are completely inactive. Although more girls are participating in a wider array of physical activities and sports than ever before, young women are twice as likely to be inactive as young men. Research is needed to identify factors that motivate girls and women to participate in sport and exercise as well as factors that lead to attrition. More research is needed to assess how ethnicity and socioeconomic status might affect the involvement of girls and women in sport and physical activity.

Several studies have correlated life stress with athletic injury. As the opportunities increase for girls and women to participate in sports at many levels (club, high school, college, professional), psychological factors associated with injury and recovery need to be explored. These psychological factors and life stresses associated with injury (moving, family death) and the psychological responses to injury and recovery (tension, depression, confusion, low self-esteem) are complex and multifactorial. The support of coaches, parents, friends, teammates, and health-care professionals can have a direct impact on the response to athletic-related injury. There is a lack of research exploring psychological response to injury in girls and women participating in sports and physical activity. Knowledge of these important factors may enhance the ability of health-care professionals and others to assist in the prevention and treatment of athletic-related injury, as well as facilitate the injured individual's return to regular physical activity.

In addition to the multitude of health benefits from participation in sports and physical activity, there exist some potential risks. The female athlete triad represents the interrelationship of disordered eating, amenorrhea, and osteoporosis that may occur individually or in combination in some physically active girls and women. Although the underlying causes of the female athlete triad have not been fully elucidated, the desire to be thin and the ongoing internal and external pressures to maintain a low body weight for competition and performance appear to contribute most significantly to the development of the triad. An increased risk for stress fractures and premature osteoporosis, a decrease in performance and well-being, and other psychological and physical repercussions may result from the triad disorders. Despite the knowledge of the related components of the triad, little is known about the prevalence, causes, optimal prevention, and treatment of each of the triad components that may occur in physically active girls and women. Research with sound methodology is needed to better define prevalence data of each component of the female athlete triad. Further study on the association of body composition and performance, as well as nutritional intake and performance parameters, is needed. In addition, research is needed on osteoporosis prevention in girls and young women, including further study on the important nutritional and hormonal factors affecting bone, as well as type and frequency of exercise that result in maximizing peak bone density and prevention of the triad disorders.

The chapters in this section emphasize the psychological and other health benefits of participation in sport and physical activity for girls and women, while discussing some of the potential health risks and consequences of unhealthy behaviors that may occur. It must be emphasized that from a public health perspective, the psychological and overall health benefits of involvement in a physically active lifestyle far outweigh the potential risks that may occur in a small percentage of individuals. Further discussion in the chapters that follow will address the biopsychosocial factors contributing to participation in sport and physical activity for girls and women, expand on the health benefits and potential risks of involvement in sports and exercise, and suggest directions for further research that may lead to increased participation in sports and physical activity as well as prevention and management of the potential risks.

Aurelia Nattiv, MD

Chapter 30

The Life of the Complete Girl: A Biopsychosocial Model of Sports Participation by Young Girls

Jerry R. May, PhD
Susan N. DiGrazia, BS
Cheryl Hug-English, MD, MPH

Developmental Differences Between Girls and Boys

Some researchers have found that girls and boys really are from two different planets. While it is far from clear just what roles nature and nurture play in creating these differences, we do know that physically and intellectually, boys and girls do not develop at the same rate.[1–4] For example, boys develop fine motor skills, such as the ability to hold a pencil, later than do girls. Boys tend to learn to read later, but they excel at gross motor skills and at visual and spatial skills. Clearly, these gender-based differences play a role in how girls and boys experience and interact with the world, including their participation in sports.

The Benefits of Physical Activities and Sports Involvement by Young Girls

Although boys and girls differ in their physical and emotional development, both can benefit from physical activity. Donna E. Shalala, Secretary of Health and Human Services, in summarizing the report of the President's Council on Physical Fitness and Sport,[5] noted that men and women of all ages can improve the quality of their lives through a lifelong practice of regular moderate physical activity. She also noted that childhood and adolescence are critical times to lay the foundation for lifelong physical activity. The good news is that more girls than ever before in the United States are participating in a wider array of physical activities and sports. However, too many young people, especially girls, are not active enough. The President's Council Report[5] and Baum[6] report that young girls are twice as likely to be inactive as young boys.

The President's Council Report[5] uses an interdisciplinary approach to investigate the impact of physical activity and sport participation on the "complete girl" (ie, her social, physical, emotional, and cultural environment). The conclusions are striking: Regular physical activity can enhance mental health, reducing symptoms of stress and depression and improving self-esteem

(Sandra Perlmutter, Executive Director President's Council on Physical Fitness and Sports, personal communication, 1997). Female athletes do better academically and have lower dropout rates than their nonathletic counterparts. Regular physical activity can reduce the risk of many chronic diseases of adulthood.

Effect on Mental Health

One of the benefits for girls who participate in sports is the positive effect on mental health, which has been reported by many researchers. Biddle[7] and Morgan[8] found that physical fitness is positively associated with mental health and well-being. Exercise and sports participation can enhance the mental health of adolescent girls by providing positive feelings about body image, improving self-esteem, increasing self-confidence, and offering tangible experiences of competency and success.[9] Three recent studies by the Melpomene Institute examined the relationship between self-esteem and physical activity in both young and teenaged girls[10–12] from diverse geographic, economic, and racial backgrounds. All 3 studies found a strong positive relationship between physical activity and self-esteem. Gill[13] reported that exercise programs, particularly weight and strength training, can enhance the self-concept of adolescent girls. Plaisted[14] and Snyder and Spreiter[15] also found that physical activity is associated with positive self-esteem and body image. Finally, the President's Council Report[5] suggests that physical activity is an effective tool for reducing the symptoms of stress and depression among girls.

Effect on Academic Achievement

Sports also are an educational asset in girls' lives. The findings of the Report show that many female high school athletes report higher grades and standardized test scores and lower dropout rates, and are more likely to go on to college than their nonathletic counterparts.[5]

Physical Health Benefits

Recognition of physical activity and sport as an effective and money-saving public health approach is growing among researchers and policy makers. Regular physical activity during adolescence can reduce girls' risk for obesity and hyperlipidemia, which have been associated with adult onset of coronary heart disease and certain cancers. In addition, active girls' high caloric expenditure decreases their risk of becoming obese.[5]

Social Benefits

Girls also benefit socially from participation in sports. Weiss and Glenn[16] found that 8- to 13-year-old children who had superior physical abilities were better accepted by their peers. Also, research indicates a correlation between exercise and sexual behavior. Several studies have shown that the greater the frequency of exercise, the older the age of first intercourse for adolescent girls.[17,18] Higher rates of athletic participation among adolescent girls were significantly associated with lower rates of both sexual activity and pregnancy.[5]

Benefits of Sports Participation

Children and adolescents often have multiple reasons for participation in organized sport, with "having fun" rated as the most important motive for both boys and girls. Other primary reasons that children play organized sports typically include improving skills, being with friends, becoming physically fit, liking the challenges, and experiencing success.[19,20]

Given the many benefits of sports and exercise, it is worth examining ways to encourage participation. Treasure[21] reports that girls and boys who perceive a climate oriented toward high mastery and moderate performance report a positive attitude toward physical education, high perceived ability, the belief that effort and ability cause success, and feelings of satisfaction. In other words, focusing on skill development rather than winning provides a more positive experience for children. Weiss and Glenn[16] found that girls who have supportive parents and peers as well as siblings, teachers, and coaches are more likely to continue their participation in sports than are individuals for whom this support is weaker.

Primary reasons for discontinuing participation include conflicts of interest, the desire to do other things, injury, lack of fun, and skills development.[19] Petlichkoff[22] placed sports withdrawal on a continuum, because many children who drop out of one sport often move on to try another sport or activity and are really "sport transfers." According to Petlichkoff, that "competition and a focus on winning may act as extrinsic motivating forces to decrease intrinsic motivation is especially likely for females." That is, if a young girl's participation in a sport depends heavily on winning, she may drop out.

Risks of Sports Participation

Unfortunately, there are potential risks involved with girls' participation in sports. The female athlete triad[23] refers to a symptom complex that is prevalent among female athletes who participate in certain sports and some girls who engage in excessive exercise. The triad includes: (1) disordered eating, (2) amenorrhea, and (3) bone loss and osteoporosis. The female athlete triad is of great concern. Compulsive and excessive exercising can lead to hormonal changes that can trigger loss of menstrual periods and osteoporosis. Continual exercise can lead to an increased number of stress fractures.

Female adolescents, in general, report greater body image disturbances and more dissatisfaction with their bodies than do males.[13,14,24] Overdorf and Gill[24] found that female adolescent athletes perceived their bodies as heavier than they actually were. Of the adolescents they sampled who were predominately within normal weight ranges, 43.8% admitted to using some form of pathogenic weight control method at least occasionally.

Estimates of female athletes with eating disorders typically range from 10% to 20%. Disturbed body images and the associated low self-esteem lay the groundwork for weight preoccupation and disordered eating. Under these conditions, participation in physical activity can often cross a very dangerous line.[25] The athlete can become obsessed with exercise and calorie counting, compulsively exercising to the point of exhaustion or physical damage. Athletes who hold unhealthy attitudes and use unhealthy weight-loss methods (eg, excessive exercise) far outnumber those with true eating disorders, but both are certainly of concern because they represent points along a continuum.[14]

Coaches can also influence an athlete's eating behavior. Griffin and Harris[26] found that coaches are more likely to encourage female athletes to lose weight but male athletes to gain weight. The authors found that coaches tended to make decisions about the need for weight control on the basis of appearance rather than more objective indicators.[2]

In spite of the many factors that contribute to disordered eating, girls can nevertheless learn positive nutritional habits through their experiences in sport and physical activity.[5]

There are also appreciable numbers of girls for whom athletic participation presents a risk to their emotional health, rather than enhancing their mental well-being. Morgan[8] found that mood states can worsen with increased training volumes. For example, healthy, nondepressed individuals may become depressed as a result of high training loads (ie, overtraining).

Barriers to Equal Access

Despite these cautions, for the overwhelming majority of female athletes, sports participation holds great benefits. Unfortunately, some girls are denied the chance to derive positive experiences from physical activity and sport because of lack of opportunity and gender stereotypes.

Access to sports participation and physical activity relates to poverty and ethnicity issues. The President's Council Report[5] found that poverty substantially limits many girls' access to physical activity and sport, especially minority girls, who are overrepresented in lower socioeconomic groups. Girls from economically disadvantaged backgrounds and girls with disabilities can face unique obstacles in relation to physical activity and sport.

For example, poor families cannot afford to invest in health club memberships, exercise machines, and sports equipment. Poor families often cannot pay user fees or costs to transport their children between home and school athletic activities. Dual-worker families or single parents (most often mothers) sometimes depend on older daughters to cook or care for smaller children after school, thus curbing their involvement with extracurricular activities.[27]

Summary

The benefits to women of exercise, sports, and physical activity are many. This must, however, be tempered by the fact that overexercising and overtraining can produce detrimental side effects. A healthy balance of varied physical activity should be encouraged.

References

1. Kantronwitz B, Kalb C: Boys will be boys. *Newsweek*, May 11, 1998.
2. Gilligan C (ed): *In a Different Voice: Psychological Theory and Women's Development*. Cambridge, MA, Harvard University Press, 1982.
3. Gurian M (ed): *The Wonder of Boys: What Parents, Mentors and Educators Can Do to Shape Young Boys Into Exceptional Men*. New York, NY, Putnam Publishing Group, 1996.
4. Weinberg MK, Tronick EZ, Cohn JF, Olson KL: Gender differences in emotional expressivity and self-regulation during early infancy. *Dev Psychol* 1999;35:175–188.
5. Bunker LK, Pradt K (eds): *Physical Activity and Sport in the Lives of Girls*. Washington, DC, President's Council on Physical Fitness and Sports, 1977.
6. Baum AL: Young females in the athletic arena. *Child Adolesc Psychiatr Clin N Am* 1998;7:745–755.
7. Biddle S: Exercise and psychosocial health. *Res Q Exerc Sport* 1995;66:292–297.
8. Morgan WP: Physical activity, fitness, and depression, in Bouchard C, Shephard RJ, Stephens T (eds): *Physical Activity, Fitness, and Health: International Proceedings and Consensus Statement*. Champaign, IL, Human Kinetics, 1994, pp 851–867.
9. McAuley E: Physical activity and psychosocial outcomes, in Bouchard C, Shephard RJ, Stephens T (eds): *Physical Activity, Fitness, and Health: International Proceedings and Consensus Statement*. Champaign, IL, Human Kinetics, 1994, pp 551–568.
10. Jaffee L, Manzer R: Girls' perspectives: Physical activity and self-esteem. *Melpomene: A Journal for Women's Health Research* 1992;11:19–26.
11. Jaffee L, Ricker S: Physical activity and self-esteem in girls: The teen years. *Melpomene: A Journal for Women's Health Research* 1993;12:14–23.
12. Jaffee L, Wu: After school activities and self-esteem in adolescent girls. *Melpomene: A Journal for Women's Health Research* 1996;15:18–25.
13. Gill DL: Psychological, sociological, and cultural issues concerning the athletic female, in Pearl AJ (ed): *The Athletic Female*. Champaign, IL, Human Kinetics, 1993.
14. Plaisted V: Gender and sport, in Morris T, Summers JJ (eds): *Sport Psychology: Theory, Applications and Issues*. Brisbane, Australia, John Wiley & Sons, 1995, pp 538–574.
15. Snyder EE, Spreiter EA: Correlates of sport participation among adolescent girls. *Res Q* 1976;47:804–809.
16. Weiss MR, Glenn SD: Psychological development and females' sport participation: An interactional perspective. *Quest* 1992;44:138–157.
17. Brown JT, Ellis L, Guerrina ML, Paxton DM, Poleno P: The relationship between the frequency of exercise and the age of onset of sexual intercourse in adolescent females. *Nurse Pract* 1997;22:16–18.

18. Miller KE, Sabo DF, Farrell MP, Barnes GM, Melnick MJ: Athletic participation and sexual behavior in adolescents: The different worlds of boys and girls. *J Health Soc Behav* 1998;39:108–123.

19. Weiss MR, Petlichkoff LM: Children's motivation for participation in and withdrawal from sport: Identifying the missing links. *Pediatr Exerc Sci* 1989;1:195–211.

20. Ewing ME, Seefeld V: Participation and attrition patterns, in *American Agency-sponsored and Interscholastic Sports: An Executive Summary*. North Palm Beach, FL, Sporting Goods Manufacturers Association, 1989. Final Report.

21. Treasure DC: Perceptions of the motivational climate and elementary school children's cognitive and affective response. *J Sport and Exerc Psychol* 1997;19:278–290.

22. Petlichkoff LM: The drop-out dilemma in youth sports, in Bar-Or O (ed): *The Child and Adolescent Athlete*. Oxford, England, Blackwell Scientific, 1996, pp 418–430.

23. Lutter JM, Jaffee L (eds): *The Bodywise Woman*, ed 2. Champaign, IL, Human Kinetics, 1996.

24. Overdorf VG, Gill KS: Body image, weight and eating concerns and use of weight control methods among high school female athletes. *Women Sport Physical Act J* 1994;3:69–79.

25. Polivy J: Physical activity, fitness, and compulsive behaviors, in Bouchard C, Shephard RJ, Stephens T (eds): *Physical Activity, Fitness and Health: International Proceedings and Consensus Statement*. Champaign, IL, Human Kinetics, 1994, pp 883–897.

26. Griffin J, Harris MB: Coaches' attitudes, knowledge, experiences and recommendations regarding weight control. *Sport Psychologist* 1996;10:180–194.

27. *The Wilson Report: Moms, Dads, Daughters and Sports*. New York, NY, Women's Sports Foundation, 1988.

Chapter 31

Psychology and Exercise in Women

Heidi Prather, DO
Anthony Margherita, MD

The female athlete has more diverse opportunities to participate in sports and exercise than in years past. This is in part due to changing legislation, attitudes, and demographics. The social and cultural influences related to athletics and athletic participation for women are different from those for men. In some sports, women have participated for generations, thereby establishing role models, behavior patterns, and social hierarchy. Others evolved as training approaches and attitudes changed. The importance and interest in exercise participation for health and social reasons has progressively become more popular. As a result, women athletes are currently in "uncharted territory" regarding their experiences in sports and exercise. Literature describing and investigating the female experience exists but is still evolving. Psychology of sports and exercise regarding women is growing rapidly. Differentiating male and female psychological issues relating to exercise and sport is important to understanding participation and injury recovery. With increasing numbers of elite athletes and women's sports receiving more media attention, new insights should be gained regarding gender and role identification regarding exercise and sports.

Socialization

Opportunities for girls and women in sports continue to increase at the school and even preschool age level. The number of girls participating in sports and exercise is growing exponentially. A 1990 survey by the Women's Sports Foundation revealed that 91% of women surveyed thought it was important for girls to participate in organized sports.[1] Studies have shown the importance of socializing influences and participation and success in sports. Young athletes report they pursue sports to improve their skills, have fun, and associate with others. The more support and positive feedback the individual receives, the more likely he or she is to continue to participate in the activity. In general a child's sense of accomplishment in sports is directly tied to the child's perception that she or he is capable of participating in the sport.[2,3] Eccles and Harold[4] reported that girls have a more negative assessment of their competence than boys. This may be due to gender-role socialization.

Women have multiple roles in today's society. Many work full-time, provide most child care, manage the family finances, and direct the activities of daily life in the family household. Finding a balance in these multiple roles is often challenging. Kopp and Ruzicka[5] examined the psychological well-being of 162 women enrolled in a community college. They showed that women occupying two or three of the roles of partner, mother, and paid employee were happier and reported a higher self-esteem than those occupying one or none. Despite having more responsibilities, women continue to want to increase their ability to exercise for both the physical and mental benefits. A survey of 400 women found that respondents thought that the "most important" benefits of exercise included cardiovascular fitness (82%), improved muscle tone (82%), firmer body (82%), weight maintenance (78%), and improved self-image (70%).[6] DiNucci and associates[7] reported that college women participating in a group sport had more positive feelings about their body weight and physical condition compared to nonathletes. It is important to note that college women have special pressures to have an attractive physical appearance.[7] Though their motives may be diverse, women are increasing their exercise participation for physical and psychological benefits.

In today's media-dominated society, young people are increasingly influenced by images in the media and through advertising. Consequently, through coverage and portrayal of sports figures, the media play an increasingly influential role. Female athletes and teams are gaining exposure through increased media coverage and endorsements. These athletes serve as role models for the sports in which these women participate. Although coverage of women's sports has increased, the amount of coverage given to women is dramatically less than that given to men. In years past, this discrepancy in coverage has implied that women are not interested in sports participation. Yet, coverage of women's sports is increasing with the attention given to the Olympic games and the renewal of professional women's basketball. However, portrayal of women in the media remains much different than that of men. Theberge[8] reported in the early 1990s that female athletes are often praised for their femininity or attractiveness. In contrast, men are described as athletic, strong, and powerful. The message sent to viewers appears to be that of trivialization of women's participation in the sport and perpetuation of gender stereotypes. Much less focus is placed on the woman's athletic accomplishment.[9] New investigations are needed to update the effect the media are having on sports and exercise promotion. With changes in media coverage in recent years, new studies are needed to identify continued differences.

Actual or perceived social role and identification play a prominent role in shaping a young woman's attitudes in adolescence and adulthood. These social roles are personally and culturally defined. Gaining acceptance of female athletes in a more prominent role means overcoming gender stereotypes. A more negative status is noted for women participating in a more masculine sport. The athlete may find herself in a "catch-22." If she exudes a more feminine appearance and/or behavior, her accomplishments may be devalued. If she assumes a more masculine appearance and/or behavior, she may suffer ridicule and social rejection. Lack of support systems may contribute to the athlete discontinuing her participation in the sport.[10,11] Adolescents are especially susceptible to stereotypes. As girls reach puberty their desire to be accepted by their peer group becomes more important than their previous support system of family. It becomes important to "fit in." As would be expected, this is also the time of greatest decline in sports participation.[11] The attrition of young athletes from sports has been found to be related primarily to the athlete becoming interested in other activities or the athlete's desire to avoid the competitiveness of a program.[12,13] Unfortunately, these reports did not compare male and female reasons for attrition. No reports have indicated what these "other interests" are.[14] Better identification of reasons for motivation to stay in sports would enable the development of improved support systems for sports and exercise participants of all ages.

Kane[2] compared social role identification of male and female high school students. When asked what role they most wanted to be remembered for, the male respondents most frequently (36.36%) answered "athlete." The female respondents most frequently (36.36%) chose "leader in activities." In fact, female students chose the role of athlete least often (9.0%). This study also reports the athlete's feelings on appropriateness of sport. When men were asked if they were to date a female athlete which sport would they choose, their first choices in response were tennis (63.64%), golf (11.57%), and volleyball (9.92%). Basketball (10.74%) was the highest sex-inappropriate sport chosen followed by softball (4.13%). Similarly, when asked who they wanted to be friends with, the females chose tennis player and golfer more often. Kane[2] concluded that to understand the status of the female athlete in high school, consideration must be given to participation and to the type of sport.

A number of studies have looked at the female athlete and role conflict.[3,15,16] Traditional female roles are often conflicting with those of the athlete. Allison[17] completed a study review and determined that role conflict continues despite women's increasing participation in sports and exercise. He concluded that athletes report low levels of role conflict. This includes athletes playing a more "masculine" type sport. Allison[17] attributed this response to the concept that the female athlete is most likely to internalize these images or that the images have a negative impact on self-concept. Female athletes endorse more masculine traits than nonathletes. Athletes have a more masculine self-concept and a more encompassing range of acceptable behavior and therefore less role conflict.[10,18,19] These traits prove to be beneficial outside of the sporting activity.

Psychological Traits

Psychological profile studies regarding athletes are abundant. Often, these profiles analyze data from only male athletes. Jackson and Marsh[3] studied psychological characteristics of female athletes versus nonathletes. They concluded that the athletes had more motivation, assertion, achievement orientation, independence, and self-sufficiency. Other studies have found similar positive effects when comparing women participating in exercise versus those who do not exercise. Those in the exercise groups were found to have a better self-concept regarding physical abilities, appearance, and self-esteem.[17,20,21] Elite athletes have been found to have higher levels of self-confidence and concentration. They have less precompetition anxiety and fewer thoughts of failure, and they tend to recover more easily after errors are made.[22] In a study of elite and nonelite runners, both groups were found to have low levels of negative mood states and to report high vigor.[23]

Competitive stress is an entity with which all competitors must contend. The ability to effectively deal with stress and anxiety emotions can have a direct effect on the athlete's success. Nideffer[24] discussed that anxiety is a result of an overaroused state. The athlete may experience increased respiration and heart rate, profuse sweating, urinary frequency, and dry mouth. The overaroused state can lead to interruption in concentration, which may lead to performance problems. Athletes who are able to control their arousal and channel the energy toward their competitive effort usually are more successful competitively.[25] Identification of an athlete who experiences significant competitive stress may not always be obvious. Signs include repeated injuries, sickness or somatic complaints unrelated to a specific injury, and the repeated inability to perform as well in competition as in practice.

Seggar and associates[26] developed the Athlete Stress Inventory that consists of 49 items. Four factors were found to relate to competitive stress and affect performance for female college athletes as compared to nonathletes. These factors included negative mood, team compatibility, physical well-being, and academic efficacy. One hundred forty-eight athletes were studied, and the validity of the scores was determined through correlation of performance of 32 athletes on three collegiate teams. Stress scores reported 4 days before competition were significantly correlated with performance for individual sports including tennis and gymnastics. However, this was not correlated with a group sport. Negative mood was not significantly correlated with any sport. The authors attributed this to the ease with which negative mood may be overcome during competition. For tennis, team compatibility, physical well-being, and academic efficacy had significant correlation with performance scores. For gymnasts, team compatibility and academic efficacy had significant correlation with performance scores. The authors noted that while negative mood may be more easily overcome, team compatibility, physical well-being, and academic efficacy are longer lasting.[26]

Comparisons by gender regarding stress management in the workplace are available in the literature. Gadzella and associates[27] found eight significant differences in stress producers between men and women. One hundred fifty-eight men and 243 women responded to a questionnaire containing statements describing 20 types of stress producers and 20 types of coping mechanisms. Women reported higher stress producer scores than men when they compared their job performance with that of others. The women were overcritical of their job responsibilities, realized personal limitations on the job, and experienced frustration with frequent interruptions. They also felt socially isolated in their jobs. Men reported higher stress scores when the work pertained to higher administrative roles. With regard to coping strategies, women reported more "let down." Women take more time for themselves when under stress and exercise but overreact to criticism. Men under stress seek support or advice from close friends.[27] Some of these stress producers and coping techniques may be inferred in the athlete. No study to date compares stress and coping strategies of female and male athletes. Further definition of these gender differences would enable more specfic intervention for stress management in female sports and exercise participants.

Response to Injury

Athletes and avid exercisers are often faced with a change in their training and performance activities as a result of injury. Time away from competition may be frustrating for the athlete. Psychosocially derived causes of injury as well as psychological responses to injury and recovery are complex and multifactorial.

Several studies have correlated life stress with injury in the athletic population. Many of these studies have included male high school and college football players. A high correlation was found between life-event stress scores and days missed due to injury.[28–30] There are few studies correlating life stress and injuries for women participating in sports. Kerr and Minden[31] reported that 83% of elite female gymnasts had sustained an injury within the previous 2 years that interfered with training. They measured that a stressful event, such as a family death or a move, in the year before the competitive season was associated with an increased risk of injury.[31] Rider and Hicks[32] did not find this same correlation. They studied 35 male and 17 female high school basketball players. Life events were assessed via questionnaires. Injuries were classified as medical problems that prevented practice or competition one day beyond the injury. Data were compared between boys and girls. No significant differences were noted. The number of days missed due to injury was not significantly related to life-event stresses. The injuries were negatively correlated with coping skills and social-support variables. These were not statistically significant.[32] A considerable problem with comparison between the female and male athletes is that 41% of the questionnaires given to female athletes from the original sample group were not completed.

Self-esteem has also been found to correlate with the relative risk for injury. Athletic injury has been negatively correlated with self-esteem. However, some coping skills may enhance consistency in completing rehabilitation for an injury.[33–35] Several studies have described the negative impact of injury on the exercise participant.[36,37] One particular problem often experienced during the recovery period is the loss of control the athlete feels during rehabilitation.[38] Wasley and Lox[39] investigated the effect of acute versus chronic injury on self-esteem and coping strategies. There were no differences between those acutely injured and chronically injured athletes in accepting responsibility. Chronically injured athletes scored higher on escape and avoidance and lower in seeking social support. Athletes with chronic injuries scored more negatively on self-esteem measures.[39] Smith and associates[40] also studied athletes' emotional responses to injury. Forty-nine male and 23 female athletes ranging in age from 12 to 54 years were studied from the time of injury up until their return to sports activity or 4 months postinjury, depending on which came first. For 69%, this was the first injury, and 31% had experienced a similar injury previously. Two standardized questionnaires, Emotional Responses of Athletes to Injury and the Profile of Mood States Test, were used to measure response to injury. Gender comparisons demonstrated no differences between male and female athletes. A significantly higher expression of anger was noted in younger athletes (younger than 18 years of age) as compared to older athletes. The athletes were also compared by length of time out of sports activity because of injury. Group 1 missed their activity less than 2 weeks, group 2 was out 2 to 6 weeks, and group three was out 6 to 24 weeks. The athletes who were out longer were found to have statistically significant postinjury mood disturbances with greater tension, depression, and confusion compared to those out from injury 6 weeks or less. The athletes restricted from participation for more than 6 weeks experienced more tension, depression, and anger and less vigor than college norms. These mood changes lasted for 1 month.[40]

In a follow-up, Smith and associates[41] prospectively studied whether preinjury and postinjury differences exist in the mood state and self-esteem in athletes. They studied 238 male and 38 female athletes participating in team sports in high school and college. Of these, 36 athletes sustained 43 injuries during the study. Postinjury increases were noted in depression and anger. Vigor was significantly less postinjury. Twenty-seven of the injuries required the athlete to miss less than 2 weeks from participation, and 9 required the athlete to miss 3 or more weeks. The only significant predictor for postinjury depression was length of time missed from participation due to the injury. The physical and psychological variables measured included level of participation, type of sport, age, previous injury, preinjury stress, gender, mood state scales, and self-esteem. Only two of these variables, level of participation and type of sport, were predictors of injury. The authors concluded that postinjury alterations in mood state more likely were attributed to the occurrence of the injury and were related to the time away from the sport as a result of injury. The injury was not predicted solely by an altered preinjury mood change.[41]

An athlete's support system has a direct impact on how the athlete is able to manage an injury. The athlete can be influenced by the reactions of friends, teammates, parents, and coaches. Coaches and health care providers may have considerable effect on how the athlete responds and copes with new circumstances of injury. Crossman and associates[42] studied 35 athletes, their coaches, and medical professionals. The study group included 9 male and 26 female athletes ranging in age from 16 to 37 years. A nonstandardized questionnaire was used to assess outcome. Athletes rated the disruptive impact of the injury significantly lower than did the medical professionals. The short-term effects were greater for athletes participating at a lower level of competition and for those who had not had an injury previously. Coaches rated the seriousness of the injury higher than the medical professionals did. The coaches also overestimated the disruptive effect for higher level athletes. In contrast, higher level athletes underestimated the impact of the injury. These contrasts may result from the idea that the loss of a higher level athlete will have a more negative impact on the team and would affect the attitude of the coach. Higher level athletes have often sustained injuries earlier in their career. The author concluded that higher level athletes may have developed good coping skills or ignored minor injuries in the past, thereby underestimating the effect of a more serious injury.[42]

Disordered Eating

Disordered eating and eating disorders have received media attention in relation to psychological issues and the female athlete. Unfortunately, the general practice of screening for such disorders is not routine or universal among health care providers. Many athletes with disordered eating may manifest behaviors that do not completely fulfill the criteria for eating disorders. Unfortunately, if these issues are not addressed, the athlete may go on to demonstrate the behaviors that meet the full description for an eating disorder. This topic is covered in detail in chapter 32. The following discussion will focus on the psychological factors and their relationship to disordered eating.

There is increasing evidence that the young female athlete is at particular risk for developing disordered eating habits as a result of her drive to excel. The prevalence of disordered eating is reported to range from 15% to 62%. Disordered eating is much more prominent in "body-aware" sports and "thin-build" sports such as dance, gymnastics, and long-distance running. In her quest to succeed in competition and maintain a low body weight, the athlete's coping skills may be overly challenged.[43]

Women with eating disorders may have grown up in a family that did not promote the development of adequate coping skills to deal with stressful situations. Root[44] studied families of women with eating disorders. These families demonstrated characteristics such as inability to resolve conflict, inability to express and tolerate negative emotions, inability to regulate appropriate intimacy, and distance with family relationships. With lack of appropriate coping skills, the women may often rely on others for a sense of self-worth. They often need compliments regarding their appearance or performance. Further stress may provoke more of the eating disorder behaviors.[43]

Disordered eating may develop as an attempt at coping with stress even in individuals with a good family support system. The athlete may lack assertiveness and become overwhelmed with stress associated with competition, academics, injury, performance, relationship with teammates and coach, financial problems, or family issues. Disordered eating may arise out of the need for control. The athlete's self-esteem and identity may be closely tied to her athletic performance. If the athlete's performance is poor or as she is ending her career, she may develop disordered eating as a means of coping with the loss.[43] Sinclair and Orlick[45] reported that there were no significant differences between female and male athlete retirement. Low self-esteem has been found to be associated with anorexia nervosa and bulemia nervosa.[20,21,46,] However, as a group athletes when compared to nonathletes have higher self-esteem.[47,48]

Another psychological trait, perfectionism, is found more commonly in athletes at risk for disordered eating. Several studies have concluded that adolescent athletes may set excessively high standards for personal achievement, which place them at greater risk than their nonathlete peers.[47,49,50] Root[44] also reported that disordered eating may develop as a result of victimization by physical or sexual abuse. This is thought to be an uncommon stimulus but should be considered in evaluation.

Overtraining and Burnout

Overtraining and burnout are other issues with which the female athlete must contend. Some athletes compete year round and may have started participating in sports at an early age. The combination of psychological demands and physical stress can lead to staleness and burnout. Overtraining has been defined as the loss of drive, physical fatigue, and a plateau in performance. The end point for this continued stress may result in burnout, which includes loss of interest in participation and physical and emotional exhaustion.[51,52] The athlete may quit participation completely. Skrinar and associates[20] reported that 47% of college athletes admitted to experiencing burnout. Long training and inadequate recovery time can contribute to the development of burnout. Other psychosocial issues such as conflict with coaches may also contribute. Individual psychological traits that promote burnout that may particularly affect the female athlete include perfectionism and lack of assertiveness.[45] Literature addressing burnout specifically in the female athlete remains unavailable. Issues regarding burnout for the female athlete likely have both similarities and contrasts with those of men.

Summary

As more girls and women participate in exercise and sports, the psychological issues relating to participation and success will become an area of increasing need for study. The literature summarized here identifies some of the significant issues with regard to psychosocial aspects of sport and physical activity for women.

References

1. Gender in athletics: Educational fact sheet. *The Insider 2*. Nassau County, NY, Women's Sports Foundation, 1993.
2. Kane MJ: The female athletic role as a status determinant within the social systems of high school adolescents. *Adolescence* 1988;23:253–264.

3. Jackson SA, Marsh HW: Athletic or antisocial? The female sport experience. *J Sport Psychol* 1986;8:198–211.
4. Eccles J, Harold RD: Gender differences in sport involvement: Applying the Eccles' expectancy-value model. *J Appl Sport Psychol* 1991;3:7–35.
5. Kopp RG, Ruzicka MF: Women's multiple roles and psychological well-being. *Psychol Rep* 1993;72:1351–1354.
6. Melpomene Institute for Women's Health Research: The bodywise woman, in *Reliable Information About Physical Activity and Health*. New York, NY, Prentice Hall Press, 1990.
7. DiNucci JM, Finkenberg ME, McCune SL, McCune ED, Mayo T: Analysis of body esteem of female collegiate athletes. *Percept Mot Skills* 1994;78:315–319.
8. Theberge N: A content analysis of print media coverage of gender, women, and physical activity. *J Appl Sport Psychol* 1991;3:36–48.
9. Duncan MC, Hasbrook C: Denial of power in televised women's sports. *Sociol Sport J* 1988;5:1–21.
10. Cann A: Gender expectations and sports participation, in Diamant L (ed): *Psychology of Sports, Exercise, and Fitness: Social and Personal Issues*. New York, NY, Hemisphere, 1991, p 187.
11. Barnett NP, Wright P: Psychological considerations for women in sports. *Clin Sports Med* 1994;13:297–313.
12. Gould D, Feltz D, Horn T, Weiss M: Reasons for attrition in competitive swimming. *J Sport Behavior* 1983a;5:155–165.
13. Orlick T: The athletic dropout: A high price for inefficiency. *Can Assoc HPERJ* 1974;41:21–27.
14. Feltz DL, Ewing ME: Psychological characteristics of elite young athletes. *Med Sci Sports Exerc* 1987;19(suppl 5):S98–S105.
15. Anthrop J, Allison MT: Role conflict and the high school female athlete. *Res Q Exerc Sport* 1983;54:104–111.
16. Sage GH, Loudermilk S: The female athlete and role conflict. *Res Q Exerc Sport* 1979;50:88–96.
17. Allison MT: Role conflict and the female athlete: Preoccupations with little grounding. *J Appl Sport Psychol* 1991;3:49–60.
18. Challip L, Villiger J, Duignan P: Sex-role identity in a selected sample of women field hockey players. *Int J Sport Psychol* 1980;11:240–248.
19. Henschen KP, Edwards SW, Mathinos L: Achievement motivation and sex-role orientation of high school female track and field athletes versus nonathletes. *Percept Mot Skills* 1982;55:183–187.
20. Skrinar GS, Bullen BA, Cheek JM, McArthur JW, Vaughan LK: Effects of endurance training on body-consciousness in women. *Percept Mot Skills* 1986;62:483–490.
21. Trujillo CM: The effect of weight training and running exercise intervention programs on the self-esteem of college women. *Int J Sport Psychol* 1983;14:162–173.
22. Williams JM, Krane V: Psychological characteristics of peak performance, in Williams JM (ed): *Applied Sport Psychology: Personal Growth to Peak Performance*, ed 2. Palo Alto, CA, Mayfield Publishers, 1993, p 137.
23. Morgan WP, O'Connor PJ, Sparling PB, Pate RR: Psychological characterization of the elite female distance runner. *Int J Sports Med* 1987;8(suppl 2):124–131.
24. Nideffer RM: Concentration and attention control training, in Williams JM (ed): *Applied Sport Psychology: Personal Growth to Peak Performance*, ed. 2. Palo Alto, CA, Mayfield Publishers, 1993, p 243.

25. Landers DM, Boutcher SH: Arousal-performance relationships, in Williams JM (ed): *Applied Sport Psychology: Personal Growth to Peak Performance*, ed. 2. Palo Alto, CA, Mayfield Publishers, 1993, p 170.
26. Seggar JF, Pedersen DM, Hawkes NR, McGown C: A measure of stress for athletic performance. *Percept Mot Skills* 1997;84:227–236.
27. Gadzella BM, Ginther DW, Tomcala M, Bryant GW: Differences between men and women on stress producers and coping strategies. *Psychol Rep* 1991;69:561–562.
28. Cryan PD, Alles WF: The relationship between stress and college football injuries. *J Sports Med Phys Fitness* 1983;23:52–58.
29. Garrick JG, Requa RK: Injuries in high school sports. *Pediatrics* 1978;61:465–469.
30. Blackwell B, McCullagh P: The relationship of athletic injury to life stress, competitive anxiety and coping resources. *Athletic Training* 1990;25:25–27.
31. Kerr G, Minden H: Psychological factors related to the occurrence of athletic injuries. *J Sport Exerc Psychol* 1988;10:167–173.
32. Rider SP, Hicks RA: Stress, coping, and injuries in male and female high school basketball players. *Percept Mot Skills* 1995;81:499–503.
33. McPherson BD, Brown BA: The structure, processes, and consequences of sport for children, in Smoll FL, Magill RA, Ash MJ (eds): *Children in Sport*, ed 3. Champaign, IL, Human Kinetics, 1988, p 265.
34. Chan CS, Grossman HY: Psychological effects of running loss on consistent runners. *Percept Mot Skills* 1988;66:875–883.
35. Udry E: Coping and social support among injured athletes following surgery. *J Sport Exerc Psychol* 1997;19:71–90.
36. McDonald SA, Hardy CJ: Affective response patterns of the injured athlete: An exploratory analysis. *Sport Psychologist* 1990;4:261–274.
37. Smith RE, Smoll FL, Ptacek JT: Conjunctive moderator variables in vulnerability and resiliency research: Life stress, social support and coping skills, and adolescent sport injuries. *J Pers Soc Psychol* 1990;58:360–370.
38. Johnson WR: Some psychological aspects of physical rehabilitation: Toward an organismic theory. *J Assoc Phys Ment Rehabil* 1962;16:165–168.
39. Wasley D, Lox CL: Self-esteem and coping responses of athletes with acute versus chronic injuries. *Percept Mot Skills* 1998;86:1402.
40. Smith AM, Scott SG, O'Fallon WM, Young ML: Emotional responses of athletes to injury. *Mayo Clin Proc* 1990;65:38–50.
41. Smith AM, Stuart MJ, Wiese-Bjornstal DM, Milliner EK, O'Fallon WM, Crowson CS: Competitive athletes: Preinjury and postinjury mood state and self-esteem. *Mayo Clin Proc* 1993;68:939–947.
42. Crossman J, Jamieson J, Hume KM: Perceptions of athletic injuries by athletes, coaches, and medical professionals. *Percept Mot Skills* 1990;71:848–850.
43. Johnson MD: Disordered eating in active and athletic women. *Clin Sports Med* 1994;13:355–369.
44. Root MPP: Persistent, disordered eating as a gender-specific, post-traumatic stress response to sexual assault. *Psychotherapy* 1991;28:96–102.
45. Sinclair DA, Orlick T: Positive transitions from high performance sport. *Sport Psychologist* 1993;7:138–150.
46. Humphries LL, Wrobel S: Bulimia: The binge eating syndrome. *South Med J* 1983;76:181–184.
47. Taub DE, Blinde EM: Eating disorders among adolescent female athletes: Influence of athletic participation and sport team membership. *Adolescence* 1992;27:833–848.

48. Snyder EE, Kivlin JE: Women athletes and aspects of psychological well-being and body image. *Res Q Exerc Sport* 1975;46:191–199.
49. Smith NJ: Excessive weight loss and food aversion in athletes simulating anorexia nervosa. *Pediatrics* 1980;66:139–142.
50. Thornton JS: Feast or famine: Eating disorders in athletes. *Phys Sportsmed* 1990;18:116–122.
51. Feigley DA: Psychological burnout in high-level athletes. *Phys Sportsmed* 1984;12:108–119.
52. Henschen KP: Athletic staleness and burnout: Diagnosis, prevention, and treatment, in Williams JM (ed): *Applied Sport Psychology: Personal Growth to Peak Performance*, ed 2. Palo Alto, CA, Mayfield Publishers, 1993, p 328.

Chapter 32

The Female Athlete Triad

Aurelia Nattiv, MD

Introduction

Participation in sports and exercise is recommended for girls and women of all ages because of the many health benefits. In some instances, however, sports participation may be associated with significant risk to the physical and psychological well-being of the female athlete. The term "female athlete triad" describes the combination of disordered eating, amenorrhea, and osteoporosis that has been recognized as a potentially serious problem for girls and women in sports worldwide.[1–3]

Since the initial Triad Consensus Conference in 1992,[3] numerous national and international task forces, health initiatives, and committees have focused their efforts on the prevention and recognition of the triad disorders in female athletes. Despite these efforts, prospective epidemiologic data assessing prevalence and causes continue to be lacking, as are outcome studies assessing the efficacy of programs to prevent and treat the triad disorders in young athletic women. This chapter presents an overview of the female athlete triad with an emphasis on current concepts and controversies, as well as recommendations for future research.

The components of the female athlete triad—disordered eating, amenorrhea, and osteoporosis—are felt to be interrelated in their pathogenesis, etiology, and consequences.[1] An attitude that emphasizes thinness and maintaining a low body weight underlies the development of the triad. Although one or more of the components of the triad can occur in girls and women in any sport, the greatest risk is for adolescents and young women training in sports that emphasize a thin physique for appearance or improved performance.[3] The triad can negatively affect the athlete's physical performance and cause significant physical and psychological morbidity as well as mortality.

Disordered Eating

Eating disorders are characterized by a serious disturbance in eating behavior, such as severe restriction of intake or binge eating, as well as excessive concern about body shape or body weight. The term "disordered eating" refers to a spectrum of abnormal eating behaviors that may not fit the Diagnostic and Statistical Manual of Mental Disorders, Fourth Edition (DSM-IV) criteria for eating disorders.[4] Only a small percent of female athletes will have frank anorexia or bulimia nervosa, but many may have a clinically significant variant associated with dissatisfaction with their body size or shape, or they may fit the

DSM-IV criteria for Eating Disorder Not Otherwise Specified.[4] Commonly used methods for weight loss include restricting food intake; fasting; self-induced vomiting; using diet pills, laxatives, or diuretics; and excessive exercise. In addition to the potentially devastating effects of disordered eating on psychological well-being, there is also significant concern about the effects on skeletal health[5] and other physiologic sequelae of restrictive eating or purging.[6–9] An athlete experiencing excessive weight loss may demonstrate dehydration, a loss of fat-free mass, and subsequent decrease in performance.[10]

Eating disorders affect an estimated 3% of young women in the general US population,[4,6] and it is likely that clinically important variants affect twice this number.[11–13] Although the exact prevalence of disordered eating in the female athlete is not known, it is clearly a significant problem that affects many young female athletes and poses a significant risk to their psychological and physical well-being.

Eating disorders most commonly affect adolescent girls or young women, although the incidence in young children is increasing,[14] and 5% to 15% of the cases of anorexia and bulimia[15] and 40% of the cases of binge-eating disorders occur in boys and men.[4] Eating disorders are most prevalent in industrialized societies, and they occur in all socioeconomic classes and major ethnic groups in the United States.[16,17]

A combination of interactive factors most likely contributes to the development of eating disorders and disordered eating behaviors, including genetic,[18,19] neurochemical,[20] sociocultural,[21,22] and psychodevelopmental factors.[23]

Although a number of studies have assessed disordered eating behaviors in the young female athlete,[24–31] many of these studies have limitations that may preclude using their findings to generalize about the prevalence of these behaviors in specific sports or in the general female athlete population. For example, many of the studies do not use validated diagnostic instruments for assessment of eating disorders, or they lack appropriate nonathlete control subjects. In addition, most have studied the collegiate female athlete, with few assessing the adolescent athlete or other age groups. Most important, the majority of these studies have assessed *symptoms* of eating disorders by using a questionnaire, such as the Eating Disorders Inventory (EDI) or the Eating Attitude Test (EAT). Most have not included an interview by a trained clinician using the DSM-IV criteria[4] to diagnose various eating disorders, or other clinical screening tools, to diagnose disordered eating behaviors. These studies assessing eating disorder symptoms are still important, however, because body image dissatisfaction, a drive for thinness, and preoccupation with weight are important risk factors for the development of eating disorders in the female athlete.[27,32] Identifying an athlete with symptoms of eating disorders may also be important because these athletes can then be screened for the other problems of the triad—menstrual dysfunction and resultant osteoporosis. It is important to recognize, however, that the presence of particular symptoms is not the same as being clinically diagnosed with an eating disorder.

A number of the studies that assess disordered eating in female athletes using validated psychometric instruments have found the female athlete to score higher on the Drive for Thinness (DFT) subscale of the EDI or EDI-2,[25,27,30] to be more dissatisfied with her body image, and to be more preoccupied with her weight than nonathlete control subjects. In these same studies, however, the athletes did not exhibit extreme scores on the EDI or EDI-2 when compared with nonathlete control subjects.[25,27,33–35] Self-reported symptoms of disordered eating may also be underestimated. O'Connor and associates[27] found that female college gymnasts can easily simulate scores on the EDI-2, and Wilmore[10] found that scores on the EDI were not related to the existence of frank eating disorders in elite female athletes.

There may be a number of reasons that the young female athlete is at additional risk for developing or perpetuating disordered eating behaviors. First, there is an underlying belief that thinness correlates with success, whether because of faster speeds or better marks from judges. Coaches, parents, judges, and others pressuring the athlete to lose weight may present an additional risk factor for disordered eating behaviors.[2,3,32,36] Although there are no specific judging guidelines that relate specifically to body size or shape, gymnasts and athletes in other sports with an aesthetic component often believe that being thin is important to their overall success.[37]

Adolescence is a time of vulnerability to physical as well as psychological injury. Height, weight, percent of body fat, and body shape often change significantly during this time as the result of puberty, and this may present a challenge to the young female athlete who is striving to stay thin. Low self-esteem and depression, which increase at this age, may also perpetuate disordered eating behaviors.

The personality type of the successful competitive female athlete—typically, a high-achieving perfectionist with a tendency to have obsessive/compulsive traits—is similar to the personality type often described in patients with eating disorders. It is unclear if female athletes with these personality traits are most attracted to and successful in sports or if involvement in sports contributes to these behaviors.

Studies have demonstrated that anorexia nervosa has profound negative effects on bone.[5] Athletes with disordered eating behaviors, especially those that result in restricted food intake and low weight, can also experience significant bone loss. However, Sundgot-Borgen and associates[38] demonstrated that normal-weight women with bulimia nervosa have normal bone mass. This may, in part, be due to the effects of body weight on bone. Low body weight and lean body mass are independent predictors of low bone mineral density (BMD). Lower dietary fat, common in the athlete who is striving for thinness, has been associated with risk for stress fractures in female track-and-field athletes.[39] More research is needed in this area.

Amenorrhea

Secondary Amenorrhea

Secondary amenorrhea is defined as the lack of menses for 3 or more consecutive months after menarche.[40,41] A variety of menstrual irregularities is often seen among athletes, with hypoestrogenic amenorrhea at one end of the spectrum and periods of oligomenorrhea (menstrual flow occuring at intervals greater than 35 days) at an intermediate point along the spectrum.[41] Oligomenorrhea may be the result of anovulation or of low estrogen and progesterone. Luteal phase dysfunction, manifested by a shortened luteal phase and inadequate progesterone production,[41] is also common in athletes. Female athletes with luteal phase dysfunction may have regular menses.

In the general female population, the prevalence of secondary amenorrhea ranges from 2% to 5%. Amenorrhea is more frequent in athletes than in sedentary women,[41–43] with a reported prevalence among athletes ranging from 15% to 66%, depending on the sport played and other factors.

Amenorrhea associated with exercise is hypothalamic in origin. Low levels of gonadotropins and ovarian steroids have been observed consistently in amenorrheic athletes.[43,44] One of the best accepted explanations for secondary amenorrhea in the female athlete is the energy availability hypothesis proposed by Loucks and associates.[45,46] This hypothesis defines energy availability as dietary energy intake minus exercise energy expenditure. Loucks and associates proposed that a reduction in luteinizing hormone and the resultant menstrual dysfunction are caused by a failure of dietary energy intake to meet the demands of the energy cost of exercise, rather than by exercise itself.

The effect of leptin on the reproductive status of the female athlete is also being studied.[47] Low leptin levels in patients with anorexia and in female athletes who exercise strenuously have been found to be closely associated with neuroendocrine abnormalities. Leptin may monitor the body's fat content and inhibit ovulation when nutritional reserves drop below a certain level.

Amenorrhea has significant consequences for skeletal health. Decreased BMD of the lumbar vertebrae[48–50] as well as low BMD at multiple skeletal sites have been noted in young female athletes with extended periods of amenorrhea.[51,52] Evidence that bone loss in former oligomenorrheic and amenorrheic athletes may be irreversible[53] is of great concern and emphasizes the importance of prevention.

Delayed Menarche

Delayed menarche is defined as the lack of menstruation by age 16 years in a girl with secondary sexual characteristics.[41] Later mean ages of menarche are commonly reported in the female athlete. Most of the data on menarcheal age in the female athlete come from retrospective studies on athletes in a variety of sports and events within a sport.[54] The actual prevalence of delayed menarche in the female athlete is not known.

The mechanisms underlying delayed menarche in the female athlete have not been fully elucidated. Premenarcheal training for sports has been indicated as a causative factor based on correlational data in a number of sports.[55] However, the association of delayed menarche and premenarcheal training does not imply causation. Data also suggest that this association is in large part familial.[56] Most likely, an interaction of environmental and genetic factors is responsible.[57]

Warren and associates[58] associated delayed menarche with stress fractures and scoliosis in ballet dancers, and Barrow and Saha[59] found that runners with delayed menarche had an increased risk for stress fractures. Bennell and associates' prospective study[39] assessing risk factors for stress fractures in track-and-field athletes found that a later age of menarche was one of the best predictors of stress fractures in women.

In the young female athlete, does a delay in menarche affect the attainment of peak bone mass? This is an important question that has not been answered. Nichols-Richardson and associates[60] have found that young artistic gymnasts (ages 8 to 13 years) have significantly higher BMD than do nongymnast control subjects, suggesting that gymnastics training in childhood may help maximize peak BMD. Whether a delay in menarche affects this increase in BMD has not been determined.

Osteoporosis

The Consensus Development Conference on Osteoporosis defines osteoporosis as a disease characterized by low bone mass, microarchitectural deterioration of bone tissue leading to enhanced skeletal fragility, and an increased risk for fracture.[61] The World Health Organization has established diagnostic criteria for postmenopausal osteoporosis using bone density measurements[62] (Outline 1). However, no similar diagnostic criteria using bone density have been established for girls or young women.

Osteoporosis is a worldwide problem affecting an estimated 75 million people in the United States, Europe, and Japan, including one in three postmenopausal women.[63] The prevalence of osteopenia and osteoporosis in female athletes is not known. What is known is that the other triad disorders, disordered eating and amenorrhea, are often precursors to the development of osteoporosis. The etiology of premenopausal osteoporosis in young athletic women is related primarily to a hypoestrogenic state resulting from hypothalamic amenorrhea.[5,48,49]

The consequences of osteopenia and osteoporosis in the female athlete are great. Studies have demonstrated bone loss at multiple skeletal sites in the athlete with amenorrhea.[52] Low bone density has been associated with an increased risk for stress fractures in the female athlete.[39,50]

Outline 1 World Health Organization diagnostic guidelines for osteoporosis

Normal Bone: BMD $\leq$ 1 SD* below the mean peak bone mass†

Osteopenia: BMD > 1 and $\leq$ 2.5 SD below the mean peak bone mass

Osteoporosis: BMD > 2.5 SD below the mean peak bone mass

Severe Osteoporosis: Osteoporosis criteria plus one or more fragility fractures

*SD = standard deviation
†These measurements are compared with the mean value of peak bone mass in normal young women

More than 90% of peak skeletal mass is likely present by 18 years of age, with skeletal ages 10 through 14 being the most important years for bone acquisition.[64] Bone loss or a decrease in bone formation during this time may affect the attainment of peak bone mass in the young female athlete, thus making her more prone to fractures later in life.

Robinson and associates,[65] Slemenda and Johnston,[66] and Wolman and associates[67] have demonstrated site-specific increases in bone density in athletes involved in higher impact sports. The most striking studies illustrating this phenomenon have involved the female gymnast. These studies have shown that, compared with female athletes in other sports, as well as with nonathlete control subjects, the female gymnast has significantly higher BMD at various weight-bearing skeletal sites.[60,65,68] This appears to be true even in the presence of delayed menarche and secondary amenorrhea. The exact mechanisms resulting in a higher BMD in these athletes have not been fully elucidated, though the effect of high-impact forces on specific skeletal sites seems to play a role. The increased fat-free soft-tissue mass in the gymnast may also be a significant factor.[60]

Medical and Psychological Assessment

The assessment and management of an athlete with the triad disorders should address the nutritional, medical, and psychological components of the problem, ideally with a multidisciplinary team that works closely together.[1–3]

History and Physical Examination

All female athletes should be screened for the 3 components of the triad disorders at the preparticipation physical examination or at the annual physical examination by their primary care physician. Another opportunity for screening is when the athlete is being evaluated for other medical problems, such as stress fractures or recurrent illness or injury, that may be suggestive of an underlying eating disorder, menstrual dysfunction, or low bone density. An athletic girl or woman who presents with one component of the triad should be screened for the other components.

A careful history of dietary patterns, weight changes, preoccupation with weight, and frequency and severity of any purging behavior should be taken. An assessment of any purging behaviors, including abuse of laxatives, enemas, or diuretics, should be reviewed with the athlete, as well as indications of excessive exercise or abuse of stimulants. A detailed menstrual history should also be obtained, including age of menarche and detailed menstrual pattern from menarche to the present. The latter is very important, as menstrual history is one of the most important predictors of current BMD.[69,70] Any history of stress fractures, low-impact fractures, or frequent injury should be assessed.

The appropriateness of the athlete's weight for height, age, and gender should be determined according to the percent of expected body weight or body mass index (BMI).[6] Typically, a weight or BMI range is used in the athletic setting to account for individual variability in body frame and other factors, as well as methodological error.[71]

A complete physical examination should be performed including an assessment of Tanner stage. The examination should include an assessment of vital signs and general nutritional status. In athletes with very low weights, bradycardia, hypotension, and hypothermia are often seen. With bulimia, weight is often normal, but electrolyte disturbances and dehydration may cause lightheadedness and hypotension. Outline 2 lists common signs and symptoms and medical complications of eating disorders.

When amenorrhea is present, a pelvic examination is helpful to assess possible aberrations in the pelvic anatomy and to help assess the etiology of the amenorrhea. Consensus is lacking regarding the age at which the initial pelvic examination should be performed on young women who are not sexually active.

The psychological assessment of patients with disordered eating should be performed by a physician, psychologist, or psychiatrist. The clinician should assess the psychosocial context of the symptoms, establish a diagnosis, and identify any concurrent psychiatric illness, as well as risk of suicide.[6] Assessment of suicidal behavior is important because suicide is one of the main contributors to the increased mortality rate among patients with anorexia nervosa.

Laboratory Studies and Electrocardiogram

Routine laboratory studies for the athlete being evaluated for disordered eating include measurements of serum electrolytes, a complete blood count, and serum glucose levels. Thyroid function tests may be obtained if symptoms suggest possible thyroid disease. Laboratory tests and findings on physical examination may be normal, especially in patients of normal weight who have bulimia nervosa.[6]

Prolongation of the Q-T interval is a concern with anorexia nervosa, even when serum electrolyte levels are normal. An electrocardiogram is therefore indicated for an athlete with clinically significant food restriction and/or purging.

An athlete who presents with amenorrhea should undergo a urine pregnancy test, as pregnancy is the most likely etiology for missed menses in the adolescent or young adult. Thyroid-stimulating hormone, follicular stimulating hormone, and prolactin levels should be obtained as well to exclude other common causes of amenorrhea. If androgen features are present or polycystic ovarian syndrome is a possibility, luteinizing hormone, free testosterone, and dihydroepiandosterone sulfate levels may be obtained.

If the athlete is osteopenic or osteoporotic, bone markers may be helpful, including a urine N-telopeptide for assessing bone resorption and a serum osteocalcin for bone formation. Other metabolic conditions that may cause bone loss, such as underlying thyroid disease, should also be assessed to rule out secondary causes.

Outline 2 Signs, symptoms, and medical complications of eating disorders

Orofacial
- Perimolysis
- Dental caries
- Cheilosis
- Enlargement of the parotid gland
- Submandibular adenopathy

Cardiovascular
- Postural and nonpostural hypotension
- Acrocyanosis
- Electrocardiographic abnormalities: low voltage, prolonged Q-T interval, prominent U waves
- Sinus bradycardia
- Atrial and ventricular arrhythmias
- Left ventricular changes: decreased mass, decreased cavity size
- Mitral-valve prolapse
- Cardiomyopathy (due to ipecac poisoning)

Gastrointestinal
- Esophagitis, hematemesis (including the Mallory-Weiss syndrome)
- Delayed gastric emptying
- Decreased intestinal motility
- Constipation
- Rectal prolapse
- Gastric dilatation and rupture
- Abnormal results on liver-function tests
- Elevated serum amylase level

Endocrine and metabolic
- Hypokalemia (including hypokalemic nephropathy)
- Hyponatremia, (rarely) hypernatremia

Endocrine and metabolic (continued)
- Hypomagnesemia
- Hyperphosphatemia
- Hypoglycemia
- Hypothermia
- Euthyroid sick syndrome
- Hypercortisolism, elevated free cortisol level in urine
- Low serum estradiol level
- Decreased serum testosterone level
- Amenorrhea, oligomenorrhea
- Delay in puberty
- Arrested growth
- Osteoporosis
- Lipid abnormalities
- Obesity

Renal
- Renal calculi

Reproductive
- Infertility
- Insufficient weight gain during pregnancy
- Low-birth-weight infant

Integumentary
- Dry skin and hair
- Hair loss
- Lanugo
- Yellow skin due to hypercarotenemia
- Hand abrasions

Neurologic
- Peripheral neuropathy
- Reversible cortical atrophy
- Ventricular enlargement

Hematologic
- Anemia, leukopenia, neutropenia, thrombocytopenia

(Reproduced with permission from Becker A, Grinspoon SK, Klibanski A, Herzog DB: Eating disorders. N Engl J Med 1999;340:1092–1098.)

Bone Density Studies

Bone loss or inadequate bone formation is a serious problem that may be a result of disordered eating, oligomenorrhea, or amenorrhea. Because 50% of women with frank anorexia nervosa have bone density measurements more than 2 standard deviations below normal, affecting both cortical and trabecular bone,[6,72] these patients should undergo assessment of bone density.

Drinkwater and associates[69] have demonstrated a linear relationship between the degree of bone loss and the degree of menstrual dysfunction. Although there are no established guidelines for assessment of bone density in the athlete with triad disorders, I recommend obtaining a bone density for patients with a history of clinically significant disordered eating, amenorrhea, or oligomenorrhea for more than 6 to 12 months.

Treatment

Disordered Eating

Treatment of disordered eating focuses on recognition of the problem, identification and resolution of psychosocial precipitants, stabilization of the medical and nutritional condition, and reestablishment of healthy eating patterns.[6] Patients with disordered eating respond to a variety of psychotherapeutic approaches, including individual, group, or family therapy, or a combination of these therapies. The use of behavioral strategies early in treatment to control symptoms is often helpful.[6] In the athletic setting, a multidisciplinary team—including a physician, psychologist, nutritionist, and, often, an athletic trainer—working closely with the athlete is recommended. In the more serious cases, a psychiatrist is consulted. Coaches and parents need to be educated about the prevention of disordered eating and be aware of signs and symptoms.

Medication is generally not helpful in treating the primary symptoms of anorexia, but fluoxetine may stabilize recovery in patients with anorexia who have attained 85% of their expected body weight.[73] In patients with bulimia, psychopharmacologic therapy is moderately effective. Fluoxetine is the only drug, however, currently approved by the US Food and Drug Administration for the treatment of bulimia. Other selective serotonin reuptake inhibitors are used routinely, but they have not been studied to date in controlled trials. Desipramine and imipramine have also been found to be helpful in the treatment of bulimia.

The majority of athletes with disordered eating can be treated as outpatients. Candidates for inpatient care include those with very low weight (75% or less of expected body weight), rapid weight loss, cardiac arrhythmias, severe electrolyte imbalances, severe or intractable purging, or suicidal ideations, and those who are not responding to adequate outpatient therapy.[6]

Amenorrhea

The goal of the treatment of amenorrhea or oligomenorrhea is to identify the underlying problem that most likely contributed to the menstrual disorder and to establish normal menstrual function. Treatment aims to optimize nutritional status and adjust exercise to maintain a positive energy balance. Often, a 3-month period of observation without pharmacologic agents is initiated,[74] especially if the athlete is not osteopenic or osteoporotic. If this initial approach does not result in normal menses, hormonal intervention should be considered for the hypoestrogenic patient. Treatment should be individualized, and the patient should be followed closely.

Estrogen therapy has not been shown to significantly affect bone density in women with anorexia nervosa; therefore, it cannot be recommended for all anorexic patients.[75]

Osteoporosis

In the female athlete with osteopenia or osteoporosis, treating the underlying problem is the initial step. There may be a need to focus on weight gain, as well as optimizing nutritional status and establishing normal menses to assist bone health. Excessive exercise should be avoided, but weight-bearing and resistive exercises may be helpful in some athletes with low bone density who participate in nonweightbearing sports, such as swimming.

If the athlete is osteopenic, serial bone densities taken 1 year (initial follow-up) or 2 years apart may be helpful to monitor treatment. In the young athlete with osteopenia and amenorrhea, oral contraceptive pills or estrogen replacement therapy may be used if the athlete is older than 16 years, although controversy exists regarding the resultant effect on bone density.[53,76–78] Prospective longitudinal data that demonstrate an increase in BMD in the athletic woman with amenorrhea are clearly lacking.

Drinkwater and associates[79] found nasal calcitonin to increase bone density in the spine and proximal femur. Other pharmacologic agents, such as the bisphosphonates, may be used in postmenopausal women but are not approved for premenopausal women of childbearing age and are not recommended in this age group because of potential teratogenic effects. For example, the selective estrogen receptor modulator raloxifene is currently approved for the prevention and treatment of osteoporosis in postmenopausal women[80] but not in premenopausal women. In fact, tamoxifen, which is also a selective estrogen receptor modulator, has been associated with a decrease in bone density in premenopausal women, although it increases bone density in postmenopausal women.[81]

Summary

Most girls and women benefit greatly from involvement in sports and exercise. For some female athletes, however, the triad of disordered eating, amenorrhea, and osteoporosis may be a significant problem that can lead to decreased performance and increased morbidity and mortality. All female athletes should be screened for the triad disorders. The presence of one component of the triad should alert the clinician to screen for the others. Prevention and recognition of the triad disorders should be a priority in those who work closely with the female athlete. Well-controlled research is presently lacking in a number of areas, including the prevalence of the triad disorders and their prevention and treatment in the athletic setting. More research is urgently needed to define the prevalence of disordered eating in athletes, as are outcome studies that identify optimal strategies for prevention and treatment.

References

1. Otis Cl, Drinkwater B, Johnson M, Loucks A, Wilmore J: American College of Sports Medicine Position Stand: The Female Athlete Triad. *Med Sci Sports Exerc* 1997;29:i–ix.
2. Nattiv A, Agostini R, Drinkwater B, Yeager KK: The female athlete triad: The inter-relatedness of disordered eating, amenorrhea, and osteoporosis. *Clin Sports Med* 1994;13:405–418.
3. Yeager KK, Agostini R, Nattiv A, Drinkwater B: The female athlete triad: Disordered eating, amenorrhea, osteoporosis. *Med Sci Sports Exerc* 1993;25:775–777.
4. American Psychiatric Association. *Diagnostic and Statistical Manual of Mental Disorders*, ed 4. Washington, DC, American Psychiatric Association, 1994.
5. Rigotti NA, Nussbaum SR, Herzog DB, Neer RM: Osteoporosis in women with anorexia nervosa. *N Engl J Med* 1984;311:1601–1606.
6. Becker AE, Grinspoon SK, Klibanski A, Herzog DB: Eating disorders. *N Engl J Med* 1999;340:1092–1098.
7. Palla B, Litt IF: Medical complications of eating disorders in adolescents. *Pediatrics* 1988;81:613–623.
8. Pomeroy C, Mitchell JE: Medical issues in the eating disorders, in Brownell KD, Rodin J, Wilmore JH (eds): *Eating, Body Weight, and Performance in Athletes: Disorders of Modern Society*. Philadelphia, PA, Lea & Febiger, 1992, pp 202–221.
9. Ratnasuriya RH, Eisler I, Szmukler GI, Russell GF: Anorexia nervosa: Outcome and prognostic factors after 20 years. *Br J Psychiatry* 1991;158:495–502.
10. Wilmore JH: Eating and weight disorders in the female athlete. *Int J Sport Nutr* 1991;1:104–117.
11. Hoek HW: The distribution of eating disorders, in Brownell KD, Fairburn CG (eds): *Eating Disorders and Obesity: A Comprehensive Handbook*. New York, NY, Guilford Press, 1995, pp 207–211.
12. Spitzer RL, Yanovski S, Wadden T, et al: Binge eating disorder: Its further validation in a multisite study. *Int J Eat Disord* 1993;13:137–153.
13. Shisslak CM, Crago M, Estes LS: The spectrum of eating disturbances. *Int J Eat Disord* 1995;18:209–219.
14. Bostic JQ, Muriel AC, Hack S, Weinstein S, Herzog D: Anorexia nervosa in a 7-year-old girl. *J Dev Behav Pediatr* 1997;18:331–333.
15. Anderson AE: Eating disorders in males, in Brownell KD, Fairburn CG (eds): *Eating Disorders and Obesity: A Comprehensive Handbook*. New York, NY, Guilford Press, 1995, pp 177–187.
16. Crago M, Shisslak CM, Estes LS: Eating disturbances among American minority groups: A review. *Int J Eat Disord* 1996;19:239–248.

17. Gard MC, Freeman CP: The dismantling of a myth: A review of eating disorders and socioeconomic status. *Int J Eat Disord* 1996;20:1–12.
18. Strober M: Family-genetic studies of eating disorders. *J Clin Psychiatry* 1991;52(suppl):9–12.
19. Kendler KS, MacLean C, Neale M, Kessler R, Heath A, Eaves L: The genetic epidemiology of bulimia nervosa. *Am J Psychiatry* 1991;148:1627–1637.
20. Brewerton TD: Toward a unified theory of serotonin dysregulation in eating and related disorders. *Psychoneuroendocrinology* 1995;20:561–590.
21. Garner DM, Garfinkel PE, Schwartz D, Thompson M: Cultural expectations of thinness in women. *Psychol Rep* 1980;47:483–491.
22. Becker AE, Hamburg P: Culture, the media, and eating disorders. *Harv Rev Psychiatry* 1996;4:163–167.
23. Bruch H (ed): *Eating Disorders: Obesity, Anorexia Nervosa, and the Person Within*. New York, NY, Basic Books, 1973.
24. Dummer GM, Rosen LW, Heusner WW, Roberts PJ, Counsilman JE: Pathogenic weight-control behaviors of young competitive swimmers. *Phys Sportsmed* 1987;15:75–86.
25. Hecht S, Nattiv A, Puffer JC: Abstract: Disordered eating in female collegiate gymnasts. *Clin J Sports Med*, in press.
26. Nattiv A, Puffer JC, Green GA: Lifestyles and health risks of collegiate athletes: A multi-center study. *Clin J Sport Med* 1997;7:262–272.
27. O'Connor PJ, Lewis RD, Kirchner EM: Eating disorder symptoms in female college gymnasts. *Med Sci Sports Exerc* 1995;27:550–555.
28. Rosen LW, Hough DO: Pathogenic weight-control behaviors of female college gymnasts. *Phys Sportsmed* 1988;16:141–146.
29. Rosen LW, McKeag DB, Hough DO, Curley V: Pathogenic weight-control behavior in female athletes. *Phys Sportsmed* 1986;14:79–86.
30. Sundgot-Borgen J: Prevalence of eating disorders in elite female athletes. *Int J Sport Nutr* 1993;3:29–40.
31. Sundgot-Borgen J, Larsen S: Nutrient intake and eating behavior of female elite athletes suffering from anorexia nervosa, anorexia athletica and bulimia nervosa. *Int J Sport Nutr* 1993;3:431-432.
32. Sundgot-Borgen J: Risk and trigger factors for the development of eating disorders in female elite athletes. *Med Sci Sports Exerc* 1994;26:414–419.
33. Benson JE, Allemann Y, Thientz GE, Howald H: Eating problems and calorie intake levels in Swiss adolescent athletes. *Int J Sports Med* 1990;11:249–252.
34. Harris MB, Greco D: Weight control and weight concerns in competitive female gymnasts. *J Sport Exerc Psychol* 1990;12:427–433.
35. Warren BJ, Stanton AL, Blessing DL: Disordered eating patterns in competitive female athletes. *Int J Eat Disord* 1990;9:565–569.
36. Johnson MD: Disordered eating in active and athletic women. *Clin Sports Med* 1994;13:355–369.
37. Hecht S, Nattiv A, Balague G, Marshall N: Gymnastics and the female athlete triad, in Marshall N (ed): *The Athlete Wellness Book*. Indianapolis, IN, USA Gymnastics, 1999.
38. Sundgot-Borgen J, Bahr R, Falch JA, Sundgot Schneider LS: Normal bone mass in bulimic women. *J Clin Endocrinol Metab* 1998;83:3144–3149.
39. Bennell KL, Malcolm SA, Thomas SA, et al: Risk factors for stress fractures in track and field athletes: A twelve-month prospective study. *Am J Sports Med* 1996;24:810–818.

40. Loucks AB, Horvath SM: Athletic amenorrhea: A review. *Med Sci Sports Exerc* 1985;17:56–72.

41. Shangold M, Rebar RW, Wentz AC, Schiff I: Evaluation and management of menstrual dysfunction in athletes. *JAMA* 1990;263:1665–1669.

42. Feicht CB, Johnson TS, Martin BJ, Sparks KE, Wagner WW Jr: Secondary amenorrhea in athletes. *Lancet* 1978;2:1145–1146.

43. Loucks AB, Mortola JF, Girton L, Yen SS: Alterations in the hypothalamic-pituitary-ovarian and the hypothalamic-pituitary-adrenal axes in athletic women. *J Clin Endocrinol Metab* 1989;68:402–411.

44. Schwartz B, Cumming DC, Riordan E, Selye M, Yen SS, Rebar RW: Exercise-associated amenorrhea: A distinct entity? *Am J Obstet Gynecol* 1981;141:662–670.

45. Loucks AB: Effects of exercise training on the menstrual cycle: Existence and mechanisms. *Med Sci Sports Exerc* 1990;22:275–280.

46. Loucks AB, Verdun M, Heath EM: Low energy availability, not the stress of exercise, alters LH pulsatility in exercising women. *J Appl Physiol* 1998;84:37–46.

47. Mantzoros CS: The role of leptin in human obesity and disease: A review of current evidence. *Ann Intern Med* 1999;130:671–680.

48. Drinkwater BL, Nilson K, Chestnut CH III, Bremner WJ, Shainholtz S, Southworth MB: Bone mineral content of amenorrheic and eumenorrheic athletes. *N Engl J Med* 1984;311:277–281.

49. Marcus R, Cann C, Madvig P, et al: Menstrual function and bone mass in elite women distance runners: Endocrine and metabolic features. *Ann Intern Med* 1985;102:158–163.

50. Myburgh KH, Hutchins J, Fataar AB, Hough SF, Noakes TD: Low bone density is an etiologic factor for stress fractures in athletes. *Ann Intern Med* 1990;113:754–759.

51. Myburgh KH, Bachrach LK, Lewis B, Kent K, Marcus R: Low bone mineral density at axial and appendicular sites in amenorrheic athletes. *Med Sci Sports Exerc* 1993;25:1197–1202.

52. Rencken ML, Chesnut CH III, Drinkwater BL: Bone density at multiple skeletal sites in amenorrheic athletes. *JAMA* 1996;276:238–240.

53. Keen AD, Drinkwater BL: Irreversible bone loss in former amenorrheic athletes. *Osteoporos Int* 1997;7:311–315.

54. Malina RM: Menarche in athletes: A synthesis and hypothesis. *Ann Hum Biol* 1983;10:1–24.

55. Frisch RE, Gotz-Welbergen AV, McArthur JW, et al: Delayed menarche and amenorrhea of college athletes in relation to age of onset of training. *JAMA* 1981;246:1559–1563.

56. Malina RM, Ryan RC, Bonci CM: Age at menarche in athletes and their mothers and sisters. *Ann Hum Biol* 1994;21:417–422.

57. Malina RM: Physical growth and biological maturation of young athletes. *Exerc Sports Sci Rev* 1994;22:389–433.

58. Warren MP, Brooks-Gunn J, Hamilton LH, Warren LF, Hamilton WG: Scoliosis and fractures in young ballet dancers: Relation to delayed menarche and secondary amenorrhea. *N Engl J Med* 1986;314:1348–1353.

59. Barrow GW, Saha S: Menstrual irregularity and stress fractures in collegiate female distance runners. *Am J Sports Med* 1988;16:209–216.

60. Nickols-Richardson SM, O'Connor PJ, Shapses SA, Lewis RD: Longitudinal bone mineral density changes in female child artistic gymnasts. *J Bone Miner Res* 1999;14:994–1002.

61. Consensus development conference: Prophylaxis and treatment of osteoporosis. *Am J Med* 1991;90:107–110.

62. Assessment of fracture risk and its application to screening for postmenopausal osteoporosis: Report of a WHO Study Group. World Health Organization Technical Report Series 843. Geneva, Switzerland, WHO, 1994.

63. Who are candidates for prevention and treatment for osteoporosis? *Osteoporosis Int* 1997;7:1–6.

64. Bonjour JP, Theintz G, Buchs B, Slosman D, Rizzoli R: Critical years and stages of puberty for spinal and femoral bone mass accumulation during adolescence. *J Clin Endocrinol Metab* 1991;73:555–563.

65. Robinson TL, Snow-Harter C, Taaffe DR, Gillis D, Shaw J, Marcus R: Gymnasts exhibit higher bone mass than runners despite similar prevalence of amenorrhea and oligomenorrhea. *J Bone Miner Res* 1995;10:26–35.

66. Slemenda CW, Johnston CC: High intensity activities in young women: Site specific bone mass effects among female figure skaters. *Bone Miner* 1993;20:125–132.

67. Wolman RL, Clark P, McNally E, Harries M, Reeve J: Menstrual state and exercise as determinants of spinal trabecular bone density in female athletes. *Br Med J* 1990;301:516–518.

68. Kirchner EM, Lewis RD, O'Connor PJ: Bone mineral density and dietary intake of female college gymnasts. *Med Sci Sports Exerc* 1995;27:543–549.

69. Drinkwater BL, Bruemner B, Chesnut CH III: Menstrual history as a determinant of current bone density in young athletes. *JAMA* 1990;263:545–548.

70. Georgiou EK, Ntalles K, Papageorgiou A, Korkotsidis A, Proukakis C: Bone mineral loss related to menstrual history. *Acta Orthop Scand* 1989;60:192–194.

71. Wilmore JH: Body weight standards and athletic performance, in Brownell KD, Rodin J, Wilmore JH (eds): *Eating, Body Weight and Performance in Athletes: Disorders of Modern Society*. Philadelphia, PA, Lea & Febiger, 1992, pp 315–329.

72. Biller BM, Saxe V, Herzog DB, Rosenthal DI, Holzman S, Klibanski A: Mechanisms of osteoporosis in adult and adolescent women with anorexia nervosa. *J Clin Endocrinol Metab* 1989;68:548–554.

73. Becker AE, Hamburg P, Herzog DB: The role of psychopharmacologic management in the treatment of eating disorders, in Dunner DL, Rosenbaum JF (eds): *Annual of Drug Therapy*. Philadelphia, PA, WB Saunders, 1998, pp 17–51.

74. Dueck CA, Matt KS, Manore MM, Skinner JS: Treatment of athletic amenorrhea with a diet and training intervention program. *Int J Sport Nutr* 1996;6:24–40.

75. Klibanski A, Biller BM, Schoenfeld DA, Herzog DB, Saxe VC: The effects of estrogen administration on trabecular bone loss in young women with anorexia nervosa. *J Clin Endocrinol Metab* 1995;80:898–904.

76. Cumming DC: Exercise-associated amenorrhea, low bone density, and estrogen replacement therapy. *Arch Intern Med* 1996;156:2193–2195.

77. Gibson JH, Mitchell A, Reeve J, Harries MG: Treatment of reduced bone mineral density in athletic amenorrhea: A pilot study. *Osteoporos Int* 1999;10:284–289.

78. Hergenroeder AC, Smith EO, Shypailo R, Jones LA, Klish WJ, Ellis K: Bone mineral changes in young women with hypothalamic amenorrhea treated with oral contraceptives, medroxyprogesterone, or placebo over 12 months. *Am J Obstet Gynecol* 1997;176:1017–1025.

79. Drinkwater BL, Healy NL, Rencken ML, Fontana D, Chesnut CH III: Abstract: Effectiveness of nasal calcitonin in preventing bone loss in young amenorrheic women. *J Bone Miner Res* 1993;8(suppl 1):S264.

80. Ettinger B, Black DM, Mitlak BH, et al: Reduction of vertebral fracture risk in postmenopausal women with osteoporosis treated with raloxifene: Results from a 3-year randomized clinical trial: Multiple Outcomes of Raloxifene Evaluation (MORE) Investigators. *JAMA* 1999;282:637–645.
81. Powles TJ, Hickish T, Kanis JA, Tidy A, Ashley S: Effect of tamoxifen on bone mineral density measured by dual-energy x-ray absorptiometry in healthy premenopausal and postmenopausal women. *J Clin Oncol* 1996;14:78–84.

Directions for Future Research

Identify factors that motivate girls' participation in sports and exercise as well as factors that lead to attrition from sport or exercise participation.

Although there is some evidence that identifies factors motivating girls to play sports, most American girls still remain sedentary. Identification of factors that might increase the appeal of sports and physical activity may result in increasing the overall numbers of active and exercising girls. Identifying reasons for attrition also could give insight into maintaining an active lifestyle through the individual's growth and development.

Define and develop strategies to overcome socioeconomic, ethnic, and/or cultural barriers to girls participating in sports and physical activity.

There is a large population of girls with barriers to sports and physical activity that relate to their poverty, as well as to ethnic and cultural issues. Future work needs to detail these issues so that strategies can be developed that foster health benefits in this population. Many mental health-related issues that have been shown to be positively modified by exercise occur in this same population.

Identify issues related to gender identification and role conflict in female sports participants.

As sports with a traditionally male-associated bias are becoming accessible to females, issues related to gender, role, and identity need to be studied.

Investigate the interaction between the coach and athlete in the following areas: (1) impact of coaching styles on the female athlete (conditional versus unconditional), and (2) impact of the coach's gender on the female athlete.

Little is known on coaching styles specific for the female athlete's involvement and performance in sports. Guidelines for coaches regarding styles that maximize involvement and performance need to be conducted. In addition, the influence of the coach's gender on the female athlete needs to be examined.

Psychological risk factors for injury in the female athlete need to be explored.

Research has begun to demonstrate that an accumulation of life events are associated with the onset of injury. Further prospective studies assessing other psychological factors (stress, depression, anxiety) and injury onset are needed.

Identify short- and long-term effects of injury on girls and women in sports and exercise.

As the opportunities for female athletes to participate in sports at collegiate and professional levels increase, career-ending injuries may result in significant short- and long-term sequelae that affect their socioeconomic status and personal identities.

Determine appropriate intervention in the management of emotional issues after injury.

Few studies have demonstrated the significant emotional impact of injury on athletes. Strategies for increasing the use of psychological counseling need to be developed in the sport-injury settings.

Investigate the relationship and influence of peers, as well as parents, and their impact on the child's participation in sports and physical activity.

As girls get older, the influences of their peers impact many of their activity decisions. Parents can play a significant role in the support system of the individual. How these support systems influence a child's development and decision to participate in sports and physical activity needs further study.

There is a need to investigate valid and reliable instrumentation for psychosocial issues relevant to participation in sports and physical activity.

Current literature uses a wide variety of tools to measure psychosocial issues. These tools are not used consistently and not all have been validated. A standard approach to identifying psychosocial issues relevant to participation in sports and physical activity will allow more appropriate interpretation and intervention across multiple health-care provider disciplines.

Identify gender differences in the psychosocial impact of sports career retirement.

Current literature describes the isolation, loss of identity, and need for control that athletes experience as their sports career ends. Issues specific to the female athlete and retirement from sports have not been clearly defined. Women's behavior in reaction to such changes may be detrimental to health and well-being and need further study.

Investigate factors that facilitate involvement as well as barriers to participation in sports and physical activity for aging women.

Motivating factors for the aging woman to participate in sports and physical activity have not been defined. Environmental and social barriers exist that may prohibit the elderly woman from participating in physical activity. These barriers have not been well defined. Identification of incentives and barriers to participation in physical activity may facilitate interventions to promote increased participation in this age group.

Explore the influence of exercise on depression in the aging woman.

Depression in the elderly is a widespread problem with both health and economical ramifications. In general, younger individuals who exercise have been found to have less stress, anxiety, and depression and higher self-esteem. Studies are needed to identify whether exercise helps reduce depression in the aging woman.

Investigations of the psychological benefits and differences of involvement in group or organized versus individual sports participation is needed.

Sports and physical activity have been shown to produce high self-esteem, confidence, a sense of mastery, and success in female participants. Studies investigating the influence of individual and team sport-specific influences and individual or group physical activities may further contribute to the understanding of the benefits of sports and physical activity.

Explore issues of vulnerability, harassment, and abuse in the woman involved in sports and physical activity.

As girls and women have increased their participation in sports and physical activity, there are reports of increased harassment and abuse. Studies investigating the incidence of coach-athlete abuse need to be conducted. Guidelines for identification, prevention, and intervention need to be determined.

Identify the impact of modality-specific physical activity on psychosocial factors (such as self-esteem and vigor).

Research has demonstrated that specific physical activities may improve self-esteem, vigor, and confidence in participants. Gender- and age-related studies in girls and women need to be conducted to establish type, frequency, intensity, and duration of activities that can contribute to general well-being in girls and women.

Identification of the biopsychosocial factors that facilitate continued participation in physical activity throughout the lifetime is needed.

A multitude of biopsychosocial factors influence participation in physical activity. These factors change with age, life events, and accessibility. More women have involved themselves in multiple roles (mother, wife, career) that may make participation in exercise more difficult. Clarification of these influential factors is important to facilitate continued participation in regular physical activity. The biopsychosocial model facilitates the understanding of the interaction of the various psychological and social parameters.

Characterize the prevalence data relating to the female athlete triad using valid and reliable instruments and appropriate control groups.

Current studies report a wide prevalence for development of the female athlete triad. Most of these studies, however, have not used valid and reliable instruments for measurement of triad disorders. Accuracy in defining the prevalence of the problem is essential in developing better interventions for prevention and treatment.

Explore the biopsychosocial factors underlying the causes of the female athlete triad.

The etiology and contributing factors for disordered eating in the athletic setting are complex and multifactorial. A biopsychosocial model needs to be applied in the athletic setting in order to get a better understanding of the multiple and unique factors involved in the development of disordered eating in the female athlete.

Explore optimal prevention and treatment strategies for each dimension of the female athlete triad.

It is presently not known what the optimal prevention and treatment strategies are for the triad disorders in the female athlete. Educational interventions leading to meaningful behavior change and prevention of disordered eating, amenorrhea, and osteoporosis need to be explored and implemented. Outcome studies assessing various treatment strategies for disordered eating, amenorrhea, and osteopenia/osteoporosis in the athletic setting need to be carefully conducted.

Develop clinical guidelines for screening, prevention, and treatment of the triad.

There has been much investigation that focuses on identification of the triad conditions. Guidelines for clinical assessment and screening, prevention, and treatment of disordered eating, amenorrhea, and osteoporosis need to be further explored and effectively implemented. Outcome studies are needed to assess the effectiveness of these guidelines.

Investigate risk factors for the development of triad disorders in various sports and in different ethnic and economic backgrounds.

Sports that emphasize body image have been determined to place individuals at greater risk for developing the female athlete triad disorders. Further investigation is needed to clarify other sport-specific issues that may contribute to preventable risks. Socioeconomic and ethnic factors that may contribute to the risk for triad disorders have not been assessed. Identification of these factors is necessary to promote appropriate prevention and intervention.

Assess the relationship of body composition and performance in sports and physical activity.

The relationship of body composition and peak performance needs to be further assessed. There are many potential health consequences that may occur for girls and women who strive to be thin or to obtain unrealistically low body weights for the sake of optimal performance. Disordered eating and the consequences of starvation and dehydration may have significant short- and long-term repercussions on these athletes' psychological and overall well-being. Furthermore, there needs to be further evaluation of present tools for measuring body composition in young women.

Explore the health risks of athlete-sport mismatch.

Further study needs to be performed on keeping athletes and their sports activity choices more balanced. As athletes grow, many of the risk-taking behaviors stem from trying to change or alter their body size and shape into the physique associated with athletes in certain sports (ie, dancers, gymnasts, etc). This "body shaping" can be detrimental to health and may be associated with disordered eating behaviors to meet the desired goals.

Assess the relationship between performance and nutritional intake in the female athlete.

The availability of energy to the exercising athlete, which incorporates the athlete's dietary intake and energy expenditure, appears to be an important component in the development of hypothalamic amenorrhea and oligomenorrhea. Studies need to assess how much energy or calories may contribute to enhancement as well as to a detriment in performance parameters in the athletic setting.

The factors contributing to peak bone mass in the growing female and in the maintenance of optimal bone health need to be evaluated prospectively.

Exercise, calcium intake, general nutrition, body weight, and estrogen status all appear to be important contibuting factors in the attainment of peak bone mass and maintenance of bone health. How much of each of these factors is needed and whether there are other factors needs further investigation. This information will help provide recommendations for girls and young women in optimizing their bone health and preventing bone loss.

Index

Page numbers in italics refer to figures or figure legends.